2015 The Year Book of VASCULAR SURGERY®

Editor-in-Chief

David L. Gillespie MD, RVT, FACS, DMCC

COL (ret), MC, USA, Chief, Department of Vascular and Endovascular Surgery, Southcoast Health Systems, Fall River, Massachusetts; Affiliated Professor of Surgery, Uniformed Services University of the Health Sciences, Bethesda, Maryland

ELSEVIER
MOSBY

ELSEVIER
MOSBY

Vice President, Global Medical Reference: Mary E. Gatsch
Associate Publisher: John Vassallo
Developmental Editor: Meredith Clinton
Production Supervisor, Electronic Year Books: Donna M. Skelton
Electronic Article Manager: Mike Sheets
Illustrations and Permissions Coordinator: Dawn Vohsen

2015 EDITION

Composition by TNQ Books and Journals Pvt Ltd, India

Editorial Office:
Elsevier
Suite 1800
1600 John F. Kennedy Blvd.
Philadelphia, PA 19103-2899

International Standard Serial Number: 0749-4041
International Standard Book Number: 978-0-323-35556-8

Associate Editors

James H. Black, III, MD, FACS

The Bertram M. Bernheim, MD Associate Professor of Surgery, Chief, Division of Vascular Surgery and Endovascular Therapy, Johns Hopkins Hospital, Baltimore, Maryland

Marc A. Passman, MD

Professor of Surgery, Section of Vascular Surgery and Endovascular Therapy, University of Alabama at Birmingham, Birmingham, Alabama

Benjamin W. Starnes, MD

Professor of Surgery and Chief, Division of Vascular Surgery; University of Washington, Seattle, Washington

Michael T. Watkins, MD

Director, Vascular Surgery Research Lab, Massachusetts General Hospital, Boston, Massachusetts

Contributors

Matthew A. Corriere, MD, MS

Assistant Professor, Department of Vascular and Endovascular Surgery, Wake Forest University School of Medicine, Winston-Salem, North Carolina

John P. Cullen, PhD

Research Associate Professor, Division of Vascular Surgery, University of Rochester School of Medicine and Dentistry, Rochester, New York

Brian G. Peterson, MD, FACS

Associate Professor of Surgery, St. Louis University School of Medicine, St Louis, Missouri

Joseph D. Raffetto, MD, FACS, FSVM

Associate Professor of Surgery, Harvard Medical School, Brigham and Women's Hospital; Chief, Vascular Surgery Division, VA Boston Healthcare System, West Roxbury, Massachusetts

Margaret Arnold, MD

Assistant Professor of Surgery, Division of Vascular Surgery, Johns Hopkins Bayview Medical Center, Baltimore, Maryland

Robert J. Feezor, MD, FACS

Assistant Professor; Program Director of Vascular Fellowship, Division of Vascular Surgery and Endovascular Therapy, Department of Surgery, University of Florida, Gainesville, Florida

Kakra Hughes, MD, FACS

Associate Professor; Director of Endovascular Surgery, Department of Surgery, Howard University and Hospital, Washington, DC

Kristine C. Orion, MD

Assistant Professor of Surgery, Yale University Medical School, New Haven, Connecticut

Brandon W. Propper, MD
Assistant Professor of Surgery USUHS; Associate Program Director for General Surgery, San Antonio Military Medical Center, Fort Sam Houston, Texas

Paul W. White MD, FACS, LTC, USARMY
DHA NCR MEDICAL DIR, Walter Reed Army Medical Center, Bethesda, Maryland

Brian G. Peterson, MD, FACS
Associate Professor of Surgery, Harvard Medical School, Brigham and Women's Hospital; Chief, Vascular Surgery Division, VA Boston Healthcare System, West Roxbury, Massachusetts

Table of Contents

Journals Represented

Journals represented in this YEAR BOOK are listed below.

American Journal of Medicine
Annals of Surgery
Annals of Thoracic Surgery
Annals of Vascular Surgery
Archives of Physical Medicine and Rehabilitation
Atherosclerosis
British Journal of Surgery
Circulation
European Journal of Internal Medicine
European Journal of Vascular and Endovascular Surgery
Injury
International Journal of Cardiology
Journal of Cardiothoracic and Vascular Anesthesia
Journal of Surgical Research
Journal of the American Medical Association
Journal of Thoracic and Cardiovascular Surgery
Journal of Vascular and Interventional Radiology
Journal of Vascular Surgery
Journal of Vascular Surgery. Venous and Lymphatic Disorders
Lancet
Metabolism Clinical and Experimental
New England Journal of Medicine
Radiologia
Spine Journal
Stroke
Surgery
Techniques in Vascular and Interventional Radiology
Thrombosis Research

STANDARD ABBREVIATIONS

The following terms are abbreviated in this edition: acquired immunodeficiency syndrome (AIDS), cardiopulmonary resuscitation (CPR), central nervous system (CNS), cerebrospinal fluid (CSF), computed tomography (CT), deoxyribonucleic acid (DNA), electrocardiography (ECG), health maintenance organization (HMO), human immunodeficiency virus (HIV), intensive care unit (ICU), intramuscular (IM), intravenous (IV), magnetic resonance (MR) imaging (MRI), ribonucleic acid (RNA), and ultrasound (US).

NOTE

The YEAR BOOK OF VASCULAR SURGERY® is a literature survey service providing abstracts of articles published in the professional literature. Every effort is made to assure the accuracy of the information presented in these pages. Neither the editors nor the publisher of the YEAR BOOK OF VASCULAR SURGERY® can be responsible for errors in the original materials. The editors' comments are their own opinions. Mention of specific products within this publication does not constitute endorsement.

To facilitate the use of the YEAR BOOK OF VASCULAR SURGERY® as a reference tool, all illustrations and tables included in this publication are now identified as they appear in the original article. This change is meant to help the reader recognize that any illustration or table appearing in the YEAR BOOK OF VASCULAR SURGERY® may be only one of many in the original article. For this reason, figure and table numbers will often appear to be out of sequence within the YEAR BOOK OF VASCULAR SURGERY®.

1 Basic Considerations

Castration of male mice prevents the progression of established angiotensin II-induced abdominal aortic aneurysms

Zhang X, Thatcher S, Wu C, et al (Saha Cardiovascular Research Ctr, Lexington, KY)

J Vasc Surg 61:767-776, 2015

Objective.—Male sex is a nonmodifiable risk factor for abdominal aortic aneurysm (AAA) development. Similar to humans, male mice are more susceptible to angiotensin II (AngII)-induced AAAs than female mice. Previous studies demonstrated that castration of males markedly reduced the formation of AngII-induced AAAs. Progression of AAA size is associated with increased risk of aneurysm rupture. In this study, we hypothesized that castration of male mice would reduce the progression of established AngII-induced AAAs.

Methods.—Male apolipoprotein E-deficient mice were infused with AngII for 1 month to induce AAA formation. Aortic diameters were measured by ultrasound imaging, and mice were stratified into two groups that underwent a sham operation or castration. AngII infusions were continued for a further 2 months. Ultrasound imaging was used to quantify lumen diameters, and excised aortas were processed for quantification of AAA size, volume, and tissue characteristics.

Results.—Sham-operated mice exhibited progressive dilation of suprarenal aortic lumen diameters during the continued AngII infusion. Aortic lumen diameters were significantly decreased in castrated mice (n = 17) compared with sham-operated mice (n = 15) at study end point (1.63 ± 0.04 vs 1.88 ± 0.05 mm; $P < .05$). However, maximal external AAA diameters were not significantly different between sham-operated and castrated mice. The vascular volume/lumen volume ratio of excised AAAs imaged by ultrasound was significantly increased by castration (9.5% ± 2.0%) vs sham operation (4.8% ± 0.9%; n = 11 per group; $P < .05$). Moreover, compared with the thin-walled AAAs of sham-operated mice, aneurysm sections from castrated mice exhibited increased smooth muscle α-actin and collagen.

Conclusions.—Removal of endogenous male hormones by castration selectively reduces aortic lumen expansion while not altering the external AAA dimensions.

Clinical Relevance.—There are no therapeutics that slow the progression of abdominal aortic aneurysms (AAAs), and as the size of an AAA increases, so does the risk of rupture and death. Male sex is a nonmodifiable risk factor for AAA development, but whether male sex hormones have a similar effect on AAA progression is unclear. Removal of male sex hormones in an established mouse model of angiotensin II-induced AAAs resulted in reduced progressive lumen dilation while not altering external AAA dimensions. Therapies that limit androgen action may provide benefit against AAA progression. Alternatively, supplemental testosterone may be contraindicated in men diagnosed with an AAA.

▶ Abdominal aortic aneurysms (AAA) are characterized by localized remodeling and vessel dilation, with an increased risk of rupture as AAA size increases. Male gender is a well-known risk factor for the development of an AAA, with a 4:1 male to female ratio. Because AAA mainly affect men, the potential relationship of male sex hormones to AAA development has been studied. Testosterone has been shown to be a primary mediator of sex differences in angiotensin II (AngII)-induced AAAs in mice. The authors investigate whether male sex hormones contribute to previously observed progressive aortic lumen dilation and vascular remodeling of established AngII-induced AAAs. In this study, they performed orchiectomy in male ApoE−/− mice with an established AAA from AngII infusion to remove effects of endogenous androgen and they quantified AAA progression. Orchiectomies were performed after 1 month of AngII infusion, when the mice had established AAAs, and the progression of these aneurysms were followed for a further 2 months, during which time AngII infusion continued. Their results demonstrated that while removal of endogenous male hormones had no effect on external AAA diameter, there was a significant decrease in aortic lumen diameter compared with sham-operated mice. In addition, there was an increase in aneurysmal expression of smooth muscle α-actin and collagen. Because the current therapy for AAA is limited to open surgical repair or endovascular repair, it is crucial that the mechanisms mediating the formation and progression of AAA are identified. The results from the present study suggest that male sex hormones markedly influence vascular wall remodeling and the progression of AAAs, and suggest that further studies should be conducted in men who have been diagnosed with an AAA and are receiving supplemental testosterone. In addition, it is possible that therapies that limit androgen action may inhibit AAA progression.

J. P. Cullen, PhD

Paclitaxel coating on the terminal portion of hemodialysis grafts effectively suppresses neointimal hyperplasia in a porcine model

Baek I, Hwang J, Park J, et al (Sungkyunkwan Univ School of Medicine, Seoul, Republic of Korea; Seoul Natl Univ, Republic of Korea)
J Vasc Surg 61:1575-1582.e1, 2015

Objective.—The local delivery of paclitaxel onto a graft has been reported to prevent neointimal hyperplasia. Because more than half of vascular stenoses occur within 3 cm of the venous anastomosis, this study tested the effectiveness of a paclitaxel coating restricted to both ends of the expanded polytetrafluoroethylene (ePTFE) graft to reduce the amount of drug delivered.

Methods.—Both ends of ePTFE grafts were coated with paclitaxel at a dose of 0.58 mg/mm^2; the total amount of paclitaxel per graft was 0.66 mg. Paclitaxel-coated hemodialysis grafts 15 cm in length were surgically implanted between the common carotid artery and external jugular vein in female Landrace pigs. The animals were sacrificed 6 weeks after graft placement. Cross sections of the anastomosis sites were analyzed histomorphometrically to measure the ratio of neointimal hyperplasia to the graft area (H/G ratio) and the percentage of luminal stenosis. The experimental results were compared between grafts coated with paclitaxel at the ends only ($n = 8$), grafts coated over the entire length ($n = 6$), and uncoated control grafts ($n = 6$).

Results.—The mean ± standard error values of the H/G ratios for the arterial anastomosis were 0.82 ± 0.13 (control), 0.41 ± 0.09 (terminal coating), and 0.21 ± 0.04 (whole coating). The values for the venous anastomosis were 0.82 ± 0.12 (control), 0.39 ± 0.11 (terminal coating), and 0.12 ± 0.03 (whole coating). Compared with the uncoated grafts, neointimal hyperplasia was suppressed effectively in the vascular grafts coated terminally with paclitaxel (artery, $P = 050$; vein, $P < .001$). However, the suppressive effect was less than that of grafts coated with paclitaxel over the entire length. The percentages of luminal stenosis showed similar tendency to the H/G ratios.

Conclusions.—Despite a reduced amount of the drug, paclitaxel coating applied to both ends of the ePTFE hemodialysis grafts effectively suppressed neointimal hyperplasia at the sites of anastomosis.

► A hemodialysis vascular graft is required by patients with end-stage renal disease in whom a native arteriovenous fistula cannot be created, especially in older and diabetic patients. Clinical trials of tissue-engineered vascular grafts have identified stenosis as the primary cause of graft failure, with 50% of grafts failing after 1 year because of stenosis followed by thrombosis as a result of neointimal hyperplasia, especially at the venous anastomosis. Neointimal hyperplasia arising at the anastomosis sites of an arteriovenous graft is characterized by the presence of smooth muscle cells and myofibroblasts, angiogenesis, and matrix deposition. Suppressing the proliferation and migration of smooth muscle cells and myofibroblasts may be a logical approach to improving vascular graft outcomes. Paclitaxel is an antiproliferative agent that interferes with the disassembly of microtubules during cell division and effectively inhibits the proliferation of vascular smooth muscle cells. The authors have previously demonstrated that paclitaxel-coated grafts markedly reduce neointimal hyperplasia in a pig model. Because minimizing the amount of paclitaxel loaded onto grafts is desirable for avoiding adverse effects of the drug, in the current study they investigated the lowest effective dose of the drug and whether coating of only a portion of the graft with the drug instead of the whole graft would prevent vessel narrowing. Using a porcine model, their results demonstrated that with less drug loaded, the paclitaxel coating on the ends of the ePTFE grafts effectively suppressed neointimal hyperplasia at the sites of graft-vessel anastomoses, although the suppressive effect was less than that of paclitaxel whole-coated grafts. As the authors state, there are several limitations in this study, including the small sample size. Further experiments are needed to determine whether, for example, the amount of paclitaxel loaded onto the expanded polytetrafluoroethylene graft is increased by extending the length of the terminal regions coated or by increasing the dose of drug per unit area of the vascular graft.

J. P. Cullen, PhD

The essential role of endothelial nitric oxide synthase activation in insulin-mediated neuroprotection against ischemic stroke in diabetes

Huang S-S, Lu Y-J, Huang J-P, et al (Chung Shan Med Univ Hosp, Taichung, Taiwan; Chang Gung Univ, Tao-Yuan, Taiwan; et al)

J Vasc Surg 59:483-491, 2014

Background.—Stroke patients with diabetes have a higher mortality rate, worse neurologic outcome, and more severe disability than those without diabetes. Results from clinical trials comparing the outcomes of stroke seen with intensive glycemic control in diabetic individuals are conflicting. Therefore, the present study was aimed to identify the key factor involved in the neuroprotective action of insulin beyond its hypoglycemic effects in streptozotocin-diabetic rats with ischemic stroke.

Methods.—Long-Evans male rats were divided into three groups (control, diabetes, and diabetes treated with insulin) and subjected to focal cerebral ischemia-reperfusion (FC I/R) injury.

Results.—Hyperglycemia aggravated FC I/R injuries with an increase in cerebral infarction and neurologic deficits, inhibition of glucose uptake and membrane-trafficking activity of glucose transporter 1, and reduction of Akt and endothelial nitric oxide synthase (eNOS) phosphorylation in the cerebrum. Insulin treatment alleviated hyperglycemia and the symptoms of diabetes in streptozotocin-diabetic rats. Insulin administration also significantly decreased cerebral infarction and neurologic deficits and increased phosphorylation of Akt and eNOS protein in the cerebrum of FC I/R-injured diabetic rats. However, the glucose uptake and membrane trafficking activity of glucose transporter 1 in the cerebrum were not restored by insulin treatment. Coadministration of the eNOS inhibitor, N-iminoethyl-L-ornithine, with insulin abrogated beneficial effects of insulin on cerebral infarct volume and neurologic deficits in FC I/R-injured diabetic rats without affecting the hypoglycemic action of insulin.

Conclusions.—These results suggest that eNOS activation is required for the neuroprotection of insulin against ischemic stroke in patients with diabetes.

▶ Stroke is a leading cause of serious long-term disability and the fifth leading cause of death in the United States, killing almost 130 000 Americans each year. Every year, more than 795 000 people in the United States have a stroke, with an estimated annual cost of $34 billion, based on health care services, medications, and missed days of work. Diabetes mellitus has been shown to aggravate brain injury induced by ischemic stroke and is associated with higher mortality, worse functional outcome, and increased frequency for recurrent stroke. The exact mechanisms of diabetes exacerbating ischemic brain injury are not fully understood. Among the various aspects of diabetic pathology, hyperglycemia is likely the most prominent contributor to excessive risk and worse outcome in stroke patients with diabetes. Nearly all of the clinical trials in diabetic patients have failed to show a reduction in cardiovascular disease (CVD) with intensive glycemic control (IGC), suggesting that the pathophysiology of the link between diabetes and CVD is complex, involving more than just hyperglycemia. In addition to its hypoglycemic effect, insulin exerts neuroprotection in diabetic rats subjected to cerebral ischemia. In the current study, the streptozotocin (STZ)-induced diabetic rat model was used to explore the possible mechanisms contributing to the neuroprotective effect of glycemic control with insulin in focal cerebral ischemia—reperfusion (FC I/R) injury. Given that impairment of endothelial nitric oxide synthase (eNOS)-dependent vascular function may contribute to a reduction of cerebral blood flow in stroke, the authors also investigated the role of eNOS signaling in hyperglycemia-associated FC I/R. The main findings of this study demonstrated that hyperglycemia exacerbated FC I/R-induced stroke size and neurologic dysfunction and that the FC I/R-induced Akt and eNOS phosphorylations were blunted in animals with diabetes. In addition, insulin increased cerebral Akt/eNOS phosphorylations and improved neurologic function in diabetes. Furthermore, inhibition of eNOS abrogated the insulin-induced neuroprotective effects of reduced cerebral infarct volume and neurologic deficits in diabetic rats without affecting insulin-induced hypoglycemia, hyperinsulinemia, and weight recovery. These exciting findings suggest that the link between diabetes and CVD is more complex than just the issue of hyperglycemia. Further research is required to support this study that demonstrates glycemic control with insulin treatment may have clinical benefits for stroke patients with diabetes, especially in those with insulinopenic diabetes. Ultimately, health care providers treating stroke patients who have diabetes may have to control hyperglycemia as early as possible; otherwise diabetes-associated endothelial dysfunction could aggravate the damage of ischemic stroke.

J. P. Cullen, PhD

Identification and characterization of microRNAs in vascular smooth muscle cells from patients with abdominal aortic aneurysms

Cheuk BLY, Cheng SWK (Univ of Hong Kong, China)

J Vasc Surg 59:202-209, 2014

Background.—The role of microRNAs (miRs) in the development of various cardiovascular diseases was recently highlighted in several studies. However, the biological role of miRs in the pathogenesis of abdominal aortic aneurysms (AAAs) is still not well defined. The present study aims to identify and characterize miR expression in the aortic explant cultures of AAA patients.

Methods.—A new microarray platform (miChip) using locked nucleic acid-modified capture probes with increased sensitivity and specificity was employed to detect the miR expression profile in human vascular smooth muscle cell cultures from AAA surgical samples. The array data were further validated by real-time quantitative reverse transcription polymerase chain reaction (qPCR) experiments with additional AAA and control aorta samples. Potential target genes of the differentially expressed miRs were predicted by bioinformatics analysis. Some of the results were confirmed by enzyme immunosorbent assay and Western blot analysis.

Results.—Total RNA extracted from the explant of six AAAs and six normal aortas exhibited notably different miR profiles. A twofold difference of miR-516a-5p and miR-1260 was expressed in AAAs compared with normal aortic cultures ($P < .05$). The expression of miR-516a-5p was more than three times higher in AAAs, and miR-1260 expression was almost four times lower, as validated by qPCR. Additional qPCR performing on an extra 10 AAAs and 10 control aortas showed similar results. The expression of three predicted targets—secretory interleukin-3, vascular endothelial growth factor A, and collagen type 1, alpha 1 proteins—was significantly elevated in aneurysmal cultures compared with normal aortic cultures ($P < .05$).

Conclusions.—This miR microarray study displayed an altered expression of miR-516a-5p and miR-1260 in AAAs compared with control aortas. Functional annotations of the two miRs via bioinformatics approaches revealed that both are highly involved in some predefined mechanisms of AAA formation. Three of their target genes were also upregulated in AAAs. The results may be critical to elucidate the functional role of miRs in diseased aorta.

▶ Until recently, RNA was thought to function exclusively within cells; however, clear evidence that RNA can act as an extracellular signal is emerging. Cells release RNA-carrying vesicles and membrane-free RNA/protein complexes into the extracellular environment and the presence of extracellular RNAs, which include microRNAs (miRs), mRNA, and long noncoding RNA, in human plasma or serum has been well documented, and recent evidence suggests that the level and composition of these circulating nucleic acids correlate well with disease or injurious conditions. With significant progress in miR microarray technology, numerous sets of miRs have been found to be highly or specifically expressed in aortic tissues with particular functions. To date, research on the biological importance of miRs in human abdominal aortic aneurysms (AAAs) is still scarce, with, for example, only 14 studies identified when using AAA and microRNA as keywords to search PubMed. The present study aimed to analyze the miR expression patterns of human vascular smooth muscle cells (VSMCs) obtained from AAA explant cultures and to compare them with control aortas using the highly sensitive and specific microarray platform. Results demonstrated a distinct miR expression profile in the diseased human VSMCs that was generated using the new miR microarray technology with high sensitivity and specificity. Increased miR-516-5p expression and decreased miR-1260 expression with the corresponding target expressions, secretory interleukin-3, vascular endothelial growth factor A, and collagen type 1, alpha 1 proteins were observed in human AAA explant cultures compared with control aortas. There are some limitations to this study that include the use of VSMCs obtained from explant cultures, a technique that may induce phenotypic changes in these cells. In addition, the tissue samples are harvested during the late stages of the human aneurysmal disease and may not truly represent the pathophysiology of the disease process. Nonetheless, these findings may be of importance in the development of novel therapeutic agents to treat AAA and therefore warrant further investigation.

J. P. Cullen, PhD

Exposure to Parental Smoking in Childhood is Associated with Increased Risk of Carotid Atherosclerotic Plaque in Adulthood: The Cardiovascular Risk in Young Finns Study

West HW, Juonala M, Gall SL, et al (Univ of Tasmania, Hobart, Australia; Univ of Turku, Finland; et al)

Circulation 131:1239-1246, 2015

Background.—The association between passive smoking exposure in childhood and adverse cardiovascular health in adulthood is not well understood. Using a 26-year follow-up study, we examined if childhood exposure to passive smoking was associated with carotid atherosclerotic plaque in young adults.

Methods and Results.—Participants were from the Cardiovascular Risk in Young Finns Study (n = 2,448). Information on childhood exposure to parental smoking was collected in 1980 and 1983. Carotid ultrasound data was collected in adulthood in 2001 or 2007. Childhood serum cotinine levels from 1980 were measured from frozen samples in 2014 (N = 1,578). The proportion of children with non-detectable cotinine levels was highest among households where neither parent smoked (84%), was decreased in households where one parent smoked (62%), and was lowest among households where both parents smoked (43%). Irrespective of adjustment for potential confounding and mediating variables, the relative risk (RR) of developing carotid plaque in adulthood increased among those where one or both parents smoked (RR = 1.7; 95% CI = 1.0-2.8; P = 0.04). Although children whose parents exercised good "smoking hygiene" (smoking parents whose children had non-detectable cotinine levels) had increased risk of carotid plaque compared with non-smoking parents (RR = 1.6; 95% CI = 0.6-4.0; P = 0.34), children of smoking parents with poor smoking hygiene (smoking parents whose children had detectable serum cotinine levels) had substantially increased risk of plaque as adults (RR = 4.0; 95% CI = 1.7-9.8; P = 0.002).

Conclusions.—Children of parents that smoke have increased risk of developing carotid atherosclerotic plaque in adulthood. However, parents who exercise good smoking hygiene can lessen their child's risk of developing plaque.

▶ Many studies have demonstrated the unfavorable effects of passive smoking, including an increased prevalence of cardiovascular disease and an increased risk of death by at least 20%. It is estimated that approximately 700 million children globally are exposed to environmental tobacco smoke. The authors have previously demonstrated that exposure to parental smoking in childhood was associated with lower endothelial-dependent flow-mediated dilatation and higher carotid-intima media thickness in adulthood. The aim of the current study was to determine whether parental smoking and smoking hygiene in childhood is related to the presence of carotid atherosclerotic plaque in adulthood. Results are reported using a 26-year follow-up study that includes parental self-reports, extensive data on potential confounding and mediating factors, and measurements of serum cotinine, an objective biomarker of exposure. Offspring exposed to parental smoking in childhood had approximately twice the risk of having a carotid atherosclerotic plaque in adulthood than did those with nonsmoking parents. However, among offspring of parents who smoked and had a detectable serum cotinine level that was indicative of poor parental smoking hygiene (eg, smoking in the presence of the child), the risk of plaque was more than doubled compared with those with no detectable cotinine. These data add to the growing body of evidence proposing that exposure to parental smoking early in life has an irreversible effect on arterial health in adulthood by demonstrating that parents who are unable to give up smoking can nonetheless lessen their child's risk of future cardiovascular burden by exercising good smoking hygiene. In addition, although both poor maternal and paternal smoking hygiene conveyed an increased risk to offspring, a stronger effect was observed for maternal smoking hygiene. The results of this study suggest that exposure to parental smoking early in life has an irreversible effect on arterial health. Although antitobacco campaigns tend to focus on fetal and neonatal effects, these data provide evidence that these campaigns should be expanded to recognize the long-term cardiovascular effects of passive smoke exposure on children and adolescents.

J. P. Cullen, PhD

CD34 affinity pheresis attenuates a surge among circulating progenitor cells following vascular injury

Harbuzariu A, Kim J, Meyer EM, et al (Univ of Pittsburgh Med Ctr, PA; Carnegie Mellon Univ, Pittsburgh, PA; Univ of Pittsburgh School of Medicine, PA; et al)
J Vasc Surg 59:1686-1694, 2014

Background.—Intimal hyperplasia (restenosis) is an exaggerated healing response leading to failure of half of vascular interventions. Increasing evidence suggests that circulating progenitor cells contribute to intimal pathology, and clinical studies have demonstrated a correlation between progenitor cells and the incidence of restenosis after cardiovascular interventions. The aims of this study were to characterize the temporal response of CD34+ progenitors following vascular injury in an ovine model and to evaluate an affinity pheresis approach to attenuate this response.

Methods.—An ovine model underwent either operative vascular injury or a nonvascular surgery (n = 3 per group). Blood was examined perioperatively over 2 weeks by flow cytometry. Next, an affinity pheresis approach to mediate systemic depletion of CD34 progenitors was designed. Custom agarose pheresis matrix with antibody affinity toward CD34 or an isotype control was evaluated in vitro. Next, following vascular injury, sheep underwent perioperative whole blood volume pheresis toward either the progenitor cell marker CD34 (n = 3) or an isotype control (n = 4) for 14 days. Animals were monitored by physical exam as well as complete blood counts. Cells recovered by pheresis were eluted and examined by flow cytometry.

Results.—Flow cytometry revealed a focal surge of circulating CD34 cells after vascular injury but not among surgical controls ($P = .05$). Toward the goal of an approach to attenuate the surge of CD34 progenitors, an evaluation of high-flow affinity matrix revealed efficacy in removal of progenitors from ovine blood in vitro. Next, a separate group of animals undergoing affinity pheresis after vascular injury was evaluated to mediate systemic depletion of CD34+ cells. Again, a surge of CD34+ cells was observed among isotype pheresis animals following vascular intervention but was attenuated over 20-fold by a CD34 pheresis approach ($P = .029$). Furthermore, an average of 77 million CD34-positive cells were eluted from the CD34 pheresis matrix. Despite multiple sessions of pheresis, complete blood counts remained essentially unchanged over 2 weeks.

Conclusions.—Despite evidence suggesting a role for CD34+ circulating progenitor cells in restenotic pathology, the temporal pattern of CD34 progenitors after vascular injury has not been previously defined. We have demonstrated a surge among circulating CD34+ cells that appears confined to procedures involving vascular injury and that this event seems to occur early after vascular injury. We further conclude that CD34 affinity pheresis attenuates the surge. This approach for direct depletion of progenitors may have important implications for the study of progenitors in vascular restenosis.

► Despite initial technical success for many vascular interventions, up to half of endovascular and open lower extremity bypasses will occlude in 5 years, half of vascular access grafts in 18 months, and 30% angiographic stenosis among bare metal coronary stents by 1 year. The underlying pathophysiology of these failures includes intimal hyperplasia and subsequent accelerated atherosclerosis. Intimal hyperplasia is characterized by proliferation of smooth muscle cells and extracellular matrix that ultimately limits luminal diameter and leads to vessel occlusion. This pathology has increased the need for both surveillance and additional interventions, contributing costs to the health care system and increasing rates of limb loss and death. Multiple studies have suggested a role of bone marrow-derived progenitors in the pathology of intimal hyperplasia. It remains unclear, however, whether mobilization of these cells is limited to surgeries involving macrovascular injury or merely a generalized injury response to surgical stress. The primary aim of the current study was to document the temporal pattern of circulating progenitor cells, using CD34, which is a marker of hematopoietic progenitor cells, after vascular injury and to compare these results with the response after a nonvascular surgery in an ovine model. Additionally, the authors evaluated a short-term affinity pheresis approach to mediate depletion of circulating progenitors and the impact, if any, on mature hematopoietic cells. The results suggest that there is a surge of CD34-positive cells limited to animals undergoing vascular injury. Given the overlap of CD34 expression on other cells such as mast cells and endothelial progenitor cells (EPC), the results were further analyzed and demonstrated similar CD34 surge trends even when CD45+ (mast cells) and CD133+ (EPC) events were excluded. It is interesting to note that despite minor vascular injuries in the control group, due to microvascular damage during surgery as well as needlestick cannulation for blood draws, there was no significant CD34 mobilization in peripheral blood compared with animals with macrovascular injury. Additional results demonstrated that the magnitude of the CD34 surge of vascular injury with isotype pheresis appears substantially higher than observed among animals who underwent vascular injury without pheresis, approaching 4-fold when comparing means on postoperative day 1. The results of this study suggest a significant progenitor mobilization event at the time of vascular injury that may represent kindling for the pathology of intimal hyperplasia. Based on reports of clinical association between restenosis in the setting of higher numbers of circulating progenitors, this approach of direct progenitor depletion may eventually have therapeutic utility.

J. P. Cullen, PhD

Acute reductions in mechanical wall strain precede the formation of intimal hyperplasia in a murine model of arterial occlusive disease

Favreau JT, Liu C, Yu P, et al (Worcester Polytechnic Inst, MA; Harvard Med School, Boston, MA; et al)

J Vasc Surg 60:1340-1347, 2014

Objective.—Intimal hyperplasia (IH) continues to plague the durability of vascular interventions. Employing a validated murine model, ultrasound biomicroscopy, and speckle-tracking algorithms, we tested the hypothesis that reduced cyclic arterial wall strain results in accentuated arterial wall IH.

Methods.—A 9-0 suture was tied around the left mouse (n = 10) common carotid artery and a 35-gauge (outer diameter = 0.14 mm) blunt mandrel. We previously showed that mandrel removal results in a ~78% reduction in diameter and ~85% reduction in flow, with subsequent delayed induction of IH by day 28. Preoperative, postoperative day-4 (before measurable IH), and postoperative day-27 circumferential wall strains were measured in locations 1, 2, and 3 mm proximal to the stenosis and in the same locations on the contralateral (nonstenosed) carotid. At postoperative day 28, arteries were perfusion fixed and arterial wall morphology was assessed microscopically in the same regions.

Results.—Strains were the same in all locations preoperatively. Wall strain was decreased in all regions proximal to the stenosis by day 4 (0.26 ± 0.01 to 0.11 ± 0.02; $P < .001$), while strains remained unchanged for the contralateral artery ($P = .45$). No statistical regional differences in mean strain or IH were noted at any time point for the experimental or contralateral artery. Based on the median, regions were divided into those with low strain (≤0.1) and high strain (>0.1). Average preoperative strains in both groups were the same (0.27 ± 0.09 and 0.27 ± 0.08). All segments in the low-strain group (n = 13) demonstrated significant IH formation by day 28, while only 31% of the high strain group demonstrated any detectable IH at day 28. (Mean low-strain intimal thickness = 32 ± 20 μm, high strain = 8.0 ± 16 μm; $P < .01$). Changes in cross-sectional area at diastole drove the reduction in strain in the low-strain group, increasing significantly from preoperatively to day 4 ($P = .04$), while lumen cross-section at systole remained unchanged ($P = .46$). Cross-sectional area at diastole and systole in the high-strain group remained unchanged from preoperatively to day 4 ($P = .67$).

Conclusions.—Early reduction in arterial wall strain is associated with subsequent development of hemodynamically induced IH.

▶ Coronary and peripheral artery diseases afflict more than 14 million Americans and remain a significant source of mortality and morbidity. Despite major advances in the endovascular treatment of such diseases, postprocedural intimal hyperplasia (IH) and pathologic wall adaptation in treated arteries limit revascularization durability. In addition to various endocrine and paracrine mediators, evidence also suggests that cellular sensing of the mechanical environment provides the cues that initiate intimal hyperplasia. The vascular wall is constantly subjected to a variety of mechanical forces including wall shear stress, wall tensile stress, and circumferential wall strain. Although a number of researchers have implicated wall shear stress as the primary factor affecting IH formation, shear stress-based explanations alone fail to predict many aspects of IH. Currently, the role of circumferential wall strain, defined as the change in wall circumference normalized to the diastolic circumference of the vessel, in the development of IH remains unclear. In the current study, the authors combine a validated murine model of IH with a recently developed method for measuring arterial wall strains in vivo, to unravel the relationship between wall strain and neointima formation. Their results demonstrate that vessels with early (4 days after acute hemodynamic perturbation) low wall strain consistently develop IH 28 days after creation of an outflow focal stenosis. Conversely, only one-third of arteries that demonstrated early high strain went on to develop a measurable amount of IH. Additionally, they demonstrate that decreases in wall strain are due primarily to early increases in the diastolic area of the vessel lumen, whereas systolic areas remain unchanged. The results also support high-frequency ultrasound as an emerging tool for quantifying arterial wall strains noninvasively in vivo. Future studies are needed to verify these biomicroscopy-based determinations by way of direct longitudinal interrogations of the mechanical qualities of the arterial wall tissues. The approaches described offer a potentially powerful tool to unravel the temporal relationships among hemodynamic perturbations, mechanical forces, and the subsequent arterial wall adaptations.

J. P. Cullen, PhD

Galectin-3, Carotid Plaque Vulnerability, and Potential Effects of Statin Therapy

Kadoglou NPE, Sfyroeras GS, Spathis A, et al (Univ of Athens, Greece; "Attikon" Univ Hosp, Athens, Greece; et al)
Eur J Vasc Endovasc Surg 49:4-9, 2015

Objectives.—Galectin-3, a member of galectines, a family of β-galactoside-specific lectins, has been reported to propagate vascular inflammation. The role of galectin-3 in carotid atherosclerosis is controversial. The aim of this study was to investigate the relationship of galectin-3 with plaque vulnerability in patients with high grade carotid stenosis.

Methods.—This was a cross sectional study of patients undergoing carotid endarterectomy (CEA). Carotid plaques obtained from 78 consecutive patients (40 symptomatic [SG], 38 asymptomatic [AG]) undergoing CEA were histologically analyzed for galectin-3, macrophages (CD68) and laminin. Pre-operatively the biochemical profile and plaque echogenicity (gray-scale median, GSM) score were determined.

Results.—There were no significant differences in clinical and demographic parameters between SG and AG ($p > .05$). The SG had a lower GSM score (44.21 ± 18.24 vs. 68.79 ± 28.79, $p < .001$) and a smaller positive stained area for galectin-3 (4.89 ± 1.60% vs. 12.01 ± 5.91%, $p < .001$) and laminin (0.88 ± 0.71% vs. 3.46 ± 2.12%, $p < .001$) than the AG. On the other hand, intra-plaque macrophage content was increased in SG ($p < .001$). For the whole cohort, symptomatic status was independently associated with intra-plaque contents of both galectin-3 (OR = 0.634, $p < .001$), and GSM score (OR = 0.750, $p < .001$). Notably, patients on long term statin treatment had elevated galectin-3 and lowered macrophage intra-plaque concentrations compared with those on short term treatment ($p < .05$).

Conclusions.—A low galectin-3 intra-plaque concentration seems to correlate with clinically and ultrasonically defined unstable human carotid plaques. Long term statin treatment may induce increase of intra-plaque galectin-3 concentration mediating plaque stabilization.

▶ Rupture and subsequent thrombosis of the vulnerable atherosclerotic plaque is the predominant pathologic substrate of acute cerebrovascular and cardiovascular events such as stroke and myocardial infarction. It is well established that carotid atherosclerosis significantly predisposes to cerebral ischemic events, and mounting evidence correlates carotid plaque texture with its stability. Galectin-3, a prominent member of the β-galactoside-specific lectins, was found to be involved in T-cell apoptosis and proliferation, neutrophil extravasation, chemotaxis, phagocytosis, and mast cell activation. In addition, galectin-3 has been reported to propagate vascular inflammation by inducing the expression of proinflammatory mediators in macrophages and the migration of monocytes into vascular walls. Despite the known interplay between atherosclerosis and inflammation, the contributory role of galectin-3 in atherogenesis progression is still controversial. Moreover, limited evidence disputes the potential role of galectin-3 in plaque destabilization. The primary aim of this study was to investigate the relationship between galectin-3 and ipsilateral neurologic symptoms and ultrasound index of carotid plaque vulnerability. The hypothesis that long-term statin therapy could favorably change concentrations of galectin-3 within atherosclerotic plaques excised from patients undergoing carotid endarterectomy was also tested. The results of this study showed a lower content of galectin-3 in symptomatic versus asymptomatic carotid plaques. Most importantly, the incidence of cerebrovascular events was independently determined by low levels of intraplaque galectin-3 and a low gray-scale median score. Long-term, preoperative therapy with statins was associated more with higher intraplaque galectin-3 levels than short-term therapy. This is the first study evaluating galectin-3 in human carotid plaques in relation to clinical criteria of plaque vulnerability. It is still the subject of debate to assume that atherosclerosis-related agents, like galectin-3, could enter the circulation and reflect ongoing activity within atherosclerotic plaques. Accordingly, serum galectin-3 levels in this study did not correlate with its respective concentration within carotid plaques, implying that circulating galectin-3 may not be a marker of carotid plaque vulnerability.

J. P. Cullen, PhD

Activation of the Proapoptotic Unfolded Protein Response in Plaques of the Human Carotid Artery

Dorweiler B, Grechowa I, Wallrath A, et al (Johannes-Gutenberg Univ, Mainz, Germany)

Eur J Vasc Endovasc Surg 48:248-257, 2014

Objective.—To analyze expression of keystone markers of apoptosis and the proapoptotic signaling pathway "unfolded protein response" (UPR) in rupture-prone plaques of the human carotid artery.

Methods.—Plaque specimens were obtained during endarterectomy for high-grade carotid stenosis, and were formalin-fixed. Ten specimens were identified that exhibited criteria of advanced rupture-prone atherosclerotic plaques, and histological and immunohistological analysis of markers of apoptosis (cleaved Caspase-3, TUNEL) and UPR (KDEL, ATF3, CHOP, CHAC-1) was performed. In addition, co-localization of apoptosis and UPR-activation was assessed by double-immunohistochemistry.

Results.—The mean size of the necrotic core was 44 ± 7% and the mean minimum/representative thicknesses of the fibrous cap were 129 ± 39 μm/280 ± 60 μm, respectively. Each specimen fulfilled at least two of the criteria for rupture-prone plaques. Semi-quantitative analysis of immunohistochemistry showed a significant increase in cleaved Caspase-3-positive (1923 ± 93 cells/mm^2) and TUNEL-positive cells (1387 ± 66 cells/mm^2) when compared with control tissue. Furthermore, expression of UPR-markers KDEL, AFT3 and CHOP was significantly increased (1175 ± 40 cells/mm^2, 1971 ± 69 cells/mm^2 and 2173 ± 120 cells/mm^2, respectively). Co-localization of UPR-activation with apoptosis was confirmed by double-immunohistochemistry, and lesional macrophages were identified as the primary cell-type involved.

Conclusion.—For the first time, activation of the proapoptotic signaling pathway UPR has been identified in advanced rupture-prone plaques of the human carotid artery. This provides additional evidence for adding UPR to the potential targets for controlling plaque apoptosis and thereby preventing plaque progression/rupture.

▶ More than 15 million people worldwide suffer strokes each year, resulting in 5 million deaths and a further 5 million individuals who are permanently disabled. In the cerebrovascular circulation, atherosclerotic plaques that rupture as a result of their thin fibrous caps and large lipid cores have been identified as being positively associated with recent transient ischemic attack (TIA) and stroke. Increased apoptosis of lesional macrophages is one of the molecular mechanisms that leads to increased size of the necrotic core and thinning of the fibrous cap. Among several triggers of apoptosis, endoplasmic reticulum (ER) stress was identified as a potent inducer of macrophage apoptosis. ER stress occurs as a consequence of a mismatch between the load of unfolded and misfolded proteins in the ER and the capacity of the cellular machinery that copes with that load and sets a compensatory mechanism, the unfolded protein response (UPR), in motion, which reduces protein load and increases folding capacity. The authors of this study analyzed the expression of keystone markers of apoptosis and the proapoptotic signaling pathway UPR in human advanced rupture-prone carotid lesions. Carotid artery specimens were obtained from patients undergoing carotid endarterectomy for high-grade stenosis of the internal carotid artery. Analysis of lesion morphology confirmed that all specimens exhibited features of rupture-prone plaques corresponding to the inclusion criteria of this study (minimum cap thickness < 200 μm, representative cap thickness < 500 μm, and necrotic core > 25%). Their results demonstrate that activation of the proapoptotic signaling pathway UPR is robust and significantly increased in plaques compared with control tissue (common femoral, common carotid, and nondiseased internal carotid artery). This is the first study examining UPR activation in human carotid plaques, and the findings fit well with results obtained from human coronary plaques and data from atherogenic mice models highlighting ER stress and the UPR as a potential and potent inducer of apoptosis of vascular cells, and thereby contributing to plaque progression and rupture. Putting the results into perspective, acute cerebrovascular events (stroke and TIA) may now be considered as the clinical events together with acute coronary syndromes that warrant intense research into development and implementation of antiapoptotic strategies. Targeting activation of UPR may serve as a potential mechanism to relieve ER-induced apoptosis, and thereby reduce acute events/plaque ruptures in cardiovascular disease.

J. P. Cullen, PhD

Predicting Carotid Artery Disease and Plaque Instability from Cell-Derived Microparticles

Wekesa AL, Cross KS, O'Donovan O, et al (Waterford Inst of Technology, Ireland; Waterford Regional Hosp, Ireland; et al)
Eur J Vasc Endovasc Surg 48:489-495, 2014

Objectives.—Cell-derived microparticles (MPs) are small plasma membrane-derived vesicles that shed from circulating blood cells and may act as novel biomarkers of vascular disease. We investigated the potential of circulating MPs to predict (a) carotid plaque instability and (b) the presence of advanced carotid disease.

Methods.—This pilot study recruited carotid disease patients (aged 69.3 ± 1.2 years [mean ± SD], 69% male, 90% symptomatic) undergoing endarterectomy ($n = 42$) and age- and sex-matched controls ($n = 73$). Plaques were classified as stable ($n = 25$) or unstable ($n = 16$) post surgery using immunohistochemistry. Blood samples were analysed for MP subsets and molecular biomarkers. Odds ratios (OR) are expressed per standard deviation biomarker increase.

Results.—Endothelial MP (EMP) subsets, but not any vascular, inflammatory, or proteolytic molecular biomarker, were higher ($p < .05$) in the unstable than the stable plaque patients. The area under the receiver operator characteristic curve for $CD31^{+}41^{-}$ EMP in discriminating an unstable plaque was 0.73 (0.56–0.90, $p < .05$). $CD31^{+}41^{-}$ EMP predicted plaque instability (OR = 2.19, 1.08–4.46, $p < .05$) and remained significant in a multivariable model that included transient ischaemic attack symptom status. Annexin V^{+} MP, platelet MP (PMP) subsets, and C-reactive protein were higher ($p < .05$) in cases than controls. Annexin V^{+} MP (OR = 3.15, 1.49–6.68), soluble vascular cell adhesion molecule-1 (OR = 1.64, 1.03–2.59), and previous smoking history (OR = 3.82, 1.38–10.60) independently ($p < .05$) predicted the presence of carotid disease in a multivariable model.

Conclusions.—EMP may have utility in predicting plaque instability in carotid patients and annexin V^{+} MPs may predict the presence of advanced carotid disease in aging populations, independent of established biomarkers.

► Carotid artery disease often has no symptoms; simple quantitation based on the degree of stenosis has limitations, and there is a need to look beyond this parameter when assessing stroke risk. The majority of cardiovascular deaths are most commonly the result of disruption or rupture of the fibrous cap of a lipid laden vulnerable atherosclerotic plaque. Consequently, atherosclerotic plaque stability is an important prognostic indicator of future cardiovascular events and therefore has become the focus of novel treatment strategies. Microparticles (MPs) are small (less than 1 mM) vesicles released by apoptotic cells with an antigen distribution that is representative of the cell membranes from which they derive. Increased levels of endothelial microparticles (EMPs), platelet microparticles (PMPs), and leukocyte microparticles have been reported in the plasma of patients with atherosclerotic diseases compared with matched controls. Only 2 studies to date have investigated MP in relation to carotid artery disease plaques. The purpose of this study was to determine the ability of EMP and PMP to predict carotid plaque instability in patients undergoing endarterectomy and the presence of advanced carotid disease in a cohort of cases and matched controls. In addition to MP, a range of more frequently measured molecular biomarkers were measured to determine the additional value that might result from including MP in multivariable prediction models. Microparticles bear phospholipids that bind to annexin V, and membrane proteins of their mother cell (eg, CD31 for EMPs). Results demonstrated that when patients with stable and unstable carotid plaques were compared, the $CD31^+$ EMP subsets were higher in the unstable plaque group. In contrast, none of the vascular inflammatory, proteolytic, or angiogenic factors measured were different between these groups. Furthermore, when biomarker concentrations in carotid artery disease cases and matched controls were compared, annexin V^+ MPs, $CD41^+$ MPs, annexin V^+ $CD41^+$ MPs, and the inflammatory marker C-reactive protein were all higher in the cases. Despite the small sample size, this study is interesting and demonstrates that measurement of specific MP subsets may help predict carotid plaque instability. As suggested by the authors, further, possibly multicenter research studies, with considerably larger sample sizes are justified.

J. P. Cullen, PhD

Associations of matrix metalloproteinase-9 and monocyte chemoattractant protein-1 concentrations with carotid atherosclerosis, based on measurements of plaque and intima–media thickness

Tan C, Liu Y, Li W, et al (Hosp of Chong Qing Med Univ, YuZhong District, China)

Atherosclerosis 232:199-203, 2014

Purpose.—To examine associations of matrix metalloproteinase-9 (MMP-9) and monocyte chemoattractant protein-1 (MCP-1) concentrations with the severity of carotid atherosclerosis, based on measurements of carotid plaque and intima–media thickness (IMT).

Methods.—This cross-sectional study included 116 stroke-free participants (45.7% males, 54.3% females; mean age, 64.73 ± 14.53 years). Serum MMP-9 and MCP-1 concentrations were measured, and plaque morphology, including total plaque score (PS), plaque stability, and

IMT, was assessed ultrasonographically. Participants were grouped according to total PS (0, 1–2, ≥3), plaque stability (no plaque, stable, unstable) and IMT tertiles (<0.8 mm, 0.8–1 mm, >1 mm). Multinomial logistic regression models were used to assess the associations of MMP-9 and MCP-1 concentrations with plaque and IMT values after adjusting for vascular risk factors.

Results.—MMP-9 quartiles (*vs.* quartile 1) were significantly associated with a greater prevalence of plaque instability [Q2: odds ratio (OR) = 5.13, 95% confidence interval (CI) = 1.01–24.9, $p = 0.042$; Q3: OR = 15.5, 95% CI = 3.1–78.1, $p = 0.001$; Q4: OR = 13.2, 95% CI = 2.7–64.97, $p = 0.001$] and high total PS (Q3: OR = 10.02, 95% CI = 1.5–65.33, $p = 0.016$; Q4: OR = 21.5, 95% CI = 3.5–132.1, $p = 0.001$). MCP-1 concentration was significantly associated with IMT (OR = 22.94, 95% CI = 2.14–245.66, $p = 0.01$).

Conclusions.—Elevated serum MMP-9 concentration was independently associated with high total carotid artery PS, plaque instability, and large IMT value. MCP-1 concentration was independently associated with IMT, but not with plaque morphology.

► Matrix metalloproteinases (MMPs) are implicated in many disease processes involving inflammation in arterial and venous pathologies. A possible mechanism is that MMPs may be involved in the vulnerability of a carotid artery plaque, and identifying which atherosclerotic plaques are unstable that could provide useful information is the stratification of patients undergoing carotid endarterectomy for asymptomatic disease. In this study, serum samples of MMP-9 (a gelatinase that is implicated in many arterial and venous diseases) and monocyte chemoattractant protein 1 (MCP-1) were evaluated in 116 asymptomatic patients and correlated to ultrasonographic morphology of the carotid plaques and the intima–media thickness (IMT). The main findings were that plaque score (0-4 based on the percent of stenosis), plaque stability (based on surface characteristics, echogenicity, and texture on ultrasound exam), and IMT to some extent were significantly associated to serum MMP-9 levels in that plaques had severe stenosis, instability, and thicker and that IMT was highly correlated to MCP-1 levels. Another interesting finding was that plaque instability was highly associated with uric acid levels and that hypertension and increasing age was significantly associated with increasing plaque score, plaque instability, and IMT. It is not known whether this study provides a cause and effect of MMP-9 and MCP-1 in the pathogenesis of vulnerable asymptomatic atherosclerotic plaques. In addition, these markers, along with uric acid, may be important in identifying patients at risk warranting early intervention to prevent plaque rupture and symptoms. Uric acid regulates inflammatory pathways in smooth muscle cells, which may be involved in the development of unstable plaques. Hypertension and age are traditional cardiovascular risk factors, and hence seen in this study to correlate with plaque instability. Further studies are necessary to evaluate whether indeed these markers, when elevated, relate to actual events and that treatment is guided on biomarkers of disease. In addition, it would be interesting to determine whether high-intensity statin therapy and antiplatelet therapy have an effect on these inflammatory markers and development of symptoms.

J. D. Raffetto, MD, FACS, FSVM

2 Epidemiology

Epidemiology of peripheral arterial disease and critical limb ischemia in an insured national population

Nehler MR, Duval S, Diao L, et al (Univ of Colorado Denver, Aurora; Univ of Minnesota Med School, Minneapolis; CPC Clinical Research, Aurora, CO; et al)

J Vasc Surg 60:686-695.e2, 2014

Background.—Critical limb ischemia (CLI) represents the most severe clinical manifestation of peripheral arterial disease (PAD) and is the major cause of ischemic amputation in the United States. Risk factors and the associated incidence and prevalence of CLI have not been well described in the general population. This study describes the risk factors for PAD progression to CLI and estimates the annual incidence and prevalence of CLI in a representative United States patient cohort.

Methods.—This was a retrospective cohort analysis of adults with commercial, Medicare supplemental, or Medicaid health insurance who had at least one PAD or CLI health care claim from January 1, 2003, through December 31, 2008, and 12 months of continuous coverage. Two subgroups of CLI presentation were identified: primary CLI (patients without any prior PAD or subsequent PAD diagnostic code >30 days after CLI diagnostic code) and secondary CLI (patients with prior PAD or subsequent PAD diagnostic codes ≤30 days of a CLI diagnostic code). Patterns of presentation, annual incidence, and prevalence of CLI were stratified by health care plan. Risk factors for progression to CLI were compared by presentation type.

Results.—From 2003 to 2008, the mean annual incidence of PAD was 2.35% (95% confidence interval [CI], 2.34%-2.36%) and the incidence of CLI was 0.35% (95% CI, 0.34%-0.35%) of the eligible study population, with primary and secondary presentations occurring at similar rates. The mean annualized prevalence of PAD was 10.69% (95% CI, 10.67% 10.70%) and the mean annualized prevalence of CLI was 1.33% (95% CI, 1.32%-1.34%) of the eligible study population, and two-thirds of the cases presented as secondary CLI. CLI developed in 11.08% (95% CI, 11.30%-11.13%) of patients with PAD. A multivariable model demonstrated that diabetes, heart failure, stroke, and renal failure were stronger predictors of primary rather than secondary CLI presentation.

Conclusions.—These data establish new national estimates of the incidence and prevalence of CLI and define key risk factors that contribute to primary or secondary presentations of CLI within a very large contemporary insured population cohort in the United States (Table 2A, Table 2B, Tables 3 and 4, Supplementary Table).

▶ The Marketscan database used in this analysis includes only those Medicare beneficiaries who also had supplemental insurance coverage, and only collects data after 100% of claims have been paid. Use of this data source therefore may have biased the incidence and prevalence estimates toward a segment of the population with a relative abundance of access to care that may not be representative of Medicare beneficiaries (or the US population) as a whole in terms of demographics or socioeconomic background. The multivariable model in this analysis identified increased risk for secondary critical limb ischemia (CLI; defined as CLI that developed in the setting of previously identified peripheral arterial disease [PAD] of lesser severity) that included diabetes,

TABLE 2.—A, Incidence Population for Peripheral Arterial Disease (*PAD*) and Critical Limb Ischemia (*CLI*) Subgroups: Baseline Demographic Characteristics and Comorbidities of the Study Population in 2004 to 2008

Demographic Characteristics	Incidence Population[a] PAD[b] (n = 228,468)	Secondary CLI[c] (n = 15,402)	Primary CLI[d] (n = 18,251)	Total[e] (N = 262,121)
Age, mean ± SD years	68.9 ± 12.5	69.3 ± 12.6	69.0 ± 13.4	68.9 ± 12.6
Age group, years, %				
40-49	6.4	6.4	7.9	6.5
50-59	19.3	19.2	20.4	19.4
60-69	25.3	23.8	22.7	25.0
70-79	12.1	12.2	10.6	12.0
80-84	24.8	25.7	23.4	24.8
≥85	12.0	12.7	15.1	12.2
Gender, %				
Male	43.7	47.8	46.1	44.1
Female	56.3	52.2	53.9	55.9
Type of health plan, %				
Commercial	28.3	20.1	28.5	27.8
Medicaid	30.5	40.6	29.5	31.0
Medicare supplemental	41.2	39.3	42.0	41.2
Patients with ≥1 comorbidity, %	94.9	95.7	91.8	94.7
Diabetes	14.7	31.6	28.5	16.7
Hypertension	72.2	70.9	66.5	71.7
Myocardial infarction	43.3	41.8	34.5	42.6
Stroke	19.7	22.0	19.0	19.8
Heart failure	21.6	30.0	25.6	22.4
Renal failure	8.9	13.3	11.0	9.3
Cancer	14.5	9.6	11.3	14.0

SD, standard deviation.
[a]Incidence population: Adults ≥40 years with a PAD or CLI International Classification of Diseases, 9th Revision (ICD-9) or Current Medical Terminology (CPT; American Medical Association, Chicago, IL) code in the MarketScan database (Thomson Reuters [Healthcare] Inc, New York, NY) between 2004 and 2008, and with continuous 12-month baseline coverage.
[b]Incident PAD defined codes without CLI codes.
[c]Incident CLI defined codes with a prior PAD diagnostic code and/or subsequent PAD code ≤30 days of CLI code.
[d]Incident CLI defined codes without a prior PAD diagnostic code or subsequent PAD code ≤30 days of CLI code.
[e]Total (PAD and CLI codes combined).

TABLE 2.—B, Prevalence Population for Peripheral Arterial Disease (*PAD*) and Critical Limb Ischemia (*CLI*) Subgroups: Baseline Demographic Characteristics and Comorbidities of the Study Population in 2004

	Prevalent Population[a]			
Demographic Characteristics	PAD[b] (n = 149,254)	Secondary CLI[c] (n = 11,563)	Primary CLI[d] (n = 7732)	Total PAD[e] (N = 168,549)
Age, mean ± SD, years	68.9 ± 12.5	69.7 ± 12.6	66.3 ± 13.9	68.9 ± 12.6
Age group, years, %				
40-49	7.2	6.4	12.6	7.4
50-59	17.7	17.1	23.3	17.9
60-69	24.3	24.0	21.9	24.2
70-79	13.4	12.9	10.2	13.2
80-84	26.5	26.5	20.1	26.2
≥85	11.0	13.2	11.7	11.1
Sex, %				
Male	46.4	52.6	48.7	46.9
Female	53.6	47.4	51.3	53.1
Type of health plan, %				
Commercial	30.4	24.7	39.5	30.4
Medicaid	20.4	27.0	19.5	20.8
Medicare supplemental	49.2	48.3	41.0	48.8
Patients with ≥1 comorbidity, %	77.9	89.9	72.1	78.5
Diabetes	13.2	42.6	20.5	15.6
Hypertension	53.7	61.5	47.1	53.9
Myocardial infarction	33.6	42.3	23.4	33.8
Stroke	14.3	20.2	11.6	14.6
Heart failure	15.0	29.6	17.2	16.1
Renal failure	2.8	8.1	3.7	3.2
Cancer	8.6	7.3	7.8	8.5

SD, Standard deviation.
[a]Prevalent population: Adults ≥40 years with a PAD or CLI International Classification of Diseases, 9th Revision (ICD-9) or Current Medical Terminology (CPT; American Medical Association, Chicago, IL) code in the MarketScan database (Thomson Reuters [Healthcare] Inc, New York, NY) in 2004 with 12 months of continuous eligible insurance coverage during the 2003 baseline period.
[b]PAD defined codes without CLI codes.
[c]CLI defined codes with a prior PAD diagnostic code or subsequent PAD code ≤30 days of CLI code, or both.
[d]CLI defined codes without a prior PAD diagnostic code or subsequent PAD code ≤30 days of CLI code.
[e]Total (PAD and CLI combined).
Reprinted from the Journal of Vascular Surgery. Nehler MR, Duval S, Diao L, et al. Epidemiology of peripheral arterial disease and critical limb ischemia in an insured national population. *J Vasc Surg*. 2014;60:686-695.e2. Copyright 2014, with permission from The Society for Vascular Surgery.

stroke, and heart failure. Smoking, however, is an important risk factor for CLI that is conspicuously absent from both the descriptive statistics and models (and presumably was therefore unavailable). In considering these results, it is also important to note that many of the International Classification of Diseases, Ninth Revision codes used to categorize clinical disease states have limited ability to discriminate between patients with asymptomatic PAD and claudication and may also incorrectly capture patients with diagnoses unrelated to PAD (eg, 707.06—"chronic ulcer of skin"; 447.1—"other disorders of arteries"; and 729.5—"pain in limb"; Supplementary Table).

Large-scale, prospective epidemiologic studies primarily focused on characterizing disease prevalence have become something of an endangered species within the current research funding environment as competition has increased and focus has shifted toward deliverables with direct impact on treatment

TABLE 3.—Incidence of Peripheral Arterial Disease (*PAD*) and Critical Limb Ischemia (*CLI*) Subgroups, Overall and by Health Insurance Plan at Each Year (2004 to 2008)

			Incidence			
Group	Year	Eligible Risk Population,[a] No.	PAD,[b] %	Secondary CLI,[c] %	Primary CLI,[d] %	Total,[e] %
Overall	2004	1,638,930	2.19	0.24	0.18	2.61
	2005	1,744,766	2.83	0.23	0.23	3.29
	2006	1,366,794	3.05	0.21	0.23	3.48
	2007	2,275,054	1.83	0.10	0.14	2.07
	2008	2,702,994	2.22	0.09	0.18	2.49
Mean (95% CI)			2.35 (2.34-2.36)	0.16 (0.16-0.16)	0.19 (0.18-0.19)	2.69 (2.68-2.70)
Commercial	2004	837,108	0.88	0.06	0.08	1.02
	2005	848,702	1.50	0.09	0.13	1.72
	2006	672,715	1.31	0.07	0.10	1.48
	2007	1,472,776	0.81	0.03	0.06	0.91
	2008	1,829,209	1.29	0.05	0.10	1.45
Medicaid	2004	278,509	4.99	0.71	0.40	6.10
	2005	364,475	3.78	0.39	0.28	4.45
	2006	318,395	5.66	0.43	0.43	6.52
	2007	247,785	4.95	0.33	0.33	5.62
	2008	251,551	4.65	0.26	0.42	5.34
Medicare supplemental	2004	523,313	2.78	0.27	0.24	3.30
	2005	531,589	4.30	0.33	0.35	4.98
	2006	375,684	3.93	0.26	0.30	4.50
	2007	554,493	3.13	0.17	0.26	3.56
	2008	622,234	3.95	0.15	0.32	4.42

CI, Confidence interval.
[a]Adults aged >40 years with commercial, Medicare supplemental, or Medicaid health insurance, without evidence of symptomatic PAD or CLI at any given year between 2004 and 2008.
[b]Total number of new PAD without CLI at a given year, divided by the eligible population at risk during the same year.
[c]Total number of individuals with first occurrence of an International Classification of Diseases, 9th Revision (ICD-9) or Current Medical Terminology (CPT; American Medical Association, Chicago, IL) CLI code who also had a pre-existing PAD code or a subsequent PAD code ≤30 days in a given year, divided by the eligible population at risk during the same year.
[d]Total number of individuals with first occurrence of an ICD-9 or CPT CLI code without a pre-existing PAD code or a subsequent PAD code ≤30 days.
[e]Total number in all three groups (PAD, primary CLI, secondary CLI) in a given year, divided by the total number of individuals without evidence of symptomatic PAD or CLI during the same year.
Reprinted from the Journal of Vascular Surgery. Nehler MR, Duval S, Diao L, et al. Epidemiology of peripheral arterial disease and critical limb ischemia in an insured national population. *J Vasc Surg*. 2014;60:686-695.e2.

TABLE 4.—Prevalence of Peripheral Arterial Disease (*PAD*) and Critical Limb Ischemia (*CLI*) Subgroups Overall and by Health Insurance Plan by Year

Group	Year	Eligible Population,[a] No.	PAD,[b] %	Prevalent PAD or CLI, or Both, in Total Population			Total CLI in PAD,[f] %
				Secondary CLI,[c] %	Primary CLI,[d] %	Total PAD,[e] %	
Overall	2003	1,106,701	11.13	1.20	0.59	12.92	13.84
	2004	1,791,587	8.33	0.65	0.43	9.41	11.45
	2005	1,952,043	10.39	0.88	0.46	11.73	11.38
	2006	1,551,643	12.17	1.01	0.50	13.67	11.02
	2007	2,547,638	11.09	0.80	0.45	12.34	10.17
	2008	3,030,517	11.01	0.83	0.45	12.29	10.46
Mean (95% CI)			10.69 (10.67-10.70)	0.86 (0.86-0.87)	0.47 (0.46-0.47)	12.02 (12.00-12.04)	11.08 (11.03-11.13)
Commercial	2003	465,613	6.34	0.52	0.40	7.27	12.70
	2004	881,759	5.14	0.32	0.35	5.81	11.53
	2005	900,071	5.90	0.39	0.33	6.62	10.87
	2006	707,813	5.93	0.37	0.29	6.58	10.01
	2007	1,575,641	7.35	0.41	0.35	8.11	9.34
	2008	1,961,237	7.28	0.45	0.35	8.09	9.94
Medicaid	2003	287,429	14.54	1.89	0.73	17.16	15.24
	2004	310,506	9.81	1.01	0.49	11.30	13.20
	2005	426,573	13.76	1.52	0.59	15.87	13.30
	2006	382,087	16.27	1.66	0.62	18.55	12.32
	2007	300,951	17.50	1.77	0.69	19.97	12.33
	2008	306,389	17.66	1.89	0.68	20.23	12.72
Medicare	2003	353,659	14.66	1.52	0.73	16.91	13.33
	2004	599,322	12.26	0.93	0.53	13.72	10.65
	2005	625,399	14.56	1.13	0.56	16.25	10.40
	2006	461,743	18.34	1.45	0.71	20.50	10.54
	2007	671,046	16.98	1.29	0.59	18.86	9.98
	2008	762,891	17.91	1.40	0.61	19.92	10.08

CI, Confidence interval.
[a]Adults aged ≤40 years with commercial, Medicare supplemental, or Medicaid health insurance, from January 1, 2003, through December 31, 2008.
[b]PAD patients without CLI in a given year, divided by the eligible population in that year.
[c]PAD patients with a prior PAD diagnostic code or subsequent PAD code ≤30 days of CLI code in a given year, or both, divided by the eligible population in that year.
[d]CLI patients without a prior PAD diagnostic code or subsequent PAD code ≤30 days of CLI code in a given year, divided by the eligible population in that year.
[e]Sum of PAD, primary CLI and secondary CLI patients, divided by the eligible population in that year.
[f]Total number of primary and secondary CLI patients, divided by the total number of PAD patients in that year.
Reprinted from the Journal of Vascular Surgery. Nehler MR, Duval S, Diao L, et al. Epidemiology of peripheral arterial disease and critical limb ischemia in an insured national population. *J Vasc Surg.* 2014;60:686-695.e2. Copyright 2014, with permission from The Society for Vascular Surgery.

SUPPLEMENTARY TABLE.—International Classification of Diseases-9th Revision (*ICD-9*) and Current Procedural Terminology (*CPT*) Codes[a] used to Identify Peripheral Arterial Disease (*PAD*) and Critical Limb Ischemia (*CLI*) Patients

Category	Diagnosis/Procedure	Associated ICD-9 or CPT Codes	Frequency of Occurrence (%)
PAD diagnosis	Other peripheral vascular disease	ICD-9: 443.1, 443.22, 443.81, 443.89, 443.9	38.29
	Atherosclerosis	ICD-9: 440.0, 440.20, 440.21, 440.29, 440.30, 440.31, 440.32, 440.4, 440.8, 440.9	18.02
	Diabetes with peripheral circulatory disorders	ICD-9: 249.70, 249.71, 250.70, 250.71, 250.72, 250.73	8.40
	Chronic ulcer of skin	ICD-9: 707.06, 707.07	3.18
	Other disorders of arteries	ICD-9: 447.1	2.99
	Atheroembolism	ICD-9: 445.02	0.08
CLI diagnosis	Pain in limb	ICD-9: (729.5)[b]	4.29
	Gangrene	ICD-9: 785.4	3.29
	Ulcer of lower limb	ICD-9: (707.1, 707.10, 707.13, 707.14, 707.15, 707.19, 707.9)[b]	3.05
	Atherosclerosis (with rest pain, gangrene, or ulceration)	ICD-9: 440.22, 440.23, 440.24	1.46
	Excision/debridement	ICD-9: (77.65, 77.66, 77.67, 77.68, 86.22, 99.10)[b]	0.30
	Postoperative wound infection	ICD-9: (998.59)[b]	0.25
	Acute osteomyelitis of lower limb	ICD-9: (730.06, 730.07)[b]	0.21
	Chronic osteomyelitis of lower Limb	ICD-9: (730.16, 730.17)[b]	0.14

Lower extremity revascularization	Percutaneous transluminal angioplasty	ICD-9: 00.40, 00.41, 00.42, 00.43, 00.44, 39.50; CPT: 354542, 35454, 35456, 35459, 35470, 35472, 35473, 35474	4.47
	Peripheral Bypass	ICD-9: 39.25, 39.29; CPT: 35500, 35521, 35533, 35537, 35538, 35539, 35540, 35541, 35546, 35548, 35549, 35551, 35556, 35558, 35563, 35565, 35566, 35583, 35585, 35587, 35621, 35623, 35646, 35647, 35651, 35654, 35656, 35661, 35663, 35665, 35666, 35671, 35681, 35682, 35700, (35683, 35686, 35571)[c]	1.60
	Stents	ICD-9: 39.90, 00.45, 00.46, 00.47, 00.48, 00.55	0.85
	Other lower extremity revascularization	ICD-9: 38.08, 39.49; CPT: 35221, 35226, 35256, 35286	0.56
	Endarterectomy	ICD-9: 38.16, 38.18, 38.38, 38.48, 38.68; CPT: 35302, 35303, 35304, 35305, 35306, 35331, 35351, 35355, 35361, 35363, 35371, 35372, 35381	0.54
	Atherectomy	CPT: 35480, 35481, 35482, 35483, 35485, 35490, 35491, 35492, 35493, 35495	0.36
	Thrombectomy, lower limbs	CPT: 35875, 35876, 35879, 35881, 35883, 35884, 35903	0.22
	Repair of blood vessel	ICD-9: 39.56, 39.57, 39.58	0.04
Lower extremity amputation	Amputation	ICD-9: 84.10, 84.12, 84.14, 84.15, 85.17, 84.3, 84.91 (84.11)[b]; CPT: 27590, 27591, 27592, 27594, 27596, 27599, 27880, 27881, 27882, 27888, 27889, 28800, 28805, 28810, 28820, 28825	2.12
	Chronic infection of amputation stump	ICD-9: (997.62)[b]	0.10
	Disarticulation	ICD-9: 84.13, 84.16, 84.18; CPT: 27295, 27598	0.03

[a]American Medical Association, Chicago, Ill.
[b]Must be accompanied by one of the following codes: 440.20, 440.21, 440.22, 440.23, 440.24.
[c]Must be accompanied by one of the following codes: 35556, 35566, 35571, 35583, 35585, 35587, 35623, 35656, 35666, 35671.

and/or value. Within this environment, our understanding of the epidemiology of vascular disease will depend more on inferences derived from administrative data rather than longitudinal cohort studies. Because administrative data sets have their limitations and cannot provide the same level of insight as a prospective study, accurately characterizing PAD epidemiology using claims data will likely require multiple sources, each providing a slightly different perspective based on a sample of the larger population of interest (potentially defined based on a geographic region, a health care system, a country, or the world).

M. A. Corriere, MD, MS

Shifting abdominal aortic aneurysm mortality trends in The Netherlands

Nelissen BGL, Herwaarden JA, Pasterkamp G, et al (Univ Med Ctr Utrecht, The Netherlands)

J Vasc Surg 61:642-647, 2015

Objective.—Mortality from abdominal aortic aneurysm (AAA) in developed countries has decreased since the late 1990s. Our objective was to get an insight of mortality trends in The Netherlands for AAA disease.

Methods.—Data of all AAA deaths (1980 to 2010) were collected from the Dutch cause of death register. Cause of death was divided in two groups: with the mention of rupture and without the mention of rupture. Data were standardized and divided into three age groups (55-69, 70-84, and ≥85 years). Mortality rates per 100,000 were analyzed for both sexes and for each age group. Significant points of change were identified using joinpoint regression analysis.

Results.—Total standardized AAA mortality increased from 1980 (1062 deaths) until 1995 (1728 deaths), followed by a decline until 2010 (930 deaths). This decline was most prominent in men. Deaths without mention of rupture showed an increase from 1980 until 2010. The age of AAA death was higher in women (79.2 in 1980 and 82.1 in 2010) than in men. This difference declined as the age of death from AAA increased from 72.1 in 1980 to 77.9 years in 2010 in men. Decline in AAA mortality was first seen in the young age group (55-69 years) and then seen consecutively older age groups.

Conclusions.—Mortality from AAA is declining due to a reduction in deaths from ruptured AAAs. This was first observed in the young age groups. Men died more often and at a lower age (Fig 1).

▶ This is a study spanning 35 years on mortality trends for abdominal aortic aneurysm (AAA) disease in the Netherlands. After an increasing mortality from 1980, a decrease in AAA deaths has been observed since the mid-1990s, which accelerated after the millennium (Fig 1). This decline was first observed in the young age groups and, in later years, in the older age groups as well; occurred in both sexes; and was mainly driven by the trends in mortality due to ruptured AAA. The prevalence of death from AAA is higher and the age

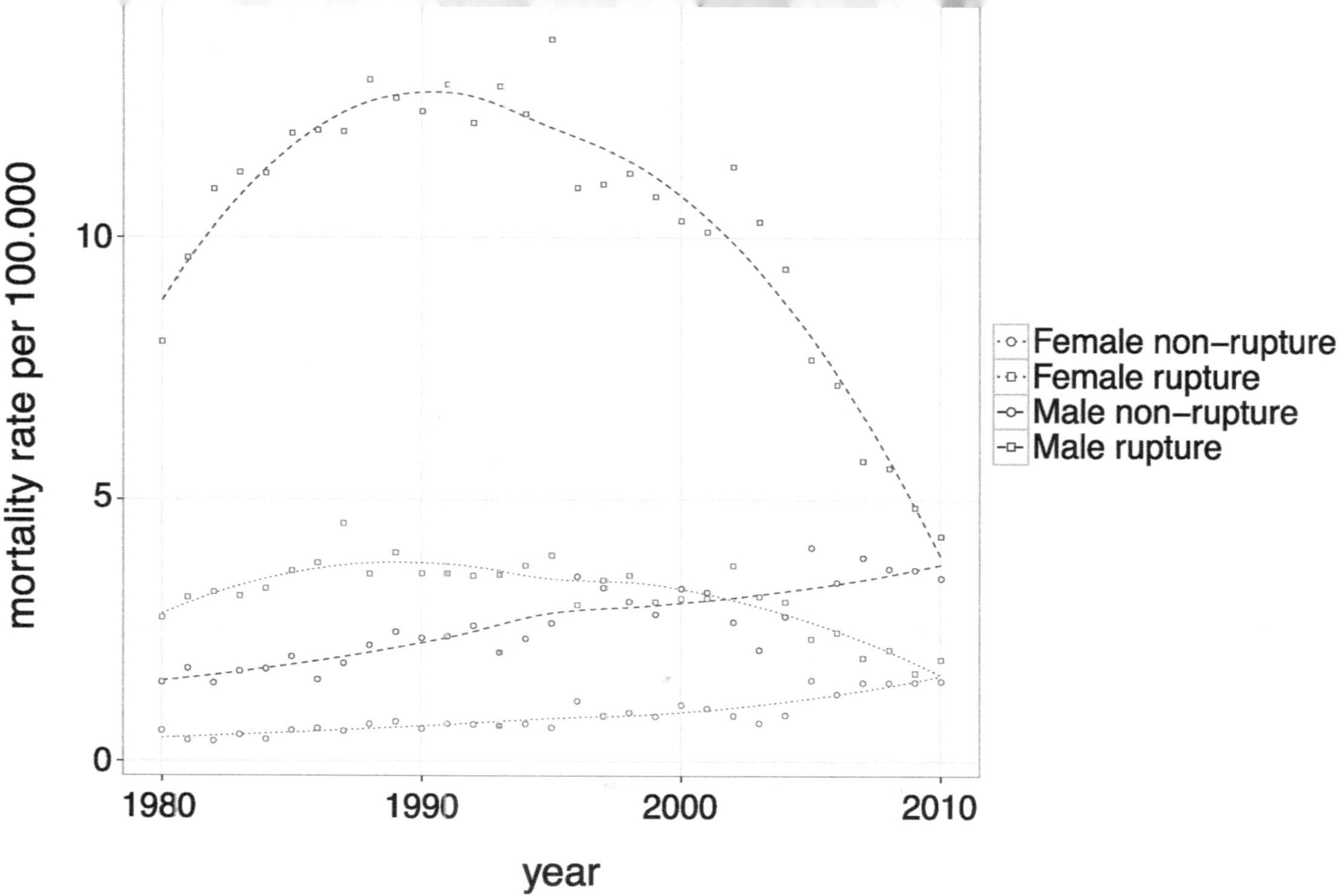

FIGURE 1.—Abdominal aortic aneurysm (AAA) standardized mortality rates in The Netherlands per 100,000 from 1980 to 2010. The year of standardization is 2010. Subgroups are made for rupture and nonrupture in men and women. For each group, a locally weighted regression curve was added for smoothing the variability in measurements. (Reprinted from the Journal of Vascular Surgery. Nelissen BGL, Herwaarden JA, Pasterkamp G, et al. Shifting abdominal aortic aneurysm mortality trends in the Netherlands. *J Vasc Surg*. 2015;61:642-647, Copyright 2014, with permission from The Society for Vascular Surgery.)

of death is lower in men than in women. However, the male-to-female ratio and the difference in age of death declined in the past decades.

These impressive trend results are likely multifactorial and involve not only better therapies including endovascular repair but also the increasing use of statins, better screening, and decreasing tobacco use. Other similar trend lines have been demonstrated in the United Kingdom.[1]

B. W. Starnes, MD

Reference

1. Anjum A, Allmen von R, Greenhalgh R, Powell JT. Explaining the decrease in mortality from abdominal aortic aneurysm rupture. *Br J Surg*. 2012;99:637-645.

3 Vascular Laboratory and Imaging

Six-minute walk test closely correlates to "real-life" outdoor walking capacity and quality of life in patients with intermittent claudication

Nordanstig J, Broeren M, Hensäter M, et al (Sahlgrenska Univ Hosp and Academy, Gothenburg, Sweden)

J Vasc Surg 60:404-409, 2014

Objective.—We used outdoor walking distance measured during 40 minutes as "real-life" outdoor walking capacity in 49 patients with intermittent claudication (IC). The outdoor walking distance was measured by a global positioning system application for a smartphone. The relationships of self-reported maximum walking distance (SR-MWD), the MWD on a graded treadmill test, and the 6-minute maximum walk distance (6MWD) vs outdoors walking capacity were investigated. Also studied were the associations of SR-MWD, MWD, and 6MWD with health-related quality of life assessed with the disease-specific instrument the Vascular Quality of Life Questionnaire (VascuQoL).

Methods.—In this prospective observational cohort study, 49 IC patients underwent an outdoor walking capacity test for 40 minutes, and MWD and 6MWD were measured. SR-MWD was recorded, and all subjects completed the VascuQoL questionnaire. Associations between the different walk estimates and outdoor walking capacity and health-related quality of life were investigated by correlation analysis (Spearman ρ).

Results.—Outdoor walking distance during 40 minutes was a median 2495 m (range, 1110-3300 m). SR-MWD correlated moderately and MWD correlated strongly to outdoor walking capacity ($r = 0.56$ and $r = 0.65$; $P < .001$, respectively). The 6MWD test showed the largest correlation to the outdoor walking capacity ($r = 0.78$; $P < .001$). The 6MWD was the only test that showed correlations with the VascuQoL sum score ($r = 0.53$; $P < .01$) and all of the domain scores, whereas SR-MWD and MWD showed weak correlations to the VascuQoL.

Conclusions.—The distance walked during the 6-minute walk test is closely correlated to outdoor walking capacity and health-related quality

TABLE 2.—Correlation Pattern (Spearman ρ) Between the Different Walking Tests and the Vascular Quality of Life (*VascuQoL*) Total and Domain Scores

	Vascuqol Scores					
Variable	Activity	Symptom	Pain	Emotional	Social	Total Sum
SR-MWD	0.40[a]	0.3	0.32	0.24	0.23	0.37[a]
MWD	0.37[a]	0.23	0.40[a]	0.27	0.2	0.34[a]
6MWD	0.57[b]	0.38[a]	0.52[b]	0.39[a]	0.38[a]	0.53[b]

6MWD, 6-minute maximum walking distance; *MWD*, maximum walking distance during graded treadmill test; *SR-MWD*, self-reported maximum walking distance.

[a]$P < .05$ level (two-tailed).

[b]$P < .01$ level (two-tailed).

Reprinted from the Journal of Vascular Surgery. Nordanstig J, Broeren M, Hensäter M, et al. Six-minute walk test closely correlates to "real-life" outdoor walking capacity and quality of life in patients with intermittent claudication. *J Vasc Surg*. 2014;60:404-409, Copyright 2014, with permission from the Society for Vascular Surgery.

of life in IC patients. Our data support the use of 6MWD for routine clinical evaluation of walking capacity in IC patients (Table 2).

▶ This study provides a valuable assessment of correlations between Global Positioning System (GPS)-based walking assessment with the Vascular Quality of Life Questionnaire and 3 different walking assessments more commonly used for clinical treatment decisions: self-reported maximum walking distance (SR-MWD), maximum walking distance (MWD), and 6-MWD. Although the authors correctly acknowledge that the SR-MWD is an important determinant for offering invasive treatment within the status quo, this measure is inconsistently obtained (frequently with extensive prompting from the provider) and often reported in variable units that may be defined based on city blocks, meters, or contextually by interference with daily activities (such as shopping, work, or recreation). This general predisposition toward bias and relatively poor correlation with quality of life (which was also observed with commonly used treadmill-based walking assessments; Table 2) certainly attest to the need for more objective and precise methods for quantifying claudication symptoms.

Several elements of GPS-based walking assessment give it unique and novel potential for quantifying PAD symptoms. Because GPS data can be obtained while patients are walking in conditions that mimic "real-world" (to use the authors' terminology) conditions, in which the patient sets his or her own pace and is able to rest intermittently, can potentially provide us with greater precision than treadmill in assessing how walking impairment impacts both activities of daily living and quality of life. Despite these potential advantages, however, GPS-based walking assessment will have to circumnavigate several barriers before widespread availability for routine clinical practice. Costs and necessary equipment (this study relied on an iPhone-based app but did not include cost data), satellite coverage, and access to a flat outdoor walking area currently make this tool unavailable for many patients. It should also be noted that symptoms in this patient cohort were mild; only 20% of participants were categorized as having Rutherford Class III (severe claudication symptoms). Further validation may therefore be necessary for patients with severe disease who experience symptoms over relatively short walking distance, and it is possible that GPS measurement may be less useful for this subgroup of patients. Additional validation may also be necessary among patients with other chronic medical conditions that may impair walking activity; although these patients were excluded from this study, patients with claudication who also have comorbidities with equal or greater potential to impair their walking (such as chronic obstructive pulmonary disease and osteoarthritis) are relatively common within the elderly PAD population. Beyond diagnosis and treatment selection, GPS also holds future promise for assessing responses to interventions in an era when interest in patient-reported outcomes is on the rise.

M. A. Corriere, MD, MS

Applicability of global positioning system for the assessment of walking ability in patients with arterial claudication

Gernigon M, on behalf of the Post-GPS Study Coinvestigators Group (Univ Hosp, Angers, France)

J Vasc Surg 60:973-981.e1, 2014

Objective.—This study determined for the first time the clinical applicability of a global positioning system (GPS)-monitored community-based walking ability assessment in a large cohort of patients with peripheral artery disease (PAD).

Methods.—A multicenter study was conducted among PAD patients who complained of intermittent claudication. Patients equipped with a GPS device performed a community-based outdoor walk. We determined the number of technically satisfactory GPS recordings (attempt No. 1). Patients with unsatisfactory GPS recordings were asked to perform a second attempt (attempt No. 2). From the satisfactory recordings obtained after attempts No.1 and No. 2, we analyzed several GPS parameters to provide clinical information on the patients' walking ability. Results are reported as median (interquartile range).

Results.—A total of 218 patients performed an outdoor walk. GPS recordings were technically satisfactory in 185 patients (85%) and in 203 (93%) after attempts No. 1 and No. 2, respectively. The highest measured distance between two stops during community walking was 678 m (IQR, 381-1333 m), whereas self-reported maximal walking distance was 250 m (IQR, 150-400 m; $P < .001$). Walking speed was 3.6 km/h (IQR, 3.1-3.9 km/h), with few variations during the walk. Among the patients who had to stop during the walk, the stop durations were <10 minutes in all but one individual.

Conclusions.—GPS is applicable for the nonsupervised multicenter recording of walking ability in the community. In the future, it may facilitate objective community-based assessment of walking ability, allow for the adequate monitoring of home-based walking programs, and for the

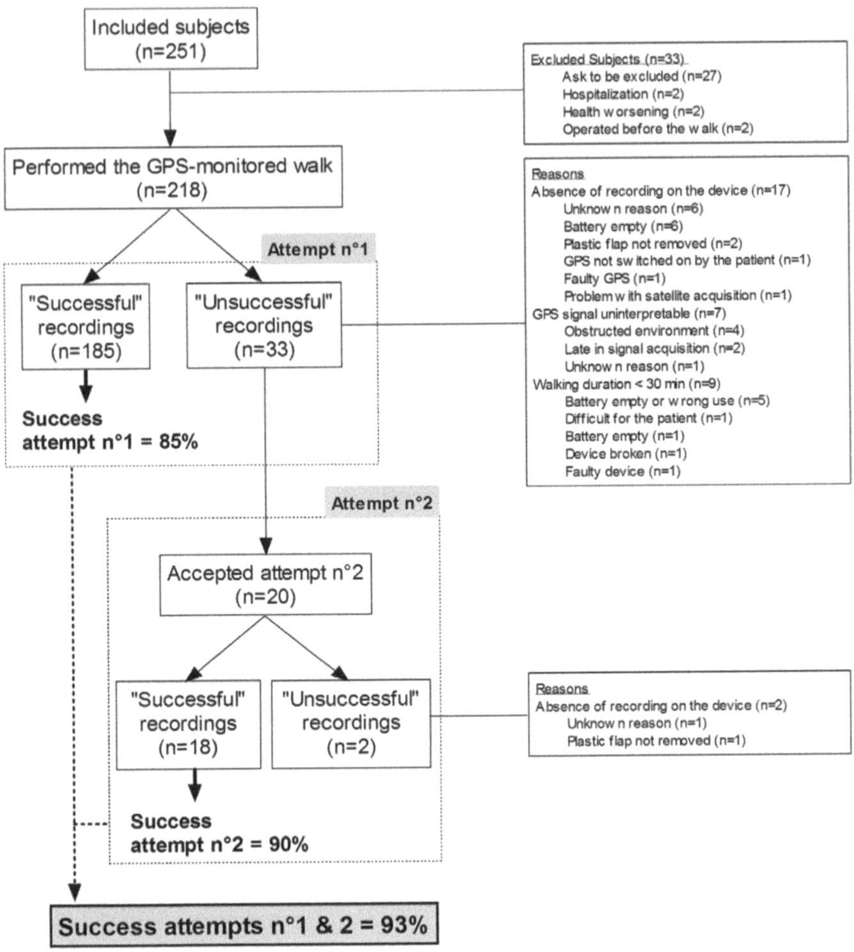

FIGURE 1.—Flow diagram shows patients through each stage of the study with the corresponding percentages of technically satisfactory global positioning system (*GPS*) recordings and causes of technically unsatisfactory GPS recordings. (Reprinted from the Journal of Vascular Surgery. Gernigon M, on behalf of the Post-GPS Study Coinvestigators Group. Applicability of global positioning system for the assessment of walking ability in patients with arterial claudication. *J Vasc Surg*. 2014;60:973-981, Copyright 2014, with permission from The Society for Vascular Surgery.)

study of new dimensions of walking in PAD patients with intermittent claudication (Fig 1, Tables 3 and 5).

▶ Beyond the specific findings and comparisons presented, it is interesting to consider the potential future impacts of global positioning system (GPS) technology on both research and clinical practice. One could envision this technology supplanting some of the on-site testing we currently use based on several potential advantages over the status quo. From a patient perspective, the

TABLE 3.—Global Positioning System (GPS) Results Among the 203 Participants with Technically Satisfactory Recordings After Attempt No. 1 and Attempt No. 2

GPS Parameters	Median (Interquartile Range)
Total distance walked during the stroll, m	2982 (2419-3622)
Whole stroll duration, minutes[a]	61.4 (58-66)
Stops per patient, No.[b]	7 (3-11)
HMD between two stops, m	678 (381-1333)
Mean walking speed, km/h	3.6 (3.1-3.9)
Mean stop duration, minutes[b]	1.3 (0.6-2.2)

HMD, Highest measured distance.
[a]Excludes the initial and final resting periods.
[b]Calculated for patients with at least one stop.
Reprinted from the Journal of Vascular Surgery. Gernigon M, on behalf of the Post-GPS Study Coinvestigators Group. Applicability of global positioning system for the assessment of walking ability in patients with arterial claudication. *J Vasc Surg*. 2014;60:973-981.e1, with permission from the Society for Vascular Surgery.

TABLE 5.—Practical Feasibility for the Patients to Perform the Outdoor Global Positioning System (GPS) Walk (n = 218)

		Level of Difficulty			
Task	No Answer, No.	Very Difficult, No. (%)	Rather Difficult, No. (%)	Rather Easy, No. (%)	Very Easy, No. (%)
Organize the walk	11	5 (2)	29 (14)	106 (51)	67 (32)
Find an appropriate flat area	9	2 (1)	22 (11)	99 (47)	86 (41)
Start the GPS device	7	4 (2)	20 (9)	79 (37)	108 (51)
Maintain a regular walking pace	9	7 (3)	110 (53)	78 (37)	14 (7)
Stroll for a minimum of 1 hour	8	64 (30)	99 (47)	42 (20)	5 (2)

Values in parentheses are percentages of available answers.
Reprinted from the Journal of Vascular Surgery. Gernigon M, on behalf of the Post-GPS Study Coinvestigators Group. Applicability of global positioning system for the assessment of walking ability in patients with arterial claudication. *J Vasc Surg*. 2014;60:973-981.e1, with permission from the Society for Vascular Surgery.

advantage is the ability to complete the test in the real world, natural environment where they experience their symptoms without the need for an appointment or the somewhat awkward and time-consuming task of walking on a treadmill in front of a technician wearing leg cuffs. GPS technology could also be used to assess responses to treatment interventions through new outcomes that are better for patients and providers because they can be obtained at the patient's discretion without the need for personnel to perform the test or collate the data. This would be a major advance over our current approach, where treadmill testing is often used to diagnose claudication, but postintervention outcome assessment is often limited to resting noninvasive studies and subjective patient reporting. It is further plausible that providing a patient with a GPS device may actually impact adherence to a structured exercise program, particularly among patients without access to supervised programs, by nature of the fact that they are aware that their walking activity is being tracked and monitored (also known as the Hawthorne effect[1]). GPS technology could, therefore, function as both a diagnostic tool and a treatment adjunct. The GPS devices used were relatively inexpensive (~$75 for the device plus antenna) when compared with the cost of a treadmill test, particularly if the GPS equipment is durable enough to be reused. From a cost perspective, it will be interesting to observe the reaction of payers to this technology, which, if covered by insurance, could foreseeably decrease costs if GPS testing was used instead of (rather than in addition to) treadmill evaluation.

If GPS technology is eventually adopted into widespread clinical use, providers will have to develop experience and familiarity with interpreting the results. Several GPS-based parameters used to quantify walking activity (or, to use the authors' preferred term, *strolls*) cannot be assessed through treadmill testing because of practical limitations, including highest measured distance (HMD), self-selected walking speed, and stop durations. This last parameter is particularly interesting to consider, as the first stop on the treadmill usually concludes the test (and has a duration that lasts until the patient dresses and walks out of the examination room). It is interesting that HMD was 2- to 3-fold higher than maximum walking distance (MWD), a treadmill-based measure that is one of the most studied parameters of walking ability in peripheral arterial disease. Correlation between these 2 measures was poor (although statistically significant), and it may be that this large-scale difference reflects differences in pacing (which is regulated by the patient for GPS measurement but by the treadmill for MWD) or other differences between testing environments. Perhaps patients are more inclined to stop walking when they are on a treadmill, with a technician observing them and a clinic appointment scheduled immediately afterward (a hypothesis that seems self-evident to the point of being unworthy of formal testing). Regardless of the explanation for the difference between these parameters, one can't help wondering whether HMD provides a more direct real-world assessment of functional impairment, as patients are walking at a self-selected speed when their symptoms bring their daily activities to a halt.

Use of GPS-based testing has several limitations, however, that may decrease its utility. The authors attributed a number of unsatisfactory recordings to uninterpretable signals or inappropriate location of the walk in an "obstructed environment" (Fig 1). This finding suggests that GPS technology may be poorly suited for use in indoor or covered areas, potentially making it impractical in geographic regions with severe climates or harsh weather. Even within temperate areas, utility of GPS testing might be subject to seasonal variation. The high rate of failure on the first attempt at GPS assessment in this study (15%) implies that there is also a learning curve for patients using the technology for the first time and further suggests that focused education and practice might be necessary to decrease rates of failure with the initial attempt. Given that 10 of 33 participants (approximately 40%) who had an unsuccessful recording after their initial attempt were willing to try a second time, it may be that a certain percentage of patients will reject this form of measurement because they find it frustrating or otherwise unacceptable (Table 5).

M. A. Corriere, MD, MS

Reference

1. Landsberger HA. *Hawthorne revisited. Management and the Worker: its Critics, and Developments in Human Relations in Industry.* Ithaca, NY: Cornell University; 1958.

Duplex ultrasound diagnosis of failing stent grafts placed for occlusive disease

Troutman DA, Madden NJ, Dougherty MJ, et al (Pennsylvania Hosp, Philadelphia)

J Vasc Surg 60:1580-1584, 2014

Objective.—We previously showed that duplex ultrasound (DU) imaging is beneficial in the diagnosis of failing vein and prosthetic grafts performed for arterial occlusive disease. The purpose of this study was to evaluate whether DU imaging can reliably diagnose failing stent grafts (ie, covered stents) placed for arterial occlusive disease.

Methods.—Between July 1, 2005, and June 30, 2013, we placed 142 stent grafts in 92 arterial segments (1.5 stent grafts/stenotic artery) for lower extremity occlusive disease in patients who also underwent at least one DU surveillance study documenting a patent stent graft. Stent grafts were placed in 29 iliac and 52 femoropopliteal arteries and in 11 failing infrainguinal bypass grafts. Stent grafts used were Viabahn (W. L. Gore and Associates Inc, Flagstaff, Ariz) in 116 (82%), Wallgraft (Boston Scientific, Natick, Mass) in 23 (16%), Fluency (C. R. Bard Inc, Tempe, Ariz) in 2 (1%), and iCast (Atrium, Hudson, NH) in 1 (1%). Mean follow-up was 16 months (range, 1 week-86 months). Postoperative DU surveillance was performed in our Intersocietal Accreditation Commission accredited noninvasive vascular laboratory at 1 week, then every 3 months the first year, and every 6 months thereafter. DU measured peak systolic velocities (PSVs) and velocity ratio of adjacent PSVs (Vr) every 5 cm within the stent graft and adjacent arteries.

Results.—We retrospectively classified the following factors as "abnormal DU findings:" focal PSVs >300 cm/s, uniform PSVs <50 cm/s throughout the graft, and a Vr >3.0. Fifteen of 20 patients with one or more of these abnormal DU findings underwent prophylactic intervention (n = 8) or occluded without intervention (n = 7), whereas only two of 72 with normal DU findings occluded (*P* =.0001). Excluding the eight patients who underwent prophylactic intervention, seven of 12 patients with abnormal DU findings occluded without intervention vs two of 72 with normal DU findings (*P* =.0001).

Conclusions.—These findings suggest that follow-up DU surveillance can predict failure of stent grafts placed for lower extremity occlusive disease. Focal PSVs >300 cm/s, Vr >3.0, and most importantly, uniform PSVs

<50 cm/s throughout the stent graft were statistically reliable markers for predicting stent graft thrombosis.

▶ Reliable duplex ultrasound (DUS) criteria for identification of stent grafts at risk for occlusion would provide a major contribution to postimplantation management, informing decisions regarding repeat intervention as well as surveillance. This study evaluated a single-center cohort of patients treated with stent grafts for occlusive peripheral arterial disease. The study cohort consisted of patients with either intermittent claudication or critical limb ischemia that were treated with either balloon or self-expanding stents for disease involving the iliac, femoral-popliteal, or vein graft occlusive disease. The authors used an aggressive standardized DUS surveillance protocol that included an early postintervention baseline study at 1 week, followed by studies every 3 months during the first year and every 6 months thereafter in the absence of findings suggesting increased risk for graft thrombosis. A combined set of DUS criteria was used to designate an abnormal duplex based on 1 or more of the following: focal peak systolic velocity (PSV) elevation >300 cm/s, low PSVs (<50 cm/s) throughout the length of the stent graft, or a velocity ratio (Vr) >3. Based on these criteria, they concluded that an abnormal duplex was associated with occlusion among patients who were not treated with prophylactic repeat intervention to maintain patency.

Sensitivity and specificity were used in this study to evaluate associations between abnormal DUS and risk of subsequent graft occlusion. This approach is somewhat unorthodox, as these statistics are commonly used to evaluate reliability of screening tests relative to a gold standard or known disease state at a single point in time based on rates of true versus false-positive and false-negative results, rather than for predicting a future outcome. It is therefore unclear why more conventional approaches (such as logistic regression, survival analysis, or proportional hazards regression) were not used, making interpretation of the results somewhat difficult in terms of relative thrombosis risk over time. These considerations aside, the analysis nonetheless provides some evidence-based criteria for identifying stent grafts at risk for occlusion and suggests a role for surveillance imaging based on the stark contrast in occlusion rates following normal versus abnormal studies.

Several additional analyses would have been of potential interest for readers considering whether bare metal stents versus stent grafts should be favored for long-segment lower extremity occlusive lesions. For example, one might expect that the symptom severity and outcomes associated with stent graft occlusion might be worse than for bare metal stents given that stent grafts occlude branch vessels (and associated collaterals) throughout the covered segment. More severe presentations associated with stent-graft occlusion might also be expected due to higher rates of distal embolization at the time of occlusion; this is a known phenomenon associated with prosthetic bypass graft occlusion that increases the risk of limb loss (as mentioned by the authors in their discussion). Characterization of the outcomes associated with prophylactic repeat intervention performed based on an abnormal DUS would also provide valuable information regarding repeat intervention resulted in postoperative DUS "normalization," allowing resumption of their standard surveillance protocols and criteria. Alternatively, lack of "normalization" following prophylactic repeat intervention would result in challenging decision making and question the rationale for this approach. Finally, given the heterogeneity of diagnoses, anatomic locations, and device types used in this study, stratified comparisons evaluating the DUS criteria based on these factors would have been interesting and perhaps would have provided information that would inform clinical management more specifically. Hopefully, we can anticipate additional analyses from this group and others that will fill these remaining evidence gaps and objectively define the role of stent grafts for treatment of lower extremity arterial occlusive disease.

M. A. Corriere, MD, MS

Calf volume changes with venous occlusion air plethysmography in assessment of patients after deep venous thrombosis

Lattimer CR, Geroulakos G, Kalodiki E (Ealing Hosp, Middlesex, UK; et al)
J Vasc Surg Venous Lymphat Disord 2:416-423, 2014

Background.—This is an analysis of the hemodynamic response of post-thrombotic legs to a sustained thigh compression and quick-release maneuver. This is an integral part of the investigation of venous occlusion plethysmography that has been promoted as a way of assessing the venous return. The aim was to quantify the venous volume changes in patients after deep venous thrombosis (DVT) and to determine whether refluxing legs differed from obstructed legs.

Methods.—The inflow and outflow air plethysmography tracings of 332 of 519 legs were examined retrospectively. These tracings from 192 patients were performed between 1989 and 1999. The median age was 51 (17-89) years; 65% of the patients were men, and 52% were left legs. The retrospective clinical class distribution (%) by the Clinical, Etiologic, Anatomic, and Pathologic (CEAP) classification was as follows: $C_0 = 5.4$, $C_2 = 3.3$, $C_3 = 68.4$, $C_4 = 13$, $C_5 = 3.6$, $C_6 = 6.3$. Inclusion criteria were a history of DVT and a duplex ultrasound examination documenting the site and type of deep venous disease. Ascending phlebography was performed in 28% of patients to complement duplex ultrasound in assessing the site of disease. Reflux was defined as reverse flow (>1 second) and obstruction as luminal narrowing, wall irregularity, or luminal echogenic material. Air plethysmography was performed in the supine position. After calibration with 100 mL of air, a thigh cuff was inflated to 80 mm Hg, and the resulting increase in calf volume was recorded by the sensor calf cuff with an ink trace on graphic paper. At the volume plateau, the thigh cuff was deflated suddenly to record the decrease in calf volume.

Results.—Reflux alone was identified in 19.6% of limbs and obstruction alone in 42.2%. Iliofemoral involvement was identified in 56.6%. The thigh compression/release maneuver caused a significant median (interquartile range) net reduction in calf volume by 9 (5-15) mL ($P < .0005$, Wilcoxon). The outflow volume was significantly greater than the inflow volume overall and also when legs were separated into categories on the basis of their site and type of disease ($P < .0005$, Wilcoxon). There was no significant difference in calf volume change in legs with iliofemoral involvement compared with those with distal disease. However, pure refluxing legs had significantly greater inflow and outflow volumes compared with legs with pure obstruction ($P < .0005$), with a median (interquartile range) reduction in calf volume of 13 (8-18) mL (reflux group) vs 7 (2-13) mL (obstruction group) ($P < .0005$, Mann-Whitney).

Conclusions.—Thigh compression significantly improves the venous return in patients after DVT evidenced by a greater absolute reduction of calf volume. This change was significantly greater in pure refluxing legs than in those with obstruction alone.

▶ Venous inflow and outflow are important basic principles that allow physiologically for normal venous inflow from the lower extremity, which exits through the iliofemoral venous system (outflow) to return to the heart. Both inflow and outflow can be altered in patients who have had deep venous thrombosis with residual obstruction (venous wall irregularity, webs, luminal stenosis, residual echogenic material) or who have no obstruction but valvular insufficiency disease, leading to severe reflux of the deep venous system. Interestingly, there was no significant difference in calf volumes of legs with iliofemoral venous system involvement compared with those with more distal (popliteal venous system) disease. However, the refluxing legs had significantly greater inflow and outflow volumes compared with those with obstruction, with a net median (interquartile range) reduction in calf volume of 13 (8-18) mL versus 7 (2-13) mL ($P < .0005$). This would indicate that patients with residual obstruction in the deep venous systems have a reduced net decrease in calf volume compared with patients with only reflux and no obstruction. Outflow fraction was significantly reduced in patients who had iliofemoral venous thrombosis compared with popliteal thrombosis. There was no difference in outflow fraction between obstructed limbs versus refluxing limbs. This information would indicate that a reduction in outflow fraction is a marker for previous deep venous thrombosis especially in the iliofemoral venous segments. It is important to discriminate whether outflow obstruction means an impairment of the flow in a major vein or a global impairment of the drainage of the leg itself. However, one could have a significant venous outflow stenosis but excellent collaterals and have a normal outflow fraction; or one could have a lesser stenosis but no collateral venous network and have symptoms and a mildly reduced outflow fraction. Future noninvasive tests are needed to delineate significant outflow obstruction that has a high positive predictive value and a low false negative rate.

J. D. Raffetto, MD, FACS, FSVM

Can and should carotid ultrasound be used in cardiovascular risk assessment? The internist's perspective

Ray A, Huisman MV, Rabelink TJ (Leiden Univ Med Ctr, The Netherlands)

Eur J Intern Med 26:112-117, 2015

Cardiovascular risk management is a major and challenging task for internists. Risk scores using algorithms based on traditional risk factors are helpful in identifying patients in whom intensive prevention strategies are warranted. However there remains a need for more accurate screening tools to allow clinicians to individualize the primary prevention programs to their patients.

Approximately 40–80% of apparently healthy, asymptomatic subjects exhibit increased thickness of the lamina intima-media of the carotid artery or have atherosclerotic carotid plaques. These abnormalities can be measured safely and at low cost by ultrasound. Subclinical carotid lesions are strongly associated with generalized atherosclerotic burden and the risk of future cardiovascular events. Although many cardiovascular risk management guidelines recommend the use of these parameters incorporation in clinical practice is still not commonplace.

Based on the current literature it can be stated that in high risk patients there is no additional value of carotid ultrasound because even in the absence of carotid lesions these patients should receive an intensive risk reduction regime. In the large low-intermediate risk group however carotid ultrasound findings carry subtle but possibly clinically relevant information about cardiovascular risk profile. The effect of treatment decisions based on carotid ultrasound parameters has not been studied. Sequential measurements to monitor progression and evaluate treatment response on an individual basis are not sufficiently reproducible.

We therefore recommend the use of carotid ultrasound in low to intermediate risk patients but emphasize the importance of interpreting the results in conjunction with all cardiovascular risk factors and avoid follow-up measurements.

▶ There are few issues in vascular surgery that generate more conversation among vascular specialists than the management of the asymptomatic carotid stenosis. This article makes a case against identifying carotid stenosis in asymptomatic patients. It is most important to note that these authors define asymptomatic carotid stenosis to mean no previous history of ipsilateral transient ischemic attack or stroke. By their definition, patients with asymptomatic carotid stenosis could have symptoms unrelated to ipsilateral carotid territory ischemia, such as dizziness, syncope, or symptoms related to coronary artery or lower-extremity arterial disease. To make their analysis, these authors refer to the 2 largest and most important multicenter randomized clinical trials that compared medical management and carotid endarterectomy in asymptomatic patients with high-grade stenosis, a North American study (the Asymptomatic Carotid Atherosclerosis Study [ACAS]) and a European study (the Asymptomatic Carotid Surgery Trial [ACST]). These authors acknowledge that in both the ACAS and the ACST, the annual risk of stroke was approximately 2% in medically managed patients and approximately 1% in patients who underwent carotid endarterectomy. They appropriately point out that because rates of perioperative stroke or death were 2% to 3%, it took approximately 2 years for the benefit of endarterectomy to begin surpassing that of medical management. The authors of this analysis take issue with the fact that selection criteria for inclusion in these trials was potentially biased and ill defined, and therefore applying these trial outcomes to specific patients in general practice may be difficult. The main component of their argument against monitoring patients for asymptomatic stenosis is based on the concept that the ACAS and ACST began more than 20 years ago, in an era of less effective and less intensive medical management. They suggest that the potential net benefit of endarterectomy for asymptomatic carotid stenosis depends substantially on the stroke rate among medically managed patients. They reference 3 studies from Europe in which the stroke rates were 1% or less annually in medically managed patients with asymptomatic carotid stenosis of 50% or greater; risks were no higher in patients with stenosis of 70% or greater than in those with stenosis of 50% to 69%. In an international study of patients with stenosis of 70% or greater, the annual stroke rate of medically managed patients was 1%. They conclude that the results of the ACAS and ACST trials probably do not apply to patients receiving current antithrombotic, antihypertensive, or lipid-lowering medications, whose stroke risk related to asymptomatic carotid stenosis is 1% per year or less. By comparison, the risk of periprocedural stroke or death after carotid endarterectomy remains between 2% and 3% in the 2 randomized clinical trials. Thus their argument against ultrasound screening for carotid disease in asymptomatic patients is quite compelling.

M. T. Watkins, MD

4 Perioperative Considerations

Preoperative smoking is associated with early graft failure after infrainguinal bypass surgery

Selvarajah S, Black JH III, Malas MB, et al (The Johns Hopkins Hosp, Baltimore, MD; Johns Hopkins Bayview Med Ctr, Baltimore, MD)

J Vasc Surg 59:1308-1314, 2014

Objective.—Smoking has been implicated as the single most important risk factor for the development of peripheral arterial disease. Whereas previous studies have found poor long-term outcomes in smokers undergoing lower extremity bypass, there is a lack of consistent reports describing the effects of persistent tobacco abuse on early outcomes after infrainguinal bypass.

Methods.—The American College of Surgeons National Surgical Quality Improvement Program database from 2005 to 2011 was queried for primary infrainguinal bypasses. A bivariate analysis was done to assess preoperative and intraoperative risk factors for the primary outcome of 30-day graft failure comparing active smokers with nonsmokers, defined as patients who did not smoke within the 12 months before surgery. Multivariable logistic regression was conducted to assess the independent association of active smoking with graft failure.

Results.—In 6614 (40.0%) active smokers and 9920 (60.0%) nonsmokers, 16,534 infrainguinal bypasses were performed. Active smokers were more likely to be younger, male, and of nonwhite race and to have a history of chronic obstructive pulmonary disease ($P < .001$, all). Nonsmokers were more likely to be functionally dependent and had significantly more comorbidities (ie, hypertension, diabetes, obesity, congestive heart failure, history of previous cardiac surgery or intervention, and dialysis; $P < .001$, all). The presence of critical limb ischemia was similar in both groups (53.1% of active smokers vs 53.5% of nonsmokers; $P = .61$). More nonsmokers received a tibial-level bypass than did active smokers (47.8% vs 33.9%; $P < .001$). There was a trend toward increased early graft failure in active smokers compared with nonsmokers (5.3% vs 4.7%; $P = .08$). With adjustment for other variables, especially bypass level and graft type, there was an independent association between active smoking and early graft failure (adjusted odds ratio, 1.21; 95% confidence interval, 1.02-1.43; $P = .03$).

Conclusions.—Although nonsmokers were significantly older, had more comorbidities, and required more distal revascularization, active smokers still had an increased risk for development of early graft failure. These results stress the need for immediate smoking cessation before lower extremity bypass. Further research is warranted to determine an optimal period of abstinence among smokers with peripheral arterial disease to reduce their risk for early graft failure (Tables 1, 2 and 4).

▶ This study based on the National Surgery Quality Improvement Project (NSQIP) participant use data file provides a useful example of the importance of comorbidity adjustment. Although an association between active smoking

TABLE 1.—Demographic and Baseline Characteristics of the Study Population, Stratified by Smoking Status

Variables	Infrainguinal bypass (NSQIP 2005-2011) Nonsmokers (n = 9920), No. (%)	Active smokers (n = 6614), No. (%)	Total (N = 16,534), No. (%)	*P*
Mean age ± SD, years	71.7 ± 11.2	62.4 ± 10.1	68.0 ± 11.7	<.001
Male sex	6169 (62.2)	4389 (66.4)	10,558 (63.9)	<.001
White	7566 (76.3)	4977 (75.3)	12,543 (75.9)	<.001
Obese	2984 (31.3)	1673 (26.1)	4657 (29.2)	<.001
Above moderate alcohol consumption	313 (3.2)	597 (9.3)	910 (5.5)	<.001
Comorbidities				
Diabetes present				<.001
Insulin independent	2115 (21.3)	1115 (16.9)	3230 (19.5)	
Insulin dependent	2996 (30.2)	1271 (19.2)	4267 (25.8)	
Cardiac				
Hypertension	8749 (88.2)	5297 (80.1)	14,046 (85.0)	<.001
Angina ≤1 month	199 (2.0)	131 (2.0)	230 (2.0)	.91
AMI ≤6 months	205 (2.1)	117 (1.8)	322 (2.0)	.18
CHF	328 (3.3)	112 (1.7)	440 (2.7)	<.001
PCS/PCI	4213 (42.5)	1976 (29.9)	6189 (37.4)	<.001
Neurologic				
TIA	737 (7.4)	428 (6.5)	1165 (7.1)	.02
Pulmonary				
COPD	978 (9.9)	1124 (17.0)	2102 (12.7)	<.001
Pneumonia	31 (0.3)	12 (0.2)	43 (0.3)	.11
Renal				
Renal failure	161 (1.6)	71 (1.1)	232 (1.4)	.003
Dialysis	1005 (10.1)	274 (4.1)	1279 (7.7)	<.001
Others				
Preoperative wound infection	4253 (42.9)	1980 (29.9)	6233 (37.7)	<.001
Thrombocytosis	750 (7.8)	511 (8.0)	1261 (7.9)	.64
Sepsis	424 (4.3)	230 (3.5)	654 (4.0)	.01
Bleeding disorder	2286 (23.0)	1545 (23.4)	3831 (23.2)	.64
PRBC transfusion <72 hours	96 (1.0)	43 (0.7)	139 (0.8)	.03
Dependent functional status	1969 (19.9)	741 (11.2)	2710 (16.4)	<.001
Any major operation in the last 30 days	668 (7.2)	363 (5.8)	1031 (6.6)	.001

AMI, Acute myocardial infarction; *CHF*, congestive heart failure; *COPD*, chronic obstructive pulmonary disease; *NSQIP*, National Surgical Quality Improvement Program; *PCS/PCI*, previous cardiac surgery/percutaneous coronary intervention; *PRBC*, packed red blood cell; *SD*, standard deviation; *TIA*, transient ischemic attack.

TABLE 2.—Presentation Characteristics and Operative Details of Patients Undergoing Infrainguinal Bypass Stratified by Smoking Status

Variables	Infrainguinal Bypass (NSQIP 2005-2011) Nonsmokers (n = 9920), No. (%)	Active smokers (n = 6614), No. (%)	Total (N = 16,534), No. (%)	*P*
CLI	5308 (53.5)	3512 (53.1)	8820 (53.3)	.61
Level of bypass				<.001
Popliteal	5177 (52.2)	4373 (66.1)	9550 (57.8)	
Tibial	4743 (47.8)	2241 (33.9)	6984 (42.2)	
Type of graft				.001
Vein	6856 (69.1)	4393 (66.4)	11,249 (68.0)	
Prosthetic	3064 (30.9)	2221 (33.6)	5285 (32.0)	
Emergency procedure	454 (4.6)	288 (4.4)	742 (4.5)	.50
Surgical specialty				.06
Vascular surgery	9426 (95.0)	6265 (94.7)	15,691 (94.9)	
General surgery	488 (4.9)	337 (5.1)	825 (5.0)	
Other	6 (0.1)	12 (0.2)	18 (0.1)	
Anesthesia				.01
General	8797 (88.7)	5980 (90.4)	14,777 (89.4)	
Epidural	365 (3.7)	197 (3.0)	562 (3.4)	
Spinal	561 (5.7)	327 (4.9)	888 (5.4)	
MAC	90 (0.9)	58 (0.9)	148 (0.9)	
Regional	94 (1.0)	48 (0.7)	142 (0.9)	
Other	12 (0.1)	4 (0.1)	16 (0.1)	
ASA class				
Life-threatening/ moribund	2187 (22.1)	1108 (16.8)	3295 (19.9)	<.001
Resident involvement	6497 (65.7)	4205 (63.8)	10,702 (64.9)	.01
Operative time, minutes, median (IQR)	212 (157-281)	198 (146-267)	206 (152-276)	<.001

ASA, American Society of Anesthesiologists; *CLI*, critical limb ischemia; *IQR*, interquartile range; *MAC*, monitored anesthesia care; *NSQIP*, National Surgical Quality Improvement Program.

and perioperative graft thrombosis following infrainguinal bypass was not identified using simple logistic regression, active smokers were older and had a higher prevalence of comorbidities (with the exception of chronic obstructive pulmonary disease; Table 1) and had a greater frequency of prosthetic graft conduit (Table 2). Active smoking was associated with increased risk in the multivariable model adjusting for these factors (Table 4). Active smoking was defined based on a 12-month period, making it somewhat challenging to apply the results to decision making within routine clinical practice. Deferring elective infrainguinal bypass until a 12-month period of smoking abstinence may seem impractical and might be unacceptable to many patients or providers, but perhaps it should be considered when symptoms are limited to intermittent claudication (which was the case for nearly half the smokers who were treated with bypass in this study). Critical limb ischemia presents a greater dilemma in which providers often lack the luxury of time to optimize modifiable risk factors due to rest pain and amputation risk.

TABLE 4.—Multivariable Logistic Regression of 30-day Graft Failure Comparing Active Smokers with Nonsmokers After Infrainguinal Bypass Surgery (N = 16,534)

Graft Failure	Odds Ratio	95% Confidence Interval	*P*
Active smoker	1.21	1.02-1.43	.03
Age	0.99	0.98-0.99	.003
Female	1.27	1.09-1.49	.001
Nonwhite race	1.21	1.02-1.43	.02
Heavy alcohol consumption	0.68	0.46-1.00	.05
CLI	1.73	1.48-2.03	<.001
Tibial-level bypass	2.17	1.84-2.56	<.001
Prosthetic graft	1.27	1.07-1.50	.006
Thrombocytosis	1.21	0.95-1.54	.13
Hypertension	0.95	0.77-1.17	.60
Diabetes	0.78	0.66-0.92	.003
Congestive heart failure	1.30	0.87-1.95	.19
PCS/PCI	0.84	0.71-0.99	.04
Dialysis	0.85	0.64-1.13	.30
Any major operation within past 30 days	1.21	0.94-1.57	.15
Preoperative wound infection	1.10	0.93-1.29	.26
Dependent functional status	1.21	1.00-1.47	.05
Emergency surgery	1.58	1.18-2.13	.002
ASA class 3-5	1.09	0.90-1.32	.35
Resident involvement	1.17	0.99-1.37	.07
Complications occurring before median time to graft failure[a]	1.43	1.17-1.75	.001

ASA, American Society of Anesthesiologists; *CLI*, critical limb ischemia; *PCS/PCI*, previous cardiac surgery/percutaneous coronary intervention.

[a]Includes any wound, cardiac, pulmonary, renal, or other complication occurring within the first 5 days after infrainguinal bypass surgery.

Social acceptability bias may lead some patients who are actively smoking to indicate otherwise, making self-reported smoking status an inherently problematic variable. Most providers who treat peripheral artery disease have met a patient who either quit smoking on the day of their clinic appointment or vows to quit smoking if a revascularization procedure is undertaken. It is somewhat artificial to treat smoking as an all-or-none phenomenon (although that is how it is defined within NSQIP and many other large datasets), ignoring the potential dose effects of pack-years before cessation. Alternatively, smoking might be more appropriately considered as a chronic disease characterized by variability in dosing and periods of both abstinence and relapse. Although this study provides an additional contribution to the large body of evidence showing the negative effects of smoking on peripheral arterial disease risk and outcomes, most providers probably would not admit a burning need for more evidence that smoking is harmful. What are needed more desperately, however, are more effective approaches to helping patients conquer smoking and ongoing societal initiatives aimed at preventing people from starting.

M. A. Corriere, MD, MS

Functional status of elderly adults before and after interventions for critical limb ischemia

Vogel TR, Petroski GF, Kruse RL (Univ of Missouri, Columbia)

J Vasc Surg 59:350-358, 2014

Objective.—The impact of interventions for critical limb ischemia (CLI) on functional status in the elderly remains unclear. Open and endovascular procedures were evaluated.

Methods.—Medicare inpatient claims were linked with nursing home assessment data to identify elective admissions for lower extremity procedures for CLI. A functional impairment score (0-28; higher scores indicating greater impairment) based on residents' need for assistance with self-care activities, walking, and locomotion was calculated before and after interventions. Hierarchical modeling determined the effect of the surgery on residents' function, controlling for comorbidity, cognition, and prehospital function.

Results.—Three hundred fifty-two and 350 patients underwent open and endovascular procedures, respectively (rest pain, 84; ulceration, 351; gangrene, 267). Hospitalization was associated with a significant worsening in function following both procedures. Disease severity was associated with the amount of initial decline but not with the rate of recovery ($P > .35$). Residents who received open surgery improved more quickly following hospital discharge ($P = .011$).

Conclusions.—In the frail elderly, open and endovascular procedures for CLI were associated with similar initial declines in functional status, suggesting that compared with open procedures, less invasive endovascular procedures were not associated with maintaining baseline function. In this select population, endovascular procedures for CLI were not associated with improved functional status over time compared with open. Six months posthospital, patients who received traditional open bypass had significantly better functional status than those who received endovascular procedures for all CLI diagnoses. Further analysis is required to assist stakeholders in performing procedures most likely to preserve functional status in the frail elderly and nursing home population.

▶ The decision for method of revascularization in a threatened limb is primarily based on anatomic factors, with considerable attention being paid to the overall health of the patient. "High-risk" patients often receive more aggressive endovascular attempts and may in fact be outrightly refused open surgical revascularization options. This critical decision reflects an appropriate concern for the immediate perioperative health of the patient. In an era of increasing concern for outcomes data, clinicians should continue to follow patients to see the eventual benefit. Not only is periprocedural safety and limb salvage important, but the benefit to the patient in terms of improvement of lifestyle and relief of symptoms should be considered. In this retrospective review of long-stay patients treated successfully with open and endovascular means, there were suggestions that the return to a more independent state was more rapid after open revascularization compared with endovascular procedure. What is missing from this Medicare database review is the hemodynamic improvement or lack thereof, as well as the resolution of the symptoms. The ultimate best therapy will be a combination of safety, efficacy, cost, and long-term benefit to the patient. In addition to the standard metrics with which vascular surgeons are intimately familiar (limb salvage, patency, mortality), we should sit with patients and families preoperatively and elucidate ultimate treatment goals such as longevity, relief of symptoms, or functional independence.

R. J. Feezor, MD, FACS

Iliofemoral complications associated with thoracic endovascular aortic repair: Frequency, risk factors, and early and late outcomes

Vandy FC, Girotti M, Williams DM, et al (Univ of Michigan Cardiovascular Ctr, Ann Arbor)

J Thorac Cardiovasc Surg 147:960-965, 2014

Background.—Risk factors and outcomes after iliofemoral complications after thoracic aortic endovascular repair remain poorly characterized. This study was performed to characterize factors influencing perioperative iliofemoral complications during thoracic aortic endovascular repair.

Methods.—All patients undergoing transfemoral thoracic aortic endovascular repair since 2005 with adequate preoperative aortoiliac 3-dimensional imaging (n = 126) were identified. Assessment of imaging was blinded with regard to occurrence of iliofemoral complications, defined as anything other than successful transfemoral device delivery and primary closure of an arteriotomy.

Results.—The complication rate was 12% (n = 15). Univariate analysis identified that female gender, preoperative ankle-brachial index, average and minimal iliac diameters, diameter difference between iliac artery and sheath size, and iliac morphology score (calculated by combining iliac tortuosity, calcification, and vessel diameter) were associated with iliofemoral complications (all $P < .05$). Multivariate analysis identified the (1) difference between average iliac diameter and sheath size ($P = .014$), (2) iliac artery morphology score ($P = .033$), and (3) ankle-brachial index ($P = .012$) as independent predictors for iliofemoral complications. Early mortality was higher in those with complications (13.3% vs 1.8%, $P = .069$). Four-year freedom from limb loss, claudication, or revascularization was 97.9%. Iliofemoral complications reduced late survival primarily as a result of increased mortality within the first year ($P = .047$).

Conclusions.—Thoracic aortic endovascular repair can be performed safely via a transfemoral approach. Alternative access in patients with high preoperative iliac artery morphology scores and device delivery size requirements over the native iliofemoral size may reduce iliofemoral complications. If early complications occur, prompt repair results in low rates of ischemic limb complications at late follow-up.

▶ Iliofemoral complications continue to account for a large portion of the morbidity and mortality encountered during thoracic endovascular aortic repair (TEVAR). By analyzing preoperative 3-dimensional imagining in 127 TEVAR cases, the authors identify 5 factors that predict iliofemoral complications. These factors are female sex, high preoperative ankle-brachial index (perhaps indicative of heavily calcified vessels), low average and small minimal iliac diameters, diameter difference between iliac artery and sheath size, and high iliac morphology score (IMS). Perhaps most importantly, although not specifically seen in this study, is the IMS component of calcification.

An iliofemoral complication rate of 12% was seen in this study (consistent with those of larger studies), and, intuitively, early mortality was significantly higher in those patients that suffered iliofemoral complications compared with those that did not experience access-related complications (13.3% vs 1.8%; $P = .069$). Although access complications have been shown to correlate with early morbidity and mortality, this study identifies those factors that most significantly lead to iliofemoral complications.

TEVAR is often referred to as a minimally invasive option for treating pathology of the thoracic aorta, as it is in this article. Perhaps *minimally invasive* isn't an appropriate term, and *less invasive* is more accurate when comparing TEVAR with open repair, as iliofemoral complications are still prevalent and can lead to devastatingly poor outcomes. Those patients who possess the risk factors identified in this study seen on preoperative 3-dimensional imaging predicting iliofemoral complications should be informed accordingly that they are at high risk for potential complications, and perhaps alternate modes of access rather than femoral access should be more liberally utilized.

B. Peterson, MD, FACS

Aspirin responsiveness safely lowers perioperative cardiovascular risk

Calderaro D, Pastana AF, Flores Da Rocha TR, et al (Univ of São Paulo Med School, Brazil)
J Vasc Surg 58:1593-1599, 2013

Introduction.—Vascular surgeries are related to high cardiac morbidity and mortality, and the maintenance of aspirin in the perioperative period has a protective effect. The purpose of this study was to evaluate the association between preoperative platelet aggregability and perioperative cardiovascular (CV) events.

Methods.—A preoperative platelet aggregation test was performed on an impedance aggregometer in response to collagen and to arachidonic acid (AA) for 191 vascular surgery patients under chronic use of aspirin. We analyzed the following CV events: acute myocardial infarction, unstable angina, isolated troponin elevation, acute ischemic stroke, reoperation, and cardiac death. Hemorrhagic events were also evaluated and classified according to the Thrombolysis In Myocardial Infarction criteria.

Results.—The incidence of CV events was 22% (n = 42). Higher platelet response to AA was associated with CV events, so that patients in the fourth quartile (higher than 11Ω) had almost twice the incidence of CV events when compared with the three lower quartiles: 35% vs 19%; $P = .025$. The independent predictors of CV events were hemodynamic instability during anesthesia (odds ratio [OR], 4.12; 95% confidence interval [CI], 1.87-9.06; $P < .001$), dyslipidemia (OR, 3.9; 95% CI, 1.32-11.51; $P = .014$), preoperative anemia (OR, 2.64; 95% CI, 1.19-5.85; $P = .017$), and AA platelet aggregability in the upper quartile (OR, 2.48; 95% CI, 1.07-5.76; $P = .034$). Platelet aggregability was not associated with hemorrhagic events, even when we compared the lowest quartile of AA platelet aggregability (0-1.00 Ω) with the three upper quartiles (>1.00 Ω; OR, 0.77; 95% CI, 0.43-1.37; $P = .377$).

Conclusions.—The degree of aspirin effect on platelet aggregability maybe important in the management of perioperative CV morbidity, without increment in the bleeding toll.

► This study demonstrating that higher levels of platelet aggregation are associated with cardiovascular complications after vascular surgery/intervention suggests that vascular patients derive significant benefit by maintenance on aspirin perioperatively. The fact that platelet aggregability (ie, aspirin responsiveness) was not associated with increased bleeding complications further indicates that aspirin is not associated with increased perioperative bleeding complications. I suspect that this gives credence to the current practice of many vascular surgeons.

The Vascular Study Group of New England recently reported that not only aspirin, but clopidogrel is also safe and not associated with major bleeding after vascular surgery. In this study of more than 10 000 patients (with more than 7000 on aspirin alone), no increased bleeding complications were identified postoperatively.[1]

It is critical, nonetheless, to mention a recent *New England Journal of Medicine* article, the POISE-2 (Perioperatie Ischemic Evaluation 2) trial which shows quite the opposite.[2] This randomized, controlled trial concludes that perioperative administration of aspirin has no significant effect on death or myocardial infarction but has an increased risk of major bleeding. This "significantly increased risk of bleeding" was 4.6% versus 3.8% ($P = .04$). In addition, only about 5% to 6% of patients in this trial were undergoing vascular surgery.

In light of the POISE-2 trial, whereas many of us will continue perioperative aspirin use in our practices, I may be forced to suspend my dogmatic proclamation, and insistence, on this practice—at least for the moment.

K. Hughes, MD, FACS

References

1. Stone DH, Goodney PP, Schanzer A. Clopidogrel is not associated with major bleeding complications during peripheral arterial surgery. *J Vasc Surg*. 2011;54: 779-784.
2. Devereaux PJ, Mrkobrada M, Sessler DI, et al. Aspirin in patients undergoing non-cardiac surgery. *N Engl J Med*. 2014;370:1494-1503.

Assessing Readmission After General, Vascular, and Thoracic Surgery Using ACS-NSQIP

Lucas DJ, Haider A, Haut E, et al (Walter Reed Natl Military Med Ctr, Bethesda, MD; The Johns Hopkins Univ School of Medicine, Baltimore, MD; et al)
Ann Surg 258:430-439, 2013

Objective.—In 2012, Medicare began cutting reimbursement for hospitals with high readmission rates. We sought to define the incidence and risk factors associated with readmission after surgery.

Methods.—A total of 230,864 patients discharged after general, upper gastrointestinal (GI), small and large intestine, hepatopancreatobiliary (HPB), vascular, and thoracic surgery were identified using the 2011 American College of Surgeons National Surgical Quality Improvement Program. Readmission rates and patient characteristics were analyzed. A predictive model for readmission was developed among patients with length of stay (LOS) 10 days or fewer and then validated using separate samples.

Results.—Median patient age was 56 years; 43% were male, and median American Society of Anesthesiologists (ASA) class was 2 (general surgery: 2; upper GI: 3; small and large intestine: 2; HPB: 3; vascular: 3; thoracic: 3; $P < 0.001$). The median LOS was 1 day (general surgery: 0; upper GI: 2; small and large intestine: 5; HPB: 6; vascular: 2; thoracic: 4; $P < 0.001$). Overall 30-day readmission was 7.8% (general surgery: 5.0%; upper GI: 6.9%; small and large intestine: 12.6%; HPB: 15.8%; vascular: 11.9%; thoracic: 11.1%; $P < 0.001$). Factors strongly associated with readmission included ASA class, albumin less than 3.5, diabetes, inpatient complications, nonelective surgery, discharge to a facility, and the LOS (all $P < 0.001$). On multivariate analysis, ASA class and the LOS remained most strongly associated with readmission. A simple integer-based score using ASA class and the LOS predicted risk of readmission (area under the receiver operator curve 0.702).

Conclusions.—Readmission among patients with the LOS 10 days or fewer occurs at an incidence of at least 5% to 16% across surgical subspecialties. A scoring system on the basis of ASA class and the LOS may help stratify readmission risk to target interventions.

▶ This timely study gives us an interesting and sophisticated look at readmissions in general, vascular, and thoracic surgery. Of specific interest to vascular surgeons is the finding that there is a 12% 30-day readmission rate and a 15% postoperative complication rate for patients undergoing vascular surgery.

The authors prove what we intuitively suspect: that readmissions are related to patient comorbidities, case complexity, and postoperative complications. Identifying American Society of Anesthesiologists class and length of stay as the 2 factors most correlated with readmission, the authors developed a predictive readmission score: length of stay/2 + American Society of Anesthesiologists score (rounded off to a single integer), and determined that a score of 4 is a cutoff, accounting for almost 80% of readmissions. This readmission score had a high specificity but poor sensitivity, that is, it was better at predicting who wound not need readmission than who would need readmission.

I commend the authors on the efforts at developing this score, and agree that this could prove potentially useful in allocating case management resources. Given that sicker patients undergoing complex, complicated operations are the ones most likely to be readmitted, it seems to me that the Centers for Medicare and Medicaid Services would do well to take into account the likelihood for readmission when deciding to financially penalize our hospitals for high readmission rates.

K. Hughes, MD, FACS

5 Grafts and Graft Complications

The use of cryopreserved aortoiliac allograft for aortic reconstruction in the United States

Harlander-Locke MP, for The Vascular Low-Frequency Disease Consortium (Univ of California Los Angeles; et al)

J Vasc Surg 59:669-674, 2014

Background.—Aortic infections, even with treatment, have a high mortality and risk of recurrent infection and limb loss. Cryopreserved aortoiliac allograft (CAA) has been proposed for aortic reconstruction to improve outcomes in this high risk population.

Methods.—A multicenter study using a standardized database was performed at 14 of the 20 highest volume institutions that used CAA for aortic reconstruction in the setting of infection or those at high risk for prosthetic graft infection.

Results.—Two hundred twenty patients (mean age, 65; male:female, 1.6/1) were treated since 2002 for culture positive aortic graft infection (60%), culture negative aortic graft infection (16%), enteric fistula/erosion (15%), infected pseudoaneurysm adjacent to the aortic graft (4%), and other (4%). Intraop cultures indicated infection in 66%. Distal anastomosis was to the femoral artery and iliac. Mean hospital length of stay was 24 days, and 30-day mortality was 9%. Complications occurred in 24% and included persistent sepsis (n = 17), CAA thrombosis (n = 9), CAA rupture (n = 8), recurrent CAA/aortic infection (n = 8), CAA pseudoaneurysm (n = 6), recurrence of aortoenteric fistula (n = 4), and compartment syndrome (n = 1). Patients with full graft excision had significantly better outcomes. Ten (5%) patients required allograft explant. Mean follow-up was 30 ± 3 months. Freedom from graft-related complications, graft explant, and limb loss was 80%, 88%, and 97%, respectively, at 5 years. Primary graft patency was 97% at 5 years, and patient survival was 75% at 1 year and 51% at 5 years.

Conclusions.—This largest study of CAA indicates that CAA allows aortic reconstruction in the setting of infection or those at high risk for infection with lower early and long-term morbidity and mortality than other previously reported treatment options. Repair with CAA is associated with low rates of aneurysm formation, recurrent infection, aortic

blowout, and limb loss. We believe that CAA should be considered a first line treatment of aortic infections.

▶ Aortic graft infections continue to be a rare but difficult problem for vascular surgeons. Opinion is split regarding the gold-standard treatment for these patients. Historically, excision and extra-anatomical bypass has been favored. However, if patient is young (average age here 65 years), these smaller bypasses may not provide adequate inflow for an active adult. Naturally, some surgeons have moved to cryopreserved allografts to maintain size of conduit while decreasing the risk of recurrent infection. Unfortunately, published evidence began to show that these allograft reconstructions were prone to aneurysmal degeneration and risk of catastrophic "blow out." Alternatively, many surgeons also perform in-line reconstruction using rifampin-soaked Dacron grafts with low early reinfection rates and less concern of graft degeneration or digestion in later phases. An ongoing concern is the class of offending organisms may be shifting compared with older reports. Traditionally, the main culprit was *Salmonella*; however, with frequent use of broad-spectrum antibiotics, this has changed. As noted herein, the most frequent microbacteria are polymicrobial, methicillin-sensitive *Staphylococcus* and methicillin-resistant *Staphylococcus*. But not far behind are the more virulent organisms. The authors herein have discerningly presented the largest series on cryopreserved aortoiliac allografts (CAA) in aortic reconstruction for infection. It is thought that modern advances in cryopreservation techniques have improved the integrity of the collagen matrix. This study allays the concern of allograft degeneration because only 14 patients (7%) developed CAA pseudoaneurysm or rupture at 5 years. Furthermore, reinfection only occurred in 8 patients (4%), which is significantly lower than the previously reported incidence in larger series: 20% for extra-anatomic bypass, 13% for neo-aortoiliac system, and 10% to 15% with prosthetic grafts. On a specific technical analysis, they also found that complete excision of the previous aortic graft had significantly improved outcomes than when only a partial graft excision was performed. Ultimately, this study proves CAA provides 1 more tool to add to our armamentarium in caring for these challenging patients for whom graft choice is one of many difficult decisions that must be considered.

J. H. Black III, MD, FACS

Defining utility and predicting outcome of cadaveric lower extremity bypass grafts in patients with critical limb ischemia

Chang CK, Scali ST, Feezor RJ, et al (Univ of Florida, Gainesville)
J Vasc Surg 60:1554-1564, 2014

Objective.—Despite poor long-term patency, acceptable limb salvage has been reported with cryopreserved saphenous vein bypass (CVB) for various indications. However, utility of CVB in patients with critical limb ischemia (CLI) remains undefined. The purpose of this analysis was to determine the role of CVB in CLI patients and to identify predictors of successful outcomes.

Methods.—A retrospective review of all lower extremity bypass (LEB) procedures at a single institution was completed, and CVB in CLI patients were further analyzed. The primary end point was amputation-free survival. Secondary end points included primary patency and limb salvage. Life tables were used to estimate occurrence of end points. Cox regression analysis was used to determine predictors of limb salvage.

Results.—From 2000 to 2012, 1059 patients underwent LEB for various indications, of whom 81 received CVB for either ischemic rest pain or tissue loss. Mean age (± standard deviation) was 66 ± 10 years (male, 51%; diabetes, 51%; hemodialysis dependence, 12%), and 73% (n = 59) had history of failed ipsilateral LEB or endovascular intervention. None had sufficient autogenous conduit for even composite vein bypass. Infrainguinal CVB (infrapopliteal target, 96%; n = 78) was completed for multiple indications including Rutherford class 4 (42%; n = 34), class 5 (40%; n = 32), and class 6 (18%; n = 15). Eleven (14%) had CLI and concomitant graft infection (n = 8) or acute on chronic ischemia (n = 3). Intraoperative adjuncts (eg, profundaplasty, suprainguinal stent or bypass) were completed in 49% (n = 40) of cases. Complications occurred in 36% (n = 29), with 30-day mortality of 4% (n = 3). Median follow-up for CLI patients was 11.8 (interquartile range, 0.4-28.4) months with corresponding 1- and 3-year actuarial estimated survival (± standard error mean) of 84% ± 4% and 62% ± 6%. Primary patency of CVB for CLI was 27% ± 6% and 17% ± 6% at 1 and 3 years, respectively. Amputation-free survival was 43% ± 6% and 23% ± 6% at 1 and 3 years, respectively, and significantly higher for rest pain (59% ± 9%, 36% ± 10%) compared with tissue loss (31% ± 7%, 14% ± 7%; log-rank, P = .04). Freedom from major amputation after CVB for CLI was 57% ± 6% and 43% ± 7% at 1 and 3 years. Multivariable predictors of limb salvage for the CVB CLI cohort included postoperative warfarin (hazard ratio = HR], 0.4; 95% confidence interval = CI], 0.2-0.8), dyslipidemia (HR, 0.4; 95% CI, 0.2-0.9), and rest pain (HR, 0.4; 95% CI, 0.2-0.9). Predictors of major amputation included graft infection (HR, 3.1; 95% CI, 1.1-9.0).

Conclusions.—In CLI patients with no autologous conduit and prior failed infrainguinal bypass, CVB outcomes are disappointing. CVB performs best in patients with rest pain, particularly those who can be anticoagulated with warfarin. However, it may be an acceptable option in patients with minor tissue loss or concurrent graft infection, but consideration should be weighed against the known natural history of nonrevascularized CLI and nonbiologic conduit alternatives, given potential cost implications (Fig 4 and Table 2).

▶ Chang et al reviewed all infrainguinal bypasses performed at their institution over a 12-year period. By focusing on outcomes associated with critical limb

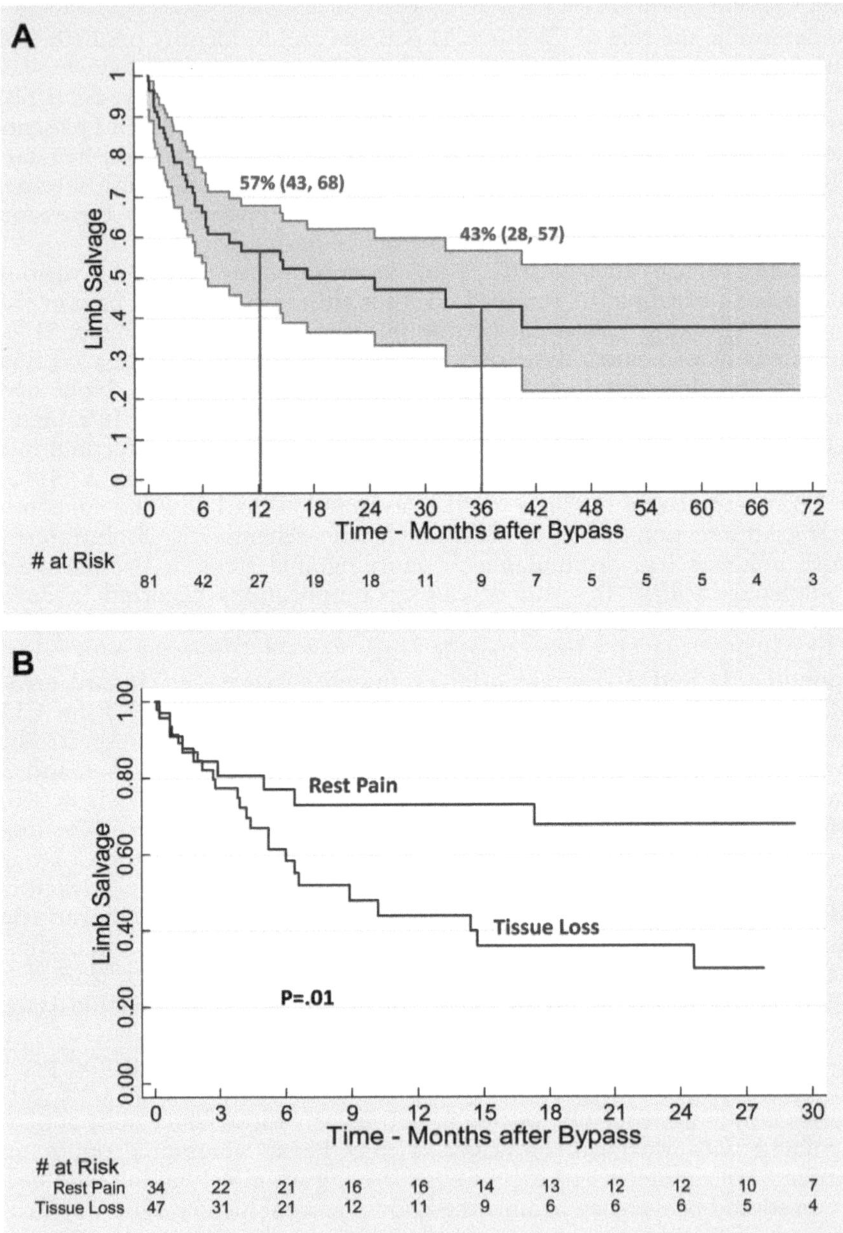

FIGURE 4.—**A**, Freedom from major (above the ankle) amputation in all critical limb ischemia (CLI) patients is demonstrated on this graph. **B**, Similar to amputation-free survival (AFS), freedom from major amputation was significantlydifferent (log-rank, P = .01) between rest pain and tissue loss patients. Notably, a significant proportion of patients in the rest pain group underwent concomitant femoral arterial or iliac inflow reconstruction at the time of their cadaveric vein bypass, which likely contributed to these findings. All displayed time intervals have <10% standard error of the mean. (Reprinted from the Journal of Vascular Surgery. Chang CK, Scali ST, Feezor RJ, et al. Defining utility and predicting outcome of cadaveric lower extremity bypass grafts in patients with critical limb ischemia. *J Vasc Surg*. 2014;60:1554-1564, Copyright 2014, with permission from The Society for Vascular Surgery.)

TABLE 2.—Operative Details and Donor Characteristics Of Critical Limb Ischemia (CLI) Patients

Operative details	N = 81, No. (%)
Bypass configuration	
Proximal anastomosis	
External iliac artery	1 (1)
Common femoral artery	76 (94)
Superficial femoral artery	3 (4)
Profunda femoris artery	1 (1)
Distal anastomosis	
Above-knee popliteal artery	3 (4)
Below-knee popliteal artery	7 (9)
Tibial artery	70 (86)
Tibioperoneal trunk	2 (2)
Posterior tibial artery	28 (35)
Anterior tibial artery	21 (26)
Peroneal artery	19 (23)
Dorsalis pedis artery	1 (1)
Conduit configuration	
Reversed greater saphenous vein	43 (53)
Nonreversed greater saphenous vein	29 (36)
Composite saphenous vein	7 (9)
Composite vein/artery	2 (4)
Adjuncts (any)	40 (49)
Inflow procedure	28 (34)
Distal anastomotic adjunct	5 (6)
Donor characteristics	*N* = 73
Age, years ± SD	38 ± 13
Male	99% (72)
Preservation time, days ± SD	196 ± 143
ABO/Rh matched	41% (55)

SD, Standard deviation.
Reprinted from the Journal of Vascular Surgery. Chang CK, Scali ST, Feezor RJ, et al. Defining utility and predicting outcome of cadaveric lower extremity bypass grafts in patients with critical limb ischemia. *J Vasc Surg*. 2014;60:1554-1564, Copyright 2014, with permission from The Society for Vascular Surgery.

ischemia (CLI; which accounted for >85% of the cohort) rather than lumping these patients together with claudicants into a single cohort, the authors avoid a common pitfall that often limits the conclusions that can be drawn from conduit-based analyses of lower extremity bypass. For the sake of comparison, however, it would have been useful to have also included prosthetic graft bypasses (acknowledged in the discussion as a lower-cost alternative that can be used in the absence of overt infection with similar patency) within this analysis. Functional status and quality of life are other relevant outcomes that could not be analyzed in this retrospective study but are often key considerations when trying to choose between treatment options. Nonetheless, the authors provide a wealth of data related to indications, disease severity, technical details (including anatomic configurations), and long-term outcomes. They report primary patency of 27% and 17% at 1 and 3 years, respectively (with similar rates of secondary patency), whereas freedom from major amputation was 51% at 1 year and 47% at 3 years. The results also suggest that anticoagulation positively impacts limb salvage rates among patients treated with cadaveric bypass and, therefore, should be considered in appropriate-risk patients.

The authors are to be commended for sharing these results, which include less than spectacular patency rates that might bias some against publication. Given the dismal long-term survival of patients with CLI (comparable to some of the least favorable cancer diagnoses[1]) and the severity of their symptoms, a strategy focused on short-term outcomes may be appropriate when options are limited and the alternatives (such as major extremity amputation) are associated with significant costs and morbidity. One, therefore, might justifiably conclude that limb preservation in approximately 50% of patients at 1 year is acceptable, particularly among patients with CLI whose previous revascularizations have failed. Value is defined by outcomes relative to cost,[2] and the worth of 1 or more years of amputation-free or pain-free survival is a key consideration when assessing whether cadaveric vein bypass is worth undertaking for CLI. As clinical decisions are increasingly approached from a cost-conscious perspective within resource-constrained environments, providers must strive to keep the patient's perspective in mind.

M. A. Corriere, MD, MS

References

1. Norgren L, Hiatt WR, Dormandy JA, Nehler MR, Harris KA, Fowkes FG. Inter-society consensus for the management of peripheral arterial disease (TASC II). *J Vasc Surg*. 2007;45:S5-S67.
2. Brook RH. The end of the quality improvement movement: long live improving value. *JAMA*. 2010;304:1831-1832.

Increased minimum vein diameter on preoperative mapping with duplex ultrasound is associated with arteriovenous fistula maturation and secondary patency

Dageforde LA, Harms KA, Feurer ID, et al (Vanderbilt Univ Med Ctr, Nashville, TN)

J Vasc Surg 61:170-176, 2015

Objective.—Autogenous arteriovenous hemodialysis accesses (arteriovenous fistulas [AVFs]) are preferred for chronic hemodialysis access. Preoperative vein mapping by duplex ultrasound is recommended before AVF creation, but there are few data correlating vein diameter with postoperative outcomes. Also, vein diameter has not been included in prior predictive models of fistula maturation. This study aims to test whether preoperative vein diameter is associated with failure of AVF maturation and long-term (secondary) patency.

Methods.—We performed a retrospective analysis of clinical variables of patients undergoing brachiobasilic or brachiocephalic AVF creation.

Kaplan-Meier and multivariate Cox regression models tested whether preoperative minimum vein diameter (MVD) and clinical covariates were associated with failure of AVF maturation and secondary patency.

Results.—The sample included 158 adults (54 ± 14 years; 45% male; 61% white; 56% diabetes; body mass index, 32 ± 8; MVD, 3.4 ± 1.1 mm; follow-up, 12 ± 9 months [range, <1-40 months]). Increased MVD was associated with decreased risk of AVF failure. More than one third of AVFs with MVD <2.7 mm failed to mature within 6 months. Multivariate models that adjusted for age, diabetes, race, gender, body mass index, and preoperative dialysis status demonstrated that increased MVD was associated with decreased risk of failure of maturation and better long-term patency overall ($P = .005$ and $P = .001$, respectively).

Conclusions.—Patients with a larger MVD on preoperative vein mapping are at lower risk for failure of fistula maturation and have increased long-term AVF patency. MVD is the only clinical or demographic factor associated with both AVF maturation and long-term patency. MVD is an important preoperative indicator of fistula success in assessment of potential AVF sites. Future predictive models of fistula maturation and patency should include MVD.

▶ Despite the routine use of duplex ultrasound scan, the failure rate of arteriovenous fistulas (AVF) remains high. Recent single-center studies still report a primary AVF failure rate of 26% to 50% and a primary 1-year patency rate of 36% to 46% for a primary AVF. Although some experts suggest a vein diameter of 2.5 mm as adequate for AVF creation, there are few published data to validate this threshold or to correlate initial vein diameter with subsequent AVF maturation. The aim of this study was to test whether after adjustment for clinical factors, vein diameter as measured by preoperative duplex ultrasound scan is associated with AVF maturation or long-term (secondary) patency in patients both with and without prior arteriovenous access. AVFs with mean vein diameter (MVD) of less than 2.7 mm were associated with a higher risk of failure of maturation and a lower long-term patency than were AVFs with MVD of greater than 3.3 mm. After controlling for age, diabetes, race, sex, coronary artery disease, peripheral vascular disease, and preoperative dialysis status, increased vein diameter was associated with an increased likelihood of maturation and better overall patency. One of the major limitations of this data analysis is that the data were obtained retrospectively and there may be day-to-day variation in MVD related to temperature, anesthesia, and the state of hydration of the patient. Unfortunately, the results of this study did not describe a definitive threshold for an MVD that is predictive of fistula maturation or long-term patency. Prospective studies designed to determine such a threshold are sorely needed.

M. T. Watkins, MD

One-year patency rate of native arteriovenous fistulas reconstructed by vascular stripping in hemodialysis patients with venous neointimal hyperplasia

Lu F-P, Liu L-P, Lu Z-X (First Hosp of Tsinghua Univ, Beijing, China)
J Vasc Surg 61:192-196, 2014

Objective.—There are limited therapeutic measures for stenosis of arteriovenous fistulas (AVFs) due to venous neointimal hyperplasia (VNH). In the current retrospective study, we reviewed the clinical data of hemodialysis patients who underwent AVF reconstruction by VNH stripping. The primary measure of interest was the secondary patency rate of the restored AVF.

Methods.—The study included hemodialysis patients who underwent AVF reconstruction by VNH stripping (group A), AVF reconstruction proximal to the original fistula (group B), or creation of a new AVF (group C). Patency was evaluated immediately after the surgery and at follow-up visits.

Results.—Of 353 patients who underwent AVF reconstructions, 327 (91.9%) were for late AVF failure. The final analysis included 305 patients: 76, 128, and 101 patients in groups A, B, and C, respectively. The three groups were comparable in age, sex, causes for AVF, AVF sites, and the artery for the AVF ($P > .05$). At 3-month follow-up, the secondary AVF patency rate was comparable across the three groups at 93.4%, 92.2%, and 92.1% in groups A, B, and C, respectively. The patency rate at 6 and 12 months was also comparable across groups A, B, and C at 89.5%, 89.8%, and 88.1% at 6 months and 84.2%, 85.9%, and 81.2% at 12 months, respectively.

Conclusions.—Reconstructing the AVF by surgically removing VNH is an effective technique for late hemodialysis access failure, with maximal preservation of blood vessels.

► A mature arteriovenous fistula (AVF) may still develop venous neointimal hyperplasia (VNH) after a period of successful use, leading to venous stenosis with or without thrombosis. Failure of an AVF vascular access can be early (failed maturation of AV anastomosis, typically < 3 months after AVF creation) or late (> 3 months after AVF creation). The most important factor causing late failure is venous stenosis, particularly perianastomotic stricture due to VNH formation. These authors recently developed an operative technique to repair AVFs by surgical stripping of VNH and AV reanastomosis. In the current retrospective study, the authors reviewed the clinical data of hemodialysis patients who had undergone AVF reconstruction by VNH stripping in 3 groups of patients each with more than 100 patients with long-term follow-up. The 3 groups studied were Group A, AVF reconstruction by VNH stripping; Group B, AVF reconstruction proximal to the original fistula; and Group C, newly created AVF. The authors have demonstrated long-term patency rates of AVFs reconstructed by surgically removing VNH and reanastomosis that are comparable with the patency rates obtained by other surgical approaches. Although the data were collected retrospectively, the same surgeon performed all 3 operations. The VNH procedure provides maximal preservation of blood vessels for long-term hemodialysis, shortens the time to restart hemodialysis therapy because the restored AVF by VNH stripping can be used for hemodialysis immediately after the operation, and waiting for several weeks for fistula maturation is not necessary because the veins have already arterialized. This is a novel approach to neointimal hyperplasia that may be applicable to a larger patient population.

M. T. Watkins, MD

6 Aortic Aneurysm

Aortic biomechanics by magnetic resonance: Early markers of aortic disease in Marfan syndrome regardless of aortic dilatation?

Teixido-Tura G, Redheuil A, Rodríguez-Palomares J, et al (Universitat Autònoma de Barcelona, Spain; Georges-Pompidou-European-Hosp, Paris, France; et al)

Int J Cardiol 171:56-61, 2014

Background.—Previous studies demonstrated the usefulness of MRI in the evaluation of aortic biomechanics in Marfan patients with aortic dilatation. However, these parameters have not been well studied in earlier stages of aortic disease. The present work aimed to study aortic biomechanics: aortic distensibility (AD) and pulse wave velocity (PWV), by MRI in Marfan patients without advanced aortic disease.

Methods.—Eighty consecutive Marfan patients were compared with 36 age- and sex-matched controls. MRI images at the level of ascending, descending and abdominal aorta were used to determine AD and PWV.

Results.—Marfan patients (27 men; age: 32.0 ± 10.5 years; mean aortic root diameter: 37.2 ± 4.6 mm) had lower AD at all levels (ascending 2.6 ± 2.1 vs. 6.2 ± 3.7 $\text{mm Hg}^{-1} \cdot 10^{-3}$, $p < 0.001$; descending 3.1 ± 2.0 vs. 8.3 ± 4.2, $p < 0.001$; and abdominal 4.5 ± 2.2 vs. 14.0 ± 5.2, $p < 0.001$), higher aortic arch PWV (8.1 ± 6.5 vs. 4.3 ± 1.8 m/s, $p < 0.01$) and ascending-to-abdominal PWV (6.1 ± 3.0 vs. 4.7 ± 1.5 m/s, $p < 0.01$) compared with controls. Thirty-five Marfan patients had a non-dilated aortic root (mean aortic root diameter: 34.5 ± 3.8 mm). In multivariable analyses, after adjustment for age, pulse pressure and aortic dimensions, AD remained lower and PWV higher in Marfan patients; even Marfan patients with non-dilated aortic root showed impaired aortic biomechanics compared with controls. Z-score for ascending AD <−3.5 distinguished Marfan patients from controls with 82.5% sensitivity and 86.1% specificity.

Conclusions.—Aortic biomechanics by MRI were abnormal in the entire aorta in Marfan patients. Moreover, Marfan patients without dilated aortic root showed clear impairment of aortic biomechanics, which suggests that they may be used as early markers of aortic involvement in these patients (Fig 4).

▶ Aortic biomechanics within the connective tissue disorder population remains an interesting dilemma, and stiffness is hypothesized to be involved in aortic degeneration in nonsyndromic patients as well. This article compared a large series (80 patients) of patients with Marfan syndrome to age-matched controls.

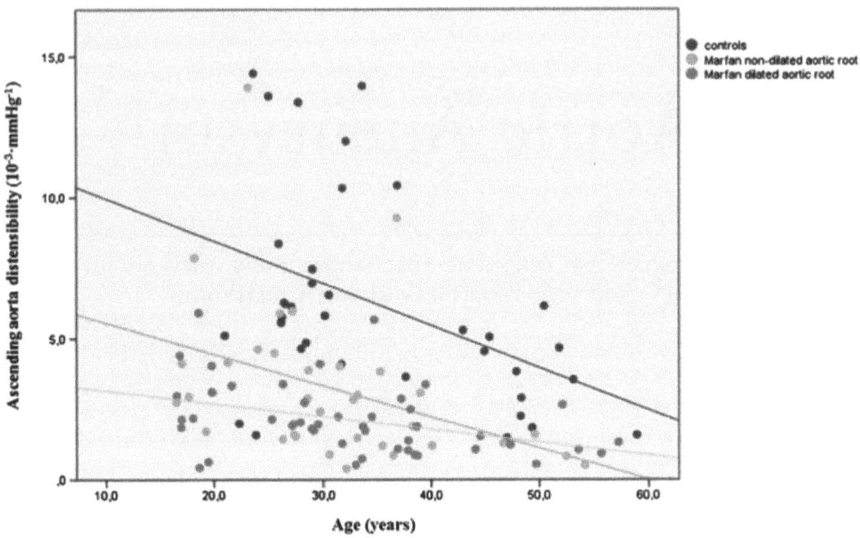

FIGURE 4.—Relationship of ascending aorta distensibility with age in controls and Marfan patients with dilated and non-dilated aortic root. (Reprinted from International Journal of Cardiology. Teixido-Tura G, Redheuil A, Rodríguez-Palomares J, et al. Aortic biomechanics by magnetic resonance: early markers of aortic disease in Marfan syndrome regardless of aortic dilatation?. *Int J Cardiol.* 2014;171:56-61, Copyright 2014, with permission from International Society for Adult Congenital Heart Disease.)

From the data presented, it is clear that lack of the fibrillin gene leads to a less distensible aorta (Fig 4). What makes this particular publication unique is that 35 patients in this series had a normal aortic root and had not progressed to aortic dilation, yet had decreased distensibility. The authors show that MRI identified changes in this subset indicating presence of disease that had not clinically manifest, but what to do with this information remains unknown—that is, can these patients be at increased risk of aortic dissection at a lower aortic diameter? Indeed, in connective tissue disorder patients, the occurrence of an aortic dissection as the first aortic surgery sets a natural history course that has multiple aortic operations likely within years after a successful Type A repair. The technology required for this type of imaging is not widely available; however, one must consider the use of dynamic MRI when available as a surveillance tool for those with known disease to avoid the catastrophic implications of an aortic dissection in its immediate and long-term time frames. Future studies hope to identify changes in aortic biomechanics that can be linked to clinical progression. Ideally, identifying these changes early can lead to earlier intervention and avoidance of dissection and acute rupture.

B. W. Propper, MD

Critical analysis of results after chimney endovascular aortic aneurysm repair raises cause for concern

Scali ST, Feezor RJ, Chang CK, et al (Univ of Florida, Gainesville)

J Vasc Surg 60:865-875, 2014

Objective.—"Chimney" techniques used to extend landing zones for endovascular aortic repair (chEVAR) have been increasingly reported; however, concerns about durability and patency remain. The purpose of this analysis was to examine midterm outcomes of chEVAR.

Methods.—All patients at the University of Florida treated with chEVAR were reviewed. Major adverse events (MAEs) were recorded and defined as any chimney stent thrombosis, type Ia endoleak in follow-up, reintervention, 30-day/in-hospital death, or ≥25% decrease in estimated glomerular filtration rate after discharge. Primary end points included chimney stent patency and freedom from MAE. Secondary end points included complications and long-term survival.

Results.—From 2008 to 2012, 41 patients (age 6 standard deviation, 73 ± 8 years; male, 66% [n = 27]) were treated with a total of 76 chimney stents (renal, n = 51; superior mesenteric artery, n = 16; celiac artery, n = 9) for a variety of indications: juxtarenal, 42% (n = 17, one rupture), suprarenal, 17% (n = 7), and thoracoabdominal aneurysm, 17% (n = 7); aortic anastomotic pseudoaneurysm, 15% (n = 6; three ruptures); type Ia endoleak after EVAR, 7% (n = 3); and atheromatous disease, 2% (n = 1). Two patients had a single target vessel abandoned because of cannulation failure, and one had a type Ia endoleak at case completion (technical success, 93%). Intraoperative complications occurred in seven patients (17%), including graft maldeployment with unplanned mesenteric chimney (n = 2) and access vessel injury requiring repair (n = 5). Major postoperative complications developed in 20% (n = 8). The 30-day mortality and in-hospital mortality were 5% (n = 2) and 7% (n = 3), respectively. At median follow-up of 18.2 months (range, 1.4-41.5 months), 28 of 33 patients (85%) with available postoperative imaging experienced stabilization or reduction of abdominal aortic aneurysm sac diameters. Nine patients (32%) developed endoleak at some point during follow-up (type Ia, 7% [n = 3]; type II, 10% [n = 4]; indeterminate, 7% [n = 3]), and one patient underwent open, surgical conversion. The estimated probability of freedom from reintervention (± standard error mean) was 96% ± 4% at both 1 year and 3 years. Primary patency of all chimney stents was 88% ± 5% and 85% ± 5% at 1 year and 3 years, respectively. Corresponding freedom from MAEs was 83% ± 7% and 57% ± 10% at 1 year and 3 years. The actuarial estimated survival for all patients at 1 year and 5 years was 85% ± 6% and 65% ± 8%, respectively.

Conclusions.—These results demonstrate that chEVAR can be completed with a high degree of success; however, perioperative complications and MAEs during follow-up, including loss of chimney patency and endoleak, may occur at a higher rate than previously reported. Elective use of chEVAR should be performed with caution, and comparison to open and fenestrated EVAR is needed to determine long-term efficacy of this technique (Fig 1).

▶ Chimney endovascular aortic repair (chEVAR) has been proposed as a method of treating patients without appropriate proximal landing in the infrarenal aorta. A retrospective review from University of Florida shows that while initial success is achieved and mortality is low, the durability over a 3-year period is poor (Fig 1). Major events occurred in up to 20% of the population, and more than 30% developed an endoleak with only half of these being a type II endoleak. This study highlights a more important characteristic of EVAR, which is aortic seal zone. Often infrarenal devices are used off instruction for use (IFU) in short or hostile necks as other options are less appealing or technically challenging. The idea of chEVAR seeks to raise the seal level to that of normal aorta. Chimney techniques remain a challenge as often long stent grafts are required to achieve fixation in renal vessels. These grafts leave "gutters" that are difficult to interpret in the setting of anticoagulation and final imaging. Balloon-expandable stent grafts, typically the standard for fenestrated repair,

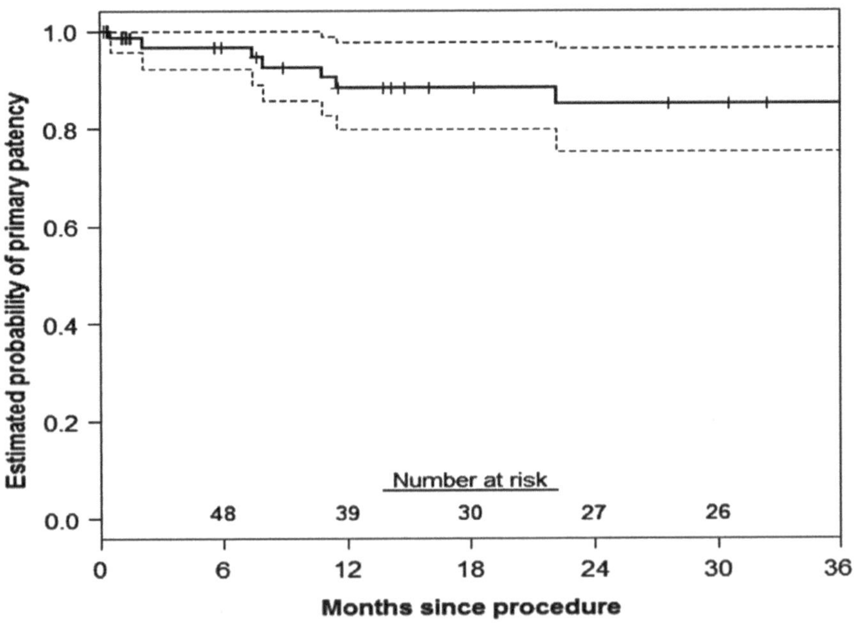

FIGURE 1.—This Kaplan-Meier curve demonstrates the estimated probability of primary stent patency up to 3 years (n = 76 stents). Overall, nine stents (one celiac, six renal, and two superior mesenteric artery) occluded. Seven of those occlusions (9%) occurred within 3 years. Accounting for patients with less than 3 years of follow-up, the estimated probability of primary patency at 3 years is 85% (95% confidence interval, 75%-95%). The standard error of the mean is <10% at all displayed intervals. (Reprinted from the Journal of Vascular Surgery. Scali ST, Feezor RJ, Chang CK, et al. Critical analysis of results after chimney endovascular aortic aneurysm repair raises cause for concern. *J Vasc Surg*. 2014;60:865-873, Copyright 2014, with permission from The Society for Vascular Surgery.)

maintain good radial force, yet flexibility is compromised. This leads to awkward angles for chimney repair and likely predisposes these grafts to kinking and thrombosis. Additionally, respiratory variation on visceral vessels creates flexion points on the distal stent potentially leading to target vessel thrombosis. Conversely, self-expanding stent grafts have weak radial force but greater flexibility. This leads to nice angulation but compression from more rigid aortic devices. The results of this particular article should be considered by aortic surgeons; data like these are often not published because they represent a "negative result." Despite the long-term results presented, chEVAR still has a role as a bailout option for unintentional visceral coverage during aortic surgery but should be considered very selectively.

B. W. Propper, MD

Family Members of Patients with Abdominal Aortic Aneurysms are at Increased Risk for Aneurysms: Analysis of 618 Probands and their Families from the Liège AAA Family Study

Sakalihasan N, Defraigne J-O, Kerstenne M-A, et al (Univ Hosp of Liège, Belgium)

Ann Vasc Surg 28:787-797, 2014

Background.—The objectives were to answer the following questions using a well-characterized population in Liège, Belgium: 1) what percentage of abdominal aortic aneurysm (AAA) patients have a positive family history for AAA, 2) what is the prevalence of AAAs among relatives of AAA patients; and 3) do familial and sporadic AAA cases differ in clinical characteristics.

Methods and Results.—Unrelated AAA patients diagnosed at the Cardiovascular Surgery Department, University Hospital of Liège, Belgium, between 1999 and 2012 were invited to the study. A detailed family history was obtained in interviews and recorded using Progeny software. In the initial interview 62 (10%) of the 618 AAA patients reported a positive family history for AAA. We divided the 618 patients into two study groups: Group I: 296 AAA patients (268; 91% males) were followed up with computerized tomography combined with positron emission tomography, and Group II: 322 AAA patients (295; 92% males) whose families were invited to ultrasonography screening. Ultrasonography screening identified 24 new AAAs among 186 relatives (≥50 years) of 144 families yielding a prevalence of 13%. The highest prevalence (25%) was found among brothers. By combining the number of AAAs found by ultrasonography screening with those diagnosed previously the observed lifetime prevalence of AAA was estimated to be 32% in brothers. The familial AAA cases were more likely to have a ruptured AAA than the sporadic cases (8% vs. 2.4%; $P < 0.0001$).

Conclusions.—The findings confirm previously found high prevalence of AAA among brothers, support genetic contribution to AAA pathogenesis and provide rationale for targeted screening of relatives of AAA patients.

▶ Abdominal aortic aneurysm (AAA) development has multiple risk factors, including environmental and genetic factors. Several studies have documented a familial pattern of AAA. This study looked at the familial pattern of AAA among a well-characterized patient population in Liege, Belgium, all of which had extensive pedigree analysis and history. Known heritable connective tissue disorder patients, such as Marfan syndrome, were excluded. They found the highest prevalence of familial AAA (FAAA) among brothers (25%). When combining this with screening, 32% of brothers were detected with AAA. This is a higher incidence than the conventional wisdom of a 20% figure for nonsyndromic aneurysms in a family. Interestingly, there was a higher rate of rupture noted in the population of FAAA versus sporadic AAA (8% vs 2.4%, $P < .0001$), further supporting the notion that familial AAA may represent a more aggressive phenotype of common AAA.

A common limitation of these studies was observed in this study as well: getting accurate and detailed family histories can be challenging. In addition, the authors noted a low participation rate in the ultrasound screening relatives. However, despite the limitations, studies like this provide the necessary background for further study into the genetic markers for AAA and have great implications for screening strategies. Indeed, the discussion of this article includes an excellent dissertation and review on the subject of the risk of AAA among relatives.

M. Arnold, MD

Hypogastric and subclavian artery patency affects onset and recovery of spinal cord ischemia associate with aortic endografting

Eagleton MJ, Shah S, Petkosevek D, et al (Cleveland Clinic Lerner College of Medicine, OH)

J Vasc Surg 59:89-95, 2014

Objective.—Spinal cord ischemia (SCI) is a devastating complication associated with aortic aneurysm repair. The aim of the current study was to evaluate factors affecting outcomes from SCI associated with endovascular aortic aneurysm repair.

Methods.—A total of 1251 patients underwent endovascular repair of aortic aneurysm as part of a device trial between 1998 and 2010 utilizing endovascular abdominal aortic aneurysm repair (n = 351), thoracic endovascular aortic aneurysm repair (n = 201), fenestrated endovascular aortic aneurysm repair (n = 227), and visceral branched endografts (n = 472). Records and imaging studies were reviewed to supplement prospective outcome data. Demographics, type of repair, collateral bed (hypogastric/subclavian) patency, clinical presentation, and outcomes were evaluated on patients with SCI. Survival was calculated using life-table analysis.

Results.—SCI occurred in 2.8% (n = 36) of patients: abdominal aortic aneurysm, 0.3%, juxtarenal, 0.4%, thoracic aortic aneurysm, 4.6%, and thoracoabdominal aortic aneurysm, 4.8%). Four (11%) required carotid-subclavian bypass prior to endografting, and two underwent coverage of the left subclavian artery. Unilateral hypogastric artery occlusion was present in 11 (31%) patients prior to endograft placement, and three had bilateral occlusions. An additional seven patients had occlusion of at least one hypogastric artery during surgery. SCI was apparent immediately in 15 (42%) patients. Immediate onset of symptoms was observed in 73% of patients with at least one occluded collateral bed but in only 24% of those with patent collateral beds ($P = .021$). Of those presenting in a delayed fashion, nine (43%) had a clear precipitating event prior to onset of SCI (hypotension, n = 6, and segmental artery drain removal, n = 3). Recovery occurred in 24 (67%) patients, most within 7 days. Immediate presentation was a negative predictor of recovery ($P = .025$), as was occlusion of at least one collateral bed ($P = .035$). Mean follow-up was 22 ± 4 months with 30-day and 1-year survival of 92 ± 4.6% and 56 ± 8.3%. Survival was only 36% at 3 months in those with permanent SCI compared with 92% ($P < .001$) in those with temporary symptoms.

Conclusions.—SCI continues to complicate aortic surgery despite the advent of endovascular therapy. Occlusion of a single collateral bed is associated with an increased risk for immediate onset of SCI and lack of recovery. These factors are harbingers of poor outcomes and increased short-term mortality. This may be prevented by preserving collateral bed patency in patients undergoing extensive endovascular procedures.

► Spinal cord ischemia (SCI), and its sequelae, is among the most feared complication after thoracic aortic intervention. Over the past half-century, numerous techniques have evolved to decrease the risk of SCI, each with incremental impact. The authors of this article not only discuss these maneuvers, but more importantly have potentially identified a high-risk group of patients in whom SCI may develop. Patients with collateral bed occlusion, unilateral/bilateral hypogastric or subclavian, seem to have an increased incidence of SCI. Of those with immediate symptoms (n = 15), 10 had 1 or 2 collateral beds occluded. Of the 21 patients with delayed symptoms, 4 patients had at least 1 collateral bed occluded. Indeed, many of these collateral bed losses are technical and planned, but preemptive procedures to revascularize the area before coverage (bypass vs transposition) should now be considered. More interesting was their finding that those patients who had a delayed onset of SCI seem to fare better than those with immediate deficits. In fact, nearly 25% of SCI patients presented after 24 hours and 33% after 48 hours. That considered, it is impractical in many patients to maintain prolonged drainage, and a selective strategy of cerebrospinal fluid drainage may be considered. Overall, the authors expertise in complex repairs is reflected in their laudatory results; a notable feature of this article was the high incidence of endoleak (31%) while maintaining a low 2.9% incidence of SCI. This may further argue for staged procedures and crafty specific adjuncts to maintain sac perfusion after definitive repair.

K. C. Orion, MD

Molecular diagnosis in vascular Ehlers-Danlos syndrome predicts pattern of arterial involvement and outcomes

Shalhub S, Black JH 3rd, Cecchi AC, et al (Univ of Washington, Seattle; The Johns Hopkins Hosp, Baltimore, MD; Univ of Texas Health Science Ctr at Houston; et al)

J Vasc Surg 60:160-169, 2014

Objective.—The management of arterial pathology in individuals with vascular Ehlers-Danlos syndrome (vEDS) remains a challenge. Here we describe the correlation between *COL3A1* gene mutation type and the clinical phenotype in individuals with vEDS.

Methods.—Individuals with confirmed molecular diagnoses of vEDS were enrolled in a multi-institutional natural history study. Data collected included demographics, clinical and family histories, arterial pathology (aneurysm, dissection, and rupture), operative details, and autopsy reports. Individuals were classified into two cohorts by the type of *COL3A1* mutations and their effect on the amount of normal collagen produced: those with mutations that lead to minimal (MIN) production (10%-15%) of normal type III collagen and those with haploinsufficiency (HI) mutations that lead to production of 50% of the normal type III collagen.

Results.—A cohort of 68 individuals (72%) from 56 families had arterial pathology (44% male) with 13% HI. The HI group was older at the time of their first vascular event (mean, 42 [range, 26-58] years vs 33 [range, 8-62] years; $P = .016$) and had a higher incidence of aortic pathology than the MIN group (56% vs 21%; $P = .025$). Visceral arterial pathology was seen in 43 arteries in 23 individuals in the MIN group vs only one artery in five individuals in the HI group. Emergency surgical procedures were more likely to be undertaken when vEDS diagnosis was not known (81% vs 41%; $P = .005$), and 81% of these procedures were open surgical repair compared with 19% endovascular repairs ($P = .019$). Open and endovascular repairs were equally used in the elective setting. Postoperative complications were highest when the diagnosis of vEDS was not known (62% vs 14%; $P < .001$) and when procedures were undertaken in an emergency setting (5% vs 55% $P < .001$). Mortality due to arterial complications was 0% in the HI cohort and 21% in the MIN cohort ($P = .132$).

Conclusions.—Arterial pathology in vEDS individuals is related to the underlying *COL3A1* mutation type. The arterial pathology in individuals with HI mutations occurs at later ages with a higher incidence of aortic disease compared with other *COL3A1* mutation types. Molecular diagnosis is recommended because diagnosis confirmation, appropriate

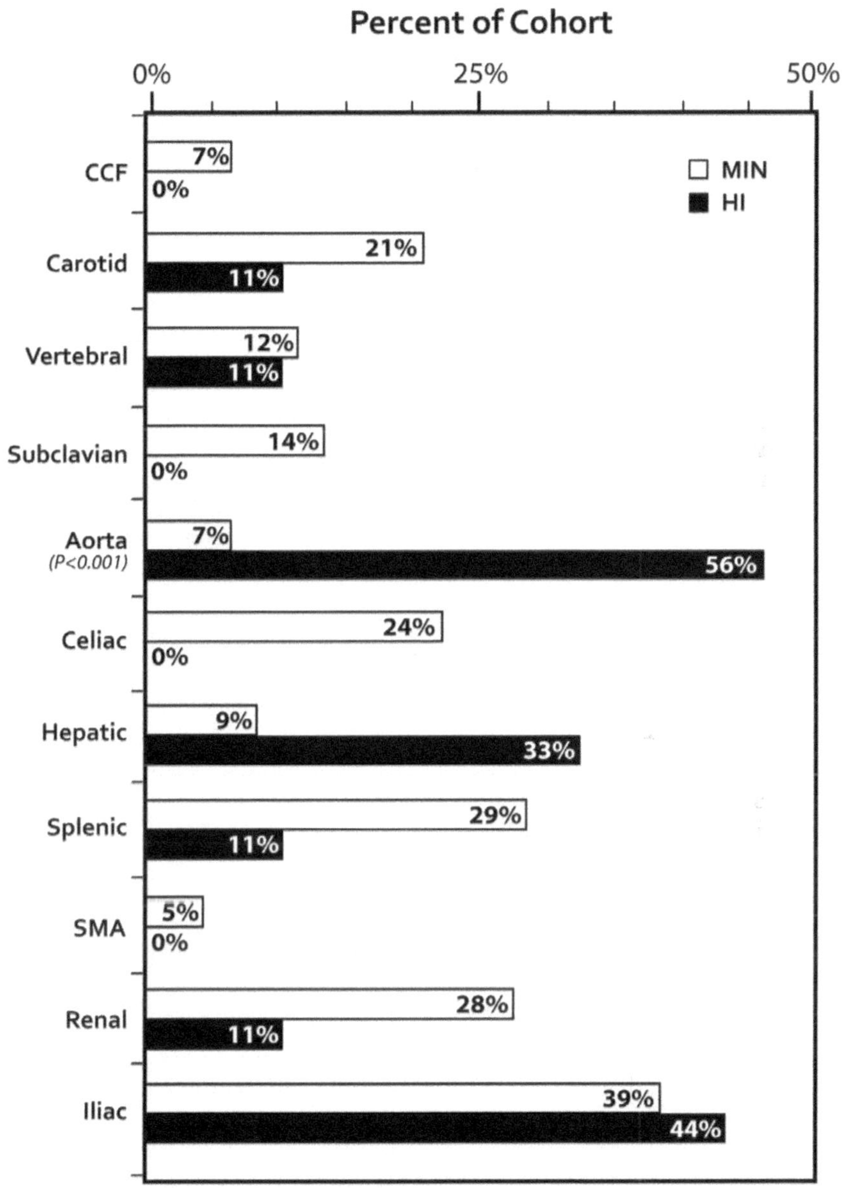

FIGURE 3.—Arterial involvement in vascular Ehlers-Danlos syndrome (vEDS) patients by *COL3A1* mutations. Although vEDS involves medium-sized arteries more commonly, there was an increased prevalence of aortic involvement in the HI cohort compared with the MIN cohort ($P = .025$). CCF, Carotid cavernous fistula; *HI*, mutations that lead to 50% normal type III collagen production; *MIN*, mutations that lead to minimal (10%-15%) normal type III collagen production; *SMA*, superior mesenteric artery. (Reprinted from the Journal of Vascular Surgery. Shalhub S, Black JH 3rd, Cecchi AC, et al. Molecular diagnosis in vascular Ehlers-Danlos syndrome predicts pattern of arterial involvement and outcomes. *J Vasc Surg*. 2014;60:160-169, Copyright 2014, with permission from The Society for Vascular Surgery.)

surveillance, and prophylactic interventions in an elective setting improve surgical outcomes (Fig 3).

▶ The treatment of patients with vascular manifestations of Ehlers-Danlos (vEDS) remains complex and challenging. The surgical outcomes, particularly with open approaches, have been considered hazardous. The authors of this report advocate for early genetic testing to establish a diagnosis of Ehlers-Danlos, but more importantly reveal the underlying mutation type. Knowledge of the specific molecular diagnosis may allow for appropriate genetic counselling, preoperative discussion that is tailored to the specifics of the disease, and modification of the surgical technique. The report raises an important distinction in vEDS, that is, those patients with a specific mutation (haploinsufficiency [HI]) tended to large vessel events versus missense mutations (MIN) in which collagen III production is minimal (Fig 3). Furthermore, HI patients suffered no mortality after intervention versus a 21% mortality rate in MIN patients. In addition, the study suggests patients with a confirmed genetic mutation should be offered periodic surveillance even in the absence of current vascular pathology. This surveillance allows the patients to be treated in an elective setting, which can greatly improve outcomes and mortality, as emergent procedures were associated with more complications. As a general rule, the authors concur that first-degree family members should also be offered counselling and testing. By establishing a diagnosis, and now even the mutation type, early, the physician and surgeon can recognize the complexities presented by vEDS, and can provide better care and outcomes for these patients.

M. Arnold, MD

Surgical Management of Aortitis with Early Aneurysmal Dilation

Lee CJ, Kibbe MR, Eskandari MK, et al (Northwestern Univ, Chicago, IL)

Ann Vasc Surg 28:568-574, 2014

Background.—Aortitis is a rare and serious condition that requires expedient surgical evaluation. Diagnosis is generally made by computed tomography (CT). Surgery is most often performed when significant aneurysmal changes have already occurred. Outcomes of early surgical management of aortitis with early aneurysmal dilation have not been reported previously.

Methods.—A retrospective review of open abdominal aortic repairs performed from 1999 to 2009 at a single center was done from a prospectively collected database. Patients with a confirmed radiographic appearance of aortitis and treated surgically were selected. Demographic, clinical, and surgical data of patients with aortitis showing early aneurysmal changes (aortic diameter <4 cm) were then analyzed. All aortitis cases with >4-cm aortic diameters and with prosthetic aortic grafts were excluded.

Results.—During the observation period, 421 open abdominal aortic repairs were performed. Of these, 10 (2.4%) were identified as having primary aortitis without significant aneurysmal changes. The mean age of the patients was 62 (range 48–77) years. There were 6 (60%) men and 4 (40%) women in the cohort. Four patients (40%) had culture-negative aortitis, whereas 6 (60%) had positive microbial cultures at the time of diagnosis. Paravisceral involvement was seen in 8 (80%) cases. All patients underwent in situ repair with aortic homografts. Mean operative time was 348 minutes and mean estimated blood loss was 2475 mL. Median follow-up time was 23.1 months with a range of 1.7–51.4 months. Operative mortality was 0%, and 1 late death occurred at 23 months postoperatively. There were 9 significant in-hospital (30-day) events occurring in 5 patients, including 3 cardiovascular events, 2 pulmonary events, 3 acute renal failures, and 1 deep surgical site infection.

Conclusions.—Aortitis is an uncommon indication for aortic repair. Infectious aortitis is most commonly confirmed by microbiologic studies, but a significant number of cases have no demonstrable microbial source. Outcomes after early surgical management for aortitis with small aneurysms demonstrated improved mortality when compared with series reviewing outcomes in aortitis patients with large mycotic aneurysms.

▶ Aortitis is a relatively complex pathology because diagnosis can be challenging, and nonsurgical treatment options are limited. Typically, treatment is reserved for patients with larger size aneurysm dilation (> 4 cm), but it is well accepted that aortitis alone is a risk factor for degeneration and rupture. This article reports excellent results when aortitis is identified early and surgical treatment is instituted before significant dilation (< 4 cm, compared with 20%–40% mortality in aneurysm). The results for treatment showed no early mortality in these patients with repair being accomplished using cryopreserved homograft. The authors contend that early repair eliminates the possibility for acute degeneration and rupture; furthermore, early repair eliminates some anatomic challenges presented by larger aneurysms. One of the ongoing challenges is when surgical repair should be pursued. These data, albeit from a small cohort, make the argument to offer repair once the diagnosis of aortitis is established. With suprarenal involvement, there is a tendency to push medical therapy, because thoracoabdominal repair carries higher surgical risk. Within this series, 80% of patients had a thoracoabdominal repairs with good outcomes in both the visceral patch repair and full replacement groups. Other groups have reported good success with repair using rifampin soaked Dacron, and any randomized series is unlikely given the rarity of disease. The authors also drive home the message that distinction of autoimmune aortitis from mycotic aneurysm development is a difficult clinical decision and cite rapid progression, fever, and distant source as key determinants of the latter.

B. W. Propper, MD

A comparison of open surgery versus endovascular repair of unstable ruptured abdominal aortic aneurysms

Gupta PK, Ramanan B, Engelbert TL, et al (Univ of Tennessee Health Science Ctr, Memphis; Univ of California, San Francisco; Univ of Wisconsin Hosp and Clinics, Madison)

J Vasc Surg 60:1439-1445, 2014

Objective.—Two randomized trials to date have compared open surgery (OS) and endovascular (EVAR) repair for ruptured abdominal aortic aneurysm (rAAA); however, neither addressed optimal management of unstable patients. Single-center reports have produced conflicting data regarding the superiority of one vs the other, with the lack of statistical power due to low patient numbers. Furthermore, previous studies have not delineated between the outcomes of stable patients with a contained rupture vs those patients with instability. Our objective was to compare 30-day outcomes in patients undergoing OS vs EVAR for all rAAAs, focusing specifically on patients with instability.

Methods.—Patients who underwent repair of rAAA were identified from the American College of Surgeons (ACS) National Surgical Quality Improvement Program (NSQIP) database (2005 to 2010). Unstable patients with rupture were identified as those who were American Society of Anesthesiologists Physical Status Classification 4 or 5 requiring emergency repair with at least one of the following: preoperative shock, preoperative transfusion of <4 units, preoperative intubation, or preoperative coma or impaired sensorium. Univariable and multivariable logistic regression analyses were performed.

Results.—Of the 1447 patients with rAAA, 65.5% underwent OS and 34.5% EVAR. Forty-five percent were unstable, and for these patients, OS was performed in 71.3% and EVAR in 28.7%. The 30-day mortality rate was 47.9% (OS, 52.8%; EVAR, 35.6%; $P < .0001$) for unstable rAAAs and was 22.4% for stable rAAAs (OS, 26.3%; EVAR, 16.4%; $P = .001$). Amongst patients with unstable rAAA, 26% had a myocardial infarction or cardiac arrest ≤30 days (OS, 29.0%; EVAR, 19.1%; $P = .006$), and 17% needed postoperative dialysis (OS, 18.7%; EVAR, 12.8%; $P = .04$). Amongst patients with stable rAAA, 13.6% had a myocardial infarction or cardiac arrest ≤30 days (OS, 14.9%; EVAR, 11.6%; $P = .20$), and 11.5% needed postoperative dialysis (OS, 13.3%; EVAR, 8.7%; $P = .047$). Multivariable analyses showed OS was a predictor of 30-day mortality for unstable rAAA (odds ratio, 1.74; 95% confidence interval, 1.16-2.62) and stable rAAA (odds ratio, 1.64; 95% confidence interval, 1.10-2.43).

Conclusions.—Approximately one-third of patients treated for rAAA undergo EVAR in NSQIP participating hospitals. Not surprisingly, unstable patients have less favorable outcomes. In both stable and unstable rAAA patients, EVAR is associated with a diminished 30-day mortality and morbidity (Table 1).

▶ There remain questions regarding the utility of endovascular aneurysm repair (EVAR) in the management of ruptured abdominal aortic aneurysms (rAAA), particularly in view of recently published randomized trials. The Amsterdam Acute Aneurysm Trial[1] was a recently published randomized, controlled trial comparing EVAR against open surgical repair (OR) in hemodynamically stable patients such that 78% of patients were excluded because of hemodynamic instability. The Immediate Management of the Patient with Rupture: Open versus Endovascular Repair (IMPROVE) trial[2] was published earlier this year comparing EVAR with OR in both stable and unstable patients. Unfortunately, unstable patients were not compared separately.

The authors of this important study compared results of 30-day mortality in patients undergoing both EVAR and OR in an unstable cohort of the National Surgical Quality Improvement Program database between 2005 and 2010.

TABLE 1.—Postoperative Events with Univariable Analysis

	Stable rAAA			Unstable rAAA		
Thirty-day Outcomes[a]	OS (n = 482)	EVAR (n = 311)	*P* Value[b]	OS (n = 466)	EVAR (n = 188)	*P* Value[b]
Wound infection						
Superficial	8 (1.7)	9 (2.9)	.32	8(1.7)	10 (5.3)	.02
Deep	3 (0.6)	2 (0.6)	.99	3 (0.6)	3 (1.6)	.4
Wound dehiscence	10 (2.1)	3 (1.0)	.27	12 (2.6)	3 (1.6)	.57
Urinary tract infection	27 (5.6)	6 (1.9)	.01	34 (7.3)	15 (8.0)	.75
Transfusion >4 units PRBC post-op	111 (23.0)	61 (19.6)	.26	138 (29.6)	58 (30.9)	.76
Pneumonia	97 (20.1)	26 (8.4)	<.0001	111 (23.8)	37 (19.7)	.25
Reintubation	57 (11.8)	20 (6.4)	.01	41 (8.8)	24 (12.8)	.13
Failure to extubate at 48 hours	215 (44.6)	48 (15.4)	<.0001	210 (45.1)	68 (36.2)	.04
Deep venous thrombosis	23 (4.8)	6 (1.9)	.04	18 (3.9)	9 (4.8)	.66
Pulmonary embolism	10 (2.1)	4 (1.3)	.58	5 (1.1)	4 (2.1)	.29
Renal insufficiency	22 (4.6)	7 (2.3)	.09	25 (5.4)	6 (3.2)	.31
Acute renal failure requiring dialysis	64 (13.3)	27 (8.7)	.047	87 (18.7)	24 (12.8)	.07
Stroke	8 (1.7)	4 (1.3)	.77	13 (2.8)	2 (1.1)	.18
Coma	9 (1.9)	0	.01	6 (1.3)	0	.19
Cardiac arrest	49 (10.2)	17 (5.5)	.02	114 (24.5)	26 (13.8)	.003
MI	26 (5.4)	21 (6.8)	.43	24 (5.2)	12 (6.4)	.53
Return to operating room	111 (23.0)	64 (20.6)	.42	98 (21.0)	45 (23.9)	.42
Hospital length of stay, days	13.8 ± 16.3	8.7 ± 13.8	<.0001	12.7 ± 16.9	12.4 ± 14.8	.87
Death	127 (26.3)	51 (16.4)	.001	246 (52.8)	67 (35.6)	<.0001

EVAR, Endovascular aortic repair; *MI*, myocardial infarction; *OS*, open surgery; *PRBC*, packed red blood cells; *rAAA*, ruptured abdominal aortic aneurysm.

[a]Categoric data are shown as number (%) and continuous data as mean ± standard deviation.

[b]The *P* value reflects univariate analysis: Pearson χ^2 test and analysis of variance *F* test comparing the preoperative variables between OS and EVAR. $P < .05$ is significant.

This unstable cohort was based on a surrogate created by the authors consisting of urgently treat patients who (1) experienced preoperative shock, (2) received greater than 4 U of preoperative transfusion, (3) required preoperative intubation, or (4) had impaired sensorium or preoperative coma.

In the stable cohort, 793 patients, EVAR was significantly better than OR (16.4% vs 26.3%; $P = .001$), and in the unstable cohort, 654 patients, EVAR was also significantly better than OR (35.6% vs 52.8% 30-day mortality; $P < .0001$; Table 1).

This study confirms my bias but should still be interpreted with caution based on the quality of the data (an unproven surrogate for instability). Nonetheless, the rate of EVAR for rAAA is increasing and is nearly 65% in the United States in 2015 (W. Robinson, Pacific Northwest Endovascular Conference, May 2015; unpublished data). In a recent panel discussion of world experts in May 2015, not a single panelist would choose OR over EVAR as a first-line strategy for an anatomically suitable rAAA patient. I think the chances of a repeat randomized, controlled trial to solve this problem are zero at this point. We all know how to treat these patients in 2015.

B. W. Starnes, MD

References

1. Reimerink JJ, Hoornweg LL, Vahl AC, et al. Endovascular repair versus open repair of ruptured abdominal aortic aneurysms: a multicenter randomized controlled trial. *Ann Surg*. 2013;258:248-256.
2. Powell JT, Sweeting MJ, Thompson MM, et al. Endovascular or open repair strategy for ruptured abdominal aortic aneurysm: 30 day outcomes from IMPROVE randomised trial. *BMJ*. 2014;348:f7661.

A novel endovascular debranching technique using physician-assembled endografts for repair of thoracoabdominal aneurysms

Anderson J, Nykamp M, Danielson L, et al (Univ of South Dakota, Sioux Falls; Sanford Res, Sioux Falls, SD; et al)
J Vasc Surg 60:1177-1185, 2014

Objective.—The objective of this study was to demonstrate a technique that uses physician-assembled endografts to make use of the benefits of parallel grafts while also providing for circumferential seal and fixation in repair of thoracoabdominal aneurysms in inoperable patients.

Methods.—A single-center all-comers retrospective analysis of 14 patients was performed that looked at the early outcomes of patients treated for thoracoabdominal aneurysms. Three Crawford type II, four type III, four type IV, and three type V thoracoabdominal aneurysms were treated. Contrast material, fluoroscopy time, length of stay, clinical success, and technical success were measured.

Results.—There was no in-hospital, 30-day, or 6-month mortality. We found two type III endoleaks in the early design. One required coil embolization. Average volume of contrast material and average fluoroscopy time were 76.9 mL and 119.1 minutes, respectively. Average length of stay was 10.5 days, and average procedure time was 251.2 minutes. Clinical success was observed in 78.6% of patients to date, and technical success was observed in 85.7% of patients.

Conclusions.—Short-term results show that this approach is safe. The device can be safely implanted, is off-the-shelf, and can treat each of the Crawford thoracoabdominal aneurysm types. Finally, the assembly of off-the-shelf components may shorten the regulatory path for this physician-assembled endograft (Figs 1-4).

▶ This study caught my eye only because it involves physician modification of commercially available stent grafts. I am a true believer that surgeons, in particular, possess the skillset to custom design a procedure and medical device to fit any patient. It is what we do.

The senior author creatively used endovascular devices from multiple device manufacturers to create his own system for managing complex thoracoabdominal aneurysms in 14 patients. Although this study was small with unknown and unreported mean follow-up, the 30-day mortality rate of 0% is remarkable. Mean fluoroscopy time for the procedures was 119.1 minutes, which is excessive but probably related to early experience.

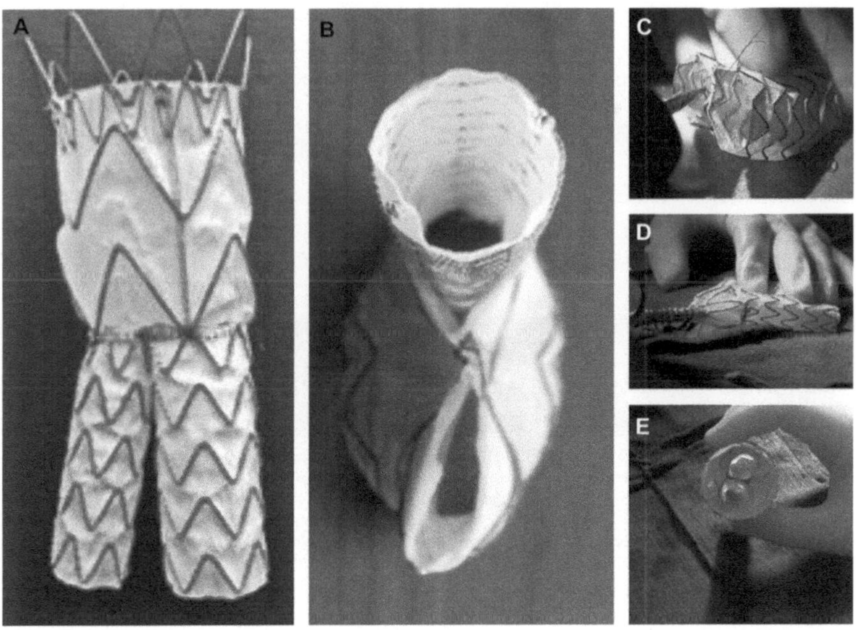

FIGURE 1.—Sequence of constructing (**A**) the thoracic bifurcation graft (early configuration shown in B), including (**C**) sewing the common seam and (**D**) sewing the end-to-end anastomosis between the Valiant and the two Endurant limbs. E, Top view of the thoracic bifurcation showing no gutters. (Reprinted from the Journal of Vascular Surgery. Anderson J, Nykamp M, Danielson L, et al. A novel endovascular debranching technique using physician-assembled endografts for repair of thoracoabdominal aneurysms. *J Vasc Surg*. 2014;60:1177-1185, Copyright 2014, with permission from The Society for Vascular Surgery.)

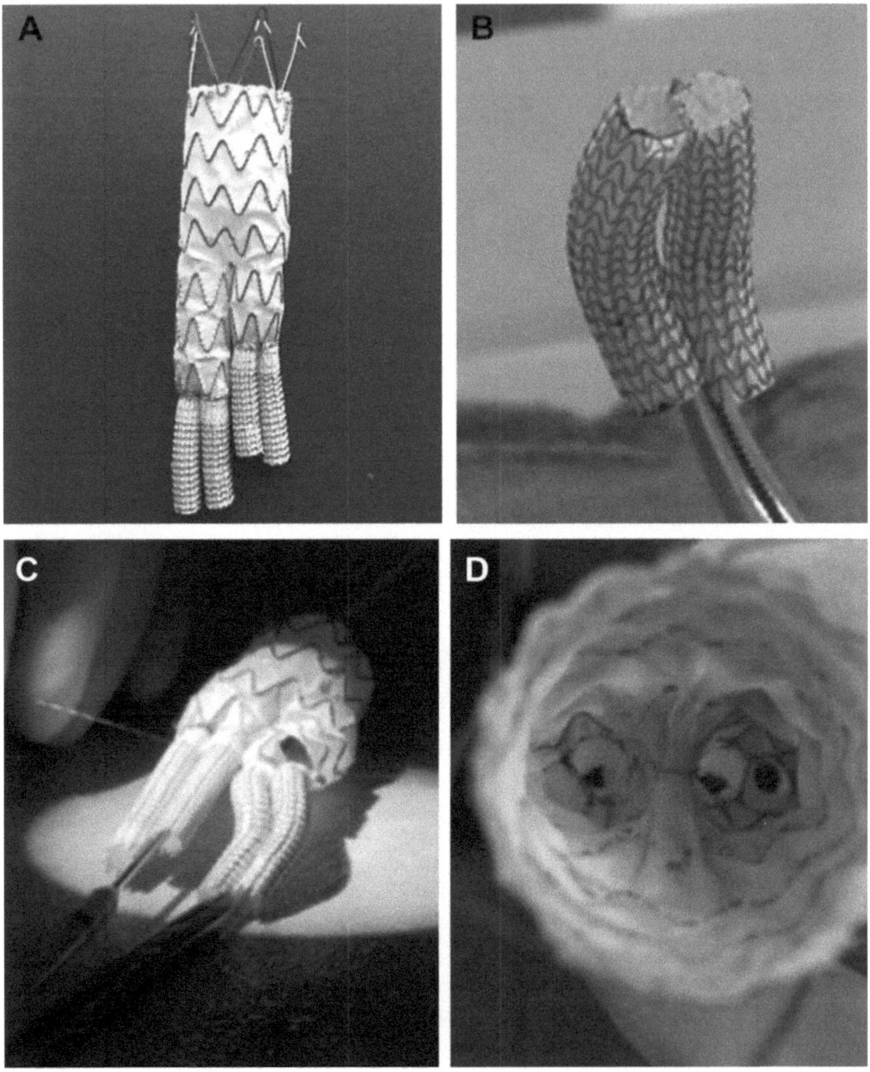

FIGURE 2.—Sequence of construction of (**A**) the visceral manifold, including (**B**) sewing a common seam between two shortened Gore Viabahns and (**C**) sewing the Gore Viabahns to the distal end of a Medtronic Endurant in an end-to-end anastomosis. **D**, Top view of the visceral manifold showing no gutters. (Reprinted from the Journal of Vascular Surgery. Anderson J, Nykamp M, Danielson L, et al. A novel endovascular debranching technique using physician-assembled endografts for repair of thoracoabdominal aneurysms. *J Vasc Surg*. 2014;60:1177-1185, with permission from The Authors.)

I think it is important to disseminate this report in the form of 4 figures (Figs 1-4), depicting the physician-modified process. The chances of this procedure ever

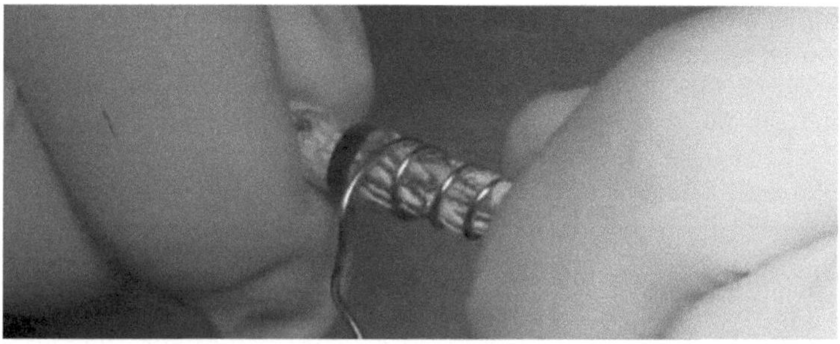

FIGURE 3.—Spiral wire re-constraining technique. (Reprinted from the Journal of Vascular Surgery. Anderson J, Nykamp M, Danielson L, et al. A novel endovascular debranching technique using physician-assembled endografts for repair of thoracoabdominal aneurysms. *J Vasc Surg.* 2014;60:1177-1185, with permission from The Authors.)

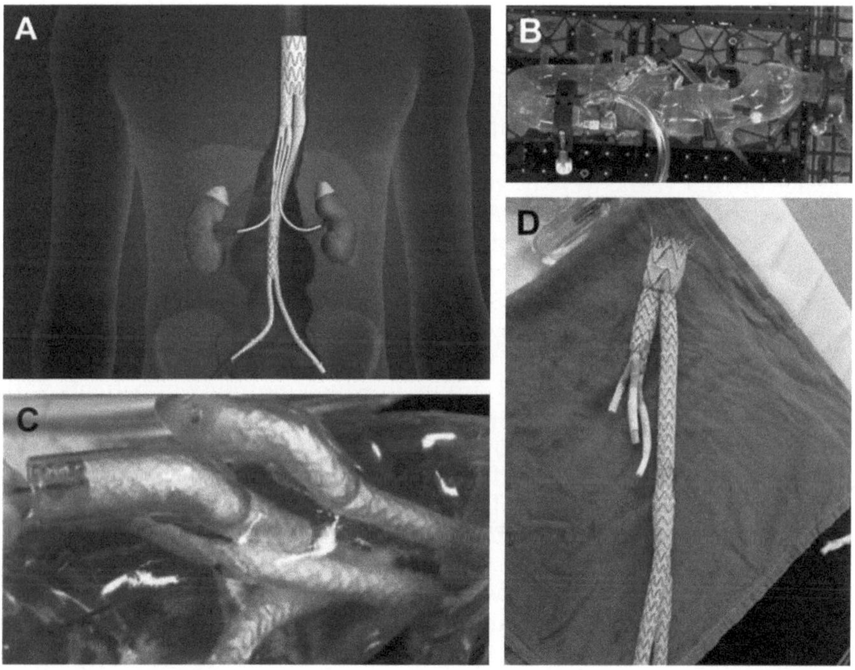

FIGURE 4.—**A**, Demonstration of early concept including an animation of the assembly in a type III thoracoabdominal aortic aneurysm (TAAA). **B**, Top view of a three-dimensional printed type III TAAA with 4 L/min water flowing to simulate in vivo use. **C**, Stents in the visceral vessels after simulated use. **D**, Assembly of all component devices as they would be deployed in vivo. (Reprinted from the Journal of Vascular Surgery. Anderson J, Nykamp M, Danielson L, et al. A novel endovascular debranching technique using physician-assembled endografts for repair of thoracoabdominal aneurysms. *J Vasc Surg.* 2014;60:1177-1185, with permission from The Authors.)

getting US Food and Drug Administration approval is miniscule but gives a hint to engineers from the device manufacture companies as to what we are looking for!

B. W. Starnes, MD

Abdominal compartment syndrome associated with endovascular and open repair of ruptured abdominal aortic aneurysms

Rubenstein C, Bietz G, Davenport DL, et al (Hadassah Hebrew Univ, Jerusalem, Israel; Peripheral Vascular Associates, San Antonio, TX; Univ of Kentucky College of Medicine, Lexington)

J Vasc Surg 61:648-654, 2015

Background.—Abdominal compartment syndrome (ACS) is a known complication of ruptured abdominal aortic aneurysm (rAAA) repair and can occur with either endovascular (EVAR) or open repair. We hypothesize that the underlying mechanism for the development of ACS may differ for patients treated with EVAR or open operation.

Methods.—All patients who presented with rAAA at a tertiary care medical center between January 2005 and December 2010 were included in the study. Demographic factors, type of repair (open vs EVAR), development of ACS, intraoperative and postoperative fluid requirements, estimated blood loss, length of stay, and morbidity and mortality were recorded. Student t-test and Fisher exact test were performed. A *P* value <.05 was considered significant.

Results.—Seventy-three patients, 62 men and 11 women with an average age of 70.5 years, were treated for rAAA. Forty-four (60%) underwent open repair; 29 (40%) had EVAR. Overall mortality was 42% (31 of 73), with mortality being 31% (9 of 29) in EVAR and 48% (21 of 44) in open repair. ACS developed in 21 patients (29%), more frequently in open repair than in EVAR (15 of 44 [34%] vs 6 of 29 [21%]; *P* = NS). Mortality was higher in patients who developed ACS compared with those without ACS (13 of 21 [62%] vs 17 of 52 [33%]; *P* =.022). This finding was especially pronounced in the EVAR group, in which mortality in patients with ACS was 83% (5 of 6) compared with 17% (4 of 23) without ACS (*P* =.005). Intraoperative fluid requirements were significantly higher in EVAR patients who developed ACS compared with those without ACS, including packed red blood cells (5600 mL vs 1100 mL; *P* < .0001), total blood products (9300 mL vs 1500 mL; *P* < .001), crystalloid (11,200 mL vs 4500 mL; *P* < .001), and estimated blood loss (5000 mL vs 660 mL; *P* =.006). In patients treated with open repair, there were no significant differences in intraoperative fluid requirements between those who developed ACS and those without ACS. However, patients who developed ACS after open repair required significantly more crystalloid on the first and second postoperative days (first postoperative day, 8300 mL vs 5600 mL [*P* =.01]; second postoperative day, 6500 mL vs 3800 mL [*P* =.004]).

Conclusions.—This study demonstrates that the development of ACS after repair of rAAA is associated with increased mortality, especially in EVAR-treated patients. The higher intraoperative blood and blood product requirements associated with ACS in EVAR patients suggest that one potential cause of early ACS is continued hemorrhage from lumbar and inferior mesenteric vessels through the ruptured aneurysm sac. Hence, open ligation of such vessels should be considered in patients developing early ACS after EVAR for rAAA (Fig 1).

▶ With the ongoing controversy over the utility of endovascular aneurysm repair (EVAR) versus open repair of ruptured abdominal aortic aneurysms, this recent report emerges as an important one describing a single center experience with managing abdominal compartment syndrome (ACS). These authors treated 73 patients who had ruptured abdominal aortic aneurysm (rAAA) over 5 years (44 open and 29 EVAR). Although a small series, the incidence of ACS was 29% and was highly lethal, particularly in the EVAR group (83% mortality rate when present in the EVAR group).

ACS, when it occurs in the setting of rAAA, is highly morbid and often lethal. These authors recommend an algorithm to treat these patients (Fig 1). I'm afraid, however, that this algorithm and the recommendations listed are incorrect for a multitude of reasons. First, there are no anatomic descriptions of the patients undergoing EVAR. We do not know if these patients were treated within the Instructions for Use (IFU) for a particular device (aortic diameter and length) or if successful seal was accomplished in all patients. We get a glimpse at how the EVAR patients were treated intraoperatively in that the authors describe only a single decompressive laparotomy performed at the time of EVAR for rAAA. What is known (and the authors recognize this) is that early

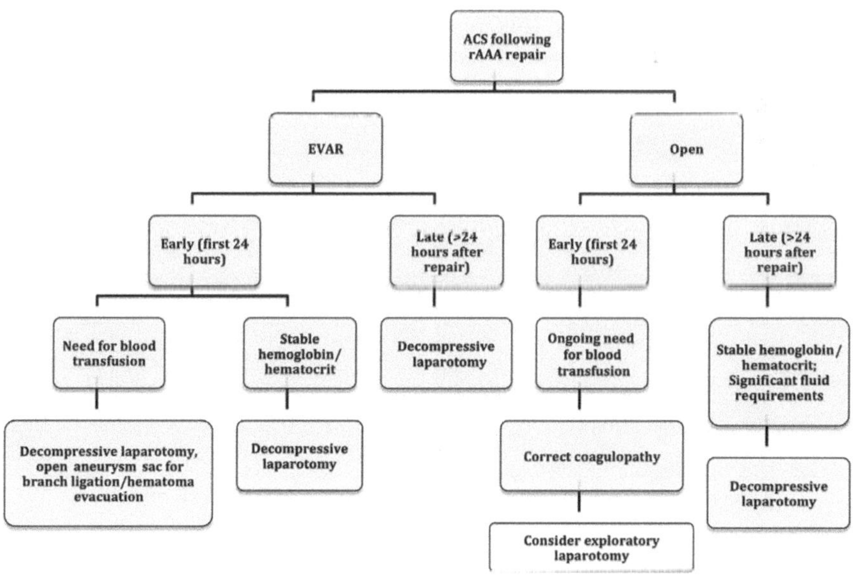

FIGURE 1.—Proposed algorithm for treatment of abdominal compartment syndrome (*ACS*) after endovascular aneurysm repair (*EVAR*) or open repair of ruptured abdominal aortic aneurysm (*rAAA*). (Reprinted from the Journal of Vascular Surgery. Rubenstein C, Bietz G, Davenport DL, et al. Abdominal compartment syndrome associated with endovascular and open repair of ruptured abdominal aortic aneurysms. *J Vasc Surg*. 2015;61:648-654, Copyright 2014, with permission from The Society for Vascular Surgery.)

diagnosis of ACS is imperative, and failure to decompress in a timely fashion is uniformly fatal.

In our own experience of more than 350 ruptured AAA's treated with an EVAR-first strategy, we have learned that treating rAAA patients who are not anatomic candidates for EVAR (short necks and neck diameters > 32 mm) with an endovascular approach results in a 100% mortality rate. In addition, decompression and vacuum-assisted wound dressings are all that are needed to manage ACS. Retroperitoneal hematoma evacuation and attempts at lumbar or inferior mesenteric artery ligation are fraught with complication and should be avoided when possible in these settings. Correct coagulopathy and decompress. If the patient is still bleeding, question the original approach at repair and if the patient was a good candidate in the first place.

B. W. Starnes, MD

Acute bilateral renal artery chimney stent thrombosis after endovascular repair of a juxtarenal abdominal aortic aneurysm

Scali ST, Feezor RJ, Huber TS, et al (Univ of Florida College of Medicine, Gainesville)

J Vasc Surg 61:1058-1061, 2015

The use of "chimney" stents to augment the proximal landing zone for endovascular aneurysm repair has been increasingly reported. Despite mounting enthusiasm for this technique, the durability of this type of repair and capability to preserve perfusion to target branches remains a

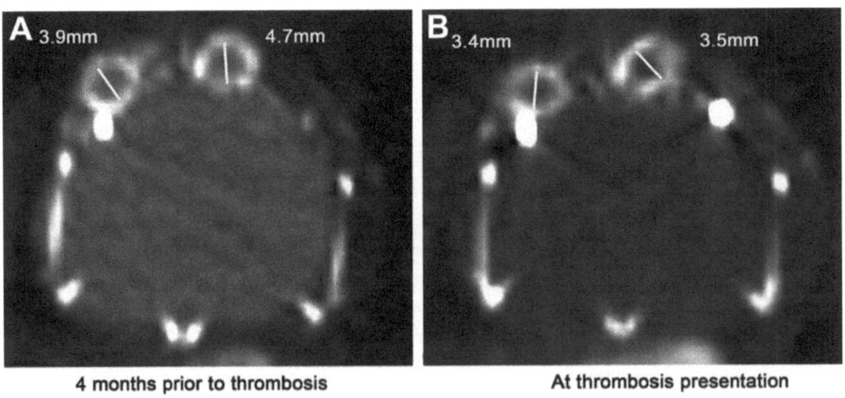

FIGURE 1.—A, Three-month post-chimney endovascular aneurysm repair (chEVAR) computed tomography (CT). B, Noncontrasted CT at time of chimney thrombosis. This figure demonstrates the pre- (A) and post- (B) chimney thrombosis axial CT scans. A, This image demonstrates that the 6-mm Atrium iCAST stents never fully expanded to their nominal size. Additionally, there are subtle changes in the conformation of the stents, as evidenced by the short axis configuration and measurements when comparing the two images. (Reprinted from the Journal of Vascular Surgery. Scali ST, Feezor RJ, Huber TS, et al. Acute bilateral renal artery chimney stent thrombosis after endovascular repair of a juxtarenal abdominal aortic aneurysm. *J Vasc Surg*. 2015;61:1058-1061, Copyright 2014, with permission from The Society for Vascular Surgery.)

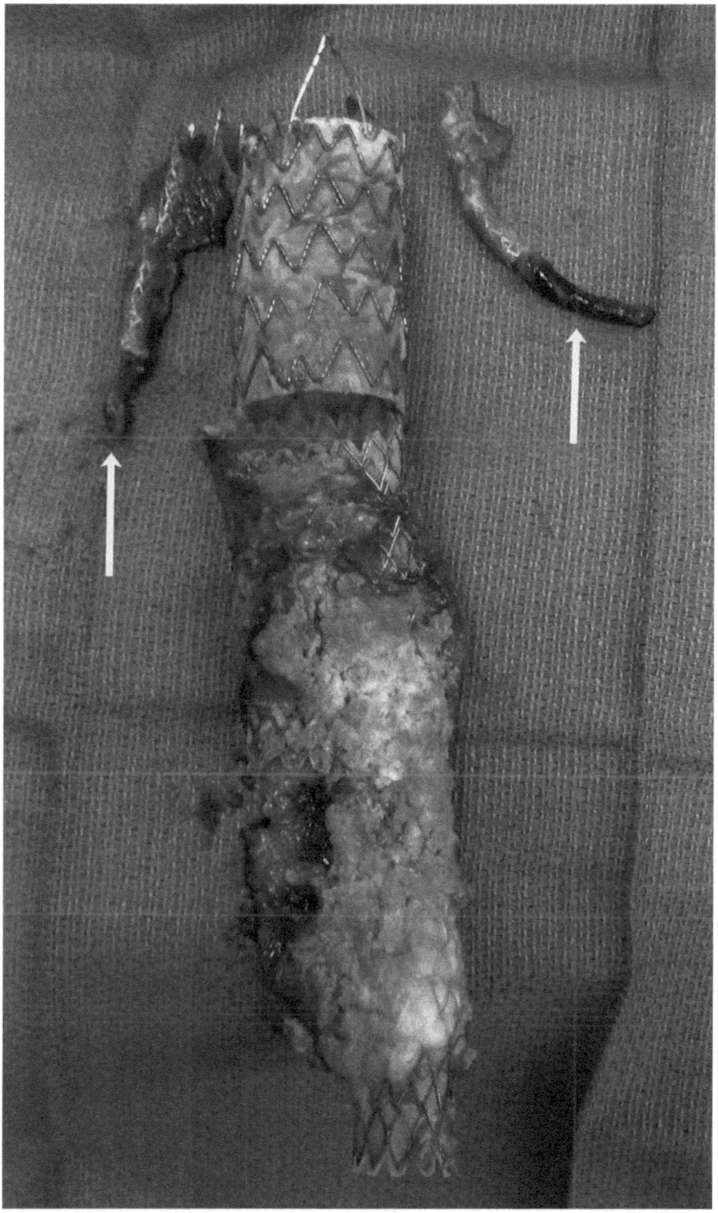

FIGURE 2.—Devices at explantation. This image demonstrates all endovascular devices explanted from the patient's aorta with thrombus within each stent extending into the renal arteries (*arrows*). (Reprinted from the Journal of Vascular Surgery. Scali ST, Feezor RJ, Huber TS, et al. Acute bilateral renal artery chimney stent thrombosis after endovascular repair of a juxtarenal abdominal aortic aneurysm. *J Vasc Surg*. 2015;61:1058-1061, Copyright 2014, with permission from The Society for Vascular Surgery.)

paramount concern. Here, we report management of a patient presenting with acute bilateral renal chimney stent thrombosis and a type Ia endoleak (Figs 1 and 2).

▶ This report should raise concern among any surgeons performing parallel grafts in the form of chimneys and snorkels. This strategy for treating juxta-renal and short-neck aneurysms is increasing with little or no validation of long-term durability. Currently, less than 150 cases are reported in the world literature, mostly consisting of small single-institution series with only short-term follow-up. Cumulative renal stent patency in these reports exceeds 90%, but these short-term results in a small group of heterogeneous patients do not establish durability of this technique for juxta-renal aneurysms.[1]

The reported case is depicted in Figs 1 and 2. Fortunately, the patient only required short-term dialysis and eventually had an uneventful outcome after explant of the grafts and open aortic reconstruction. This case highlights the potential pitfalls of chimney and snorkel grafts. In the era of evolving fenestrated technology and excellent long-term outcomes of both fenestrated and open juxta-renal aneurysm repair, elective parallel endografting should be used with caution. I applaud the authors for taking the time to publish this case report, as all of the negative outcomes are underreported.

B. W. Starnes, MD

Reference

1. Moulakakis KG, Mylonas SN, Avgerinos E, et al. The chimney graft technique for preserving visceral vessels during endovascular treatment of aortic pathologies. *J Vasc Surg*. 2012;55:1497-1503.

Acute kidney injury defined according to the 'Risk,' 'Injury,' 'Failure,' 'Loss,' and 'End-stage' (RIFLE) criteria after repair for a ruptured abdominal aortic aneurysm

van Beek SC, Legemate DA, Vahl A, et al (Univ of Amsterdam, The Netherlands; Onze Lieve Vrouwe Gasthuis, Amsterdam, The Netherlands)
J Vasc Surg 60:1159-1167, 2014

Objective.—Acute kidney injury (AKI) is a serious complication after repair of a ruptured abdominal aortic aneurysm (RAAA). In the present Society for Vascular Surgery (SVS)/International Society for CardioVascular Surgery (ISCVS) reporting standards patients are classified as no dialysis (grade I), as temporary dialysis (grade II), and as permanent dialysis or fatal outcome (grade III). However, AKI is a broad clinical syndrome including more than the requirement for renal replacement therapy. The recently introduced 'Risk,' 'Injury,' 'Failure,' 'Loss,' and 'End-stage' (RIFLE) classification for AKI comprises three severity categories based on serum creatinine and urine output ('Risk,' 'Injury,' and 'Failure'). The objective of the present study was to assess the incidence of AKI using the RIFLE criteria (AKI_{RIFLE}). Secondary objectives were to assess the incidence of AKI as defined using the SVS/ISCVS reporting standards ($AKI_{SVS/ISCVS}$) and the association between AKI_{RIFLE} and death.

Methods.—This was an observational cohort study in 362 consecutive patients with an RAAA in three hospitals in Amsterdam (The Netherlands) between 2004 and 2011. The end points were the incidence of AKIRIFLE, of $AKI_{SVS/ISCVS}$, and the combined 30-day or in-hospital death rate. A multivariable logistic regression model was made to assess the association between AKI_{RIFLE} and death after adjustment for preoperative shock profile (Glasgow Aneurysm Score) and postoperative shock profile (Acute Physiology and Chronic Health Evaluation [APACHE] II score, use of vasopressors, and fluid balance during the first 24 hours after intervention).

Results.—AKI_{RIFLE} occurred in 74% (267/362; 95% confidence interval [CI], 69%-78%), with 27% of these patients categorized as 'Risk' (71/267; 95% CI, 22%-32%), 39% categorized as 'Injury' (104/267, 95% CI, 33%-45%), and 34% categorized as 'Failure' (92/267; 95% CI, 29%-40%).

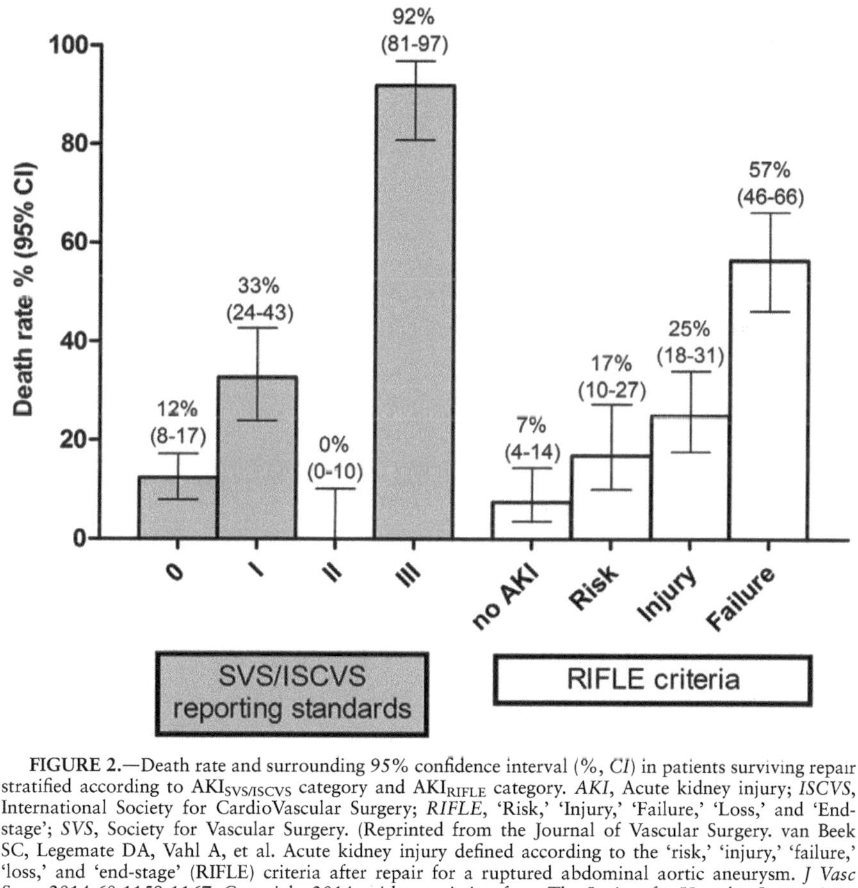

FIGURE 2.—Death rate and surrounding 95% confidence interval (%, *CI*) in patients surviving repair stratified according to $AKI_{SVS/ISCVS}$ category and AKI_{RIFLE} category. *AKI*, Acute kidney injury; *ISCVS*, International Society for CardioVascular Surgery; *RIFLE*, 'Risk,' 'Injury,' 'Failure,' 'Loss,' and 'End-stage'; *SVS*, Society for Vascular Surgery. (Reprinted from the Journal of Vascular Surgery. van Beek SC, Legemate DA, Vahl A, et al. Acute kidney injury defined according to the 'risk,' 'injury,' 'failure,' 'loss,' and 'end-stage' (RIFLE) criteria after repair for a ruptured abdominal aortic aneurysm. *J Vasc Surg*. 2014;60:1159-1167, Copyright 2014, with permission from The Society for Vascular Surgery.)

TABLE 1.—The 'Risk,' 'Injury,' 'Failure,' 'Loss,' and 'End-stage' (RIFLE) Criteria and the Society for Vascular Surgery/International Society for CardioVascular Surgery (SVS/ISCVS) Reporting Standards for Acute Kidney Injury (AKI)[5,8]

Category	RIFLE SCr Criteria[a]	RIFLE Urine Output Criteria
Risk	Increase ≥1.5 times from baseline or GFR decrease >25%	<0.5 mL/kg/h ≥6 hours
Injury	Increase ≥2 times from baseline or GFR decrease >50%	<0.5 mL/kg/h ≥12 hours
Failure	Increase ≥ 3 times from baseline or GFR decrease >75% or ≥354 µmol/L with an acute increase ≥44 µmol/L from baseline	<0.3 mL/kg/h ≥24 hours or anuria ≥12 hours
Loss	Complete loss of kidney function >4 weeks	
End-stage	Complete loss of kidney function >3 months	
	SVS/ISCVS Reporting Standards	*SVS/ISCVS Reporting Standards in the Present Study*
I	No dialysis	SCr >159 µmol/L within 7 days after admission
II	Temporary dialysis, prolonged hospitalization, permanently reduced renal function	Temporary dialysis
III	Permanent dialysis, transplant, or fatal outcome	Permanent dialysis or temporary dialysis with fatal outcome

Editor's Note: Please refer to original journal article for full references.

GFR, Glomerular filtration rate; *SCr*, serum creatinine.

For the RIFLE criteria, only one criterion (SCr or urine output) has to be fulfilled to qualify for a category. Patients are classified based on the criterion that places them in the worst category.

[a]Based on change between two SCr values within 7 days after admission.

$AKI_{SVS/ISCVS}$ occurred in 48% (175/362; 95% CI, 43%-53%), with 53% of these categorized as 'grade I' (92/175; 95% CI, 45%-60%), 19% as 'grade II' (34/175; 95% CI, 14%-26%), and 28% as 'grade III' (49/175; 95% CI, 22%-35%). After multivariable adjustment for shock profiles the risk of dying in patients categorized as AKI_{RIFLE} 'Failure' was greater than in patients without AKI_{RIFLE} (adjusted odds ratio, 6.360; 95% CI, 2.231-18.130).

Conclusions.—The incidence of AKI defined according to the RIFLE criteria (74%) was greater than defined using the SVS/ISCVS reporting standards (48%) and patients categorized as 'Failure' using the RIFLE criteria had a greater risk of dying than patients without AKI. These results indicate that the problem of AKI is much bigger than previously anticipated and that minimizing injury to the kidney could be an important focus of future research on reducing the death rate after RAAA repair (Fig 2 and Table 1).

▶ In ruptured abdominal aortic aneurysm (RAAA) studies, renal replacement therapy (dialysis) is often used as an endpoint based on Society for Vascular Surgery (SVS)/International Society for CardioVascular Surgery (ISCVS) reporting standards. However, acute kidney injury is a very broad clinical syndrome including more than the requirement for dialysis. In 2004, the Acute Dialysis Quality Initiative group introduced the Risk, Injury, Failure, Loss, End-Stage (RIFLE) criteria for acute kidney injury based on serum creatinine and urine output criteria (Table 1).[1] In daily practice, the RIFLE criteria can be used to identify high-risk patients.

One of the main purposes of this study was to see if the RIFLE criteria could be applied to a population of patients presenting with RAAA and help predict mortality risk better than current standards. A direct comparison between RIFLE criteria and the SVS/ISCVS reporting standards is inappropriate. The RIFLE criteria can be used to improve risk stratification for clinical and research purposes, and the existing reporting standards are only used to score severe complications for research purposes only. In this important study, death rate did positively correlate with the RIFLE criteria (Fig 2).

This study shows that most surgically treated RAAA patients do subsequently have acute kidney injury defined using the RIFLE criteria—more so than previously reported. The RIFLE criteria identified a large group of patients with an increased risk of dying after adjustment for shock profile. Finally, these results indicate that the problem of acute kidney injury is much larger than previously reported and could, therefore, be an important focus of future research on reducing the rate of death after RAAA.

B. W. Starnes, MD

Reference

1. Bellomo R, Ronco C, Kellum JA, Mehta RL, Palevsky P. Acute renal failure - definition, outcome measures, animal models, fluid therapy and information technology needs: the Second International Consensus Conference of the Acute Dialysis Quality Initiative (ADQI) Group. *Crit Care.* 2004;8:R204-R212.

Ambulatory percutaneous endovascular abdominal aortic aneurysm repair

Dosluoglu HH, Lall P, Blochle R, et al (Veterans Affairs Western New York Healthcare System, Buffalo; State Univ of New York at Buffalo; et al)
J Vasc Surg 59:58-64, 2014

Objective.—Percutaneous endovascular abdominal aortic aneurysm repair (PEVAR) has been associated with fewer groin wound complications and shorter operative times, but same-day discharge (SDD) has not been reported. The goal of our article is to assess the feasibility and safety of ambulatory PEVAR and identify patient characteristics that are eligible for this approach.

Methods.—Consecutive patients who underwent elective endovascular abdominal aortic aneurysm repair (EVAR) between March 2011 and December 2012 were reviewed. SDD was discussed during the preoperative visit with patients who were functionally independent, without significant comorbidities, and had favorable anatomy. These patients were given the option to be discharged in the evening of the PEVAR after 6 hours of bed rest if the procedure was uneventful. Causes for discharge delay and early outcomes were analyzed.

Results.—During the study period, 79 patients underwent abdominal aortic aneurysm (AAA) repair, 64 of whom (mean age, 70.2 ± 9.9; range, 59-97) had elective EVAR (3 ruptures, 5 acute presentations, 3 fenestrated EVARs, 4 elective open AAA repairs were excluded). Fifty-three patients (83%) had bilateral percutaneous access, seven had unilateral percutaneous (11%) access, and the remaining four (6%) had bilateral femoral endarterectomies. The percutaneous closure success rate was 96% in 113 attempts (three conversions for inadequate hemostasis, one for inability to deploy device). Mean length of stay was 1.3 ± 1.4 days (median, 1 day) with no 30-day mortality. Twenty-one patients (33%) were discharged the same day (SDD group), 24 (37%) on postoperative day (POD) 1, 16 (25%) on POD 2/3, and 3 (5%) stayed ≥4 days. One patient in the SDD group was readmitted on POD 3 after EVAR for severe postimplantation syndrome. Of the 23 patients who were discharged on POD 1, 10 were kept overnight due to severe chronic obstructive pulmonary disease, coronary artery disease, or advanced age, three transportation issues, two inability to void, two patient preference, two for renal protection, and four due to unplanned femoral cutdown. Patients in the SDD group were significantly younger (66.5 ± 5.4 years vs 72.0 ± 10.6 years; $P = .029$), had smaller AAAs (5.3 ± 0.5 cm vs 5.9 ± 1.0 cm; $P = .013$), less blood loss (115 ± 90 mL vs 232 ± 198 mL; $P = .012$), and shorter operating time (79 ± 24 minutes vs 121 ± 73 minutes; $P = .013$). There were fewer American Society of Anesthesiologists 4 patients in the SDD group (24% vs 48%; $P = .056$). The majority (81%) of patients in all groups had general anesthesia (86% vs 79% SDD vs others; $P = .523$).

Conclusions.—Ambulatory PEVAR was found to be feasible and safe in one-third of patients undergoing elective EVAR who did not have excessive medical risk, had good functional capacity, and underwent an uneventful procedure. The impact of SDD on cost-effectiveness needs to be further assessed and may not be feasible in hospitals reimbursed based on admission status.

▶ I have long been a champion for totally percutaneous endovascular abdominal aortic aneurysm repair (PEVAR) as I believe it to be safe and particularly less morbid than surgical cut-down for a majority of patients requiring endovascular abdominal aortic aneurysm repair (EVAR). Dr Dosluoglu and colleagues report their experience with same-day discharge (SDD) for a small cohort of patients undergoing PEVAR. Because device costs are somewhat fixed, decreasing intensive care and overall hospital lengths of stay and wound complications should theoretically further reduce the cost of EVAR.

During the 21-month study period, 79 patients were treated with a variety of EVAR techniques. Twenty-one patients (33%) were discharged on the same day. These patients were younger, had smaller aneurysms, less estimated blood loss, shorter operative times, and all were done using a totally percutaneous technique. The majority, 86%, had general anesthesia, and only 1 patient was readmitted on postoperative day 3 with postimplantation syndrome. All percutaneous closure failures (n = 4) were identified in the operating room, and all of these patients were kept in the hospital. Interestingly, 15 patients (23% of the entire cohort) in this series developed postimplantation syndrome manifested by fever, pain, and leukocytosis. All were managed expectantly with hydration and antipyretics, suggesting that this syndrome should not be a barrier to SDD as long as patients can be educated for signs, symptoms, and treatment strategies.

This study is essentially a validation of the PEVAR technique. One potential concern for sending patients home on the same day is life-threatening bleeding or limb ischemia after discharge. In this experience, all percutaneous failures occurred in the operating theater with no patient returning to the operating room in the early or late postoperative period.

The current study was conducted at a Veterans Administration hospital, and hospital reimbursement was not affected by a patients' ambulatory status. This is currently impossible in the private sector because it would result in a financial loss to the hospital. Until the Centers for Medicare and Medicaid Services allows coding for these devices in an outpatient setting, ambulatory PEVAR will not be feasible in private sector hospitals.

B. W. Starnes, MD

Biomechanics and gene expression in abdominal aortic aneurysm

Reeps C, Kehl S, Tanios F, et al (Technische Universität, Munich, Germany)

J Vasc Surg 60:1640-1647, 2014

Objective.—The aim of the study was to detect inter-relations between the mechanical conditions and material properties of abdominal aortic aneurysm (AAA) wall and the underlying local gene expression of destabilizing inflammatory, proteolytic, and structural factors.

Methods.—During open surgery, 51 tissue samples from 31 AAA patients were harvested. Gene expression of collagen types I and III, inflammatory factors CD45 and MSR1, proteolytic enzymes matrix metalloproteinases 2 and 9, and tissue inhibitor of matrix metalloproteinase 1 was analyzed by reverse transcription-polymerase chain reaction. Material properties of corresponding AAA tissue samples were assessed by cyclic sinusoidal and destructive testing. Local mechanical conditions of stress and strain were determined by advanced nonlinear finite element analysis based on patient-specific three-dimensional AAA models derived from preoperative computed tomography data.

Results.—In the AAA wall, all parameters analyzed were significantly expressed at the messenger RNA level. With respect to mechanical properties of the aneurysmatic wall, expression of collagen III correlated with the stiffness parameter α ($r = -0.348$; $P = .017$), and matrix metalloprotease 2 correlated with the stiffness parameter β and wall strength ($r = -0.438$ and -0.593; $P = .005$ and $P < .001$). Furthermore, significant relationships were observed between local AAA diameter and the expression of CD45, MSR1, and tissue inhibitor of matrix metalloproteinase 1 ($r = 0.285$, 0.551, 0.328; $P < .05$). However, we found no inter-relation of local calculated wall stresses and strains with gene expression.

Conclusions.—Our results show for the first time that gene expressions of destabilizing factors within AAA tissue might be correlated to geometric and mechanical properties of the AAA wall. However, we found no influence of local mechanical conditions on gene expression of these factors. Therefore, these preliminary results are still ambiguous (Supplementary Table).

▶ The impact of inflammatory and proteolytic processes on the strength and constitutive properties of the abdominal aortic aneurysm (AAA) wall have never been supported by mechanical testing of AAA tissue samples. Furthermore, mechanical quantities such as wall stresses and strains and their influence on the expression of inflammatory or proteolytic processes in the aneurysm wall have never been investigated. From what I can gather in this study, computed tomography (CT) data sets were used to obtain 3-dimensional reconstructions of AAA geometries including intraluminal thrombus with commercial segmentation software. Images of these reconstructions (51 human subjects) were used during surgery to indicate the exact sample excision site by the surgeon. The most important results of this study were the interdependencies between mechanical conditions, AAA geometry, gene expression, and material properties of the aneurysm wall (Supplementary Table).

What is most interesting about all of this is that the methodology has been described fusing CT data sets with actual tissue stress and strain analysis and local gene expression and inflammatory mediator production within the aortic

SUPPLEMENTARY TABLE.—Selected Examples of Corresponding Biomechanical Parameters, Histologic Features, and Expression Analysis

	Age, Years	Thrombus, mm	Max AAA Diameter, mm	Biomechanical Parameters: Radius (Mechanics), mm	von Mises Strain, kPa	von Mises Stress, kpa	Max Tension, N/mm	Strength, N/mm²	α, N/mm²	β, N/mm²	Biomechanical Parameters: Wall Thickness, mm	Histology[a]: Infiltrates	Neovascularization	Expression Analysis[b]: CD45	MSR1	TIMP-1	ColI A2	ColIII A1	MMP-2	MMP-9
Sample 1	69	6.95	61.0	25.15	0.152	175.6	1.247	0.594	0.094	1.84	2.10	+++	++/+++	4.58	0.45	4.69	1.51	1.60	0.93	0.51
Sample 2	69	1.64	56.5	16.46	0.174	241.2	1.703	1.064	0.073	1.97	1.60	++	++	2.96	0.16	1.45	1.06	1.43	1.05	0.08
Sample 3	50	0.00	73.0	34.89	0.221	315.4	0.717	0.360	0.069	1.14	1.99	+++	++/+++	5.12	0.21	3.75	1.40	1.07	1.23	1.74
Sample 4	69	19.95	56.5	26.22	0.109	94.7	1.306	0.637	0.048	1.38	2.05	++/+++	++	1.02	0.43	1.04	0.41	0.93	0.95	0.09
Sample 5	62	13.95	52.5	25.75	0.131	123.6	1.582	0.676	0.170	3.49	2.34	+/++	+/++	17.78	0.98	0.93	1.10	0.00	0.56	0.92
Sample 6	59	2.99	59.0	25.27	0.177	220.4	2.278	0.945	0.212	8.87	2.41	+++	++/+++	2.89	0.19	1.80	0.21	0.12	0.26	0.32
Sample 7	64	6.25	56.0	25.51	0.161	177.1	1.803	1.244	0.129	5.44	1.45	+++	++/+++	20.25	0.71	0.84	0.57	0.60	0.62	3.68
Sample 8	80	17.10	67.5	32.96	0.112	101.6	2.613	0.860	0.069	2.49	2.84	++	+	6.83	0.43	0.63	0.26	0.15	0.58	0.52
Sample 9	79	22.77	51.5	24.48	0.106	91.4	2.046	2.181	0.114	15.41	1.34	+/++	+/−	7.91	0.14	0.42	0.25	0.16	0.13	0.14
Sample 10	75	0.00	63.0	20.48	0.206	280.7	1.573	0.837	0.030	3.28	1.88	++/+++	+/++	0.98	0.09	0.51	0.19	0.18	0.12	0.10

AAA, Abdominal aortic aneurysm; *Col*, collagen; *MMP*, matrix metalloproteinase; *TIMP-1*, tissue inhibitor of matrix metalloproteinase 1.

[a]Semiquantitative grading: −, no inflammatory cells, no neovessels; +, few scattered inflammatory cells or a minority of neovessels; ++, moderate amount of inflammatory cells or neovessels; +++, strong appearance of inflammatory cells, frequently in clusters, and high number of neovessels.

[b]Expression analysis at mRNA level by reverse transcription–polymerase chain reaction from formalin-fixed tissue samples adjacent to the histologic specimens. All values show relative expression of the individual factors related to the expression of glyceraldehyde 3-phosphate dehydrogenase (eg, 4.58 means a 4.58-fold higher expression than that of glyceraldehyde 3-phosphate dehydrogenase).

wall. Future research directed at symptomatic or ruptured aneurysms may provide novel imaging targets to potentially help us predict rupture.

B. W. Starnes, MD

Castration of male mice prevents the progression of established angiotensin II-induced abdominal aortic aneurysms

Zhang X, Thatcher S, Wu C, et al (Univ of Kentucky, Lexington)

J Vasc Surg 61:767-776, 2015

Objective.—Male sex is a nonmodifiable risk factor for abdominal aortic aneurysm (AAA) development. Similar to humans, male mice are more susceptible to angiotensin II (AngII)-induced AAAs than female mice. Previous studies demonstrated that castration of males markedly reduced the formation of AngII-induced AAAs. Progression of AAA size is associated with increased risk of aneurysm rupture. In this study, we hypothesized that castration of male mice would reduce the progression of established AngII-induced AAAs.

Methods.—Male apolipoprotein E-deficient mice were infused with AngII for 1 month to induce AAA formation. Aortic diameters were measured by ultrasound imaging, and mice were stratified into two groups that underwent a sham operation or castration. AngII infusions were continued for a further 2 months. Ultrasound imaging was used to quantify lumen diameters, and excised aortas were processed for quantification of AAA size, volume, and tissue characteristics.

Results.—Sham-operated mice exhibited progressive dilation of suprarenal aortic lumen diameters during the continued AngII infusion. Aortic lumen diameters were significantly decreased in castrated mice (n = 17) compared with sham-operated mice (n = 15) at study end point (1.63 ± 0.04 vs 1.88 ± 0.05 mm; $P < .05$). However, maximal external AAA diameters were not significantly different between sham-operated and castrated mice. The vascular volume/lumen volume ratio of excised AAAs imaged by ultrasound was significantly increased by castration (9.5% ± 2.0%) vs sham operation (4.8% ± 0.9%; n = 11 per group; $P < .05$). Moreover, compared with the thin-walled AAAs of sham-operated mice, aneurysm sections from castrated mice exhibited increased smooth muscle α-actin and collagen.

Conclusions.—Removal of endogenous male hormones by castration selectively reduces aortic lumen expansion while not altering the external AAA dimensions.

Clinical Relevance.—There are no therapeutics that slow the progression of abdominal aortic aneurysms (AAAs), and as the size of an AAA increases, so does the risk of rupture and death. Male sex is a nonmodifiable risk factor for AAA development, but whether male sex hormones have a similar effect on AAA progression is unclear. Removal of male sex hormones in an established mouse model of angiotensin II-induced AAAs resulted in reduced progressive lumen dilation while not altering

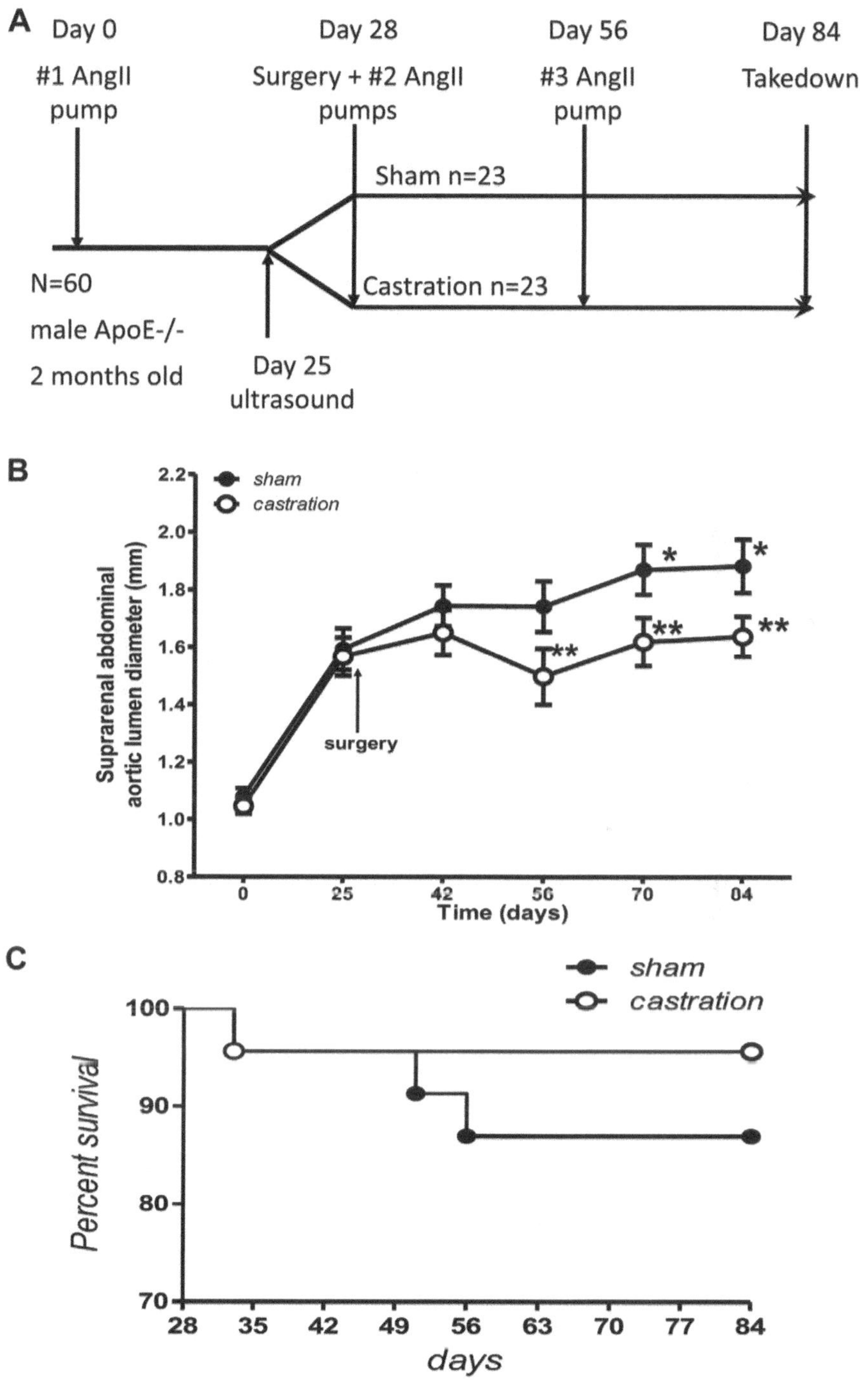

FIGURE 1.—Castration reduces abdominal aortic lumen dilation in angiotensin II (*AngII*)-infused mice. **A**, Experimental design for quantifying effects of castration on the progression of established AngII-induced abdominal aortic aneurysms (AAAs). **B**, Suprarenal aorta lumen dilation at various time points after AngII infusion in sham-operated (n = 20) and castrated (n = 22) mice. The *arrow* indicates sham-operation or castration surgery. **C**, Percentage survival of mice is shown in each group from day 28 to day 84 of AngII infusion. The *error bars* show the standard error of the mean. *ApoE*$^{-/-}$, apolipoprotein E-deficient. *$P < .05$ compared with day 28 of AngII infusion; **$P < .05$ compared with sham. (Reprinted from the Journal of Vascular Surgery. Zhang X, Thatcher S, Wu C, et al. Castration of male mice prevents the progression of established angiotensin II-induced abdominal aortic aneurysms. *J Vasc Surg*. 2015;61:767-776, Copyright 2014, with permission from The Society for Vascular Surgery.)

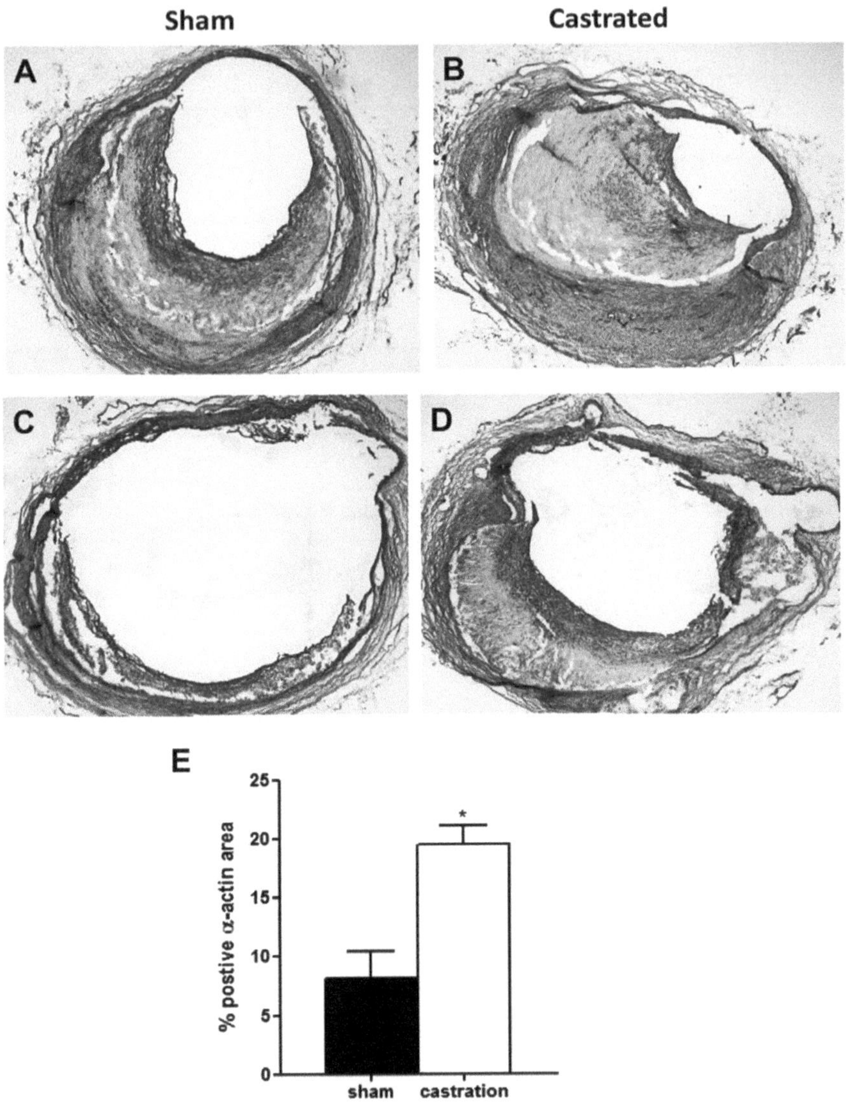

FIGURE 4.—Abdominal aortic aneurysm (AAA) sections from castrated mice have increased smooth muscle α-actin immunostaining. AAA sections from (**A** and **B**) the proximal to (**C** and **D**) the distal end of AAA tissue sections from (**A** and **C**) sham-operated and (**B** and **D**) castrated mice were immunostained for smooth muscle α-actin. E, Quantification of α-actin immunostaining in AAA sections from each group exhibiting the largest luminal dilation. Data are mean ± standard error of the mean (*error bars*) from six AAAs per group. *$P < .05$ compared with sham. (Reprinted from the Journal of Vascular Surgery. Zhang X, Thatcher S, Wu C, et al. Castration of male mice prevents the progression of established angiotensin II-induced abdominal aortic aneurysms. *J Vasc Surg*. 2015;61:767-776, Copyright 2014, with permission from The Society for Vascular Surgery.)

external AAA dimensions. Therapies that limit androgen action may provide benefit against AAA progression. Alternatively, supplemental testosterone may be contraindicated in men diagnosed with an AAA (Figs 1 and 4).

▶ One cannot go a single day in the year 2015 without hearing or seeing at least 1 advertisement on the news or on talk radio related to male sexual performance. Phrases such as "low T" and "ED" (erectile dysfunction) are repeated casually while our families sit to watch the evening news. Viagra, Cialis, men's health centers and clinics—all with the seemingly singular intent of preserving "maleness" for as long as humanly possible and making a lot of money along the way. Well, here may be a valid reason for us to dissuade our male patients harboring aortic aneurysms from this sort of behavior.

Several studies have demonstrated that male sex is one of the strongest nonmodifiable risk factors for human abdominal aortic aneurysm (AAAs).[1-3] The results of this mouse study demonstrate that male sex hormones markedly influence vascular wall remodeling and the progression of AAAs (Fig 1). In addition, castration of male mice prevented progressive lumen dilation of established angiotensin II–induced AAAs in male mice. AAAs from castrated mice exhibited smaller lumen diameters with thickened vascular walls with more pronounced smooth muscle alpha actin and collagen immunostaining (Fig 4).

While castration seems a little excessive for the male patient with an AAA, avoidance of testosterone therapies may be prudent!

B. W. Starnes, MD

References

1. Lederle FA, Johnson GR, Wilson SE. Abdominal aortic aneurysm in women. *J Vasc Surg*. 2001;34:122-126.
2. Best VA, Price JF, Fowkes FG. Persistent increase in the incidence of abdominal aortic aneurysm in Scotland, 1981–2000. *Br J Surg*. 2003;90:1510-1515.
3. Acosta S, Ogren M, Bengtsson H, Bergqvist D, Lindblad B, Zdanowski Z. Increasing incidence of ruptured abdominal aortic aneurysm: a population-based study. *J Vasc Surg*. 2006;44:237-243.

Comparative safety of endovascular and open surgical repair of abdominal aortic aneurysms in low-risk male patients

Siracuse JJ, Gill HL, Graham AR, et al (Weill Cornell Med College, NY)
J Vasc Surg 60:1154-1158, 2014

Objective.—The prevalence of significant comorbidities among patients with abdominal aortic aneurysms (AAAs) has contributed to widespread enthusiasm for endovascular AAA repair (EVAR). However, the advantages of EVAR in patients at low risk for open surgical repair (OSR) remain unclear. The objective of this study was to assess perioperative outcomes of EVAR and OSR in low-risk patients.

Methods.—Patients undergoing EVAR and OSR for infrarenal AAAs were identified in the 2007 to 2010 National Surgical Quality Improvement Program data sets. AAA-specific risk stratification, by the Medicare aneurysm scoring system, was used to create matched low-risk (score <3) cohorts. Perioperative morbidity and mortality were assessed by crude comparisons of matched groups and regression models.

Results.—Of 11,753 elective patients undergoing EVAR, 4339 (37%) were deemed low risk (score <3). A matched cohort of 1576 low-risk patients was developed from a total of 3804 (41%) undergoing OSR. The low-risk cohorts included only male patients and those <75 years of age, without significant cardiac, pulmonary, or vascular comorbidities. Mean age in both low-risk groups was 67 ± 6 years ($P = NS$). EVAR patients had higher rates of obesity (40% vs 33%; $P < .001$), diabetes (16% vs 13%; $P = .005$), history of cardiac intervention (24% vs 19%; $P < .001$), cardiac surgery (23% vs 20%; $P = .02$), steroid use (4% vs 2%; $P = .002$), and bleeding disorders/anticoagulation (9% vs 6%; $P = .001$) compared with OSR patients. There were no other differences between the matched cohorts. EVAR was associated with reduced 30-day mortality (0.5% vs 1.5%; $P < .01$) and reduced rates of major complications, including the following: sepsis (0.7% vs 3.2%; $P < .01$), unplanned intubation (1.0 vs 5.4%; $P < .001$), pneumonia (0.8% vs 6.1%; $P < .001$), acute renal failure (0.4% vs 2.7%; $P < .001$), and early reoperation (3.7% vs 6.0%; $P < .001$). Furthermore, EVAR was associated with reduced perioperative morbidity across organ systems, including venous thromboembolism (0.1% vs 0.3%; $P = .001$), transfusion requirement of more than 4 units (2.0% vs 13.0%; $P < .001$), cardiac arrest (0.2 vs 0.8; $P = .001$), neurologic deficits (0.2% vs 0.5%; $P = .032$), and urinary tract infections (1.2% vs 2%; $P = .02$).

Conclusions.—Our results demonstrate that even among those male patients at low risk for OSR on the basis of comorbidities, EVAR is associated with reduced perioperative mortality and major complications. Whereas clinical decisions must account for safety and long-term effectiveness, the short-term benefit of EVAR is evident even among male patients at the lowest risk for OSR (Tables 1 and 3).

▶ Vascular specialists continue to debate the appropriateness of endovascular aneurysm repair (EVAR) in patients who are suitable candidates for open surgical repair who could be expected to tolerate open repair. In fact, low-risk patients may be preferentially offered open repair, particularly if surgeons believe the favorable durability of open repair overshadows any short-term benefit of EVAR in patients at low risk for postoperative complications. Using the American College of Surgeons National Surgical Quality Improvement Program database between 2007 and 2010, the authors identified 15 557 patients undergoing elective repair (11 753 EVAR and 3804 open). Abdominal aortic aneurysm-specific risk stratification, by the Medicare aneurysm scoring system, was used to create matched low-risk cohorts (Table 1). In this scoring system, a score of 3 or less is considered low risk. Interestingly, female sex in the model is

TABLE 1.—Medicare Aneurysm Scoring System[10]

Risk Factor	Score
Age >80 years	11
Age 76-80 years	6
Age 71-75 years	1
Female	4
ESRD	9
CRI, no dialysis	7
CHF	6
PVD or CBVD	3

CBVD, Cerebrovascular disease; *CHF*, congestive heart failure; *CRI*, chronic renal insufficiency; *ESRD*, end-stage renal disease; *PVD*, peripheral vascular disease.

High risk, >11; moderate risk, 3-11; low risk, <3.

Editor's Note: Please refer to original journal article for full references.

TABLE 3.—Systemic Complications

Complications	Total, No. (%)	EVAR, No. (%)	OSR, No. (%)	*P* Value
Total	5527	4068	1459	N/A
Mortality, 30-day	46 (0.8)	24 (0.5)	22 (1.5)	.001
Return to the OR within 30 days	239 (4.3)	151 (3.7)	88 (6.0)	<.001
Deep venous thrombosis	30 (0.5)	14 (0.3)	16 (1.1)	.001
Graft complications	35 (0.6)	29 (0.7)	6 (0.4)	.21
Postoperative blood transfusion	28 (0.5)	8 (0.2)	20 (1.4)	<.001
Myocardial infarction	39 (0.7)	18 (0.4)	21 (1.4)	<.001
Cardiac arrest	20 (0.4)	8 (0.2)	12 (0.8)	<.001
Neurologic deficit	16 (0.3)	8 (0.2)	8 (0.5)	.032
Stroke	8 (0.1)	5 (0.1)	3 (0.2)	.48
Acute renal failure	54 (1.0)	15 (0.4)	39 (2.7)	<.001
Postoperative intubation >48 hours	130 (2.4)	26 (0.6)	104 (7.1)	<.001
Pulmonary embolism	16 (0.3)	10 (0.2)	6 (0.4)	.31
Unplanned reintubation	120 (2.2)	41 (0.1)	79 (5.4)	<.001

EVAR, Endovascular aneurysm repair; *N/A*, not applicable; *OR*, operating room; *OSR*, open surgical repair.

assigned a score of 4, no female patients are considered low risk; therefore, this analysis only included male patients.

Of the patients treated during the study period, 4339 patients (37%) undergoing EVAR were low risk, whereas 1576 patients (41%) undergoing open repair were low risk. Once matched, EVAR was associated with a strikingly lower 30-day mortality rate (0.5% vs 1.5%; $P < .01$) compared with open repair. Moreover, EVAR was associated with reduced perioperative morbidity across all organ systems (Table 3). This finding reaffirms the superior short-term outcomes of EVAR. This finding should be useful for all vascular specialists counseling low-risk patients when considering the risk of death perioperatively is 3 times higher in those undergoing open repair!

B. W. Starnes, MD

Custom fenestration templates for endovascular repair of juxtarenal aortic aneurysms

Leotta DF, Starnes BW (Univ of Washington, Seattle)
J Vasc Surg 61:1637-1641, 2015

Physician-modified endovascular grafts, with fenestrations added to accommodate major branch vessels, provide a means for endovascular treatment of abdominal aortic aneurysms that are adjacent to the renal arteries. Manual measurements of vessel origin locations from computed tomography images, however, take time and can lead to errors in the positions of the fenestrations. To make the fenestration process faster and more accurate, we have developed a procedure to create custom templates that serve as patient-specific guides for graft fenestration. We use a three-dimensional printer to create a clear rigid sleeve that replicates the patient's aorta and includes holes placed precisely at the locations of the branch vessels. The sleeve is slipped over the graft, the locations of the openings are marked with a pen, and the fenestrations are created after the sleeve is removed. Custom fenestration templates can potentially

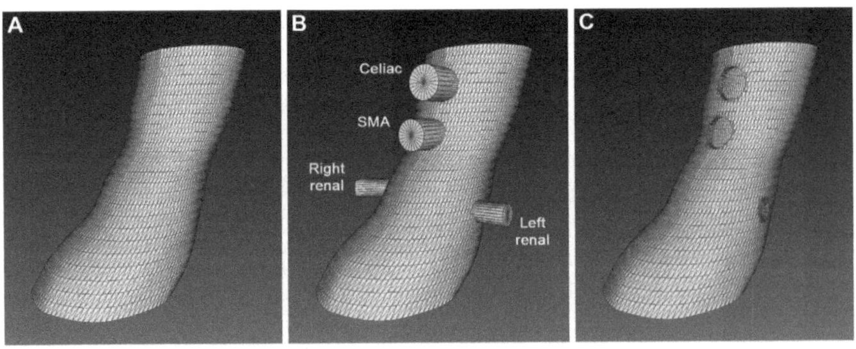

FIGURE 2.—Fenestration template computer-assisted design model. The lumen contours shown in Fig 1 were converted to a solid model format compatible with a three-dimensional (3D) printer. **A,** Polygon model of the aneurysm proximal neck. **B,** Combined display of the proximal neck model and cylinders at each of the branch vessel origins. The cylinder diameters are set to match the branch vessel opening diameters as measured from the original computed tomography (CT) images. SMA, Superior mesenteric artery. **C,** The result of the Boolean difference between the proximal neck object and each cylinder is a hole in the aorta model at the location of each of the branch vessel origins. (Reprinted from the Journal of Vascular Surgery. Leotta DF, Starnes BW. Custom fenestration templates for endovascular repair of juxtarenal aortic aneurysms. *J Vasc Surg*. 2015;61:1637-1641, Copyright 2014, with permission from The Society for Vascular Surgery.)

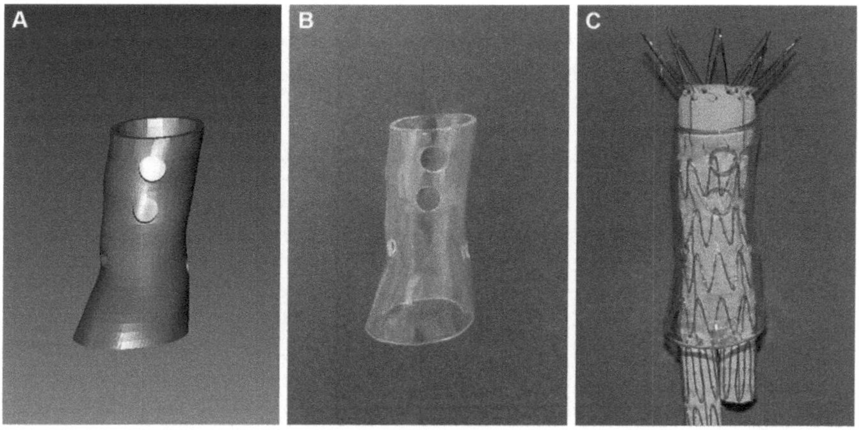

FIGURE 3.—Three-dimensional (3D)-printed fenestration template. **A,** Computer model of the template. **B,** Solid printed model of the template created using a stereolithography 3D printer with clear resin. **C,** An endovascular graft inserted in the template. (Reprinted from the Journal of Vascular Surgery. Leotta DF, Starnes BW. Custom fenestration templates for endovascular repair of juxtarenal aortic aneurysms. *J Vasc Surg*. 2015;61:1637-1641, Copyright 2014, with permission from The Society for Vascular Surgery.)

save procedural costs and make minimally invasive aortic aneurysm repair available to more patients (Figs 2 and 3).

► There is certainly a conflict of interest here, but I believe that this report has an important impact in breaking down the barriers to wide adoption of fenestrated endovascular techniques for repair of all intact abdominal aortic aneurysms. The primary barrier is the expertise in and time required for planning. The actual procedure, in my mind, is very easy. This publication is the first to describe use of CT data sets to physically print the subject's perivisceral aorta to perfectly localize target vessel fenestrations prior to implantation (Figs 2 and 3). This is true customization of any graft to fit the patient.

Imagine a day in the future when a patient is being transferred from an outside hospital with a ruptured aortic aneurysm. You look at the CT and find that there is a short neck for endovascular aneurysm repair. A 3-dimensional (3-D) template is easily and rapidly printed using customized software, sterilized, and then used to guide on-table customization of the stent graft. By the time the patient arrives, they have a graft that has been customized to fit their anatomy with 4 to 5 cm of healthy aortic seal. That day will come. It could happen today with current 3-D printing technology that is 100 times faster than standard 3-D printers. Eventually, the day will come when many if not all implanted medical devices are customized and 3-D printed to fit the patient.

B. W. Starnes, MD

Debate: Whether evidence supports reducing the threshold diameter to 5 cm for elective interventions in women with abdominal aortic aneurysms

Vavra AK, Kibbe MR, Bown MJ, et al (Northwestern Univ, Chicago, IL; Univ of Leicester, UK; Imperial College London, UK)

J Vasc Surg 60:1695-1701, 2014

Current practice guidelines recommend repair of asymptomatic abdominal aortic aneurysms once they reach the 5.5-cm-diameter threshold and are based on information from randomized controlled trials. However, because aneurysms are more common in men, women are underrepresented in these trials, and questions persist about whether this repair threshold should apply to them. In addition, women have smaller aortas to begin with and in most aneurysm cohorts are older, have more atherosclerotic risk factors, are less likely to be anatomic candidates for endovascular repair, and do poorer after emergency or elective repair of their aneurysm. These are just some of the issues that our discussants address in determining whether the repair threshold should be at a smaller diameter for women (Fig 2).

▶ The topic of this Trans-Atlantic Debate could not be more timely. With the lowest mortality risk for elective aneurysm repair in decades, the idea of fixing smaller aneurysms earlier, especially in women, is resurfacing. Two well-

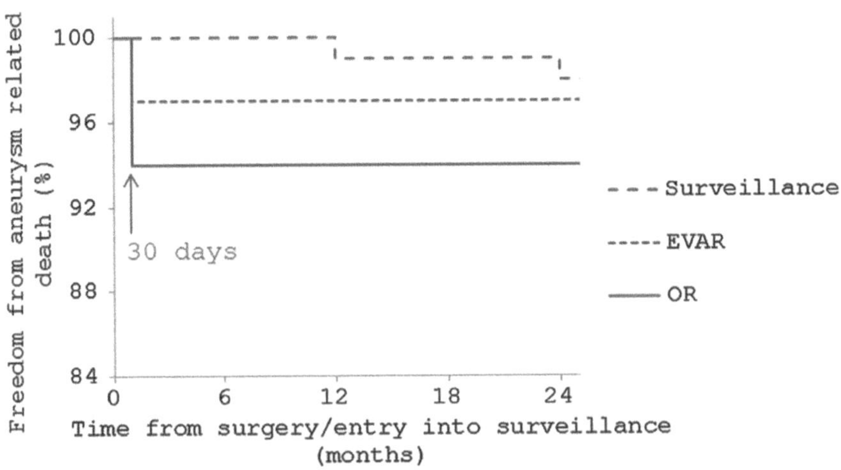

FIGURE 2.—Best evidence available statistical simulation of short-term and medium-term outcomes for aneurysm-related mortality or rupture in women with a small (5.0-cm) abdominal aortic aneurysm (AAA) based on best available evidence. Errors of estimates are not shown, and aneurysm-related postoperative events and mortality are not included in endovascular aneurysm repair (*EVAR*) or open repair (*OR*) models due to lack of data. (Reprinted from the Journal of Vascular Surgery. Vavra AK, Kibbe MR, Bown MJ, et al. Debate: whether evidence supports reducing the threshold diameter to 5 cm for elective interventions in women with abdominal aortic aneurysms. *J Vasc Surg*. 2014;60:1695-1701, Copyright 2014, with permission from The Society for Vascular Surgery.)

respected groups make their arguments in favor or against repair of smaller aortic aneurysms in women.

The maximum diameter of any aortic aneurysm has consistently been shown to be the most predictive measure of rupture risk. That said, both groups of debaters clearly acknowledge that women rupture at smaller diameters and experience worse outcomes and higher mortality than men when presenting with rupture.[1-5] With 1 figure, I respectfully hand the debate to the Brits. Fig 2 depicts the best available evidence and simulation of aneurysm-related death in women over the midterm. All of the risk for both endovascular aneurysm repair and open repair occurs within the first 30 days and then flattens out. Surveillance eventually catches up but not for at least 2 years. In the end, all factors must be considered before offering elective repair to a woman with a smaller aneurysm. Both strategies, early repair and surveillance, have strong arguments behind them.

B. W. Starnes, MD

References

1. United Kingdom Small Aneurysm Trial Participants. Long-term outcomes of immediate repair compared with surveillance of small abdominal aortic aneurysms. *N Engl J Med.* 2002;346:1445-1452.
2. Mortality results for randomised controlled trial of early elective surgery or ultrasonographic surveillance for small abdominal aortic aneurysms. The UK Small Aneurysm Trial Participants. *Lancet.* 1998;352:1649-1655.
3. Lederle FA, Wilson SE, Johnson GR, et al. Immediate repair compared with surveillance of small abdominal aortic aneurysms. *N Engl J Med.* 2002;346:1437-1444.
4. Ouriel K, Clair DG, Kent KC, Zarins CK; Positive Impact Of Endovascular Options For Treating Aneurysms Early (PIVOTAL) Investigators. Endovascular repair compared with surveillance for patients with small abdominal aortic aneurysms. *J Vasc Surg.* 2010;51:1081-1087.
5. Cao P; Caesar Trial Collaborators. Comparison of surveillance vs aortic endografting for small aneurysm repair (CAESAR) trial: study design and progress. *Eur J Vasc Endovasc Surg.* 2005;30:245-251.

Durability and survival are similar after elective endovascular and open repair of abdominal aortic aneurysms in younger patients

Lee K, Tang E, Dubois L, et al (Univ of Western Ontario, London, Canada)
J Vasc Surg 61:636-641, 2015

Objective.—The role of endovascular repair (EVAR) of aortic aneurysms in young patients is controversial. The purpose of this study was to determine the long-term outcomes and reintervention rates in patients 60 years of age or younger who underwent elective open or endovascular repair of an abdominal aortic aneurysm.

Methods.—Retrospective review of a prospectively collected vascular surgery database at a university-affiliated medical center was performed to identify all patients who underwent elective repair of an abdominal aortic aneurysm between 2000 and 2013 and were 60 years of age or younger at the time of the repair. Preoperative anatomic measurements were performed and compared with instructions for use (IFU) criteria for the endografts.

Results.—The study cohort comprised 169 patients 60 years of age or younger (mean age, 56.7 ± 2.8 years) who underwent elective repair (119 open repair, 50 EVAR). Patients treated with open repair and EVAR had similar comorbidities, except that EVAR patients were more likely to have hypertension ($P = .03$) and poor left ventricular function ($P = .04$). The open repair group had significantly larger suprarenal ($P = .004$) and infrarenal ($P = .005$) neck angles, shorter neck lengths ($P < .001$), and larger maximum aneurysm diameter ($P = .02$) compared with the EVAR group. Only five patients (13%) in the EVAR group did not meet all IFU criteria. The overall in-hospital mortality rate was 1.8% (0% EVAR, 2.5% open repair; $P = .56$). Overall mean life expectancy was 11.5 years (9.8 years EVAR, 11.9 years open repair; $P = .09$). The 1-year (98% EVAR, 96% open repair), 5-year (86% EVAR, 88% open repair), and 10-year (54% EVAR, 75% open repair) survival did not differ between EVAR and open repair ($P = .16$). Long-term survival (78% EVAR, 85% open repair; $P = .09$) and reintervention rates (12% EVAR, 16% open repair; $P = .80$) did not differ. No late aneurysm rupture or aneurysm-related deaths were observed. The most common causes of long-term mortality were malignant disease and cardiovascular events. Reinterventions in the open repair group were exclusively laparotomy related (incisional hernia repairs), whereas all reinterventions in the EVAR group were aortic related, including one conversion to open repair.

Conclusions.—After elective aneurysm repair, younger patients have a moderate life expectancy related to malignant disease and cardiovascular health. EVAR offers durability and long-term survival similar to those with open repair in these younger patients as long as aneurysm anatomy and IFU are adhered to.

▶ This is an important study and resonates the point of one of the earlier reports I reviewed this year from Siracuse et al.[1] Since the beginning of the endovascular era, the holdouts have long questioned the management of "young patients" with aortic aneurysms decrying that open repair was more durable and long lasting and should be the preferred method in this cohort of patients. We must remember that most of these young patients harboring aortic aneurysms are anything but healthy. They typically have a longstanding history of smoking and other cardiovascular risk factors. In my mind, the fact that they developed an aortic aneurysm at such a young age speaks to the accelerated aspect of the disease in this patient population!

This report is another single-institution series reporting an important message. Twenty-five percent to 50% of these young patients are dead within 10 years regardless of the method of treatment of their aortic aneurysm and usually because of cancer or cardiovascular disease. These authors looked at 169 patients younger than 60 years who underwent either endovascular repair (EVAR; $n = 50$) or open repair ($n = 119$). In-hospital mortality was zero for

EVAR and 2.5% for open repair (*P* value, not significant because of small sample size). The 1-, 5-, and 10-year survival did not differ between groups.

The findings of this retrospective study show that patients 60 years of age or younger do equally well after elective EVAR or open repair, with similar chances of survival during the perioperative period. These young aneurysm patients have a moderate life expectancy primarily related to malignant disease and cardiovascular events but similar chances of long-term survival regardless of the method of initial repair. The message is again: EVAR should be the method of repair in anatomically suitable young patients, with similar outcomes expected at 5 and 10 years compared with open repair.

B. W. Starnes, MD

Reference

1. Siracuse J, Gill H, Graham A, et al. Comparative safety of endovascular and open repair of abdominal aortic aneurysms in low risk male patients. *J Vasc Surg*. 2014; 60:1154-1158.

Early and delayed rupture after endovascular abdominal aortic aneurysm repair in a 10-year multicenter registry

Candell L, Tucker L-Y, Goodney P, et al (Univ of California, San Francisco, Oakland; Kaiser Permanente, Oakland, CA; Dartmouth-Hitchcock Med Ctr, Lebanon, NH; et al)

J Vasc Surg 60:1146-1153, 2014

Objective.—Rupture after abdominal endovascular aortic aneurysm repair (EVAR) is a function of graft maintenance of the seal and fixation. We describe our 10-year experience with rupture after EVAR.

Methods.—From 2000 to 2010, 1736 patients with abdominal aortic aneurysm (AAA) from 17 medical centers underwent EVAR in a large, regional integrated health care system. Preoperative demographic and clinical data of interest were collected and stored in our registry. We retrospectively identified patients with postoperative rupture, characterized as "early" and "delayed" rupture (≤30 days and >30 days after the initial EVAR, respectively), and identified predictors associated with delayed rupture.

Results.—The overall follow-up rate was 92%, and the median follow-up was 2.7 years (interquartile range, 1.2-4.4 years) in these 1736 EVAR patients. We identified 20 patients with ruptures; 70% were male, the mean age was 79 years, and mean AAA size at the initial EVAR was 6.3 cm. Six patients underwent initial EVAR for rupture (n = 2) or symptomatic presentation (n = 4). Of the 20 post-EVAR ruptures, 25% (five of 20) were early, all occurring within 2 days after the initial EVAR. Of these five patients, four had intraoperative adverse events leading directly to rupture, with one type I and one type III endoleak. Of the five early ruptures, four patients underwent endovascular repair and one received repair with open surgery, resulting in two perioperative deaths. Among the remaining 15 patients, the median time from initial EVAR to rupture was 31.1 months (interquartile range, 13.8-57.3 months). Most of these delayed ruptures (10 of 15) were preceded by AAA sac increases, including three patients with known endoleaks who underwent reintervention. At the time of delayed rupture, nine of 15 patients had new endoleaks. Among all 20 patients, six patients did not undergo repair (all delayed patients) and died, nine underwent repeated EVAR, and five had open repair. For patients who underwent repair for delayed rupture, mortality at 30 days and 1 year were 44.4% and 66.7%, respectively. Multivariable Cox regression analysis identified age 80 to 89 (hazard ratio, 3.3; 95% confidence interval, 1.1-9.4; $P = .03$), and symptomatic or ruptured initial indication for EVAR (hazard ratio, 7.4; 95% confidence interval, 2.2-24.8; $P < .01$) as significant predictors of delayed rupture.

Conclusions.—Rupture after EVAR is a rare but devastating event, and mortality after repair exceeds 60% at 1 year. Most delayed cases showed late AAA expansion, thereby implicating late loss of seal and increased endoleaks as the cause of rupture in these patients and mandating vigilant surveillance (Table 4).

▶ I had the opportunity of serving as the primary discussant for this article when it was presented at the Western Vascular Society meeting in 2013. As I read this article and my discussion, I thought it was worthy of reprinting here. Highlighted are some of the major weaknesses of large registry datasets:

Dr Benjamin Starnes (Seattle, Washington)

Good morning. So here we are together again, in Jasper, Alberta. Thanks to the society for allowing me to discuss this paper. Congratulations to Dr Candell on a nice presentation. I had several initial impressions when reading this manuscript. Much like some of the work from the Vascular Study Group of New England, and actually with a co-author from a member of the VSGNE, we have yet another example of a large Integrated Regional Health Care System collecting their experience to provide a large number of patients and present information that would potentially help guide therapy. Unfortunately, I don't feel as if this study really adds much to what we already know there were 1736 patients treated with endovascular aortic aneurysm repair (EVAR) over a 10-year period at 17 Kaiser sites. When you do the math, that is 10 EVARs per year per site—a modest experience at best. Delayed rupture occurred in only 20 patients, with six of those patients being treated for rupture or symptoms to begin with. That left only 15 patients with delayed rupture after 30 days for an incidence of 0.8%. So, we know that this is indeed a rare event! We also see that patients who experienced delayed rupture were old and the majority of their sacs increased in size over time, leading to multiple reinterventions. The authors sought to define what factors, if any, contributed to this rare event. Sadly, no data on device, instructions for use (IFU) adherence, oversizing, or anatomical suitability features were collected All we can gather from this data set is that old age and rupture at presentation were associated with increased risk of delayed rupture. We already knew that!

TABLE 4.—Demographic and Clinical Characteristics and Mortality in Patients With Delayed Aneurysm Ruptures After Surgery

Patient No.	EVAR Time Periods[a]	EVAR Device[a]	Time Until Rupture, Months[b]	Time From Last Study to Rupture, Months	Aneurysm Size Expansion[b]	Previous Endoleak	Previous Reintervention	Endoleak Type[c]	Repair Type[c]	Reintervention Successful	Mortality at End of Follow-up
6	2000-2005	Medtronic	31.1	4.1	No	None	No	None	EV	N/A	Died within 30 days
7	2006-2010	Gore	2.9	2.5	No	I or II	Yes	I and II	None	No	Died within 30 days
8	2000-2005	Medtronic	86.5	20.4	Yes	None	No	I and III[c]	EV	N/A	Died within 1 year
9	2000-2005	Medtronic	87.0	1.3	No	None	No	III	EVN/ AAlive		
10	2000-2005	Zenith	18.2	2.1	Yes	II	Yes	I and II	OR	No	Died within 30 days
11	2006-2010	Medtronic	49.1	5.9	Yes	None	No	I[b]	EV	N/A	Alive
12	2006-2010	Gore	20.3	8.0	No	None	No	I	None	N/A	Died within 30 days
13	2000-2005	Zenith	57.3	9.7	Yes	None	No	I	None	N/A	Died within 1 year
14	2006-2010	Zenith	30.7	0.1	Yes	II	Yes	II and III	OR	No	Died within 1 year
15	2000-2005	Zenith	13.8	3.5	No	None	No	I	None	N/A	Died within 30 days
16	2000-2005	Medtronic	60.4	4.1	Yes	None	No	N/A	None	N/A	Died within 30 days
17	2000-2005	Medtronic	39.7	4.5	Yes	None	No	I	EV	N/A	Alive
18	2006-2010	Zenith	2.4	0.6	Yes	None	No	N/A	None	N/A	Died within 30 days
19	2000-2005	Zenith	6.9	1.4	Yes	None	No	III	OR	N/A	Died within 30 days
20	2000-2005	Medtronic	42.6	20.7	Yes	None	No	I[b]	OR	N/A	Died within 30 days

AAA, Abdominal aortic aneurysm; *EV*, endovascular; *EVAR*, endovascular aortic aneurysm repair; *N/A*, not applicable; OR, open repair.
Most EVARs (93.2%) in the entire cohort were performed with Cook Zenith (48.4%; Cook Inc, Bloomington, Ind), Medtronic Aneurx (19.5%; Medtronic Vascular, Santa Rosa, Calif), or low-permeability Gore Excluder (25.2%; W. L. Gore & Associates, Inc, Flagstaff, Ariz).
[a]At initial EVAR.
[b]From initial EVAR to AAA rupture.
[c]At time of AAA rupture.
Reprinted from the Journal of Vascular Surgery. Candell L, Tucker LY, Goodney P, et al. Early and delayed rupture after endovascular abdominal aortic aneurysm repair in a 10-year multicenter registry. *J Vasc Surg*. 2014;60:1146-1153, Copyright 2014, with permission from by The Society for Vascular Surgery.

The conclusion is that we need to follow our patients and be diligent. Okay. So, does that mean that you're not going to treat old people or those presenting with rupture? Thankfully, according to this dataset, 99% of patients will not experience this morbid and potentially mortal event. Another interesting finding from this decade-long experience was that no ruptures were due to type II endoleaks, sustaining our belief that most type IIs are benign AND when associated with an increase in sac size, probably really aren't type IIs and are more likely types I and III. So, I have the following three questions for the authors:

1. How will this information be used to change practice within the Kaiser system? After all, isn't that why we do these studies? Is this outcome data available to ALL vascular interventionists within the Kaiser system?! In other words, how does this information get back to the guy in the trenches so that he or she can change his or her own practice?
2. With an average of only 10 EVARs per site per year, has there been any discussion about regionalization of care for EVAR in Northern California? Were some event rates higher at certain sites suggesting treatment outside of device IFUs by some "aggressive" physicians? Three of 15 delayed rupture patients had additional procedures at the index operation including snorkels and cuffs for type I endoleaks; this suggests that treatment outside the device IFU for short neck aneurysms was associated with a higher delayed rupture event rate.
3. Finally, you must tell us what the graft types and anatomical features were for all that had delayed rupture. It is astonishing to me that these data were not reported with Kaiser's reputation of such a thorough electronic medical record! Come on, guys; it's only 20 patients! I realize that you don't have this information, but this would indeed be useful data. What was the frequency of delayed rupture over time? Has this decreased over the past decade in the authors' experience? Thank you for sending me the manuscript at least 1 week before the meeting, and I look forward to your comments.

Response: Dr Leah Candell

Thank you, Dr Starnes, for your interesting comments, which speak to many issues regarding a retrospective registry. It is our goal to understand outcomes within our integrated health system. In order to do so, we must improve our data acquisition to inform our conclusions. With respect to your first comment about the modest experience across facilities: in Kaiser Permanente's early experience with EVAR, sites and clinicians were clustered around the neighboring academic centers. As experience was gained, the case volume and number of operating surgeons increased greatly throughout the second half of the study period. This is reflected in the mean follow-up of 2.7 years despite our 10 years of experience. Second, our device registry, created more than a decade ago, did not require anatomic information to be collected other than abdominal aortic aneurysm size. Although we had some promising data about IFU adherence from a subset of patients, this was by no means standard and comprehensive, which limited our ability to analyze this important topic. This is something we will address with our new national stent registry. We appreciate your comments about the observation of type II leaks, and we agree that they may represent a benign occurrence after EVAR. We looked into this in more detail and presented these findings at the VESS meeting in Boston, in June 2014. Our responses to your three specific questions follow:

1. We agree that registry information should be used for practice improvement. This is central to any system's mission to provide efficient and safe care. Currently, Kaiser Permanente registry reports are tabulated quarterly with several outcomes reported at the national, regional, and more granular levels. In addition, clinicians may request a breakout report of certain characteristics or outcomes. Similar to what is done in other registry domains, we are utilizing this ability to establish more-efficient surveillance protocols, to more appropriately select patients for intervention, and to improve processes such as percutaneous access.
2. As stated above, currently most sites that perform EVAR have higher operative volumes than they did in the early era of EVAR. There has been an evolution into a spoke-hub model in which complex thoracic and abdominal aortic interventions are performed in a few selected centers. This is certainly true with the hybrid endovascular procedures as well as fenestrated EVAR.
3. We agree that information on graft type and anatomical features is vital for understanding the rare phenomenon of delayed rupture. This content was removed from the original manuscript due to privacy concerns, but after further discussion, was added into the final manuscript that will be published. The limited availability of archived computed tomography data allowed us to make only general statements about IFU adherence and was not sufficient to enable us to comment on graft and anatomic interactions.

We thank Dr Starnes for his review of our paper and his thoughtful comments.

B. W. Starnes, MD

Early versus late experience in fenestrated endovascular repair for abdominal aortic aneurysm

Sveinsson M, Sobocinski J, Resch T, et al (Univ Hosp, Malmö, Sweden; Hôpital Cardiologique, CHRU Lille, France)

J Vasc Surg 61:895-901, 2015

Objective.—The objective of this study was to evaluate operative results and 1-year outcomes in early vs late experience after fenestrated endovascular aortic repair.

Methods.—All patients treated in Malmö, Sweden, and in Lille, France, with fenestrated endovascular repair for abdominal aortic aneurysm were prospectively enrolled in a computerized database. Early experience was defined as the first 50 patients treated at each center. Data from early and late experience were retrospectively analyzed and compared for differences in operative results and 1-year outcomes.

Results.—Early experience covered 4.7 years in Malmö and 4.5 years in Lille; late experience covered 5.6 years in Malmö and 3.7 years in Lille. A total of 288 patients were included. In the later phase, stent graft configuration was more complex because of increased number of fenestrations/scallops incorporated in the graft design (2.7 ± 0.8 vs 3.2 ± 0.7; $P < .001$). Despite this, volume of contrast material and radiation time decreased by 27% and 20%, respectively, whereas procedure time remained unchanged. At 1 year, a trend toward decreasing abdominal aortic aneurysm diameter was observed in the late group, but no differences were found in mortality, endoleaks, or target vessel patency between the groups.

Conclusions.—With increasing experience, fenestrated endovascular aneurysm repair design has become more complicated, with more visceral vessels targeted for better proximal seal, while operative risk still remains low. Simultaneously, radiation time and volume of contrast material have been reduced, with possible long-term benefits for the patient (Figs 1 and 2).

▶ This is a nice combined series of fenestrated endovascular aortic repair (EVAR) experience highlighting a couple of important points. With experience, technical

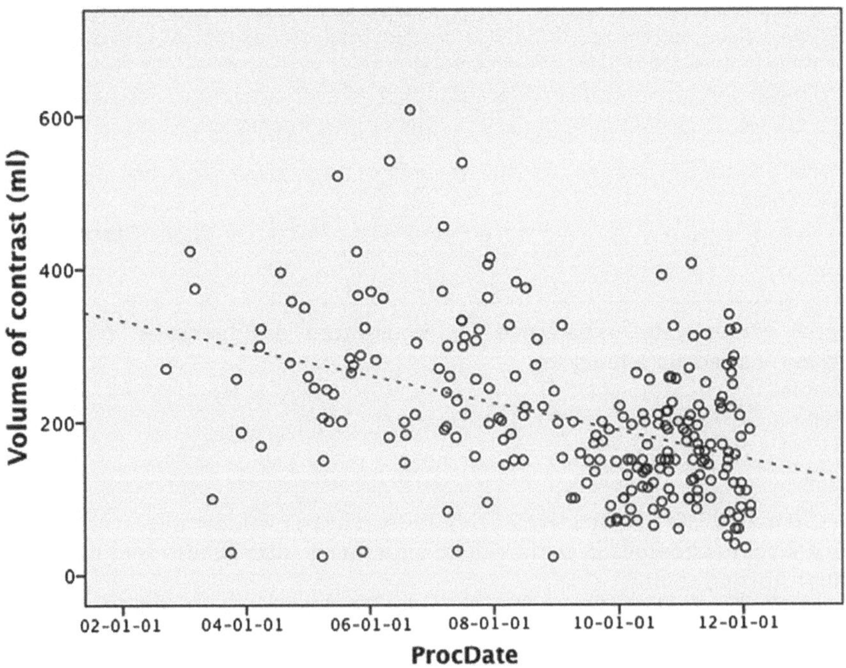

FIGURE 1.—A scattergram showing the volume of contrast material used during procedures, illustrating the reduction of volumes with growing experience. Dates are in the form of yy-mm-dd. (Reprinted from the Journal of Vascular Surgery. Sveinsson M, Sobocinski J, Resch T, et al. Early versus late experience in fenestrated endovascular repair for abdominal aortic aneurysm. *J Vasc Surg*. 2015;61:895-901, Copyright 2014, with permission from The Society for Vascular Surgery.)

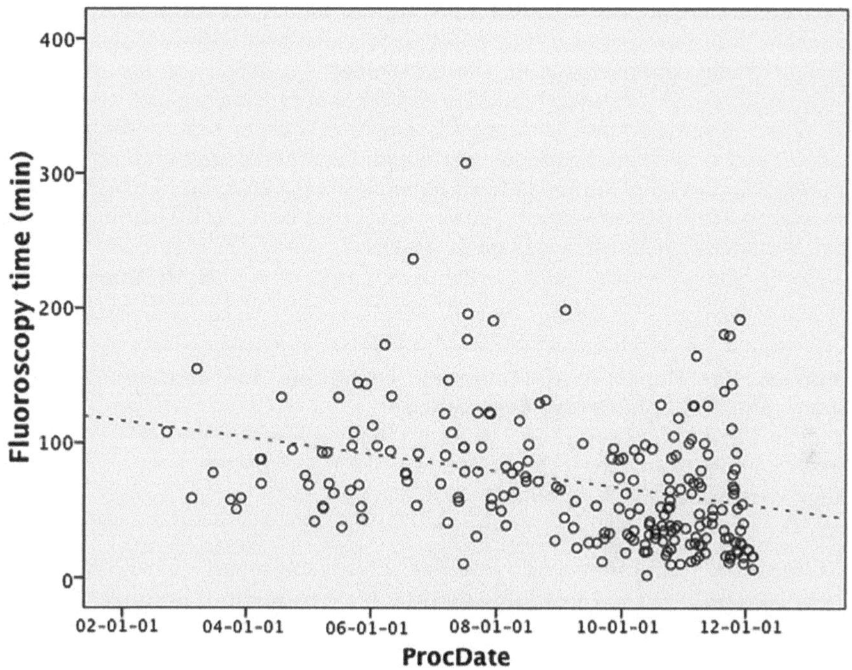

FIGURE 2.—A scattergram showing the reduction in intraoperative radiation time with more experience. Dates are in the form of yy-mm-dd. (Reprinted from the Journal of Vascular Surgery. Sveinsson M, Sobocinski J, Resch T, et al. Early versus late experience in fenestrated endovascular repair for abdominal aortic aneurysm. *J Vasc Surg.* 2015;61:895-901, Copyright 2014, with permission from the Society for Vascular Surgery.)

proficiency improves. In this series, the authors defined early experience with fenestrated EVAR (FEVAR) as the first 50 cases in each institutional experience. The late experience was everything after the first 50 cases. In short, the authors noted that their contrast use and fluoroscopy times decreased by 27% and 20%, respectively, between the 2 time periods (Figs 1 and 2). They also noted that as they became more experienced and were able to assess short-term outcomes of their early patients, they became more comfortable going higher and higher into healthier segments of the aorta. This was reflected by average number of fenestrations going from 2.7 ± 0.8 to 3.2 ± 0.7; $P < .001$. Interestingly, procedure times remained exactly the same at ~280 minutes or 4.7 hours.

I continue to question, however, the recommendation of stenting all target vessels. The authors noted that there was little attention paid to positioning of scallops over the SMA in their early experience. It was just assumed that if the device was planned right and the renal fenestrations were successfully stented, the scallop would automatically line up. This was not the case, and they noticed partial "shuttering" effects of this practice and some target vessel occlusions. They and others, therefore, recommended that all fenestrations be stented. This has not been our experience. We have learned that if the device is perfectly planned, SMA fenestrations do not require stenting with resultant excellent long-term patency. Presented at Vascular and Endovascular Surgery Society (VESS) annual meeting, Chicago June 17, 2015.

The future of EVAR rests in reliable and durable proximal seal. A seal length of 15 mm is not enough! Give me 40 mm to 50 mm of seal length in every patient, and I will show you long-term durability of aortic endografting without late-term failure. Therefore, nearly all patients should undergo FEVAR to repair any abdominal aortic aneurysm. The key to success is in precise planning. If the graft is perfectly planned, these cases are easy.

B. W. Starnes, MD

Endovascular Repair with Chimney Technique for Juxtarenal Aortic Aneurysm: A Single Center Experience

XiaoHui M, Wei G, ZhongZhou H, et al (General Hosp of People's Liberation Army, Beijing, China; Med Ctr Tsinghua Univ, Beijing, China)
Eur J Vasc Endovasc Surg 49:271-276, 2015

Objective.—Chimney endovascular aneurysm repair (Ch-EVAR) is a cheap and immediately available method for treatment of juxtarenal aortic aneurysms (JRAAs). The aim of this study was to report experiences and results with balloon expandable stent (BES) for Ch-EVAR.

Methods.—From January 2008 to June 2013 (mean time, 26 ± 13 months), 42 patients who underwent Ch-EVAR were retrospectively reviewed. All patients were thought to be at high risk for open surgery and were unsuitable (because of financial issues and fear of delays) for fenestrated endovascular aneurysm repair (FEVAR).

Results.—42 patients (35 males; mean age 71 ± 7 years) underwent chimney procedures for 56 renal arteries with 70 BESs (59 hippocampus and 11 genesis). Median follow up was 26 months (range 6—64 months). Primary technical success was 100%. Thirty day mortality was 0%. Completion angiography showed that eight cases (19%) had a type I endoleak. The 6 month follow up CT scans demonstrated three cases with complete regression of endoleak, two cases without aneurysmal growth, and three cases with an increase in aneurysmal diameter of less than 10 mm. Three patients had contrast induced nephropathy (CIN) after Ch-EVAR, two of whom had acute renal failure (ARF) and continue to require hemodialysis. Two deaths occurred during follow up, both unrelated to the aorta: one with a hemispheric stroke at 6 months and one with respiratory failure at 12 months. Therefore, the overall follow up mortality was 5%. Occlusion of one chimney stent occurred 3 months after the procedure, meaning renal artery patency rate was 98%. The aneurysm diameter reduced from 74 ± 9 mm to 64 ± 10 mm during follow up ($p < .05$).

Conclusion.—Ch-EVAR can be used to treat JRAAs with suitable anatomical conditions. However, complications of type I endoleak were not uncommon, and, therefore, further studies are required to prove its efficiency for JRAAs (Fig 1).

► Anyone who knows me well will tell you that I am heavily biased against parallel endografting, also known as *chimney and snorkel endografting* (Fig 1). This report is yet another that supports that bias. This group from Beijing reports their experience with 42 patients and 56 renal artery chimney stents (1.3 stents per branches preserved per patient). As with all other similar types of reports, their technical success was 100% and the follow-up was limited.

What strikes me about this series is that after completion angiography, there was a 31% rate of Type 1a endoleak! And after aggressive ballooning in a kissing fashion, that endoleak rate decreased to 19%. But a 19% rate of type 1a endoleak intraoperatively? In the United States, if this was a pivotal trial assessing a new endograft and the investigators reported a 19% type 1a endoleak rate, the trial would be stopped.

There are several reasons that I believe the results were as they were. An average of 1.3 stents was used per case. In fact, 28 patients had unilateral renal stents only. The fact that the authors were only treating one renal artery in most patients means they were only extending their neck length (mean 7 ± 3 mm) a few millimeters for effective seal. The biggest lesson learned in contemporary fenestrated experiences is that the higher one goes into healthier aortic neck, the better the result with extremely low incidences of type 1a endoleak.

Until we have a controlled trial with granular data to include effective length of seal and degree of oversizing of components, this strategy remains a free for all (as it apparently is in the Wild, Wild East). I just hope that when I develop my

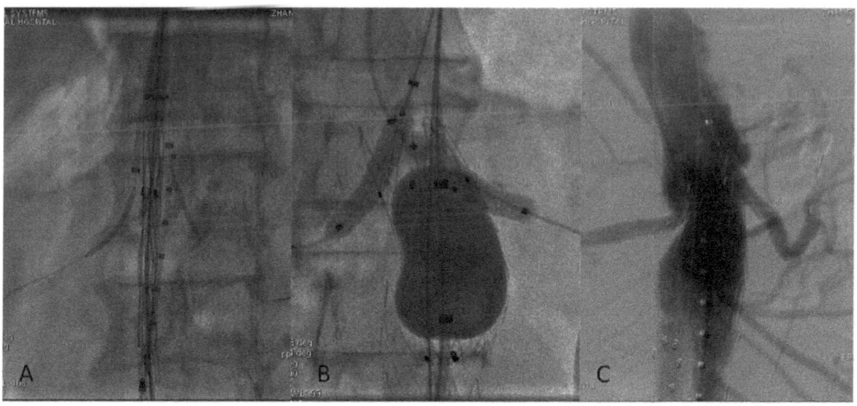

FIGURE 1.—The procedures with chimney technique for juxtarenal aortic aneurysms (JRAAs). (A) Balloon expandable stents were placed as chimneys in the right and left renal arteries. (B) The proximal "kissing balloon" (the aortic endograft and the chimney stents were ballooned simultaneously) technique is shown. (C) Completion angiogram showed the patency of chimney stents without endoleak for the aortic endograft. (Reprinted from the European Journal of Vascular and Endovascular Surgery. XiaoHui M, Wei G, ZhongZhou H, et al. Endovascular repair with chimney technique for juxtarenal aortic aneurysm: a single center experience. *Eur J Vasc Endovasc Surg*. 2015;49:271-276, Copyright 2014, with permission from The European Society for Vascular Surgery.)

juxtarenal aneurysm, I'm in Seattle and still practicing so I can do a fenestrated endovascular aneurysm repair on myself with 50 mm of effective seal.

B. W. Starnes, MD

Failure to rescue trends in elective abdominal aortic aneurysm repair between 1995 and 2011

Ilonzo N, Egorova NN, McKinsey JF, et al (Icahn School of Medicine at Mount Sinai, NY)

J Vasc Surg 60:1473-1480, 2014

Objective.—Factors affecting mortality after abdominal aortic aneurysm (AAA) repair have been extensively studied, but little is known about the effects of the shift to endovascular aneurysm repair (EVAR) vs open repair on failure to rescue (FTR). This study examines the impact of treatment modalities on FTR for elective AAA surgery during the years 1995 to 2011.

Methods.—Data for 491,779 patients undergoing elective AAA surgery were collected from Medicare files. Patient demographics, comorbidities, hospital volume, and repair type were collected. Primary outcome was FTR: the percentage of deaths in patients who had a complication within 30 days of surgery. Data were analyzed by univariate and multivariate analysis.

Results.—Patients undergoing AAA surgery have become progressively more complex, with 84.96%, 89.33%, 93.76%, and 95.72% presenting with one or more comorbidities in 1995, 2000, 2005, and 2011, respectively. Despite this, overall FTR after AAA surgery was stable from 1995 to 2000 ($P = .38$) and decreased from 2.68% to 1.58% between 2000 and 2011 ($P < .001$). In addition, FTR in EVAR decreased from 1.70% to 0.58% from 2000 to 2006 ($P = .03$) and then stabilized at 0.88% ± 0.9% after 2007 ($P = .45$). Unlike for EVAR, FTR for open repair remained stable at 3.06% ±0.17% to 2.74% ± 0.16% from 1995 to 2000 ($P = .38$) but increased to 4.51% 6 0.21% in 2011 ($P < .001$). Mortality was highest after transfusion (20.86%), prolonged ventilation (17.37%), and respiratory complications (29.78%) for all AAA surgeries. Of note, high-volume hospitals had lower FTR rates than low-volume hospitals for both open (2.73% vs 5.66%; $P < .001$) and endovascular (0.7% vs 1.69%; $P < .001$) repair. Multivariate analysis showed that high annual volume hospital status (odds ratio, 0.6; confidence interval, 0.58-0.63) and endovascular repair (odds ratio, 0.3; confidence interval, 0.28-0.31) were associated with decreased FTR.

Conclusions.—The success in AAA surgery of rescuing patients from 30-day mortality after a complication is associated with increased volume of EVAR. This increased success can also be attributed to the improved

FTR outcomes and complication rates when surgeries are performed at high-volume hospital centers (Figs 1-4).

► "Failure to rescue" (FTR) is a measure of a hospital's ability to successfully treat patients who have had a complication after surgery. It is defined as the 30-day mortality rate in patients with 2 or more complications. To calculate the FTR, the number of deaths is divided by the number of abdominal aortic aneurysm cases with complications. FTR has emerged as a useful tool for assessing surgical quality since its original definition by Silber in 1992.[1] This study analyzes the trend in FTR between 1995 and 2011 in open and endovascular AAA repair. It seeks to identify factors associated with increased success in AAA surgery.

Elective repair was performed in 491 779 patients over the study period. Among them, 295 851 underwent open repair, and 195 928 underwent endovascular repair. The percentage of endovascular repairs versus open repairs performed annually is depicted in Fig 1.

Notably, there was increased success in preventing deaths after complications among patients undergoing EVAR. FTR in these patients decreased from 1.7% to 0.58% from 2000 to 2006 ($P = .03$) and then stabilized at 0.58% 0.08% to 0.88% 0.9% after 2007 ($P = 0.45$; Fig 3). Trends in complications for either method of repair are depicted in Fig 2.

One of the most important messages from this study is the difference in FTR among low, mid- and high-volume hospitals. Low volume is described as 4

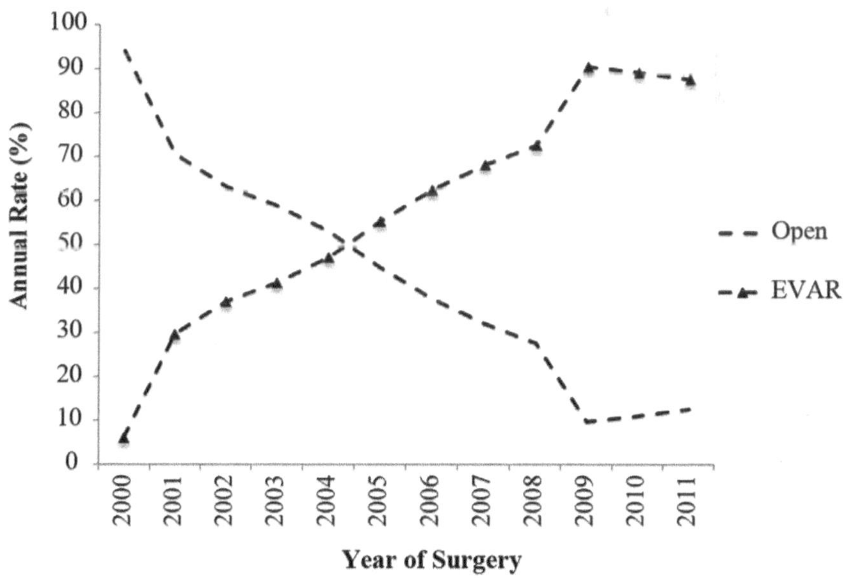

FIGURE 1.—Percentage of endovascular aneurysm repair (*EVAR*) ($P < .001$) vs open repair ($P < .001$) performed annually. (Reprinted from the Journal of Vascular Surgery. Ilonzo N, Egorova NN, McKinsey JF, et al. Failure to rescue trends in elective abdominal aortic aneurysm repair between 1995 and 2011. *J Vasc Surg*. 2014;60:1473-1480, Copyright 2014, with permission from The Society for Vascular Surgery.)

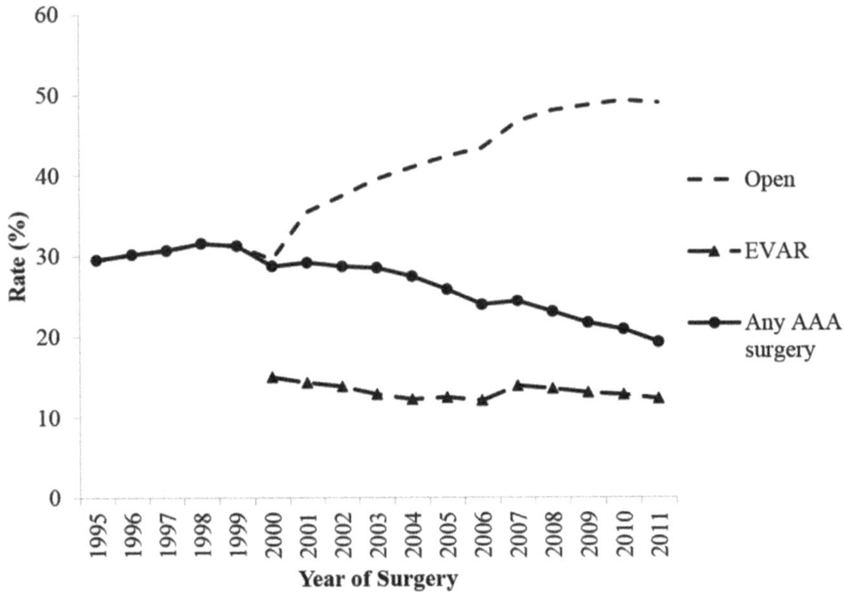

FIGURE 2.—Trend in complications during index hospitalization after open repair ($P < .001$), endovascular aneurysm repair (*EVAR*) ($P = .06$), or any abdominal aortic aneurysm (*AAA*) surgery ($P < .001$). (Reprinted from the Journal of Vascular Surgery. Ilonzo N, Egorova NN, McKinsey JF, et al. Failure to rescue trends in elective abdominal aortic aneurysm repair between 1995 and 2011. *J Vasc Surg*. 2014;60:1473-1480, Copyright 2014, with permission from The Society for Vascular Surgery.)

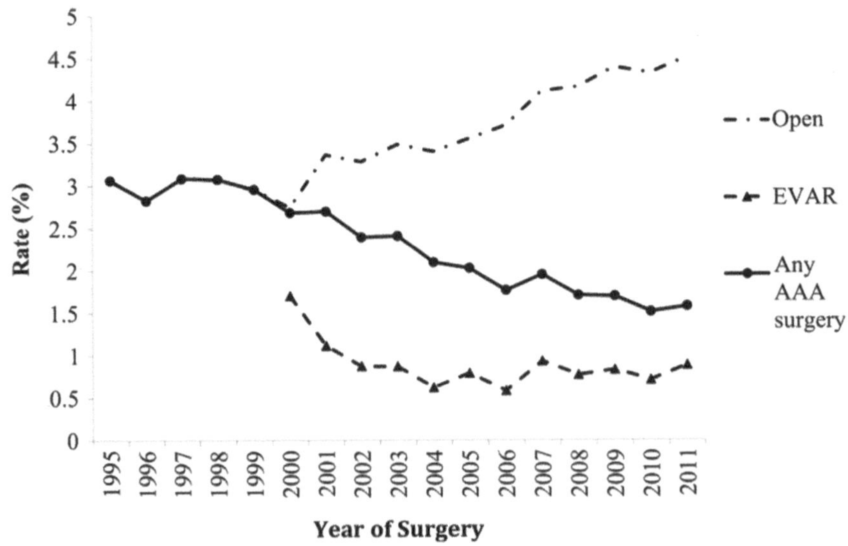

FIGURE 3.—Trend in failure to rescue (FTR) from open repair ($P = .38$, 1995-2000; $P < .001$, 2000-2011), endovascular aneurysm repair (*EVAR*) ($P = .03$, 2000-2006; $P = .45$, 2008-2011), or any abdominal aortic aneurysm (*AAA*) surgery ($P = .38$, 1995-2000; $P < .001$, 2000-2011). (Reprinted from the Journal of Vascular Surgery. Ilonzo N, Egorova NN, McKinsey JF, et al. Failure to rescue trends in elective abdominal aortic aneurysm repair between 1995 and 2011. *J Vasc Surg*. 2014;60:1473-1480, Copyright 2014, with permission from The Society for Vascular Surgery.)

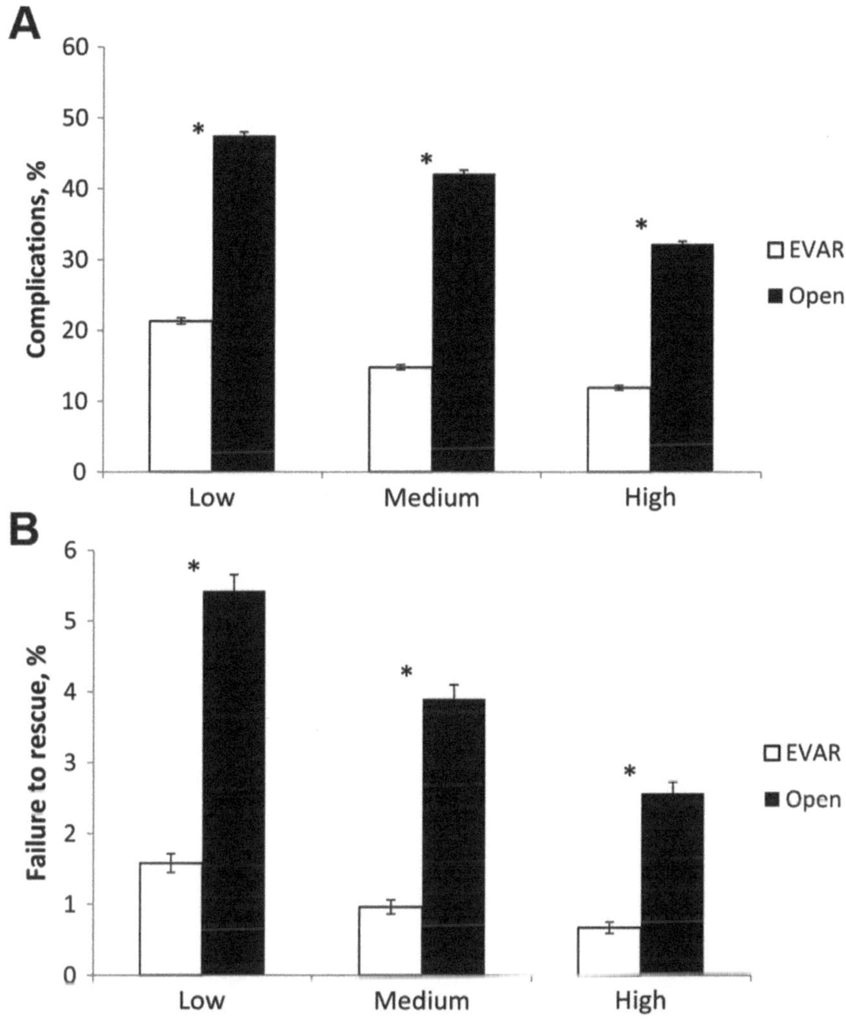

FIGURE 4.—Complication rates (A) and failure to rescue (FTR) rates (B) for endovascular aneurysm repair (*EVAR*) and open procedures performed between 1995 and 2011 in low-, medium-, or high-volume hospitals. **P* < .001. (Reprinted from the Journal of Vascular Surgery. Ilonzo N, Egorova NN, McKinsey JF, et al. Failure to rescue trends in elective abdominal aortic aneurysm repair between 1995 and 2011. *J Vasc Surg*. 2014;60:1473-1480, Copyright 2014, with permission from The Society for Vascular Surgery.)

EVARs or less, mid between 5 and 17 EVARs, and high between 18 and 177 EVARs. There has been much debate about how hospital volume and patient characteristics affect complication rates and mortality after major surgical procedures. This study of a half a million patients and 17 years of data showed a definitive relationship between hospital volume and complication rates, with hospitals of high volume having fewer complications (Fig 4).

B. W. Starnes, MD

Reference

1. Silber JH, Williams SV, Krakauer H, Schwartz JS. Hospital and patient characteristics associated with death after surgery. A study of adverse occurrence and failure to rescue. *Med Care.* 1992;30:615-629.

Fate of Patients Unwilling or Unsuitable To Undergo Surgical Intervention for a Ruptured Abdominal Aortic Aneurysm

van Beek SC, on behalf of the Amsterdam Acute Aneurysm Trial Collaborators (Academic Med Ctr, Amsterdam, The Netherlands; et al)

Eur J Vasc Endovasc Surg 49:163-165, 2015

Introduction.—The primary objective of this study was to assess the duration of in-hospital survival in 57 patients with ruptured abdominal aortic aneurysms (RAAA) who did not undergo surgical intervention.

Report.—Two hours after registration in the emergency room, 58% (95% CI 45–71) of patients were still alive. The median survival was 2.2 hours (interquartile range 1–18). In a subgroup including 26 haemodynamically stable patients, survival after 2 hours was 96% (95% CI 89–100).

Conclusion.—In patients with an RAAA without surgical intervention, the duration of in-hospital survival is limited. However, a group of haemodynamically stable patients can be identified in whom survival is much longer (Fig 1).

▶ I recall a story that my colleague, Mark Meissner, MD, told me when I first arrived to the University of Washington in 2007. It was about an old man of 82 years who presented years before the endovascular era with a ruptured abdominal aortic aneurysm (AAA) diagnosed by CT scan. The patient and the family chose to have nothing done, and he was made comfortable and placed in a quiet ward room at the end of the hall. The family asked how long it would take him to die, and the consulting surgeons responded that "they really had no idea, but it wouldn't take long."

The next day, the patient was still alive and feeling a bit better. He asked for some food to eat. To make a long story short, the patient survived and was discharged to go home with his family having survived his ruptured AAA. On the way home, there was an automobile crash and the patient did not survive. This just goes to show you that when your time is up, your time is up!

The information presented in this article is valuable. It reports the duration of in-hospital survival in 57 patients with a ruptured AAA who did not undergo surgical intervention. After 2 hours, only 58% of patients were still alive, and

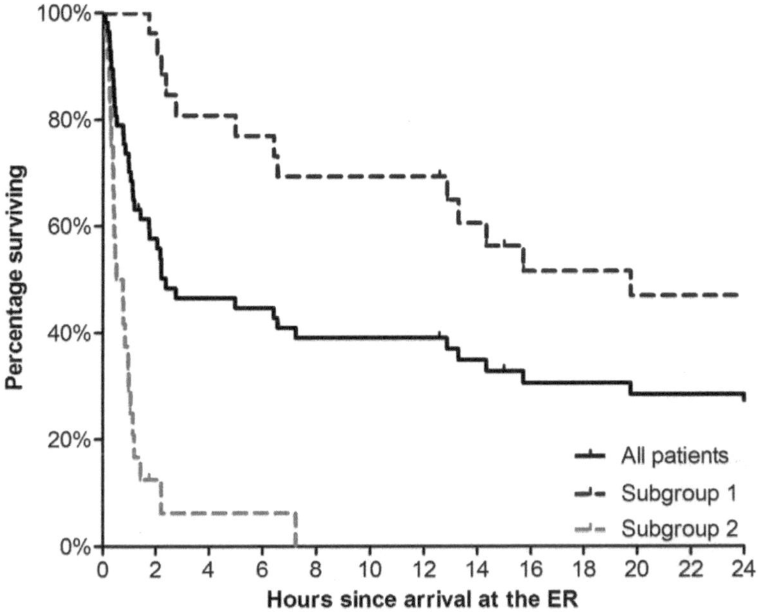

No. at risk													
All patients	57	31	25	24	20	20	20	17	14	14	13	13	13
Subgroup 1	26	25	21	20	17	17	17	14	11	11	10	10	10
Subgroup 2	24	2	1	1	0								

FIGURE 1.—Survival analysis of the first 24 hours from arrival in the ER of 57 patients with an RAAA not undergoing surgical intervention. Subgroup 1 included patients not treated because of patient decision, comorbidity, age, or aortic anatomical considerations, and subgroup 2 included patients with cardiopulmonary resuscitation (CPR) and patients with shock as reason for not intervening. (Reprinted from the European Journal of Vascular and Endovascular Surgery. van Beek SC, on behalf of the Amsterdam Acute Aneurysm Trial Collaborators. Fate of patients unwilling or unsuitable to undergo surgical intervention for a ruptured abdominal aortic aneurysm. *Eur J Vasc Endovasc Surg*. 2015;49:163-165, Copyright 2014, with permission from the European Society for Vascular Surgery.)

the median survival was 2.2 hours (interquartile range, 1–18 hours). However, in hemodynamically stable patients, survival after 2 hours was 96%. The message is that in these hemodynamically stable patients, it seems to be justified to moderately increase transfer time to reach a specialized tertiary hospital. CT scanning seems justified for diagnosis in all patients suspected of harboring a ruptured AAA.

Fig 1 shows the survival in hours of all patients (dark solid line) and 2 cohorts of subgroup 1 (hemodynamically stable) and subgroup 2 (hemodynamically unstable or with cardiopulmonary resuscitation).

B. W. Starnes, MD

Fenestrated endovascular repair of abdominal aortic aneurysms is associated with increased morbidity but comparable mortality with infrarenal endovascular aneurysm repair

Glebova NO, Selvarajah S, Orion KC, et al (The Johns Hopkins Hosp, Baltimore, MD; et al)

J Vasc Surg 61:604-610, 2015

Objective.—A recent prospective study found that fenestrated endovascular abdominal aortic aneurysm (AAA) repair (FEVAR) was safe and effective in appropriately selected patients at experienced centers. As this new technology is disseminated to the community, it will be important to understand how this technology compares with standard endovascular AAA repair (EVAR). The goal of this study was to compare the outcomes of FEVAR vs EVAR of AAAs.

Methods.—The American College of Surgeons-National Surgical Quality Improvement Program database from 2005 to 2012 was queried for AAAs (International Classification of Diseases, Ninth Revision code 441.4). Patients were stratified according to procedure (FEVAR vs EVAR). A bivariate analysis was done to assess preoperative and intraoperative risk factors for postoperative outcomes. Thirty-day postoperative mortality and complication rates were described for each procedure type. Multivariable logistic regression was performed to assess the association between the type of procedure and the risk of postoperative complications.

Results.—A total of 458 patients underwent FEVAR and 19,060 patients underwent EVAR for AAA. Patients undergoing FEVAR were older ($P = .02$) and less likely to have a bleeding disorder ($P = .046$). Otherwise, the incidence of comorbidities in both groups was similar. FEVAR was associated with increased median operative time (156 vs 137 minutes; $P < .001$), and average postoperative length of stay (3.3 vs 2.8 days; $P = .03$). There was a statistically significant increase in overall complications (23.6% vs 14.3%; $P < .001$) and postoperative transfusions (15.3% vs 6.1%, $P < .001$) and trends toward increased cardiac complications (2.2% vs 1.3%; $P = .09$) and the need for dialysis (1.5% vs 0.8%; $P = .08$) in the FEVAR group. Mortality (2.4% vs 1.5%; $P = .12$) was not statistically different. On multivariable analysis, FEVAR remained independently associated with the need for postoperative transfusions when operative time was <75th percentile (adjusted odds ratio, 1.72; 95% confidence interval, 1.09-2.72; $P = .02$) as well as when operative time was >75th percentile for respective procedures (adjusted odds ratio, 5.33; 95% confidence interval, 3.55-8.00; $P < .001$).

Conclusions.—Patients undergoing FEVAR are more likely than patients undergoing EVAR to receive blood transfusions postoperatively and are more likely to sustain postoperative complications. Although mortality was similar, trends toward increased cardiac and renal complications may suggest the need for judicious dissemination of this new technology.

Future research with larger number of FEVAR cases will be necessary to determine if these associations remain (Fig 1).

▶ I thought this was a great article and a nice snapshot of current data from initial experience with fenestrated endovascular abdominal aortic aneurysm (FEVAR) in America. This report was another evaluation of the American College of Surgeons-National Surgical Quality Improvement Program data from 2005 to 2012 and compared postoperative outcomes between FEVAR and endovascular abdominal aortic aneurysm (EVAR). During the study period, there were 458 FEVARs and 19 060 EVARs reported. FEVAR represented only 2.4% of all endovascular aneurysm repairs and was associated with more postoperative complications and a significantly higher need for blood transfusions in the perioperative period.

Interestingly, FEVAR was only 19 minutes longer on average than standard EVAR. Not surprisingly, higher operating times were associated with increased risk and increased need for blood transfusion. The 75th percentile for operating times was established to be 227 minutes. For patients with FEVAR operating times shorter than that (< 75th%), there was a 2.5-fold increased risk of receiving greater than 4 U of packed red blood cells than standard EVAR (adjusted odds ratio [AOR], 2.46; 95% confidence interval [CI], 1.46–4.13; $P < .001$). For patients with FEVAR operating times longer than the 75th percentile, there was a 5.4-fold greater likelihood of transfusion (AOR, 5.38; 95% CI, 3.33–8.71; $P < .001$; Fig 1).

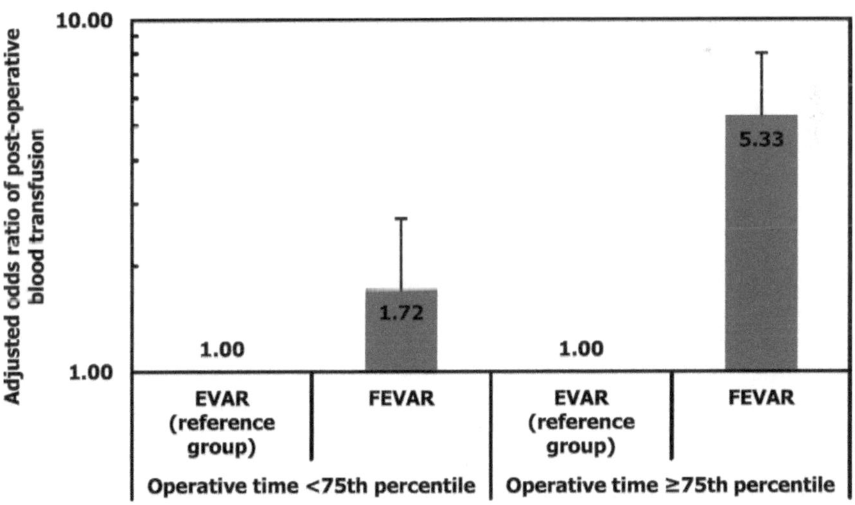

FIGURE 1.—Adjusted odds ratios (AORs) of postoperative blood transfusion in fenestrated endovascular aneurysm repair (*FEVAR*) compared with endovascular aneurysm repair (*EVAR*) stratified by operative time. The range bars indicate the standard deviation. Adjusted for age, sex, race, smoking status, diabetes, dialysisdependence, congestive heart failure, hypertension, thrombocytopenia, bleeding disorder, preoperative functional status, American Society of Anesthesiologists (ASA) class, brachial exposure, emergency procedure, and the interaction term between operative time and type of procedure. (Reprinted from the Journal of Vascular Surgery. Glebova NO, Selvarajah S, Orion KC, et al. Fenestrated endovascular repair of abdominal aortic aneurysms is associated with increased morbidity but comparable mortality with infrarenal endovascular aneurysm repair. *J Vasc Surg*. 2015;61:604-610, Copyright 2014, with permission from The Society for Vascular Surgery.)

In our own experience with nearly 200 FEVARs reported, we have noticed a similar trend of increased complication with longer procedures. Long procedures are typically related to poor planning of the fenestrated endograft to begin with and speak to the need for more streamlined and accurate planning methods. Sheath dwell times are probably responsible for the increased blood loss requiring subsequent transfusion. These results will only improve with wider penetration of this technology.

B. W. Starnes, MD

Finite Element Analysis in Asymptomatic, Symptomatic, and Ruptured Abdominal Aortic Aneurysms: In Search of New Rupture Risk Predictors

Erhart P, Hyhlik-Dürr A, Geisbüsch P, et al (Ruprecht-Karls Univ Heidelberg, Germany; et al)

Eur J Vasc Endovasc Surg 49:239-245, 2015

Objectives.—To compare biomechanical rupture risk parameters of asymptomatic, symptomatic and ruptured abdominal aortic aneurysms (AAA) using finite element analysis (FEA).

Study Design.—Retrospective biomechanical single center analysis of asymptomatic, symptomatic, and ruptured AAAs. Comparison of biomechanical parameters from FEA.

Materials and Methods.—From 2011 to 2013 computed tomography angiography (CTA) data from 30 asymptomatic, 15 symptomatic, and 15 ruptured AAAs were collected consecutively. FEA was performed according to the successive steps of AAA vessel reconstruction, segmentation and finite element computation. Biomechanical parameters Peak Wall Rupture Risk Index (PWRI), Peak Wall Stress (PWS), and Rupture Risk Equivalent Diameter (RRED) were compared among the three subgroups.

Results.—PWRI differentiated between asymptomatic and symptomatic AAAs ($p < .0004$) better than PWS ($p < .1453$). PWRI-dependent RRED was higher in the symptomatic subgroup compared with the asymptomatic subgroup ($p < .0004$). Maximum AAA external diameters were comparable between the two groups ($p < .1355$). Ruptured AAAs showed the highest values for external diameter, total intraluminal thrombus volume, PWS, RRED, and PWRI compared with asymptomatic and symptomatic AAAs. In contrast with symptomatic and ruptured AAAs, none of the asymptomatic patients had a PWRI value >1.0. This threshold value might identify patients at imminent risk of rupture.

Conclusions.—From different FEA derived parameters, PWRI distinguishes most precisely between asymptomatic and symptomatic AAAs. If elevated, this value may represent a negative prognostic factor for asymptomatic AAAs (Fig 3, Table 2).

▶ In routine clinical practice, the maximum aortic diameter is the criterion most often used for abdominal aortic aneurysm (AAA) repair. Some societal

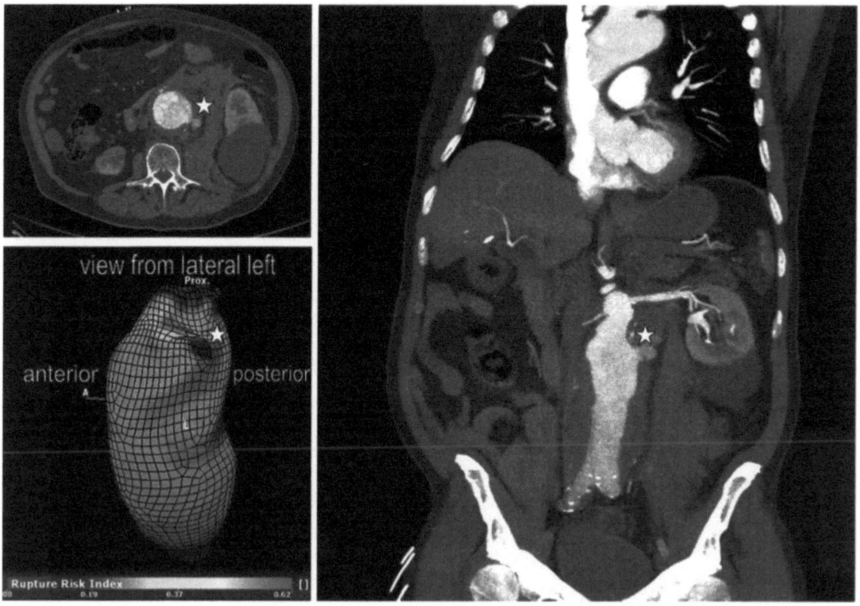

FIGURE 3.—FEA of a ruptured AAA with contrast extravasation. The rupture site was infrarenal and on the left lateral portion of the aneurysm (asterisk). FEA analyzing software precisely identified the rupture location. This region was devoid of vessel wall; therefore local rupture risk was zero (blue color). For interpretation of the references to color in this figure legend, the reader is referred to the web version of this article. (Reprinted from the European Journal of Vascular and Endovascular Surgery. Erhart P, Hyhlik-Dürr A, Geisbüsch P, et al. Finite element analysis in asymptomatic, symptomatic, and ruptured abdominal aortic aneurysms: in search of new rupture risk predictors. *Eur J Vasc Endovasc Surg*. 2015;49:239-245, Copyright 2014, with permission from The European Society for Vascular Surgery.)

TABLE 2.—Biomechanical Parameters From FEA of AAA Subgroups

	Asymptomatic AAAs ($n = 30$)	Symptomatic AAAs ($n = 15$)	Ruptured AAAs ($n = 15$)
Peak wall stress (in kPa)	202 ± 34 (138–253)	222 ± 84 (158–511)	317 ± 69 (213–413)
Peak wall rupture risk index	0.46 ± 0.11 (0.27–0.73)	0.62 ± 0.22 (0.41–1.36)	0.83 ± 0.48 (0.51–2.01)
Max AAA diameter (in mm)	59 ± 10 (50–89)	65.3 ± 19 (43–127)	84 ± 18 (66–134)
Total AAA lumen volume (in cm^3)	93 ± 33 (37–160)	118 ± 57 (58–289)	144 ± 122 (66–358)
Volume of intraluminal thrombus (in cm^3)	67 ± 72 (16–327)	71 ± 193 (13–800)	134 ± 96 (6–401)
Rupture risk equivalent diameter (in mm)	53 ± 10 (42–76)	68 ± 18 (49–124)	84 ± 38 (61–178)

Median values ± standard deviation, (lowest-highest values) are shown.

Reprinted from the European Journal of Vascular and Endovascular Surgery. Erhart P, Hyhlik-Dürr A, Geisbüsch P, et al. Finite element analysis in asymptomatic, symptomatic, and ruptured abdominal aortic aneurysms: in search of new rupture risk predictors. *Eur J Vasc Endovasc Surg*. 2015;49:239-245, Copyright 2014, with permission from The European Society for Vascular Surgery.

guidelines report an exponentially increasing annual rupture risk for patients exceeding diameters of 5.0 to 5.5 cm.[1] However, this sole parameter does not necessarily reflect the true risk of rupture in each patient.

This study of 60 patients with AAA (30 asymptomatic, 15 symptomatic, and 15 ruptured) showed that retrospective finite element analysis (FEA) found biomechanical differences in these subgroups (Fig 3). Peak wall rupture risk index and rupture risk equivalent diameter appeared to be the most sensitive parameters to differentiate asymptomatic and symptomatic AAAs (Table 2). Individual AAA rupture risk estimation based on FEA alone is still undetermined; however, these preliminary results provide further success in model verification.

It won't be long before imaging will help us better guide timing of therapy or intervention with regard to aortic aneurysm rupture risk!

B. W. Starnes, MD

Reference

1. Moll FL, Powell JT, Fraedrich G, et al. Management of abdominal aortic aneurysms clinical practice guidelines of the European society for vascular surgery. *Eur J Vasc Endovasc Surg*. 2011;41:S1-S58.

Geometry and respiratory-induced deformation of abdominal branch vessels and stents after complex endovascular aneurysm repair

Ullery BW, Suh G-Y, Lee JT, et al (Stanford Univ, CA)

J Vasc Surg 61:875-885, 2015

Objective.—This study quantified the geometry and respiration-induced deformation of abdominal branch vessels and stents after fenestrated (F-) and snorkel (Sn-) endovascular aneurysm repair (EVAR).

Methods.—Twenty patients (80% male; mean age, 75.2 ± 7.4 years; mean aneurysm diameter, 6.2 ± 1.8 cm) underwent computed tomography angiography during inspiratory and expiratory breath hold protocols after F-EVAR (n = 11) or Sn-EVAR (n = 9). Centerlines for the aorta and visceral vessels were extracted from three-dimensional models. Branch angles were computed relative to the orthogonal plane at the branch ostia, and end-stent angles of the left renal artery (LRA) and right renal artery (RRA) were computed relative to the distal stent orientation. The radius of peak curvature was defined by the circumscribed circle at the highest curvature.

Results.—Sn-renal branches were more downward-angled than F-renal branches ($P < .04$). At the distal ends of the RRA stents, Sn-RRAs were angled greater than F-RRAs ($P < .03$) and had a smaller radius of peak curvature ($P < .03$). With expiration, the end-stent angle of Sn-LRAs increased by 4° ± 4° ($P < .02$) and exhibited a significant reduction of radius of curvature ($P < .04$). The unstented celiac arteries were more downward-angled ($P < .02$, inspiration), with a smaller radius of curvature

($P < .00001$), than the unstented superior mesenteric arteries. With expiration, the celiac arteries angled upwards by 9° ± 9° ($P < .0005$), which was greater than the superior mesenteric arteries ($P < .03$). At a median postoperative follow-up of 12.6 months (range, 1.0-37.1 months), branch vessel patency was 100%, serum creatinine levels remained stable, and one reintervention was required for a type III endoleak at the main body-LRA stent interface.

Conclusions.—Sn-renals were angled more inferiorly at the branch and more angulated at the stent end than F-renals due to stent placement strategies. Sn-LRAs exhibited a significant change in end-stent angle and curvature during respiration, a finding that may compromise long-term durability for parallel stent graft configurations. Further investigation is warranted to better optimize anatomic, patient, and branch vessel stent

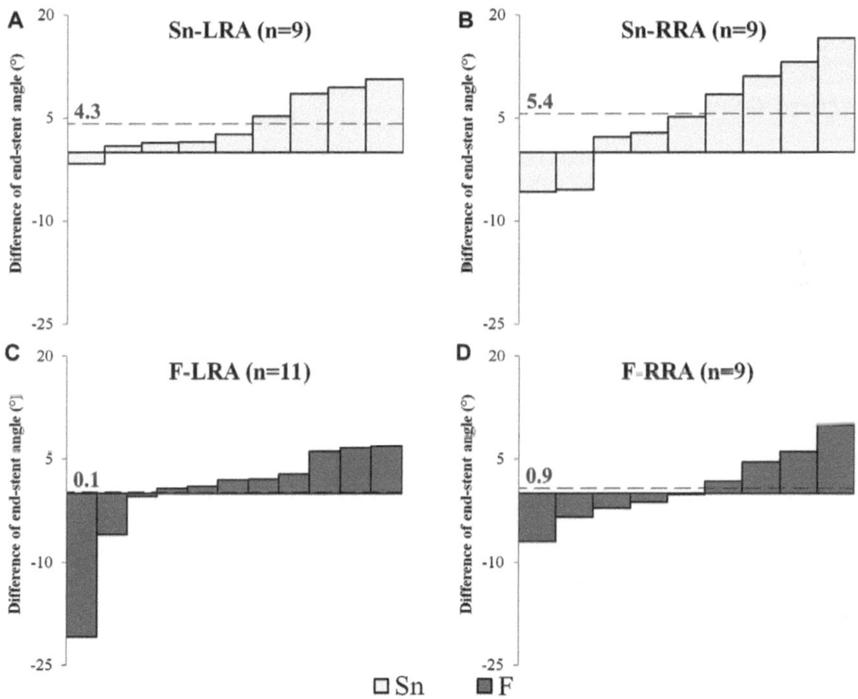

FIGURE 4.—Distribution of end-stent angle change (expiration−inspiration) for (A) snorkel-left renal artery (*Sn-LRA*), (B) Sn-right renal artery (*Sn-RRA*), (C) fenestrated-LRA (*F-LRA*), and (D) F-RRA groups. The end-stent angle change was sorted from lowest to highest. The mean value of end-stent angle change is depicted with a *dashed line*. (Reprinted from the Journal of Vascular Surgery. Ullery BW, Suh G-Y, Lee JT, et al. Geometry and respiratory-induced deformation of abdominal branch vessels and stents after complex endovascular aneurysm repair. *J Vasc Surg*. 2015;61:875-885, Copyright 2014, with permission from The Society for Vascular Surgery.)

selection between fenestrated and snorkel strategies and their relationship to long-term patency (Fig 4).

▶ Despite the promising early results with complex endovascular aneurysm repair (EVAR), long-term visceral artery patency and durability of branch vessel stents are just now becoming known. Optimal stent graft design, stent choice, and deployment approaches and strategies are in a constant state of evolution. This study adds to the paucity of literature addressing potential failure mechanisms in complex EVAR but also suggests the potential for a sustained advantage of fenestrated EVAR over snorkeled EVAR because of a more favorable branch vessel stent configuration capable of less respiratory-induced deformation, particularly on the left side (Fig 4).

Essentially, these authors looked at a small number of patients who underwent either fenestrated or snorkeled EVAR and did rapid phase CT scans with maximum inspiration and maximum expiration, judging the impact of the respiratory cycle on visceral artery movement and deformation. Branch vessels in association with fenestrated EVAR seemed to be much more resistant to respiratory-induced deformation. Long-term follow-up studies will be the final judge of which technique is more durable. I am personally biased toward a fenestrated approach.[1]

B. W. Starnes, MD

Reference

1. Mastracci TM, Greenberg RK, Eagleton MJ, Hernandez AV. Durability of branches in branched and fenestrated endografts. *J Vasc Surg*. 2013;57:926-933.

In patients stratified by preoperative risk, endovascular repair of ruptured abdominal aortic aneurysms has a lower in-hospital mortality and morbidity than open repair

Ali MM, Flahive J, Schanzer A, et al (Univ of Massachusetts Med School, Worcester)

J Vasc Surg 61:1399-1407, 2015

Objective.—Previous studies have reported that endovascular repair (EVAR) of ruptured abdominal aortic aneurysms (RAAAs) has lower postoperative mortality than open repair (OR). However, comparisons involved heterogeneous populations that lacked adjustment for preoperative risk. We hypothesize that for RAAA patients stratified by a validated measure of preoperative mortality risk, EVAR has a lower in-hospital mortality and morbidity than does OR.

Methods.—In-hospital mortality and morbidity after EVAR and OR of RAAA were compared in patients from the Vascular Quality Initiative (2003-2013) stratified by the validated Vascular Study Group of New

England RAAA risk score into low-risk (score 0-1), medium-risk (score 2-3), and high-risk (score 4-6) groups.

Results.—Among 514 patients who underwent EVAR and 651 patients who underwent OR of RAAA, EVAR had lower in-hospital mortality (25% vs 33%, $P = .001$). In risk-stratified patients, EVAR trended toward a lower mortality in the low-risk group (n = 626; EVAR, 10% vs OR, 15%; $P = .07$), had a significantly lower mortality in the medium-risk group (n = 457; EVAR, 37% vs OR, 48%; $P = .02$), and no advantage in the high-risk group (n = 82; EVAR, 95% vs OR, 79%; $P = .17$). Across all risk groups, cardiac complications (EVAR, 29% vs OR, 38%; $P = .001$), respiratory complications (EVAR, 28% vs OR, 46%; $P < .0001$), renal insufficiency (EVAR, 24% vs OR, 38%; $P < .0001$), lower extremity ischemia (EVAR, 2.7% vs OR, 8.1%; $P < .0001$), and bowel ischemia (EVAR, 3.9% vs OR, 10%; $P < .0001$) were significantly lower after EVAR than after OR. Across all risk groups, median (interquartile range) intensive care unit length of stay (EVAR, 2 [1-5] days vs OR, 6 [3-13] days; $P < .0001$) and hospital length of stay (EVAR, 6 [4-12] days vs OR, 13 [8-22] days; $P < .0001$) were lower after EVAR.

Conclusions.—This novel risk-stratified comparison using a national clinical database showed that EVAR of RAAA has a lower mortality and morbidity compared with OR in low-risk and medium-risk patients and that EVAR should be used to treat these patients when anatomically

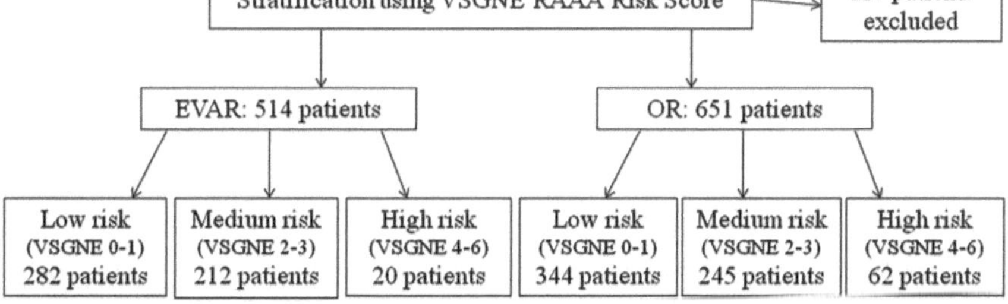

FIGURE 1.—Risk stratification of patients with ruptured abdominal aortic aneurysm (*RAAA*) from the Vascular Quality Initiative (*VQI*) who underwent endovascular repair (*EVAR*) and open repair (*OR*). *VSGNE*, Vascular Study Group of New England. (Reprinted from the Journal of Vascular Surgery. Ali MM, Flahive J, Schanzer A, et al. In patients stratified by preoperative risk, endovascular repair of ruptured abdominal aortic aneurysms has a lower in-hospital mortality and morbidity than open repair. *J Vasc Surg*. 2015;61:1399-1407, Copyright 2014, with permission from The Society for Vascular Surgery.)

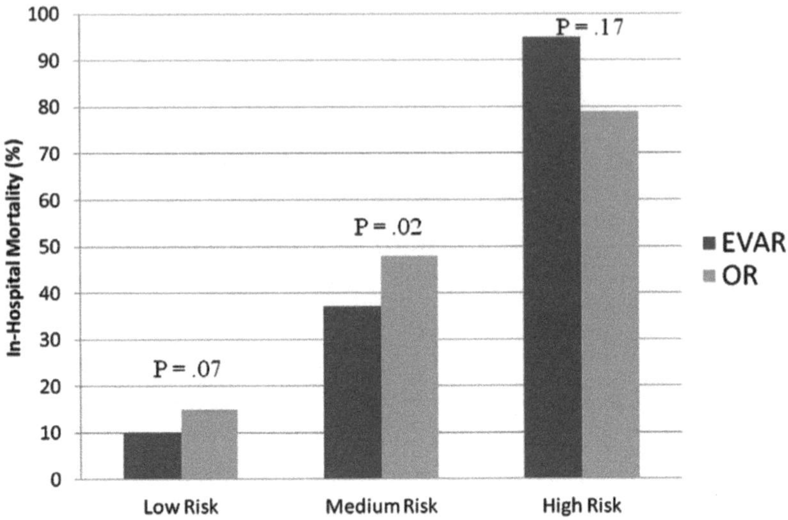

VSGNE RAAA Risk Score	0 – 1	2 – 3	4 – 6
N	626	457	82

FIGURE 2.—Comparison of in-hospital risk-stratified mortality for endovascular aneurysm repair (*EVAR*) and open repair (*OR*) in patients with ruptured abdominal aortic aneurysm (*RAAA*). *VSGNE*, Vascular Study Group of New England. (Reprinted from the Journal of Vascular Surgery. Ali MM, Flahive J, Schanzer A, et al. In patients stratified by preoperative risk, endovascular repair of ruptured abdominal aortic aneurysms has a lower in-hospital mortality and morbidity than open repair. *J Vasc Surg.* 2015;61:1399-1407, Copyright 2014, with permission from The Society for Vascular Surgery.)

feasible. For RAAA patients at the highest preoperative risk, there is no benefit to using EVAR compared with OR (Figs 1 and 2).

▶ Risk stratification for this study is listed in Fig 1. Among 514 patients who underwent endovascular aneurysm repair (EVAR) and 651 patients who underwent open repair (OR) of ruptured abdominal aortic aneurysms (RAAAs), EVAR had lower in-hospital mortality than did OR (EVAR, 25% vs OR, 33%; $P = .001$). In risk-stratified analysis, there was a trend toward lower in-hospital mortality after EVAR in the low-risk group ($n = 626$; EVAR, 10% vs OR, 15%; $P = .07$), significantly lower mortality after EVAR in the medium-risk group (n = 457; EVAR, 37% vs OR, 48%; $P = .02$), and no difference in mortality between EVAR and OR in the high-risk group (n = 82; EVAR, 95% vs OR, 79%; $P = .17$; Fig 2).

On the basis of this first risk-stratified comparison using a national clinical database, EVAR should be used to treat patients with RAAA when anatomically feasible. For RAAA patients at the highest preoperative risk, there is no benefit in using EVAR compared with OR. However, additional study is needed to account for anatomic factors in determining preoperative mortality risk.

B. W. Starnes, MD

Intra-operative Cone Beam Computed Tomography can Help Avoid Reinterventions and Reduce CT Follow up after Infrarenal EVAR

Törnqvist P, Dias N, Sonesson B, et al (Skåne Univ Hosp Malmö, Sweden)

Eur J Vasc Endovasc Surg 49:390-395, 2015

Objective/Background.—Re-interventions after endovascular abdominal aortic aneurysm repair (EVAR) are common and therefore a strict imaging follow up protocol is required. The purpose of this study was to evaluate whether cone beam computed tomography (CBCT) can detect intra-operative complications and to compare this with angiography and the 1 month CT follow up (computed tomography angiography [CTA]).

Methods.—Fifty-one patients (44 men) were enrolled in a prospective trial. Patients underwent completion angiography and CBCT during infrarenal EVAR. Contrast was used except when pre-operative renal insufficiency was present or if the maximum contrast dose threshold was reached. CBCT reconstruction included the top of the stent graft to the iliac bifurcation. Endoleaks, kinks, or compressions were recorded.

Results.—CBCT was technically successful in all patients. Twelve endoleaks were detected on completion digital subtraction angiography (CA). CBCT detected 4/5 type 1 endoleaks, but only one type 2 endoleak. CTA identified eight type 2 endoleaks and one residual type I endoleak. Two cases of stent compression were seen on CA. CBCT revealed five stent compressions and one kink, which resulted in four intra-operative adjunctive manoeuvres. CTA identified all cases of kinks or compressions that were left untreated. Two of them were corrected later. No additional kinks/compressions were found on CTA. Groin closure consisted of 78 fascia sutures, nine cut downs, and 11 percutaneous sutures. Seven femoral artery pseudoaneurysms (<1 cm) were detected on CTA, but no intervention was needed.

Conclusion.—CA is better than CBCT in detecting and categorizing endoleaks but CBCT (with or without contrast) is better than CA for detection of kinks or stentgraft compression. CTA plus CBCT identified all significant complications noted on the 1 month follow up CTA. The use of intra-operative CA and CBCT could replace early CTA after standard EVAR thus reducing overall radiation and contrast use. Technical development might further improve the resolution and usefulness of CBCT (Fig 3).

► In my mind, this article presents an inevitability. Eventually, our intraoperative imaging will be just as good and in many ways better than any other imaging currently available. This unique study indicates that intraoperative technical problems with endovascular aneurysm repair (EVAR) such as kinks and stent graft compression are better detected with cone-beam CT than with conventional angiography (Fig 3). This provides the ability of intraoperative correction, thus removing the need for secondary interventions.

Also, clinically relevant endoleaks are equally well seen between the 2 intraoperative imaging methods. Endoleaks found on early follow-up computed

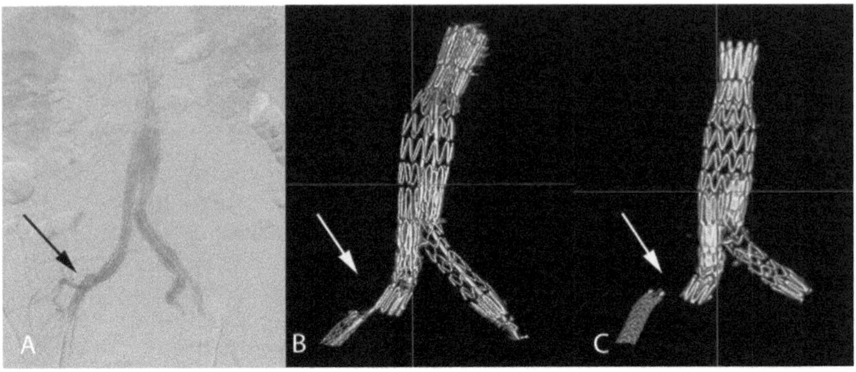

FIGURE 3.—Mis-alignment between the stents in the right iliac. (A) Completion angiography. The black arrow displays the area of interest. (B) Cone beam computed angiography (CBCT). The white arrow clearly shows kink between the iliac limb and the native artery. (C) Follow up computed tomography angiography (FU CTA) displays the same finding as the intra-operative CBCT. Note the effect of the absent guidewire when comparing CBCT and FU CTA. (Reprinted from the Journal of Vascular Surgery. Törnqvist P, Dias N, Sonesson B, et al. Intra-operative cone beam computed tomography can help avoid reinterventions and reduce CT follow up after infrarenal EVAR. *Eur J Vasc Endovasc Surg*. 2015;49:390-395, Copyright 2014, with permission from The European Society for Vascular Surgery.)

tomography angiography (CTA) were all type 2 and did not lead to further intervention. Early follow-up CTA did not add any additional information about stent graft configuration. The present results question the relevance of routine early CTA if intraoperative cone-beam CT is used. This could potentially reduce overall contrast and radiation exposure in the peri-operative setting.

One word of caution: Only 39% of patients undergoing standard EVAR were treated within the Instructions for Use (IFU) for the given device. This likely caused the event rate to be higher in the study. My belief is that this practice is best reserved for complex EVAR (fenestrated) for improving outcomes. I think it may be overkill for straightforward EVAR.

B. W. Starnes, MD

Outcomes of endovascular abdominal aortic aneurysm repair in high-risk patients

Lim S, Halandras PM, Park T, et al (Loyola Univ Chicago, Maywood, IL; Yonsei Univ, Seoul, Korea)

J Vasc Surg 61:862-868, 2015

Objective.—Although the endovascular aneurysm repair trial 2 (EVAR-2) demonstrated no benefit of EVAR in high-risk (HR) patients, EVAR is still performed widely in this patient cohort. This study compares the mid-term outcomes after EVAR in HR patients with those in normal-risk (NR) patients. In turn, these data are compared with the EVAR-2 data.

Methods.—A retrospective review from January 2006 to December 2013 identified 247 patients (75 HR [30.4%], 172 NR [69.6%]) who underwent elective EVAR for infrarenal aortic aneurysm in an academic tertiary institution and its affiliated Veterans Administration hospital. The same HR criteria used in the EVAR-2 trial were employed. Overall survival, graft-related complications, and reintervention rates were estimated by the Kaplan-Meier method. HR group outcomes were compared with the EVAR-2 data.

Results.—HR patients had a larger abdominal aortic aneurysm size and had a higher prevalence of cardiac disease ($P < .01$), chronic obstructive pulmonary disease ($P = .02$), renal insufficiency ($P < .01$), and cancer ($P < .01$). Use of aspirin (63% HR vs 66% NR; $P = .6$), statin (83% HR vs 72% NR; $P = .2$), and beta-blockers (71% HR vs 60% NR; $P = .2$) was similar; in the EVAR-2 trial, the corresponding use of these medications was 58%, 42%, and not available, respectively. Perioperative mortality (0% HR vs 1.2% NR; $P = 1.0$) and early complication rates (4% HR vs 6% NR; $P = .8$) were similar. In contrast, perioperative mortality in the EVAR-2 trial was 9%. At a mean follow-up of 3 years, the incidence rates of delayed secondary interventions for aneurysm- or graft-related complications were 7% for HR patients and 10% for NR patients ($P = .5$). The 1-, 2-, and 4-year survival rates in HR patients (85%, 77%, 65%) were lower than those in NR patients (97%, 97%, 93%; $P < .001$), but this was more favorable compared with a 36% 4-year survival in the EVAR-2 trial. No difference was seen in long-term reintervention-free survival in HR and NR patients ($P = .8$). Backward stepwise logistic regression analysis identified five prognostic indicators for post-EVAR death: age, chronic kidney disease stages 4 and 5, congestive heart failure, home oxygen use, and current cancer therapy.

Conclusions.—EVAR can be performed in patients unfit for open surgical repair with excellent early survival and long-term durability. These outcomes in the HR group compare more favorably to the EVAR-2 trial data. However, not all HR patients for open surgical repair derive the benefit from EVAR. The decision to proceed with EVAR in HR patients should be individualized, depending on the number and severity of risk factors (Fig 1 and Table 6).

▶ There has been an exponential increase in the number of endovascular aneurysm repairs (EVARs) being performed worldwide. Naturally, this popularity has been extended to high-risk patients with AAA who are medically unfit to undergo open surgical repair. This study illustrates that EVAR can be performed safely in high-risk patients with perioperative mortality and morbidity rates comparable to those in normal risk patients and that the results are more favorable than in the EVAR2 Trial (Fig 1).[1]

The findings in the present study mimic those of earlier studies to a great extent; 5 prognostic indicators for late post-EVAR mortality in descending order of importance were current cancer therapy, home oxygen dependency, advanced age, chronic kidney disease stage 4 or 5, and compromised ejection fraction. A new and important finding that has not been previously reported is

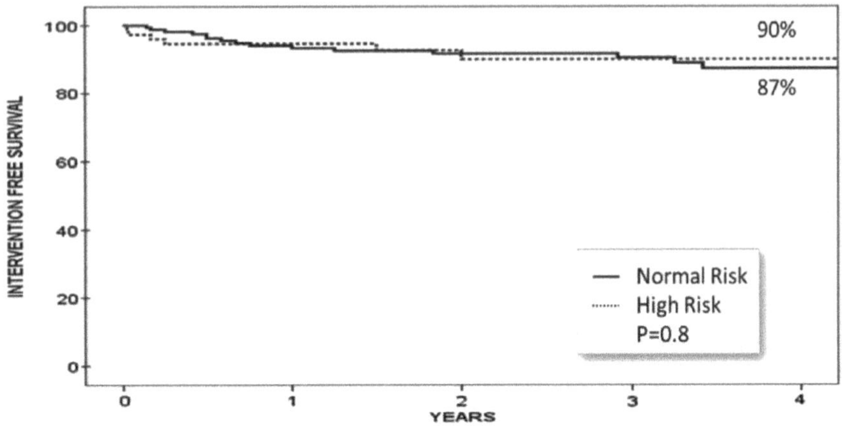

	0 yr	1 yr	2 yr	3 yr	4 yr
NR	172	126	99	68	42
HR	75	52	35	22	15

FIGURE 1.—Kaplan-Meier estimate for reintervention-free survival. *HR*, High risk; *NR*, normal risk. (Reprinted from the Journal of Vascular Surgery. Lim S, Halandras PM, Park T, et al. Outcomes of endovascular abdominal aortic aneurysm repair in high-risk patients. *J Vasc Surg*. 2015;61:862-868, Copyright 2014, with permission from The Society for Vascular Surgery.)

TABLE 6.—Predictors of Mortality After Endovascular Aneurysm Repair (EVAR)

	Hazard Ratio	95% CI	*P* Value
Age 70-80 years	3.1	1.26-7.47	.01
Age ≥80 years	5.8	2.11-13.72	<.01
Ejection fraction 20%-40%	2.9	1.03-7.19	.04
Ejection fraction ≤20%	3.6	1.03-12.82	.04
CKD stage 4-5	3.9	1.24-12.50	<.02
COPD and oxygen dependency	7.0	2.72-17.92	<.01
Current cancer treatment	11.3	3.59-35.62	<.01

CI, Confidence interval; *CKD*, chronic kidney disease; *COPD*, chronic obstructive pulmonary disease.

Reprinted from the Journal of Vascular Surgery. Lim S, Halandras PM, Park T, et al. Outcomes of endovascular abdominal aortic aneurysm repair in high-risk patients. *J Vasc Surg*. 2015;61:862-868, Copyright 2014, with permission from The Society for Vascular Surgery.

that current cancer therapy was not only a determinant of poor late outcomes but had the greatest impact (Table 6). These factors have their own weight and are additive in their impact on mortality. Current cancer therapy should be a strong deterrent to offering elective EVAR.

B. W. Starnes, MD

Reference

1. Greenhalgh RM, Brown LC, Powell JT, Thompson SG, Epstein D. Endovascular repair of aortic aneurysm in patients physically ineligible for open repair. *N Engl J Med.* 2010;362:1872-1880.

Outcomes of fenestrated endovascular repair of juxtarenal aortic aneurysm

Kristmundsson T, Sonesson B, Dias N, et al (Skåne Univ Hosp, Malmö, Sweden)

J Vasc Surg 59:115-120, 2014

Objective.—To evaluate late outcomes after fenestrated endovascular aortic repair (f-EVAR) in a tertiary European referral center.

Methods.—In 2009, we published short- and midterm results after f-EVAR in the first 54 patients treated with this technique at our center between September 2002 and June 2007. In this paper, we provide long-term follow-up of the same patient cohort with the main focus on target vessel (TV) patency, renal function, reinterventions, and survival.

Results.—A total of 54 patients were included in this study. Median age was 72 years (interquartile range [IQR], 68-76 years) at primary operation, and 85% were men. Median preoperative aneurysm diameter was 60 mm (IQR, 53-66 mm). One hundred thirty-four vessels were targeted (mean, 2.5 per patient), and 96 TV stents were placed. The median clinical follow-up was 67 months (IQR, 37-90 months), and computed tomography follow-up was 60 months (IQR, 35-72 months). Aneurysm diameter decreased ≥5 mm in 39% ± 7% at 12 months, 64% ± 8% at 36 months, and 71% ± 8% at 60 months. Primary TV patency was 94% ± 2% at 12 months, 91% ± 3% at 36 months, and 90% ± 3% at 60 months. Glomerular filtration rate decreased by 17% at 59 months (IQR, 26-73 months) follow-up (60 [IQR, 46-79] vs 50 [IQR, 38-72] mL/min/1.73 m^2; $P < .001$), and one patient became dialysis-dependent secondary to a renal stent occlusion. Reintervention-free survival was 88% ± 5% at 12 months, 69% ± 7% at 36 months, and 56% ± 5% at 60 months. At least one reintervention was done in 37% of patients, of which 29% were endoleak-related, 26% TV-related, 13% graft-limb-related, and 32% due to other causes. The majority of reinterventions (68%) were based on complications detected on routine follow-up. Estimated overall survival was 93% ± 4% at 12 months, 76% ± 6% at 36 months, and 60% ± 7% at 60 months. In total, 54% of the patients died during the 10-year study period, where 9% died of aneurysm-related causes.

Conclusions.—Long-term mortality after f-EVAR is high, but most patients die from nonaneurysmal causes. Aneurysm-related mortality is associated with technical complications that can be reduced with increased experience. Reinterventions are common, and most complications are detected on routine follow-up (Fig 2).

▶ This study provides useful long-term data on a small cohort of patients undergoing fenestrated endovascular aneurysm repair (FEVAR) from a previously reported cohort.[1] Half of patients are dead at 5 years and die most commonly of conditions not related to the aneurysm or anything device related.

Target vessel patency is excellent. At 1 year, estimated primary patency of all target vessels was 94% ± 2% and primary assisted patency was 96% ± 2%, which compares well to earlier reports of fenestrated and branched devices (Fig 2).

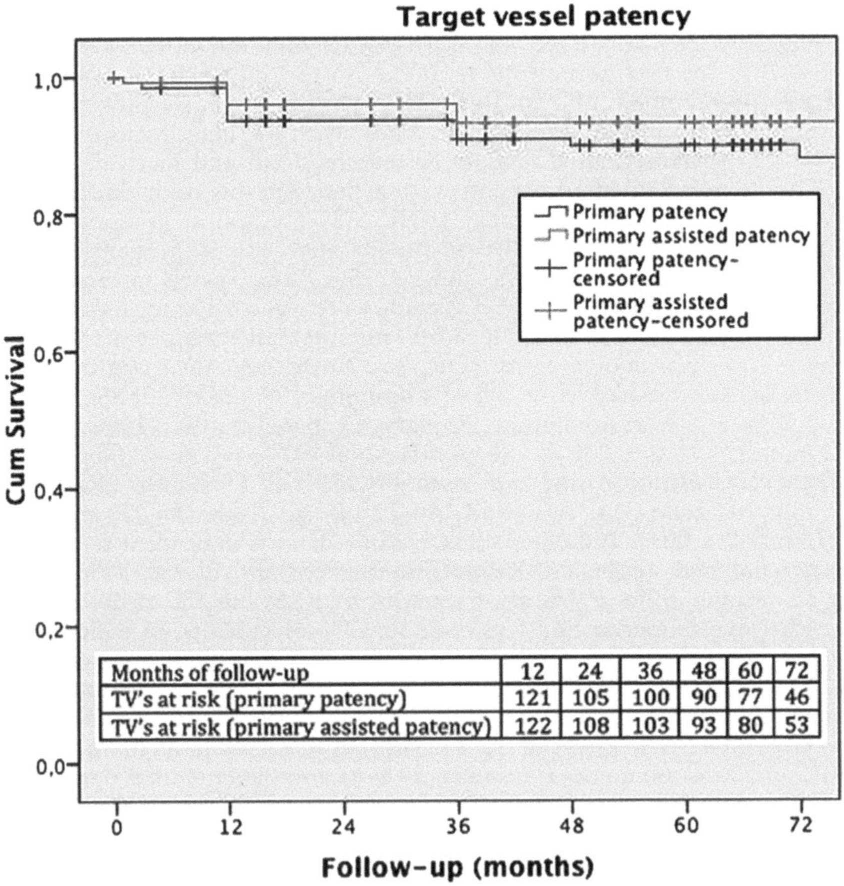

Months of follow-up	12	24	36	48	60	72
TV's at risk (primary patency)	121	105	100	90	77	46
TV's at risk (primary assisted patency)	122	108	103	93	80	53

FIGURE 2.—Kaplan-Meier Estimate of Primary and Primary-Assisted Target Vessel (*TV*) Patency Over Time. (Reprinted from the Journal of Vascular Surgery. Kristmundsson T, Sonesson B, Dias N, et al. Outcomes of fenestrated endovascular repair of juxtarenal aortic aneurysm. *J Vasc Surg*. 2014;59:115-120, Copyright 2014, with permission from The Society for Vascular Surgery.)

The authors report that aneurysm-related mortality is associated with technical complications that can be reduced with increased experience and better understanding of the stent graft behavior. This will of course be borne out in future, more mature series. We and others have recently reported the learning curve for FEVAR to be between 50 and 60 cases. This series of an initial 54 patients falls right into that zone meaning that we can expect the results to only get better.

B. W. Starnes, MD

Reference

1. Kristmundsson T, Sonesson B, Malina M, Bjorses K, Dias N, Resch T. Fenestrated endovascular repair for juxtarenal aortic pathology. *J Vasc Surg*. 2009;49: 568-574.

Part One: For the Motion. EVAR Offers No Survival Benefit over Open Repair for the Treatment of Ruptured Abdominal Aortic Aneurysms

Dubois L (Western Univ, London, Ontario, Canada)

Eur J Vasc Endovasc Surg 49:116-119, 2015

Background.—Endovascular aortic aneurysm repair (EVAR) is associated with less perioperative mortality compared to open aneurysm repair in a patient population characterized as elective and nonruptured. The risk of 30-day mortality is reduced about 50% using EVAR compared to open repair (OR) in elective abdominal aortic aneurysm (AAA) cases. It may not be as advantageous for high-risk patients. Discrepancies between observational studies and randomized controlled trials (RCTs) were discussed.

Comparing Findings.—Observational literature shows that EVAR performs better than OR, with mortality rates of 16% to 35% with EVAR but 37% to 63% with OR. Large administrative database studies also document these findings. Specific benefits accompanying EVAR for patients with a ruptured AAA include reduced physiological stress, ability to carry out the procedure under local anesthesia, reduced hypothermia, and less blood loss. With this support, some authors believe RCTs comparing the two approaches are unnecessary and possibly unethical.

The RCTs to date show no difference in early mortality between EVAR and OR in patients who have ruptured AAAs. Most involve small numbers of patients, but the IMPROVE trial is larger and more appropriately powered. It is designed pragmatically, including all patients who come for treatment with a suspected diagnosis of ruptured AAA. This ensures generalizability of the results, which indicated an equivalent 30-day mortality for EVAR and OR.

Analysis.—Observational studies suffer from several inherent biases that tend to favor EVAR. Most have a severe selection bias, with surgeons offering EVAR to ruptured patients who are sufficiently stable to undergo imaging and who have a favorable anatomy–both factors that are related to better postoperative morbidity rates. This would then favor the EVAR group. Patients with short necks and challenging anatomy would undergo OR; these features are riskier for patients whether they have EVAR or OR. In the IMPROVE trial, mortality was associated with aortic neck length regardless of the procedure done. Those with longer aortic neck lengths had lower mortality than those with short aortic neck lengths.

Other factors limiting the usefulness of observational studies are their errors in diagnostic coding, missing data on key confounding factors, and lack of information on the volume and experience of the surgeons who are performing the interventions. Observational studies also tend to overestimate the benefit of new interventions compared to RCTs.

Consequences.—If EVAR were the only option for ruptured AAA repair, patients with challenging anatomy could suffer devastating consequences. All of the patients in the IMPROVE trial who were converted from EVAR to OR because of misjudged anatomy died. Long-term, EVAR is associated with a high risk of repeat interventions associated with poor anatomy. Endoleakage and sac enlargement are more common in these patients as well. An aggressive EVAR policy would apply this approach for patients who are so moribund that they will not survive regardless of what treatment is given. Such a futile exercise wastes health care resources.

Conclusions.—Overemphasizing the perceived mortality benefits of EVAR for patients with ruptured AAAs may apply the technique too liberally. As a result, patients may be subjected to repeated interventions, higher mortality rates, and greater health care costs.

▶ This is the most up-to-date review of the controversial topic of endovascular aneurysm repair (EVAR) versus open repair (OR) for ruptured abdominal aortic aneurysm (rAAA). The conclusions of this "For the Motion" are worthy of reprint here: "Although most observational and administrative database studies suggest a reduction in mortality with EVAR for patients with a rAAA, randomized clinical trials have found equivalent early mortality when compared with OR. The observational literature suffers from selection bias, with EVAR generally reserved for those with favorable anatomy and hemodynamic stability."

The IMPROVE trial has shown that EVAR results in a reduced length of hospital stay and a higher proportion of home discharges. These benefits should be acknowledged, but a misinterpretation of the literature resulting in an aggressive "EVAR-only" policy may lead to increased short- and long-term morbidity and mortality if the procedure is attempted in those with unfavorable anatomy. The level I evidence suggests that the same care and attention that goes into selecting anatomically and physiologically suitable candidates for EVAR in the elective setting should also be applied to the ruptured patient. If patients are found to be poor anatomic candidates for EVAR, then they are likely best served with an expeditious OR.

B. W. Starnes, MD

Part Two: Against the Motion. EVAR Offers No Survival Benefit over Open Repair for the Treatment of Ruptured Abdominal Aortic Aneurysms

Mayer D, Rancic Z, Veith FJ, et al (Univ Hosp of Zurich, Switzerland)

Eur J Vasc Endovasc Surg 49:119-127, 2015

Background.—Considerable controversy surrounds the use of endovascular aneurysm repair (REVAR) versus open repair (ROR) for ruptured abdominal aortic aneurysm (rAAA). Four European randomized controlled trials (RCTs) compare REVAR with ROR, finding no significant difference in short-term (30-day) mortality between the two approaches. A critical appraisal of the RCTs assessed their methodologies and whether they offer trustworthy findings compared to other sources of data.

Methodological Issues.—The single-center UK Nottingham trial analyzed on an intention-to-treat (ITT) basis and recruited 103 patients, 32 of whom were randomized. The 30-day mortality was 53% for both REVAR and ROR. The trial's flaws include small size, number of excluded patients, and having just 15 patients undergo REVAR.

The multicenter French ECAR trial randomized only stable patients with suitable EVAR morphology and found no significant statistical difference in 30-day mortality between REVAR and ROR. Both had low mortality rates, but only 35% to 63% of patients were eligible for randomization.

The multicenter AJAX trial from the Netherlands randomized 22% of their patients and analyzed results on an ITT basis. No significant differences between the two approaches were noted for primary composite end of death and/or severe complications rates or mortality. Drawbacks include low proportion of randomized patients, imperfect interobserver agreement on computed tomographic (CT) diagnosis of rupture, and no transfer of suitable but unstable patients to centers where REVAR was an option as well as ROR. A high intraoperative conversion rate to ROR was attributed to access failure, type I endoleaks, and inexperience of the REVAR operators.

The UK IMPROVE trial was designed to be pragmatic and have a "real world design." Six hundred twenty-three patients clinically diagnosed with rAAA received either REVAR or ROR, with randomization followed by CT angiography. Patients allocated to REVAR were sometimes switched to ROR but remained in the REVAR strategy group for ITT analysis. Overall the 30-day mortality was 35% for REVAR and 37% for ROR groups. Mortality was significantly lower for women allocated to REVAR than for those in the ROR group (37% versus 57%, respectively). Patients having REVAR had significantly shorter critical care and hospital stays and were able to return home more often than those receiving ROR. Thirty-day mortality and costs were similar between the two groups.

Non-RCT Evidence.—Observational studies have some advantages over RCTs, including lower cost, greater timeliness, and a broader range of patients. Treatment effects in comparisons of REVAR and ROR find

TABLE 1.—Methodology and Limitations of Four European Randomized Controlled Trials.

Study	Country	Centers (n)	Start	End Suspected	End Definitive	Randomization	Patients Planned (*n*)	Patients Recruited (*n*) Total	REVAR	ROR	Limitations
Nottingham[1]	UK	1	Sep 2002	NA	Dec 2004	Unclear	100	32	15	17	Inclusion: high exclusion rate (69%) Team availability
ECAR[5]	France	14	Dec 2007	Dec 2010	Jan 2013	Per week, if stable (*after* CTA)	160	107	56	51	Patient selection: stable patients only Operator experience: 15 elective EVAR
AJAX[6]	the Netherlands	3[a]	Apr 2004	Oct 2007	Feb 2011	Block by computer (*after* CTA)	80 (2004) 112 (2008)	116	57	59	Patient selection: only stable patients could be referred to three trial centers Rupture diagnosis: moderate interobserver agreement (kappa = .59) Anatomic suitability: fair interobserver agreement (kappa = .39) Study: possibly underpowered
IMPROVE[7]	UK	30	Sep 2009	Mar 2013	Jul 2013	Block per telephone (*before* CTA)	600	613	316	297	Team availability: 66% of the week Team experience: 20 EVAR, five REVAR done Inclusion before CTA: inclusion of nonsuitable patients or non-rAAA

Editor's Note: Please refer to original journal article for full references.

Note. REVAR = ruptured endovascular aneurysm repair; ROR = ruptured open repair; NA = not applicable; CTA = computed tomographic angiography; EVAR = endovascular aneurysm repair; rAAA = ruptured abdominal aortic aneurysm.

[a]Of the 10 centers involved in AJAX, only three centers (the "trial centers") offered both REVAR and ROR.

Reprinted from the European Journal of Vascular and Endovascular Surgery. Mayer D, Rancic Z, Veith FJ, et al. Part two: against the motion. EVAR offers no survival benefit over open repair for the treatment of ruptured abdominal aortic aneurysms. *Eur J Vasc Endovasc Surg*. 2015;49:119-127, Copyright 2014, with permission from The European Society for Vascular Surgery.

similar outcomes. In addition, in centers that adhere to an "EVAR-whenever-possible protocol" REVAR has shown a 30-day mortality of 19.7% versus 36.3% for ROR. Observation also shows that an EVAR-only protocol should be accompanied by several adjunctive procedures and available materials. The Zurich algorithm identified five key points that contribute to success: hemodynamics, imaging, procedure, abdominal compartment syndrome, and teamwork.

Systematic reviews and meta-analyses have indicated that REVAR is not inferior to ROR, and several indicate REVAR is the superior approach. Five registries indicate that REVAR outperforms ROR.

Conclusions.—Provided the skills and materials to perform REVAR are available, REVAR should offer the best treatment option for patients with rAAA. The RCTs that have been performed are misleading in their conclusions because of methodological issues. Resources should be directed toward developing endovascular skill and team training to ensure better outcomes rather than expended in planning and performing more RCTs (Table 1).

▶ This is the second part of the debate from a reputable group in Switzerland putting forth the "against the motion" position.

Ideally, ruptured endovascular aneurysm repair (REVAR) is carried out by an interdisciplinary team of vascular surgeons, radiologists, anesthetists, and specialized scrub nurses. A standardized patient pathway for ruptured abdominal aortic aneurysms (rAAA) management and a reliable/experienced multidisciplinary team are the keys to improving patient outcomes. REVAR team training using high-fidelity simulation may be helpful in allowing less experienced colleagues to learn, practice, rehearse, improve, and maintain team-based knowledge, technical and human factor skills, and team attitudes to manage REVAR successfully.

To this group, REVAR is clearly the best treatment option for patients with a rAAA, provided the skills and materials to do it are available. Randomized controlled trials (RCTs) comparing REVAR and ruptured open repair are difficult to do, and those that have been published are misleading. It is our opinion that resources would be better directed toward developing endovascular skills and team training, rather than planning for further RCTs.

A useful summary of the 4 randomized control trials is listed in Table 1.

B. W. Starnes, MD

Prospective Evaluation of Post-implantation Inflammatory Response After EVAR for AAA: Influence on Patients' 30 Day Outcome

Arnaoutoglou E, Kouvelos G, Papa N, et al (Univ of Ioannina, Greece)

Eur J Vasc Endovasc Surg 49:175-183, 2015

Objectives.—The aim was to prospectively evaluate post-implantation syndrome (PIS) after elective endovascular aneurysm repair (EVAR) of abdominal aortic aneurysms (AAAs) and to investigate its association with clinical and laboratory parameters and the clinical outcome of the patients.

Methods.—From January 2010 till June 2013, 214 consecutive patients treated electively by EVAR for AAA were prospectively included. PIS was defined according to systemic inflammatory response syndrome criteria. Adverse events included any major adverse cardiovascular events (MACE), acute renal failure, re-admission and death from any cause.

Results.—PIS was diagnosed in 77 (34%) patients. Pre-operative white blood cell (WBC) count values ($p < .001$), endograft material (polyester) ($p < .001$), and heart failure ($p = .03$) were independent predictors of PIS. Mean post-operative temperature ($p < .001$), length of hospital ($p < .001$) and intensive care unit ($p = .008$) stay, as well as maximum post-operative WBC count ($p < .001$) and hs-CRP values ($p < .001$) were significantly higher in the PIS group. Post-operative hs-CRP ($p = .001$) and duration of fever ($p = .02$) independently predicted the occurrence of MACE. Post-operative hs-CRP ($p = .004$), maximum temperature ($p = .03$), and the presence of PIS ($p = .01$) were independent predictors of an adverse event during the first 30 days. A threshold of post-operative hs-CRP value of 125 mg/L was highly associated with the occurrence of MACE, with a sensitivity of 82% and specificity of 75%.

Conclusions.—A systematic inflammatory response is observed in a significant number of patients after EVAR. The type of endograft material seems to play a significant role in this inflammatory process. The intensity of inflammation, as assessed mainly by the post-operative hs-CRP values, correlates with the presence of a cardiovascular or any other adverse event during the first 30 days after the procedure (Fig 1).

▶ This unique, prospective study shows that postimplantation syndrome (PIS) affects nearly one-third of patients after endovascular aneurysm repair (EVAR) for abdominal aortic aneurysm (AAA). The reported incidence of PIS in the literature varies widely between 14% and 60%, and the lack of a universally accepted definition probably accounts for this variation. This group has proposed a definition of the syndrome according to systemic inflammatory response syndrome (SIRS) because PIS fulfills at least 2 of the SIRS criteria (fever and leukocytosis). In this study, PIS was defined as the presence of fever (> 38°C) and leukocytosis (> 12 000/uL). High-sensitivity C-reactive protein (hs-CRP) values were strongly related to the presence of PIS and emerged as an important predictor of 30-day outcome. A cutoff value of hs-CRP of 125 mg/dL in the immediate postoperative period could probably distinguish those patients who need extended surveillance. Such a policy could lead to early identification of any cardiovascular or other adverse event that would then be adequately treated.

Finally, another finding from this study that has been previously reported is that the type of endograft material (polyester) seems to play a significant role

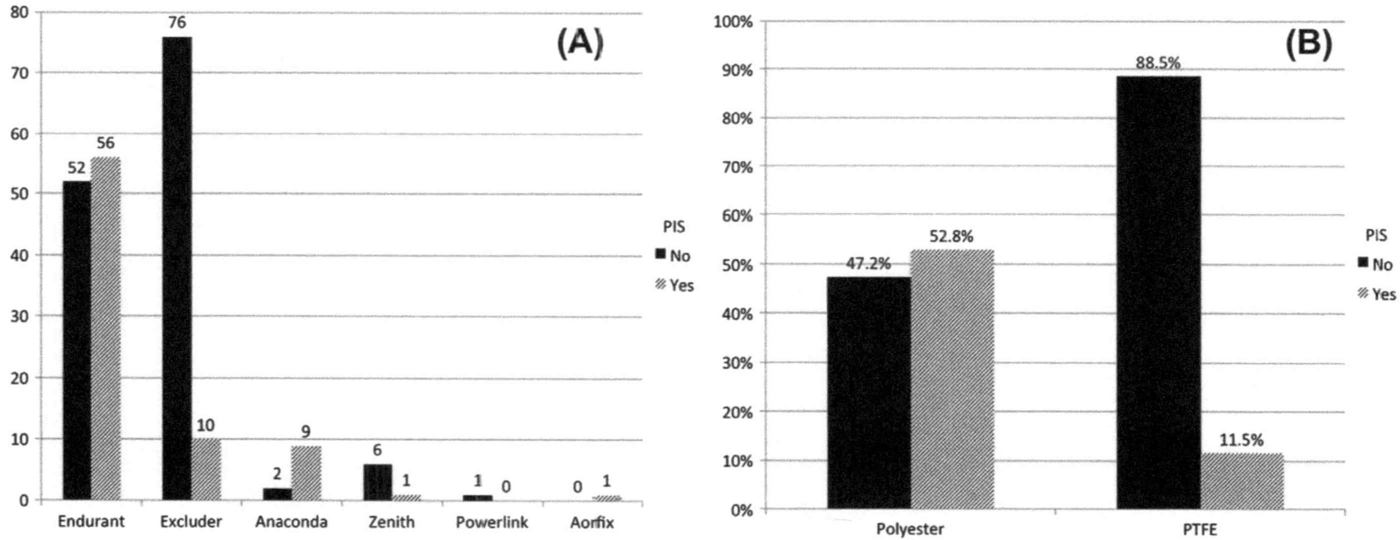

FIGURE 1.—(A) The relation between the different endografts deployed and the occurrence of post-implantation syndrome (PIS). (B) The material the endografts made and its relation to PIS. (Reprinted from the European Journal of Vascular and Endovascular Surgery. Arnaoutoglou E, Kouvelos G, Papa N, et al. Prospective evaluation of post-implantation inflammatory response after EVAR for AAA: influence on patients' 30 day outcome. *Eur J Vasc Endovasc Surg*. 2015;49:175-183, Copyright 2014, with permission from the European Society for Vascular Surgery.)

in this inflammatory process. Better bio-materials in the future may help reduce the incidence of PIS and thus potentially improve 30-day outcomes.

B. W. Starnes, MD

Readmissions after complex aneurysm repair are frequent, costly, and primarily at nonindex hospitals

Glebova NO, Hicks CW, Taylor R, et al (Univ of Colorado Denver, Aurora; Johns Hopkins Hosp, Baltimore, MD; Johns Hopkins Health System, Baltimore, MD)

J Vasc Surg 60:1429-1437, 2014

Objective.—Readmissions after complex vascular surgery are not well studied. We sought to determine the rate of readmission after thoracic and thoracoabdominal aortic aneurysm repair (TAA/TAAAR) at our institution and to identify risk factors for and costs of readmission.

Methods.—Using a prospectively collected institutional database in conjunction with a Maryland statewide database, we reviewed index admissions and early readmissions for all patients who underwent TAA/TAAAR between 2002 and 2013 at the Johns Hopkins Hospital. Only Maryland residents were included to capture readmissions to any Maryland hospital.

Results.—We identified 115 Maryland residents (58% men; mean age, 65 ± 1.2 years) undergoing TAA/TAAAR (57% open repair). Early readmissions were frequent and occurred in 29% of patients. Of the readmitted patients, 79% ($P < .001$) were not readmitted to the index hospital where their operation was performed. Readmitted patients were not significantly different from nonreadmitted patients in age, gender, race, aneurysm type, and index length of stay. They were not different in preoperative comorbidities (including coronary artery disease, diabetes mellitus, smoking, renal insufficiency, and pulmonary disease), postoperative neurologic, renal, and cardiovascular complications, or 30-day or 5-year mortality. Multivariable analysis showed that significant risk factors for readmission were open repair (odds ratio, 3.12; 95% confidence interval, 1.12-9.54; $P = .03$) and postoperative pneumonia (odds ratio, 4.31; 95% confidence interval, 1.28-15.4; $P = .02$). Readmitted patients had significantly lower average income compared with the nonreadmitted cohort (U.S. $62,000 ± $4000 vs $73,000 ± $3000; $P = .04$). Striking differences were seen between patients readmitted to the index hospital where the operation was performed, and those who were readmitted to a nonindex hospital: patients readmitted to the index hospital were readmitted mainly for aneurysm-related surgical issues, whereas patients readmitted to the nonindex hospital were readmitted for medical morbidities. An aneurysm-related intervention was required in 75% of patients readmitted to the index hospital vs in 9% of patients readmitted to the nonindex hospital. Readmissions to a nonindex hospital cost significantly less than to the index hospital (U.S. \$20,000 ± \$4400 vs \$42,000 ± \$8800; $P = .03$) and were not associated with increased overall mortality.

Conclusions.—Early readmissions after TAA/TAAA repair are frequent and often occur at hospitals other than the index institution. Risk factors for readmission include open repair and postoperative pneumonia but not

TABLE 4.—Characteristics of Patients Readmitted to the Index Hospital vs Nonindex Hospitals

Characteristics	Index Hospital	Readmitted To Nonindex Hospital	*P* Value
Patients	7 (21)	26 (79)	
Age, years	62.9 ± 3.9	69.7 ± 2.0	.12
Male sex	5 (71)	16 (62)	.63
Race			
White	4 (57)	20 (77)	.36
Black	3 (43)	6 (23)	
Income by zip code, U.S.\$	69,000 ± 12,000	59,000 ± 20,000	.28
Medicare/Medicaid payment source	3 (43)	14 (54)	.61
Distance from patient home zip code to JHH, miles	49.6 ± 19.4	30.6 ± 6.5	.24
Comorbidities			
Coronary artery disease	2 (29)	8 (31)	.91
Diabetes mellitus	3 (43)	3 (12)	.06
Smoking	5 (71)	16 (62)	.63
Hypertension	7 (100)	25 (96)	.60
Peripheral vascular disease	2 (29)	4 (15)	.58
Chronic renal insufficiency	2 (29)	2 (8)	.19
Chronic obstructive pulmonary disease	1 (14)	5 (19)	.76
Total number of comorbidities	3.14 ± 0.54	2.38 ± 0.28	.22
HSCRC			
Complexity score	2.71 ± 0.30	3.31 ± 0.15	.08
Mortality risk	3.43 ± 0.31	3.31 ± 0.16	.73
Type of aneurysm			
TAAA	0 (0)	14 (54)	.01
TAA	7 (100)	12 (46)	
Pathology			
Type B dissection	3 (43)	9 (35)	.69
Atherosclerosis	4 (57)	17 (65)	
Aneurysm size, cm	5.73 ± 0.49	6.54 ± 0.24	.15
Symptomatic presentation	6 (86)	13 (50)	.09
Urgent vs elective admission	13 (71)	31 (19)	.29
Repair type			
Open	2 (29)	11 (42)	.51
Endovascular	5 (71)	15 (58)	
Length of stay, days			
Index ICU	3.0 ± 4.2	8.0 ± 2.2	.30
Index overall	10.6 ± 12	15.4 ± 2.3	.39
Index discharge to			
Rehabilitation facility	1 (14)	13 (50)	.09
Home	6 (86)	13 (50)	

HSCRC, Health Services Cost Review Commission; *ICU*, intensive care unit; *JHH*, Johns Hopkins Hospital; *TAA*, thoracoabdominal aneurysm; *TAAA*, thoracoabdominal aortic aneurysm; *U.S.*, United States.

Continuous data are presented as mean ± standard error of the mean and categorical data as number (%).

Reprinted from the Journal of Vascular Surgery. Glebova NO, Hicks CW, Taylor R, et al. Readmissions after complex aneurysm repair are frequent, costly, and primarily at nonindex hospitals. *J Vasc Surg*. 2014;60:1429-1437, Copyright 2014, with permission from The Society for Vascular Surgery.

pre-existing patient comorbidities. Readmissions to nonindex hospitals were related to medical morbidities that were associated with fewer interventions and lower costs compared with the index hospital. Focusing on preoperative risk factors in this group of patients may not lead to reduction in readmissions. Minimizing nonsurgical complications may reduce post-TAA/TAAAR readmissions and the high costs associated with repeat care. (Table 4).

▶ Readmissions in vascular surgical patients will likely be the focus of attention in the near future. In the Medicare population, the readmission rate of vascular surgical patients is 24% overall.[1] These readmissions cost more on a per-readmission basis than any other condition studied, including coronary bypass surgery.

Readmissions are becoming an increasingly important problem as health care reimbursement schemes adjust to account for changes in federal policies. To date, minimal data exist on readmissions after complex vascular surgery. This analysis of readmissions after thoracic and thoracoabdominal aortic aneurysm repair (TAA/TAAAR) at a single tertiary care referral center identified a high early readmission rate of 29%, with only 21% of the readmitted patients returning to the index hospital where the aneurysm repair was actually performed and 79% of readmitted patients being rehospitalized at nonindex hospitals. Risk factors for readmission included poor socioeconomic status, open repair, and postoperative complications, such as pneumonia and wound infection, but not preoperative comorbidities (Table 4). Readmitted patients showed a trend toward higher 1-year mortality but had similar long-term mortality compared with nonreadmitted patients.

I think the important message here is that focusing on preoperative risk factors in this group of patients is unlikely to lead to a reduction in readmission rates. Minimizing nonsurgical complications and aggressively pursuing endovascular options for aneurysm repair, when anatomically feasible, may reduce readmissions after TAA/TAAAR and the high costs associated with repeat care.

B. W. Starnes, MD

Reference

1. Jencks SF, Williams MV, Coleman EA. Rehospitalizations among patients in the medicare fee-for-service program. *N Engl J Med.* 2009;360:1418-1428.

Results of the United States multicenter prospective study evaluating the Zenith fenestrated endovascular graft for treatment of juxtarenal abdominal aortic aneurysms

Oderich GS, on behalf of the Zenith Fenestrated Study Investigators (Mayo Clinic, Rochester, MN; et al)

J Vasc Surg 60:1420-1428, 2014

Objective.—This study reports the results of a prospective, multicenter trial designed to evaluate the safety and effectiveness of the Zenith fenestrated endovascular graft (Cook Medical, Bloomington, Ind) for treatment of juxtarenal abdominal aortic aneurysms (AAAs).

Methods.—Sixty-seven patients with juxtarenal AAAs were prospectively enrolled in 14 centers in the United States from 2005 to 2012. Custom-made fenestrated stent grafts were designed with one to three fenestrations on the basis of analysis of computed tomography data sets. Renal alignment was performed with balloon-expandable stents. Follow-up included clinical examination, laboratory studies, mesenteric-renal duplex ultrasound, abdominal radiography, and computed tomography imaging at hospital discharge and at 1 month, 6 months, and 12 months and yearly thereafter up to 5 years.

Results.—There were 54 male and 13 female patients with a mean age of 74 ± 8 years enrolled. Mean aneurysm diameter was 60 ± 10 mm. A total of 178 visceral arteries required incorporation with small fenestrations in 118, scallops in 51, and large fenestrations in nine. Of these, all 118 small fenestrations (100%), eight of the scallops (16%), and one of the large fenestrations (11%) were aligned by stents. Technical success was 100%. There was one postoperative death within 30 days (1.5%). Mean length of hospital stay was 3.3 ± 2.1 days. No aneurysm ruptures or conversions were noted during a mean follow-up of 37 ± 17 months (range, 3-65 months). Two patients (3%) had migration ≥10 mm with no endoleak, both due to cranial progression of aortic disease. Of a total of 129 renal arteries targeted by a fenestration, there were four (3%) renal artery occlusions and 12 (9%) stenoses. Fifteen patients (22%) required secondary interventions for renal artery stenosis/occlusion in 11 patients, type II endoleak in three patients, and type I endoleak in one patient. At 5 years, patient survival was 91% ± 4%, and freedom from major adverse events was 79% ± 6%; primary and secondary patency of targeted renal arteries was 81% ± 5% and 97% ± 2%, freedom from renal function deterioration was 91% ± 5%, and freedom from secondary interventions was 63% ± 9%.

Conclusions.—This prospective study demonstrates that endovascular repair of juxtarenal AAAs with the Zenith fenestrated AAA stent graft is safe and effective. Mortality and morbidity are low in properly selected patients treated in centers with experience in these procedures (Supplementary Tables 3 and 5).

► A total of 195 patients underwent imaging review by the planning center to determine eligibility. Of these, 128 patients (66%) were excluded because of the stringent anatomic criteria listed in Supplementary Table 3. Of the excluded 128 patients, the most common exclusion criterion was inadequacy of infrarenal aortic neck (<4 mm or >15 mm in length) in 60 patients (47%). This is a point that cannot be emphasized more. Two-thirds of patients were rejected due to anatomic criteria.

Rate of renal stent occlusion or stenosis was not significantly different for bare-metal stents (13%, 15 of 115) compared with covered stents (5%, 1 of 20; $P = .23$), although most experts only use covered stents for renal stenting.

SUPPLEMENTARY TABLE 3.—Reasons for Anatomic Exclusion From Participation in the Cook Zenith Fenestrated Abdominal Aortic Aneurysm (AAA) Endovascular Graft Trial

Criteria[a]	No.
Proximal neck <4 mm or >15 mm in length	60
Proximal neck diameter change over the length of the proximal seal zone >4 mm	37
Proximal neck >31 mm or <19 mm in diameter	34
Unsuitable arterial anatomy	33
Iliac artery diameter <0.5 mm at any point along access length	32
Proximal neck angulation >45 degrees relative to the long axis of the aneurysm	14
Significant occlusive disease, tortuosity, or calcification	12
Suprarenal neck angulation >45 degrees relative to the immediate infrarenal neck	9
Nonbifurcated segment of any artery to be stented <15 mm in length	9
Renal artery stenosis >50%	8
Ipsilateral iliac artery fixation site diameter <9.0 mm	7
Proximal seal site with circumferential thrombus/atheroma above the renal arteries	6
Inability to maintain at least one patent hypogastric artery	6
Iliac artery distal fixation site <30 mm in length	5
Aortic or aortoiliac aneurysm with diameter of ≤5 cm	4
Iliac artery diameter >21 mm at distal fixation site	4
Artery to be stented with a maximum diameter <3 mm or >8 mm at the vessel ostium	2
Total number of patients excluded	128

[a]A patient may meet more than one exclusion criterion.

Reprinted from the Journal of Vascular Surgery. Oderich GS, on behalf of the Zenith Fenestrated Study Investigators. Results of the United States multicenter prospective study evaluating the Zenith fenestrated endovascular graft for treatment of juxtarenal abdominal aortic aneurysms. *J Vasc Surg*. 2014;60:1420-1428, Copyright 2014, with permission from The Society for Vascular Surgery.

Freedom from renal artery occlusion was 98% 1% at 1 year and 97% 2% at 5 years (Supplementary Table 5). At 1 and 5 years, primary renal artery patency was 95% ± 2% and 81% ± 5%, respectively, and secondary renal artery patency was 98% ± 1% and 97% ± 2%, respectively. These results are certainly convincing and supportive of the long-term durability of renal stents after fenestrated endografting.

This study represents the updated and current results of the first prospective, multicenter analysis of endovascular repair with a fenestrated stent graft to treat juxtarenal abdominal aortic aneurysms. The Zenith fenestrated stent graft is based on a known platform, and the data presented in this study extend our confidence in this technique regarding its longer-term durability through 5 years. The observations of high technical success (100%), low 30-day mortality (1.5%), no conversion or rupture, only 1 (1.5%) type I and no type III endoleak, and high secondary target renal stent patency (97%) support the safety, effectiveness, and durability of the Zenith fenestrated stent graft and will thus serve as a benchmark for comparison with other devices or alternative endovascular techniques to treat similar anatomy.

A few technical lessons should be emphasized from the experience accumulated in this trial and from the well-written article. Renal artery motion is higher distal to the middle third of the renal arteries, indicating that stents should be kept as short in length (<2 cm) as possible. In our own series of more than

SUPPLEMENTARY TABLE 5.—Kaplan-Meier Estimates of Freedom From Renal Adverse Events in the Cook Zenith Fenestrated Abdominal Aortic Aneurysm (AAA) Endovascular Graft Trial

Examination Period	Freedom From Adverse Event, Kaplan-Meier Estimate (Standard Error)			
	Renal Infarct[a]	Renal Function Deterioration[b]	Dialysis[c]	Renal Artery Occlusion
1-month	0.895 (0.037) (n = 59) (e = 7) (c = 0)	1.000 (0) (n = 66) (e = 0) (c = 0)	1.000 (0) (n = 66) (e = 0) (c = 0)	1.000 (0) (n = 66) (e = 0) (c = 0)
12-month	0.880 (0.040) (n = 56) (e = 8) (c = 2)	1.000 (0) (n = 62) (e = 0) (c = 4)	1.000 (0) (n = 62) (e = 0) (c = 4)	0.969 (0.022) (n = 61) (e = 2) (c = 3)
24-month	0.880 (0.040) (n = 43) (e = 8) (c = 15)	0.981 (0.019) (n = 47) (e = 1) (c = 18)	1.000 (0) (n = 48) (e = 0) (c = 18)	0.937 (0.031) (n = 45) (e = 4) (c = 17)
36-month	0.880 (0.040) (n = 28) (e = 8) (c = 30)	0.947 (0.038) (n = 28) (e = 2) (c = 36)	1.000 (0) (n = 30) (e = 0) (c = 36)	0.937 (0.031) (n = 27) (e = 4) (c = 35)
48-month	0.880 (0.040) (n = 18) (e = 8) (c = 40)	0.912 (0.050) (n = 16) (e = 3) (c = 47)	1.000 (0) (n = 19) (e = 0) (c = 47)	0.937 (0.031) (n = 18) (e = 4) (c = 44)
60-month	0.880 (0.040) (n = 14) (e = 8) (c = 44)	0.912 (0.050) (n = 11) (e = 3) (c = 52)	1.000 (0) (n = 14) (e = 0) (c = 52)	0.937 (0.031) (n = 14) (e = 4) (c = 48)

c, Cumulative censored; *e*, cumulative events; *n*, patients at risk.
[a]As reported by sites, regardless of whether confirmed by core laboratory.
[b]Increase in serum creatinine >2 mg/dL and >30% from baseline in two or more tests.
[c]Dialysis in patients with normal preoperative renal function.
Reprinted from the Journal of Vascular Surgery. Oderich GS, on behalf of the Zenith Fenestrated Study Investigators. Results of the United States multicenter prospective study evaluating the Zenith fenestrated endovascular graft for treatment of juxtarenal abdominal aortic aneurysms. *J Vasc Surg*. 2014;60:1420-1428, Copyright 2014, with permission from The Society for Vascular Surgery.

200 patients, by far the most commonly used stent size is 7 × 22 with at least 4 to 5 mm of stent protruding into the aortic flow channel. The posterior orientation of a renal artery, especially on the right, may predispose to kinks distal to the stent edge, which can be difficult to detect on completion angiography. In these cases, a short flexible self-expandable stent extension may be added as a bridge between the rigid balloon expandable stent and the native artery. Debate continues about the need to place alignment stents in the superior mesenteric artery (SMA) or renal scallops. Although there were no instances of occlusion in the Zenith fenestrated trial, others have noted shuttering of the SMA by the fabric of single-width scallops, which may lead to bowel ischemic complications. In addition, placement of the distal bifurcated component can result in damage to alignment stents, which can be avoided by protection of the stent by inflation of an angioplasty balloon during advancement and retrieval of the distal device cannula.

In my opinion, the most important aspect of these cases revolves around the planning. Success increases with increasing experience but the learning curve is gradual with 60 cases of fenestrated endovascular aneurysm repair needed for mastery.[1]

B. W. Starnes, MD

Reference

1. Starnes BW, Arthurs Z, Singh N, Caps M. Learning Curve for Fenestrated EVAR. Presented at Vascular Annual Meeting, Vascular and Endovascular Surgery Society, June 17, 2015

Role of type II endoleak in sac regression after endovascular repair of infrarenal abdominal aortic aneurysms

Kray J, Kirk S, Franko J, et al (Mercy Med Ctr and Iowa Heart Ctr, Des Moines)
J Vasc Surg 61:869-874, 2015

Objective.—Endovascular repair (EVAR) of infrarenal aortic aneurysms (AAA) is increasingly used in patients with suitable aortic morphology conforming to device-specific instructions for use. Despite improvements in graft design, type II endoleak (EL-2) from the inferior mesenteric artery (EL-IMA) or the lumbar artery (EL-LA) remains the Achilles' heel of EVAR. The objective of this study was to evaluate the natural history of the AAA sac after EVAR. We hypothesized that persistent EL-2 would be associated with inferior AAA sac volume regression.

Methods.—A retrospective analysis was performed on all nonruptured AAA treated by elective EVAR using Food and Drug Administration-approved endografts from January 2005 to December 2008 in our facility. Review of medical records and preoperative and follow-up computed tomography angiograms at 1, 6, and 12 months was performed. Patients with type I, III, and IV endoleaks were excluded, as were those lost to all follow-up. AAA size and volume were analyzed using TeraRecon software (Aquarius Intuition, Foster City, Calif). Change in AAA sac volume was compared in patients with and without EL-2, and with an occluded vs patent IMA.

Results.—The study cohort comprised 191 patients (161 men, 30 women) with a mean age of 74 years. The mean preoperative AAA diameter was 5.5 cm (range, 4-11 cm), and mean volume was 137.45 cm^3. EL-2 was present in 24% at completion of EVAR and in 9% at a mean follow-up of 6 months (range 4-8 months). Completion angiography at 1 month showed 63% of EL-2 had resolved. Those with EL-2 present at 1 month had statistically inferior sac regression compared with those who did not (23% reduction vs 2% increase at 1 year; $P = .002$). Preoperatively, the IMA was occluded by coils or was chronically occluded in 82 patients vs 109 patients who had a patent IMA. At the 6-month follow-up, patients with an occluded IMA had an EL-2 rate of 2.4% vs 14.7% in those with a patent IMA ($P = .005$ by *t*-test). Sac volume regression was 21.8% in those with an occluded IMA vs 13.2% in those with a patent IMA ($P = .004$ by *t*-test). Regression in AAA sac volume was highly significant in patients with occluded IMA, at 30% vs 16% at 1 year ($P = .0018$ by two-sided *t*-test).

Conclusions.—The presence of persistent EL-2 after EVAR results in inferior AAA sac regression. A preoperatively patent IMA is associated with increased rates of EL-2 and inferior AAA sac regression. Consideration should be given to preoperative occlusion of a patent IMA before EVAR (Fig 4).

▶ Follow-up data were available for 191 patients (161 men, 30 women) for up to 12 months and formed the basis of this analysis. Complications for the entire cohort were < 6%, and there were no in-hospital deaths and no late ruptures. No secondary interventions were performed for type 2 endoleak (EL-2) within the first 6 months of follow-up. Beyond 6 months, the secondary intervention rate was 3.7% (3 of 82) in patients with an occluded inferior mesenteric artery (IMA; either intentionally or chronically) versus 9.2% (10 of 109) in patients with a patent IMA ($P = .15$), giving an overall secondary intervention rate of

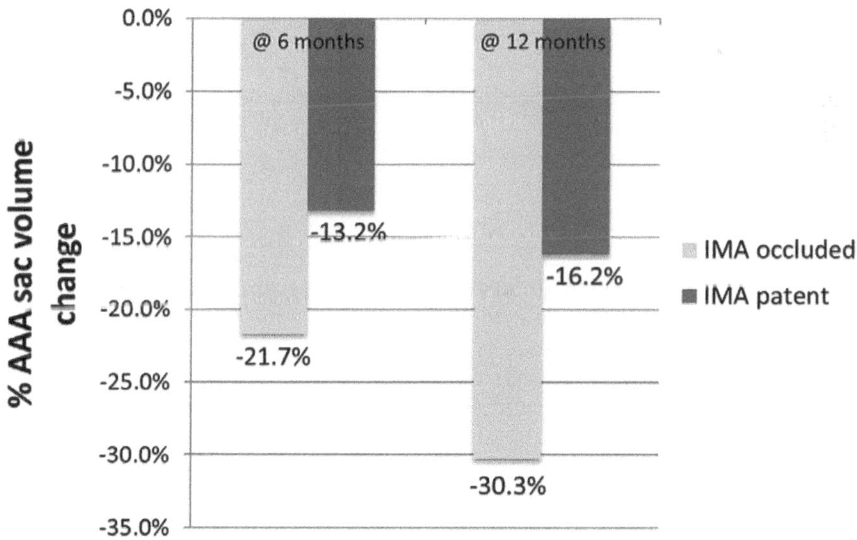

FIGURE 4.—Abdominal aortic aneurysm (*AAA*) volume change is shown by inferior mesenteric artery (*IMA*) status at 6 and 12 months. (Reprinted from the Journal of Vascular Surgery. Kray J, Kirk S, Franko J, et al. Role of type II endoleak in sac regression after endovascular repair of infrarenal abdominal aortic aneurysms. *J Vasc Surg*. 2015;61:869-874, Copyright 2014, with permission from The Society for Vascular Surgery.)

6.8%. All secondary interventions were performed for abdominal aortic aneurysm (AAA) sac enlargement.

Patency of the IMA at baseline had a significant effect on the presence of EL-2 at 6 months. When the IMA was occluded before endovascular repair (EVAR) (n = 82), 2 EL-2 were detected at 6 months (2.4%) versus 16 EL-2 (14.7% of 109 patients with a patent IMA; $P = .005$). Furthermore, EL-2 at 6 months due to both IMA and lumbar arteries (LAs) were significantly more common among those patients with a patent IMA at baseline compared with those with an initially occluded IMA (8.8% vs 1.2%; $P = .044$). Patency of the IMA at baseline also significantly influenced the degree of AAA sac shrinkage at 6 months and 12 months after EVAR (Fig 4). At 6 months, the mean AAA sac volume was reduced more in patients with an occluded IMA than in patients with a patent IMA, at 21.7% ± 18.4% versus 13.2% ± 15.8% ($P = .01$), which corresponded to an average volume reduction of 33 ± 39 mL versus 17 ± 22 mL ($P = .003$). At 12 months, mean AAA sac volume in patients with an occluded IMA at baseline was reduced by 30.3% ± 21.8% versus 16.2% ± 19.2% in patients with patent IMA ($P = .003$).

To my knowledge, this study is the first to demonstrate that a preoperatively occluded IMA is associated with significantly less EL-2 of any type (IMA and LA) and leads to a significantly greater degree of AAA sac volume reduction on follow-up. This is something I may start doing based on this study.

B. W. Starnes, MD

Rupture rates of untreated large abdominal aortic aneurysms in patients unfit for elective repair

Parkinson F, Ferguson S, Lewis P, et al (Royal Gwent Hosp, Newport, UK; et al)

J Vasc Surg 61:1606-1612, 2015

Background.—Elective abdominal aortic aneurysm (AAA) surgery relies on balancing the risk of the intervention against the risk of the aneurysm causing death. Although much is known about intervention at 5.5 cm, little is known about the fate of the patient unfit for elective surgery at this threshold. Medical therapy and endovascular surgery have revolutionized management of aortic aneurysms in the last 20 years and are thought to have affected rupture rates.

Methods.—MEDLINE via PubMed, EMBASE, and the Cochrane Library Database were searched for studies reporting follow-up of untreated large AAA approach from inception to January 2014. Data were pooled using random-effects analysis with standardized mean differences and 95% confidence intervals (CIs) reported. The primary end points were rupture rates and all-cause mortality per year by AAA size.

Results.—The search strategy identified 1892 citations, of which 11 studies comprising 1514 patients experiencing 347 ruptured AAA were included. The overall incidence of ruptured AAA in patients with AAA >5.5 cm was 5.3% (95% CI, 3.1%-7.5%) per year. This represented cumulative yearly rupture rates of 3.5% (95% CI, −1.6% to 8.7%) in AAAs 5.5 to 6.0 cm, 4.1% (95% CI, −0.7% to 9.0%) in AAAs 6.1 to 7.0 cm, and 6.3% (95% CI, −1.8% to 14.3%) in AAAs >7.0 cm. There was no heterogeneity between studies ($I^2 = 0\%$). Only 32% of these patients were offered repair on rupturing an AAA, with a perioperative mortality of 58% (95% CI, 32%-83%). The risk of death from causes other than AAA was higher than the risk of death from rupture.

Conclusions.—Rupture rates of untreated AAA were lower than those currently quoted in the literature. Non-AAA-related mortality in this group of patients is high (Figs 1 and 2).

▶ I've always wondered why we sometimes see giant aortic aneurysms (my personal record is 19 cm transverse diameter) in asymptomatic patients. How in the hell did it get that large? I've also questioned why some 4-cm aneurysms rupture when the risk is quoted to be so low. This study is interesting and gives us current clean data on rupture risk for a variety of aneurysm sizes. The methodology for this study is listed in Fig 1.

Elective abdominal aortic aneurysm (AAA) surgery relies on careful risk balancing. The risk of aneurysm rupture and death needs to be balanced against perioperative risk and an expectation of individual long-term survival. Without accurate numbers for this risk, the decision to intervene for a specific patient is flawed and runs the danger of being of higher risk than not treating the AAA with surgery.

The overall incidence of ruptured AAA in patients with an AAA greater than 5.5 cm was 5.3% (95% confidence interval, 3.-7.5) per year (Fig 2). Pooled risk of rupture was 3.5% for AAAs 5.5 to 6.0 cm, 4.1% for AAAs 6.1 to 7.0 cm, and 6.3% for AAAs greater than 7.0 cm. Quoted yearly rupture rates are cumulative, that is, a 7.5-cm AAA would have a 63% 10-year risk of rupture.

The results here fit with recent trends in the literature. The most recent analysis of rupture rates of small AAAs was between 0% and 1.61%,[1] roughly half of the rate at 5.5 to 6.0 cm in this analysis. A recent population-based study found the perioperative mortality in both medically fit and unfit patients for rupture was 53%, lower than that seen here, as would be expected. These findings have several practical implications. Multidisciplinary teams denying patients repair at 5.5 cm because of fitness for surgery can reassure patients that their risk of rupture, at 3.5% per year, is probably lower than they expect. Continued surveillance and reconsidering repair if the aneurysm size increases may be worthwhile. Attrition in this patient group from non-AAA causes will be high. A refusal of elective repair does not necessarily preclude a patient from successful emergency repair, and a frank discussion and documentation of this decision

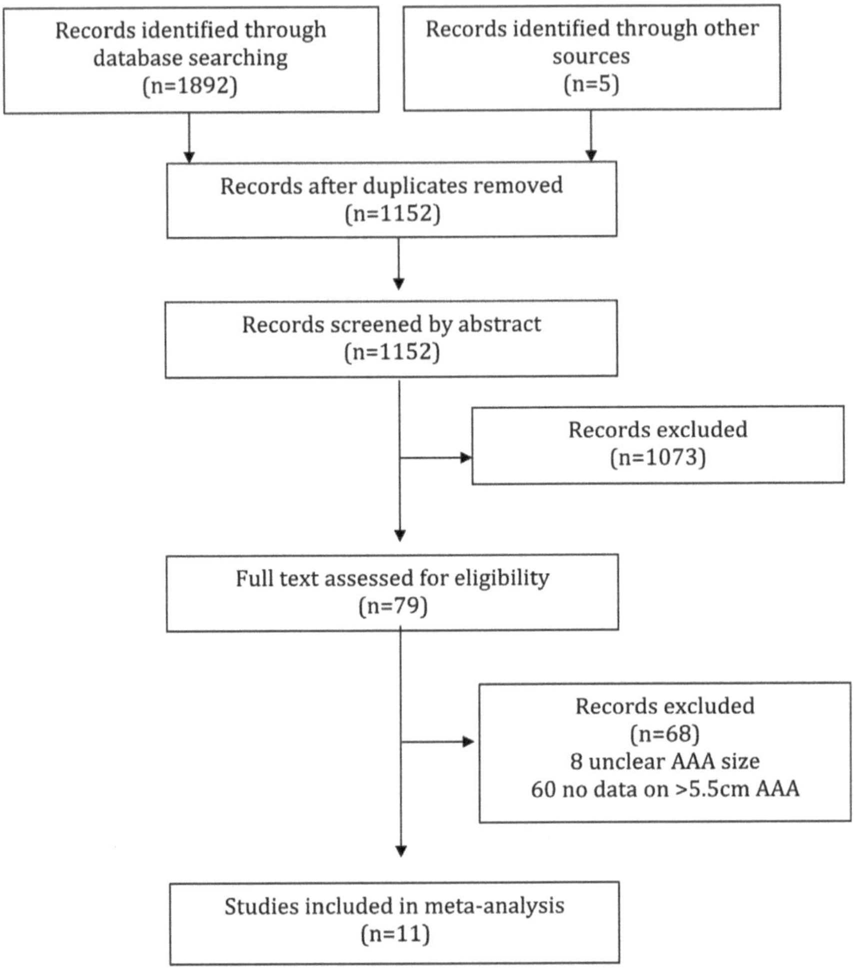

FIGURE 1.—Identification process for eligible studies. *AAA*, Abdominal aortic aneurysm. (Reprinted from the Journal of Vascular Surgery. Parkinson F, Ferguson S, Lewis P, et al. Rupture rates of untreated large abdominal aortic aneurysms in patients unfit for elective repair. *J Vasc Surg*. 2015;61:1606-1612, Copyright 2014, with permission from The Society for Vascular Surgery.)

should be separate from denying the patient an elective repair. Units performing emergency repair in these patients can expect a higher mortality than those routinely turning them down, which is another argument toward publishing elective and emergency turndown rates as surgeon level data reporting continues to expand. Large, population-based data with good postmortem or hospital-based diagnosis of ruptured AAA are required for more robust reporting.

The conclusions from this meta-analysis were that the rupture rate in patients with large aneurysms unfit for elective repair is lower than is commonly quoted. All-cause mortality in this group remains high. Outcomes following repair of

Study or Subgroup	Weight	Std. Mean Difference IV, Random, 95% CI
Tanquilut 2002	2.4%	2.60 [−11.51, 16.71]
Western 2013	8.7%	2.80 [−4.65, 10.25]
Conway 2001	10.2%	3.50 [−3.36, 10.36]
Brown 1999	11.5%	3.80 [−2.67, 10.27]
Jones 1998	4.3%	4.50 [−6.08, 15.08]
Lederle 2002	14.9%	4.50 [−1.18, 10.18]
Tambyraja 2003	4.5%	4.80 [−5.59, 15.19]
Noronen 2013	8.7%	6.00 [−1.45, 13.45]
Aziz 2004	6.2%	6.10 [−2.72, 14.92]
EVAR 2	10.2%	7.30 [0.44, 14.16]
Brown 2003	18.5%	7.90 [2.80, 13.00]
Total (95% CI)	**100.0%**	**5.28 [3.09, 7.47]**

Heterogeneity: Tau² = 0.00; Chi² = 2.54, df = 10 (P = 0.99); I² = 0%
Test for overall effect: Z = 4.72 (P < 0.00001)

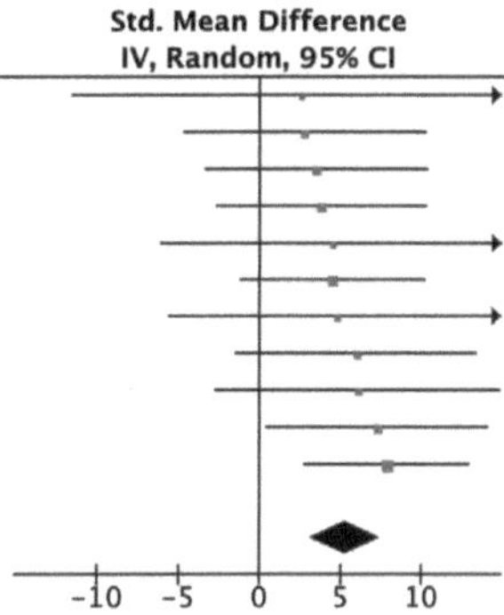

FIGURE 2.—Forest plot shows the rate of large abdominal aortic aneurysms (AAAs) in patients unfit for surgery. The *solid squares* indicate the mean difference and are proportional to the weights used in the meta-analysis. The *solid vertical line* indicates no effect. The *diamond* indicates the weighted mean difference and the lateral tips of the diamond indicate the associated confidence intervals (*CIs*) The *horizontal lines* represent the 95% CIs. *EVAR 2*, Endovascular Aneurysm Repair and Outcome in Patients Unfit For Open Repair of Abdominal Aortic Aneurysm; *IV*, inverse variance; *SE*, standard error. (Reprinted from the Journal of Vascular Surgery. Parkinson F, Ferguson S, Lewis P, et al. Rupture rates of untreated large abdominal aortic aneurysms in patients unfit for elective repair. *J Vasc Surg*. 2015;61:1606-1612, Copyright 2014, with permission from The Society for Vascular Surgery.)

rupture in patients turned down for elective surgery are worse than for all patients undergoing ruptured AAA repair.

B. W. Starnes, MD

Reference

1. Powell JT, Gotensparre SM, Sweeting MJ, Brown LC, Fowkes FG, Thompson SG. Rupture rates of small abdominal aortic aneurysms: a systematic review of the literature. *Eur J Vasc Endovasc Surg*. 2011;41:2-10.

The compatibility of p-branch "off-the-shelf" fenestrated endovascular graft in Asian patients with juxtarenal aortic aneurysm

Ou J, Cheng SWK, Chan YC, et al (The Univ of Hong Kong)

J Vasc Surg 61:1417-1423, 2015

Objective.—The Zenith pivot branch (p-branch) fenestrated endovascular graft (Cook Medical, Bloomington, Ind) is a new "off-the-shelf" device to treat patients with juxtarenal aortic aneurysms (JRAs). Two options are currently available, which appear to suit >70% of white patients. This study investigates the anatomic applicability of the p-branch fenestrated graft in a cohort of Asian patients with JRA.

Methods.—Computed tomography images of 51 consecutive Asian patients with JRA (43 men; mean age, 76.8 years) were analyzed on an Aquarius workstation (TeraRecon, San Mateo, Calif) and matched to two current configurations of the p-branch (options A and B: single superior mesenteric artery [SMA] and two renal fenestrations, and a celiac axis scallop). With use of the SMA as reference, the anatomic positions of both renal arteries and the celiac axis were figured together with their diameters on a template generated on MATLAB (MathWorks, Natick, Mass), and then they were matched with two graft configurations. The renal artery origins were assessed for three classes of "closeness of fit" based on diameter: perfect match, marginal match, and mismatch, respectively, defined as the renal artery origins being located entirely inside, partially inside, and completely outside their corresponding fenestrations. The suitability of the p-branch graft design to the aneurysms was then evaluated.

Results.—A total of 31 JRA patients (60.8%) were regarded as suitable candidates for one or both p-branch stent grafts (20 with option A, 22 with option B, and 11 with both options). In 35 patients (68.6%), both renal arteries could be aligned with the fenestrations. Among them, 16 patients (31.4%) were perfectly matched, whereas 19 patients (37.2%) were only marginally suitable. The major reason for exclusion was the misalignment of the renal fenestrations. In 16 patients with unsuitable renal fenestrations, 8 were attributed to the right renal origins being located too distally compared with their corresponding fenestrations. Another reason for exclusion was the position of the celiac axis scallop in four patients (7.84%), and insufficient aortic length for the graft was encountered in another four. If the right renal fenestration of option B was adjusted to 20 mm caudal to the SMA fenestration (level with the left fenestration), the match of renal fenestration could reach 78.4% (40 of 51).

Conclusions.—The present design of the p-branch off-the-shelf fenestrated graft is feasible for a good proportion of JRA patients in Asia. Further refinement of design may improve the anatomic match, especially a lower right renal artery origin (Fig 1).

▶ The p-branch fenestrated graft, manufactured by Cook Medical, has been introduced for treatment of juxtarenal aneurysms in some parts of the world (Fig 1). Two designs based on the anatomy of Caucasian patients with regard to the position of fenestrations and scallops are available. Two previous studies used a simple clock-face positioning of the renal origins on 1 standard graft design and reported that the anatomic suitability of this graft could exceed 70%. However, whether this can be translated to Asian patients, who have smaller renal arteries and aorta diameters, remains unknown. The aim of this study was to assess the applicability of the p-branch graft in Asian patients with juxtarenal aneurysms, taking into account the actual diameter of the renal artery origin as well as the final size of the stent graft to achieve a better match.

This study revealed that only 60.8% of Asian patients with juxtarenal aneurysms could be regarded as suitable candidates for the p-branch graft, about 10% less than their Caucasian counterparts. Even with the 15-mm pivot design, the renal fenestration was still the main reason for exclusion. In this cohort of patients, the mismatch of the right renal fenestration was particularly evident.

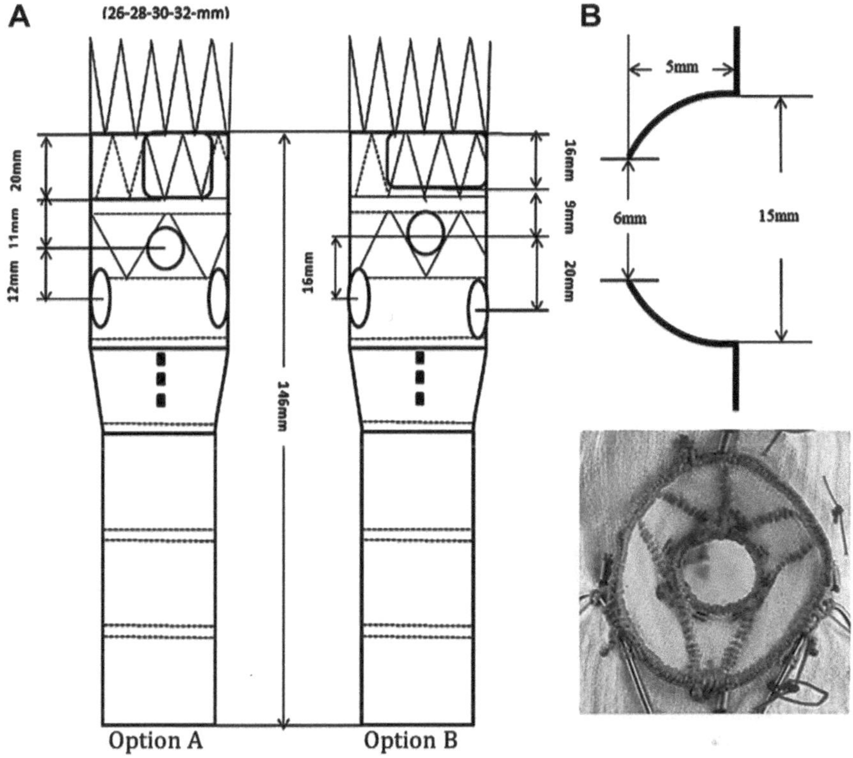

FIGURE 1.—The design of the Zenith p-branch endovascular graft. **A**, Two versions of p-branch graft (*left*, option A; *right*, option B). **B**, Renal p-branch, lateral view and outside view. (Reprinted from the Journal of Vascular Surgery. Ou J, Cheng SWK, Chan YC, et al. The compatibility of p-branch "off-the-shelf" fenestrated endovascular graft in Asian patients with juxtarenal aortic aneurysm. *J Vasc Surg*. 2015;61:1417-1423, Copyright 2014, with permission from The Society for Vascular Surgery.)

The authors found no significant differences of the relative distances from the superior mesenteric artery between the right and left renal arteries.

However, the right renal pivot of option B is placed in a higher position than the left. A simple readjustment of the right pivot fenestration in option B to a lower level in line with the left fenestration would result in an approximate 10% improvement in graft compatibility.

Even among the 68.6% of patients considered suitable for both renal fenestrations, more than half (37.2%) were marginally matched. In these marginally suitable patients, the renal stent may be subjected to higher deformation forces, leading to stent fractures or occlusions. Because all the fenestrations of the stent graft must be stented, further investigation into the long-term effects on the stents in this marginally matched condition is necessary. Whereas the position of the celiac axis scallop appeared to fit most of these Asian patients, a certain proportion of celiac trunks were partially covered by the edge of the stent graft, producing a "shuttering" effect. Once this is observed, the partially covered celiac trunk might be stented to preserve long-term patency. In this regard, the applicability could increase further by 6% because 3 celiac trunks of unsuitable patients were partially misaligned and could be stented. The length of the graft is also an important factor to consider in Asians with shorter stature. The authors stated that shortening the graft by 2 cm may expand the suitable patients with shorter abdominal aortas and allow treatment of patients with previous prosthetic or endovascular aneurysm repairs.

B. W. Starnes, MD

Type Ia endoleaks after fenestrated and branched endografts may lead to component instability and increased aortic mortality

O'Callaghan A, Greenberg RK, Eagleton MJ, et al (Cleveland Clinic Foundation, OH)

J Vasc Surg 61:908-914, 2015

Objectives.—Fenestrated and branched endografts allow for proximal sealing zone extension into or above the visceral aorta to optimize landing in healthy aorta. We describe the incidence, causes, and implications of proximal endoleak development in patients undergoing complex endovascular aortic aneurysm repair.

Methods.—All patients undergoing a fenestrated/branched repair were entered onto a prospective database, and this analysis included all those with at least one postoperative contrast computed tomography scan. Preoperative and postoperative three-dimensional imaging was reanalyzed to characterize morphology and identify endoleak. A blinded assessor used the preoperative imaging to resize the repairs in the endoleak group and a matched cohort of patients without endoleak. The outcome measures were proximal endoleak development, mortality, and component stability, and a comparison was made with all patients undergoing complex aortic repair.

Results.—From 2001 to July 2013, 969 patients underwent repair in a physician-sponsored investigational device exemption trial. Excluded were 24 emergency patients and 21 patients without requisite imaging, leaving 924 available for analysis. A proximal type Ia endoleak developed in 26 patients (2.8%). Poor choice of landing zone was implicated in most cases, with an area of sealing in the visceral aorta, compared with the thoracic aorta, being significantly associated with endoleak development ($P < .01$). Aortic-related mortality was significantly higher in the endoleak group (26.9%) than in the group without endoleak (6.2%; $P = .001$). These patients also experienced a higher incidence of component instability of 30.8% compared with 9.6% in patients without type Ia endoleak ($P < .01$).

Conclusions.—Fenestrated/branched endovascular repair has a low incidence of sealing zone failure despite the increased complexity. However, development of a proximal endoleak destabilizes the repair and leads to increased mortality. Increasing complexity of design seems to improve

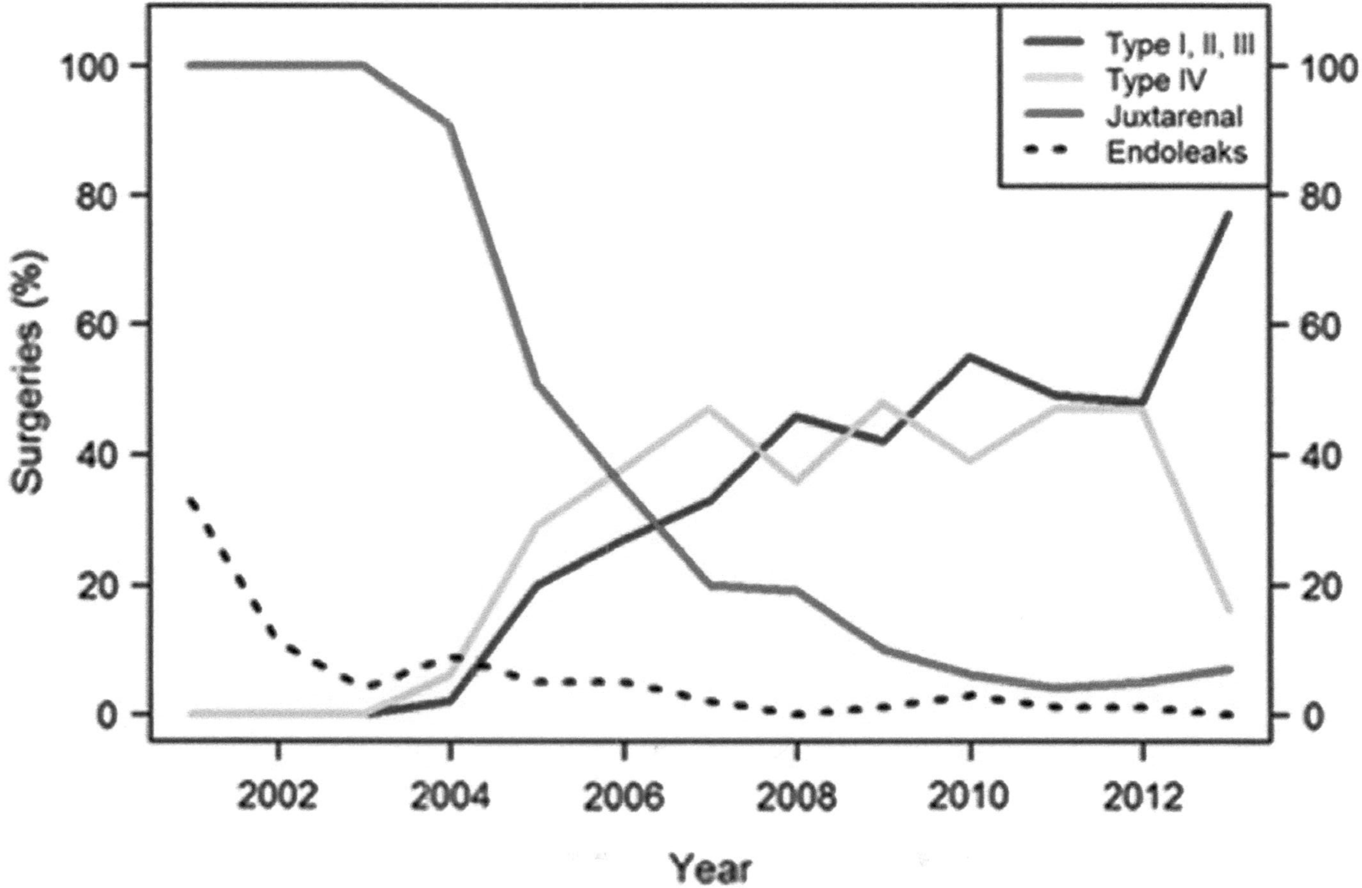

FIGURE 3.—This line graph shows how our practice has changed over the life of the study to include more of the visceral aorta in the repair to achieve a healthier sealing zone. There has been a consequent decrease in the number of juxtarenal repairs. (Reprinted from the Journal of Vascular Surgery. O'Callaghan A, Greenberg RK, Eagleton MJ, et al. Type Ia endoleaks after fenestrated and branched endografts may lead to component instability and increased aortic mortality. *J Vasc Surg*. 2015;61:908-914, Copyright 2014, with permission from the Society for Vascular Surgery.)

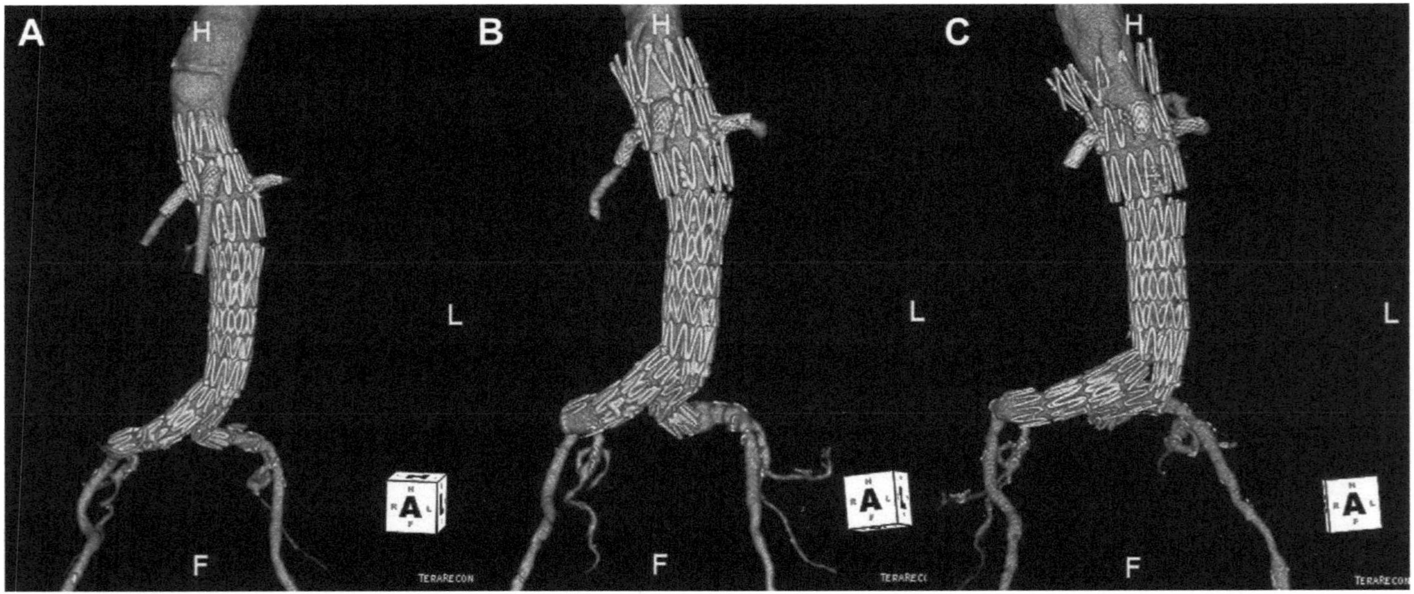

FIGURE 4.—Example of patient progression over the years shown by (A) a postimplant computed tomography (CT) scan, (B) a CT scan at 3 years, and (C) a CT scan at 6 years, with endoleak, proximal stent fracture, and branch dislocation. This patient refused further intervention. (Reprinted from the Journal of Vascular Surgery. O'Callaghan A, Greenberg RK, Eagleton MJ, et al. Type Ia endoleaks after fenestrated and branched endografts may lead to component instability and increased aortic mortality. *J Vasc Surg*. 2015;61:908-914, Copyright 2014, with permission from the Society for Vascular Surgery.)

the long-term outcome for patients requiring complex aortic repair (Figs 3 and 4).

► I recently took part as a panelist of experts discussing the proper length of seal for successful endografting. I personally believe that 15 mm of seal is simply not enough. My response on the panel was that I believed every patient undergoing endovascular aneurysm repair (EVAR) should have a minimum of 4 cm of seal length to achieve durable repair. Yes, this means that the majority of patients harboring an abdominal aortic aneurysm should have fenestrated repair. This article completely supports that bias.

This is the largest series in the literature with the longest term follow-up, and there are many important lessons here. These authors, including the late Roy Greenberg, have been pioneers in this area and impart to us that durability of EVAR is dependent on proximal seal.

Fig 3 shows the rate of juxtarenal repairs declining as the rate of more complex repairs rapidly increased over the study period at the Cleveland Clinic. This was associated with a lower type 1 endoleak rate and less component instability (Fig 4). Amazingly, the rate of proximal type 1a endoleak was only 2.8% in the entire cohort!

This analysis is the first to characterize the causes of proximal endoleaks in the fenestrated population. The authors findings of increased aortic mortality and component instability underscore the need to obtain a durable seal at the first procedure, irrespective of any resultant obligation to incorporate additional branch vessels in the repair. Branch vessel patency as described by these authors is excellent and should not be a barrier to endovascular repair.[1]

When it comes time for me to have my aneurysm repaired with EVAR, give me 4 cm of seal length ... please.

B. W. Starnes, MD

Reference

1. Mastracci TM, Greenberg RK, Eagleton MJ, Hernandez AV. Durability of branches in branched and fenestrated endografts. *J Vasc Surg*. 2013;57:926-933.

7 Nonatherosclerotic Conditions

The United States Registry for Fibromuscular Dysplasia: New Findings and Breaking Myths

Sharma AM, Kline B (Univ of Virginia School of Medicine, Charlottesville)
Tech Vasc Interv Radiol 17:258-263, 2014

Fibromuscular dysplasia (FMD) is a nonatherosclerotic, noninflammatory arterial disease predominantly seen in women. Most FMD cases are classified as medial fibroplasia, which has the appearance of a string of beads on angiography. Until recently, FMD was thought to be seen in women in their 20s and 30s, with more than 60%-75% of cases occurring in the renal artery and 25% of cases in the carotid artery. Hypertension was regarded as the primary symptom seen in these patients followed by a small number of patients presenting with intracranial aneurysms with subarachnoid hemorrhage. The United States Registry of FMD, a patient registry, has broken many preconceived notions as well as provided more in-depth knowledge of this uncommon disorder. In this review, we discuss the findings of this registry and its use in understanding this disorder. In addition to the registry, we review other recent studies and future directions in the diagnosis and management of this disorder (Table 2).

▶ In 2008, 7 medical centers formed a large, multicenter fibromuscular dysplasia (FMD) registry in the United States. This has since expanded to include 14 centers, and more than 1000 patients have enrolled. This article reviews some of the important findings to come out of the registry. The authors set out to clarify several aspects related to the diagnosis, management, and outcome of patients with FMD. Most patients in the registry are women (91%), and the mean age of patients was 51.9 years, which is older than the previously described age range of 20s to 30s. Renal artery FMD was more common in men (89.7% vs 74.1%; $P = .032$) and extracranial carotid FMD was more common in women (74.9% vs 44.1%; $P = .00043$). In addition, patients present with a wide variety of symptoms. The authors note that the presence of symptoms has a high predictive value for FMD, but the lack of symptoms was a poor predictor of its absence.

About management, most asymptomatic patients were treated with antiplatelet agents (71.8% of renal FMD patients and 80.6% of cerebrovascular patients). In the registry, 46.4% of patients underwent therapeutic procedures, including angioplasty, stenting, or bypass. Most of these procedures were for

TABLE 2.—Clinical Pearls Provided by the United States Registry for Fibromuscular Dysplasia

1. FMD is a polyvascular disease, often seen in vascular beds other than renal arteries especially cerebrovascular arteries. In patients with known FMD at one time, imaging of vascular beds from head to pelvis should be considered.
2. FMD can be present with a heterogenous group of symptoms or just hypertension. Patients with FMD often present with other symptoms such as headaches, pulsatile tinnitus, dizziness, neck pain, chest pain, abdominal pain, aneurysms, or dissections without or with hypertension.
3. Patients with known renal artery FMD often have cerebrovascular FMD and vice versa.
4. Overall, 1 of 5 patients with FMD will have dissections and 1 of 5 patients will have aneurysms.
5. Although FMD is less common in men, it is more aggressive in them and is associated with higher incidence of dissections and aneurysms.
6. Presence of physical findings such as bruits or Horner syndrome has a high positive predictive value in diagnosing FMD; however, a lack of them is a poor predictor of absence of FMD.
7. Angioplasty or other procedures for renal FMD are more likely to assist with reduction or cure of hypertension than those with atherosclerotic renal artery stenosis. Angioplasty of renal FMD for cure of hypertensionis is likely to be more effective in younger patients than those with recent-onset hypertension, and those with focal FMD.
8. FMD may have a genetic association and could be an inherited vasculopathy.
9. Lastly, the delay in diagnosis identifies the lack of medical community in recognizing symptoms of FMD and providing timely diagnosis and treatment.

renal artery disease (67.6%) with a smaller number being done for other vascular territories. Accordingly, the most frequent procedural indication was hypertension. This finding would not be a surprise when considering that the onset of essential hypertension can be in the 50- to 60-year age range; thus, FMD would be "discovered" by evaluation.

The authors included a table of clinical "pearls" (Table 2) that are highly relevant for the clinician and serve as a useful resource for the management of FMD. One fact noted by the article, that there is an average 3.6-year delay in the diagnosis of FMD, highlights the need for registries and further study of FMD.

M. Arnold, MD

Major adverse maternal cardiovascular-related events in those with aortopathies. What should we expect?

Bradley EA, Zaidi AN, Goldsmith P, et al (Nationwide Children's Hosp, Columbus, OH; et al)

Int J Cardiol 177:229-234, 2014

Major adverse maternal cardiovascular-related events (MAMCRE) in aortopathy patients undergoing pregnancy are poorly defined. The aim was to assess for MAMCRE in pregnant patients with aortopathy or aortic enlargement in conotruncal defects (CTD), and determine if there are differences between groups.

We conducted a single-center retrospective review of pregnant women (2000–2013) with hereditary vascular disease (HVD: BAV, COA), heritable fibrillinopathies (HF: MFS, EDS, LDS, FTAAS), and CTD with aortic dilatation (TOF, d-TGA, DORV). MAMCRE included: aortic dissection/surgery, therapeutic abortion, change in mode of delivery, and aortic growth >0.5 cm within 1 year.

We identified 73 patients/97 pregnancies (39/50 HVD, 15/20 HF, and 19/27 CTD). There were 14 MAMCRE (14%); 85% (n = 12) occurred in HV and HF patients and was associated with higher baseline cross-sectional-to-height (CSA/Ht) ratio (6.6 ± 2.5 vs. 5.1 ± 1.3, $p = 0.005$). There was more aortic surgery in the HF (vs. HV) (RR 3.9, $p = 0.12$). Only 2 MAMCRE (aortic growth) occurred in CTD. Overall and emergent C-section was higher than the general population (52% vs. 29%, $p < 0.001$ and 16% vs. 3%, $p < 0.001$) as was postpartum hemorrhage (PPH) (6% vs. 1.5%, $p < 0.001$).

We describe the largest series of pregnant women with aortopathy and found a substantial incidence of MAMCRE, which was associated with higher pre-pregnancy CSA/Ht ratio. Rates of C-section and PPH were higher than the general population. Our data suggest that larger, multicenter studies are needed to define risks that predict MAMCRE/obstetric events in women with aortopathies, allowing optimal medical care during pregnancy.

▶ Pregnant patients with aortopathy have a substantial increased risk of major adverse maternal cardiovascular-related events (MAMCRE). Although the cohort of patients with these pathologies is small, the effects can be devastating. The authors present the largest single-center series of pregnant women with aortopathy and share their recommendations for evaluation and treatment from before conception through delivery. Ideally, patients should have a baseline study to measure the size of the aorta preconception. Beta-blocker therapy should be used throughout pregnancy if tolerated. Decision about method of delivery (cesarian, vaginal, etc) should be discussed and carried out by a multidisciplinary group of practitioners. When counseling the patient about the risks of delivery, potential higher rates of cesarean delivery and postpartum hemorrhage should be included along with the cardiovascular complications. From the vascular surgeon's viewpoint, only 2 acute aortic dissections were captured in the series, both type A tears. Thus, the article may not guide the critical decision making for type B dissection patients, wherein hemodynamic control for the mother may run counter to fetal uterine demands. For the pregnant patient with type B dissection, the study leaves us short of guidance. On the other hand, the study did not show a statistically significant difference in MAMCRE between hereditary vascular disease and heritable fibrillinopathy, which may reassure those patients with connective tissue disorders who elect to proceed with childbirth, albeit the small number of patients may represent a selection bias. They did find a substantial rate of MAMCRE with a significant cross-sectional area of the aorta to height ratio difference (CSA/Ht). They suggest that routine aortic evaluation by this simple method may help risk stratify patients. With further study, larger multicenter data will need to be compiled to generate evidence-based protocols for optimizing management.

M. Arnold, MD

8 Thoracic Aorta

Endovascular strategies for treatment of embolizing thoracoabdominal aortic lesions

Jeyabalan G, Wallace JR, Chaer RA, et al (Univ of Pittsburgh Med Ctr, PA)

J Vasc Surg 59:1256-1264, 2014

Objective.—Aortic sources of peripheral and visceral embolization remain challenging to treat. The safety of stent graft coverage continues to be debated. This study reports the outcomes of stent coverage of these complex lesions.

Methods.—Hospital records were retrospectively reviewed for patients undergoing aortic stenting between 2006 and 2013 for visceral and peripheral embolic disease. Renal function, method of coverage, and mortality after stent grafting were reviewed.

Results.—Twenty-five cases of embolizing aortic lesions treated with an endovascular approach were identified. The mean age was 65 ± 13 years (range, 45-87 years), and 64% were female. Sixteen (64%) patients presented with peripheral embolic events, six with concomitant renal embolization. Five patients presented with abdominal or flank pain, and two were discovered incidentally. Three patients had undergone an endovascular procedure for other indications within the preceding 6 months of presentation. Nineteen patients had existing chronic kidney disease (stage II or higher), but only three had stage IV disease. Of the eight patients tested, four had a diagnosed hypercoagulable state. Eight of the patients had lesions identified in multiple aortic segments, and aortic aneurysm disease was present in 24%. Coverage of both abdominal and thoracic sources occurred in eight patients, whereas 17 had only one segment covered. Minimal intraluminal catheter and wire manipulation was paired with the use of intravascular ultrasound in an effort to reduce embolization and contrast use. Intravascular ultrasound was used in the majority of cases and transesophageal echo in 28% of patients. Two patients with stage IV kidney disease became dialysis-dependent within 3 months of the procedure. Noother patients had an increase in their postoperative or predischarge serum creatinine levels. No embolic events were precipitated during the procedure, nor were there any recurrent embolic events detected on follow-up. The 1-year mortality rate was 25%.

Conclusions.—Endovascular coverage of atheroembolic sources in the aorta is feasible and is safe and effective in properly selected patients. It does not appear to worsen renal function when performed with the use of specific technical strategies.

▶ Embolizing thoracoabdominal aortic lesions consist of 2 distinct patient populations: isolated aortic thrombus and multisegment embolizing atheroma. Historically, the former are more likely to undergo an open procedure if medically fit, and, without solid evidence for benefit, the majority of the latter are often placed on anticoagulation. What we struggle with are those patients who are not candidates for open surgery or those who continue to clinically embolize despite medical treatment. Endovascular coverage of aortic segments suspicious for embolizing etiology is an attractive avenue. Certainly, this mode has been tempered by fear of causing further emboli. Here a large series of patients successfully undergo endograft coverage without subsequent embolic events. Furthermore, the authors were presented with a high number of patients with underlying chronic renal disease. This was most likely a result of long-standing previous emboli, and perhaps indicative of the chronic insult, those with stage IV disease continued to progress to dialysis, despite successful coverage of the offending lesion. By using intravascular ultrasound (IVUS) or echocardiography, the operators were able to minimize the use of contrast and therefore mitigate further renal impairment. IVUS is a vital component of this strategy to identify the specific portion of the atherosclerotic aorta that contain mobile elements and therefore minimize the total aortic coverage. Additionally, previous reports show a mortality rate of 17% to 60% for patients with this difficult problem. And although this series has a 25% 1-year mortality, only 1 patient of the 5 deaths (n = 25) may have had a recurrent event; the rest died of unrelated causes. This is not a surprise to the reviewers because those with such severe aortic atherosclerosis are often severely affected in coronary and carotid territories. Accordingly, the endovascular solution is the clear, preferred strategy for this condition, and the technical notes of the study and figures are helpful for those considering interventions.

K. C. Orion, MD

A clinical decision model for selecting the most appropriate therapy for uncomplicated chronic dissections of the descending aorta

Hogendoorn W, Hunink MGM, Schlösser FJV, et al (Yale Univ School of Medicine, New Haven, CT; Univ Med Ctr, Utrecht, The Netherlands; et al)
J Vasc Surg 60:20-30, 2014

Objective.—The optimal treatment for patients with uncomplicated chronic Stanford type B aortic dissections (chTBADs) is still matter of debate. The purpose of this study was to design a decision tool to guide the surgeon in determining the preferred treatment option.

Methods.—A Markov decision-analysis model compared chTBAD patients treated with initial open surgical repair (OSR), thoracic endovascular aortic repair (TEVAR), and optimal medical therapy (OMT), followed during follow-up by OSR (OMT-OSR) or TEVAR (OMT-TEVAR), if indicated. Procedural risks, aortic growth and rupture rates, outcomes, and quality of life values were derived from the best available evidence in the literature. A chTBAD treatment strategy decision tool was developed, including the four key variables of age, sex, surgical risk, and maximum initial aortic diameter. Primary outcome was quality-adjusted life-years (QALYs).

Results.—For the reference patient cohort, 55-year-old men with chTBAD with a maximum aortic diameter of 5.0 cm, medium risk for surgery, and a threshold for surgery of 6.0 cm during follow-up, OSR yielded higher QALYs, with 10.06 QALYs (95% credibility interval [CI], 9.52-10.56 QALYs) vs 9.92 QALYs (95% CI, 9.23-10.58 QALYs) after TEVAR and 9.64 QALYs (95% CI, 9.38-9.88 QALYs) and 9.40 QALYs (95% CI, 9.11-9.69 QALYs) for OMT-OSR and OMT-TEVAR. The difference between OSR and OMT-OSR was 0.42 QALYs (95% CI, 0.01-0.81 QALYs) and between TEVAR and OMT-TEVAR was 0.52 QALYs (95% CI, 0.04-0.68 QALYs). This showed that intervention is preferred over OMT. A change of the four variables resulted in a change of preferred treatment. In general, OSR was the preferred treatment in younger patients with a larger aortic diameter and in low-risk patients. TEVAR was preferred in elderly patients with large aortic diameter and if the aortic diameter threshold for repair decreased. OMT was the optimal therapy in high-risk patients, elderly patients, or in patients with small aortic diameters.

Conclusions.—This decision-analysis model shows that there is no "one-size-fits-all" treatment for uncomplicated chTBADs. For the reference patient cohort, intervention is preferred over OMT. Age is the most important deciding factor, followed by initial aortic diameter. Immediate OSR is the preferred treatment option in younger patients with a large initial aortic diameter and in low-risk patients. Immediate TEVAR is preferred in elderly patients with a large initial aortic diameter and in patients with a lower threshold for OSR. OMT should be considered in high-risk patients, in patients with small initial aortic diameters, and in patients aged >80 years, unless their initial aortic diameter is >5.5 cm. However, the differences in some patient groups are clinically insignificant, allowing a major role for patient preferences and hospital-specific considerations. This clinical decision model may guide chTBAD treatment (Fig 3).

▶ This article highlights the challenges encountered when determining treatment for a chronic type B aortic dissection. The patients selected are all patients with age-related disease because connective tissue disorder patients were not included. This is an important point to emphasize because the decision treat for those with connective tissue disorders is likely quite different. From the article, it is clear that at approximately age 60, open surgical repair is essentially abandoned except in few very low-risk patients (Fig 3). After age 60, thoracic endovascular aortic repair becomes the suggested method for those that

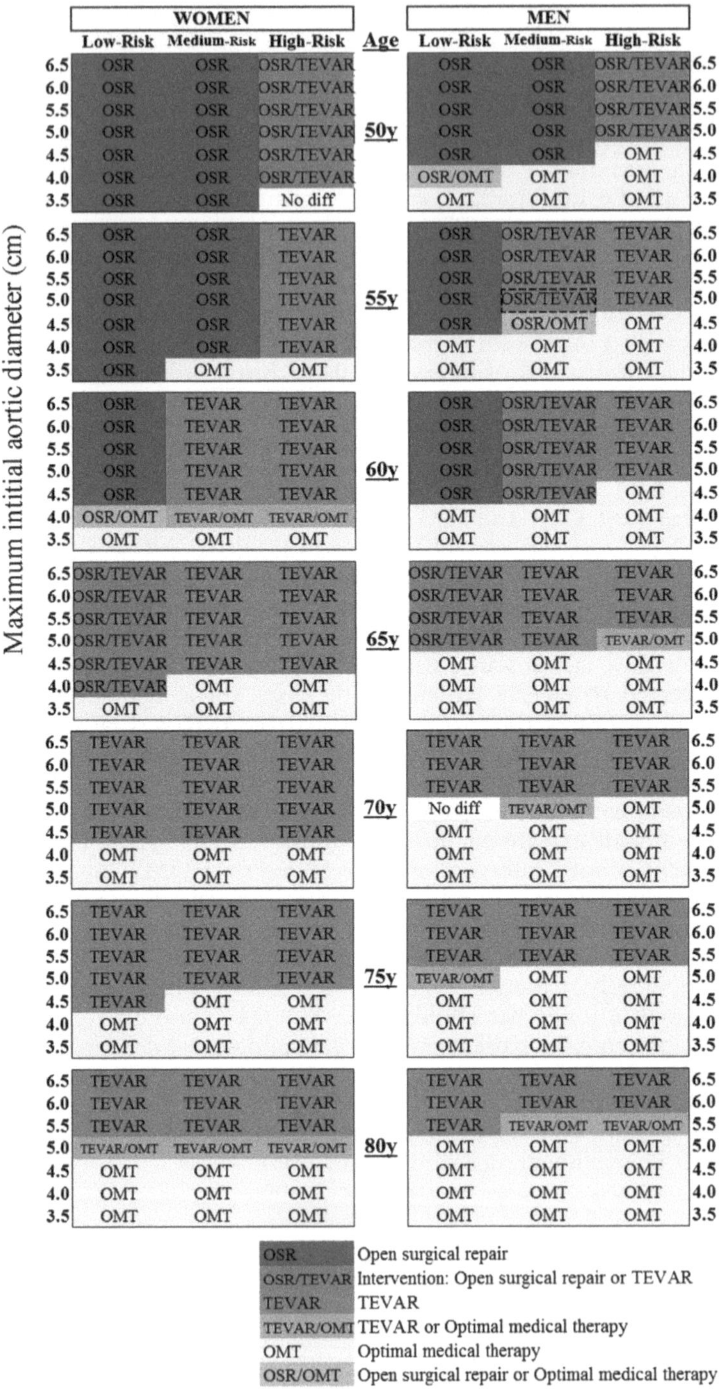

FIGURE 3.—This treatment strategy decision chart indicates optimal treatment strategy on the basis of four basic characteristics: age, sex, surgical risk profile, and maximum initial aortic diameter. Two treatment strategies in the same cell (OSR/TEVAR, TEVAR/OMT, and OSR/OMT) indicate a difference of <2 months in quality-adjusted life-years (QALYs). No *diff* indicates a difference of <2 months for all the treatment groups. The *dotted box* is the reference case. TEVAR, Thoracic endovascular aortic repair. (Reprinted from the Journal of Vascular Surgery. Hogendoorn W, Hunink MGM, Schlösser FJV, et al. A clinical decision model for selecting the most appropriate therapy for uncomplicated chronic dissections of the descending aorta. *J Vasc Surg.* 2014;60:20-30, Copyright 2014, with permission from The Society for Vascular Surgery.)

progress to large aortic diameters. The article also illustrates that as patients age, the threshold for intervention should increase including continued medical therapy in octogenarians until the aortic diameter is over 5 cm. Lastly, it is important to note that this article only outlines a treatment algorithm for chronic dissection and should not be applied to those with acute disease. Overall, the message that resonates is to consider each patient's comorbid conditions and develop an individualized plan for treatment.

B. W. Propper, MD

Aortic remodeling after endovascular treatment of complicated type B aortic dissection with the use of a composite device design

Lombardi JV, on behalf of the STABLE Investigators (Cooper Univ Hosp, Camden, NJ; et al)

J Vasc Surg 59:1544-1554, 2014

Objective.—The purpose of this study is to report updated clinical and aortic remodeling results from the Study for the Treatment of complicated Type B Aortic Dissection using Endoluminal repair (STABLE) trial, a prospective, multicenter study evaluating safety and effectiveness of a pathology-specific endovascular system (proximal stent graft and distal bare metal stent) for the treatment of complicated type B aortic dissection.

Methods.—All 86 enrolled patients (mean age, 59 years; 73.3% men) were treated within 90 days of symptom onset (55 with acute dissections and 31 with nonacute dissections). Inclusion criteria were branch vessel obstruction/compromise, impending rupture as evidenced by periaortic effusion/hematoma, resistant hypertension, persistent pain/symptoms, or aortic growth ≥5 mm within 3 months (or transaortic diameter ≥40 mm). Remodeling of the dissected aorta, including thrombosis of the false lumen and changes in the true lumen, false lumen, and transaortic diameter, were assessed in patients with available computed tomographic imaging through 2 years.

Results.—The 30-day mortality rate was 4.7% (4/86) in the overall patient group (5.5% in acute patients and 3.2% in nonacute patients). Freedom from all-cause mortality was 88.3% at 1 year and 84.7% at 2 years (no significant difference between acute and nonacute patients). From baseline to 2 years, the true lumen diameter increased significantly in the descending thoracic aorta and the more distal abdominal aorta, along with a decrease in the false lumen diameter in both aortic segments. A majority of patients had either a stable or shrinking transaortic diameter in the thoracic (80.3% at 1 year and 73.9% at 2 years) or abdominal aorta (79.1% at 1 year and 66.7% at 2 years). Transaortic growth (>5 mm) occurred predominantly in acute dissections. Consistently, a shorter time from symptom onset to treatment was found to predict transaortic growth in the abdominal aorta ($P = .03$).

Conclusions.—Endovascular repair of complicated type B aortic dissection with the use of a composite construct demonstrates favorable early

clinical outcomes and aortic remodeling. However, patients treated in the acute setting may be prone to aortic growth and may require close observation. Follow-up through 5 years is ongoing.

▶ This study reports the 2-year follow-up of 86 patients enrolled in the STABLE trial, focusing specifically on the remodeling of the aorta after stenting for complicated type B dissection. The composite device design is a modular system comprising the Zenith TX2 stent graft proximally and the Zenith endovascular bare metal stent distally. The second component was performed at the discretion of the physician if branch vessel obstruction or false lumen perfusion persisted. They separated the cohort into acute (< 2 weeks from symptoms to intervention) and nonacute (> 2 weeks). Their overall mortality compares favorably with the literature. Although there were 5 subsequent ruptures and 3 retrograde dissections, this reflects the fact that complicated B aortic dissections (cTBAD) are extremely high-risk and difficult patients to treat, and interestingly, many of these complications occurred over 30 days after device deployment.

Approximately half of the patients achieved complete false lumen (FL) thrombosis at 2 years using this technique. Therefore, half of patients had incomplete thrombosis, and persistent flow into the abdominal false lumen was even more prevalent. The authors briefly queried if more extensive coverage of the thoracic aorta with endograft rather than bare metal stent would result in better FL thrombosis. Perhaps more important than thrombosis of the FL is the cessation of aortic degeneration in terms of size for most surgeons and their patients. To this point, in the acutely treated patients, the dissected abdominal aorta diameter distal to the thoracic endovascular aneurysm repair increased at 2 years. Interestingly, this growth was not based only on persistent FL flow because a large portion of patients with incomplete FL thrombosis did not grow their respective aortic segments. This suggests that there is another component, possibly a pathophysiological condition of the dissected aorta in the acute phase. We do note that the acute group has significantly less hypertension than the nonacute dissection group that may or may not play a factor in these findings. What is true is the authors' declaration that endovascular therapy describes more of initial "management" rather than definitive treatment of patients as they evolve to chronic TBAD. Although in the authors' assessment, the acutely treated patient may be prone to continued abdominal aortic growth, potentially because of anatomical factors that lend them complicated TBADs (malperfusion, impending rupture, resistant hypertension, persistent pain, or rapid growth), these patients are unlikely to wait 2 weeks for the delayed intervention. Thus, from a decision-making standpoint, in patients with complicated acute TBAD, most surgeons would be hard-pressed to stand by. Nonetheless, endovascular repair is still a lifesaving procedure for these patients and certainly preferable over open repair of an acute aortic dissection, which is wrought with morbidity and mortality. Ultimately, after TEVAR for cTBAD, the study underscores our responsibility to follow these patients for surveillance of their entire aorta and the ongoing complexity of the dissection management.

K. C. Orion, MD

Diabetics Are Less Likely to Develop Thoracic Aortic Dissection: A 10-Year Single-Center Analysis

Theivacumar NS, Stephenson MA, Mistry H, et al (King's College Hosp, London, UK)

Ann Vasc Surg 28:427-432, 2014

Background.—Diabetes mellitus (DM) is an acknowledged risk factor for atherosclerosis, and diabetics are more likely to have hypertension. Atherosclerosis and hypertension are risk factors for aortic dissection. However, recent studies have shown that DM is associated with changes in aortic wall collagen. In this retrospective study we assess the relationship between DM and thoracic aortic dissection (TAD).

Methods.—Patients with a diagnosis of thoracic aortic dissection during the last 10 years were identified from our hospital records. The prevalence of DM in Stanford type A and B TAD was compared with that of two age- and gender-matched control groups. For every diabetic dissection case, 10 controls were selected from the hospital data.

Results.—Two hundred nineteen patients (median age 61 years, male:female ratio 145:74) were identified with TAD, comprising 131 type A dissections and 88 type B dissections. Only 3 of 131 (2.3%) type A aortic dissections were diabetics, whereas, in control group 1, 241 of 1310 (18.4%) were diabetics and, in control group 2, 116 of 1310 (8.9%) were diabetics [odds ratios: 0.1 (0.03–0.32) and 0.24 (0.07–0.76), respectively] ($P = 0.0001$ and 0.007, respectively). Similarly, only 2 of 88 (2.3%) type B aortic dissections were diabetics, whereas 228 of 880 (26.0%) and 102 of 880 (11.6%) were diabetics in groups 1 and 2 [odds ratios: 0.07 (0.02–0.27) and 0.18 (0.04–0.73), respectively] ($P = 0.0001$ and 0.0035, respectively). All these odds ratios were statistically significant ($P < 0.01$).

Conclusions.—Patients with thoracic aortic dissection are less likely to be diabetic. Although we identified association only, not causality, it is possible that DM, or its treatment, has a protective effect against aortic dissection.

▶ Because diabetes mellitus (DM) is a risk factor for atherosclerosis and hypertension is more prevalent (and often more difficult to control) in the DM population, conventional wisdom held that the DM population should be at higher risk for thoracic aortic dissection (TAD). Recent studies have begun to challenge this assumption. This article sought to assess the relationship between TAD and DM through a retrospective study. The authors had a unique study design in that they compared patients admitted to the hospital with TAD (both type A and B) with 2 different control groups. Control group 1 was all patients admitted to the hospital for any reason; group 2 was only those patients admitted for orthopedic procedures. The rationale behind this was that group 1 had an overrepresentation of patients with DM, whereas the number of patients with DM in group 2 was more reflective of the general prevalence of DM in the population at large. The authors found that only 2.3% of patients with type A TAD had DM (3:131) and only 2.3% of patients with type B TAD had DM (2:88). When compared with their control groups, this was statistically significant. They conclude that the presence of DM may confer a direct or indirect protective effect against TAD. The mechanism behind this effect is unknown at this time but could provide interesting avenues for further study. One would generally surmise diabetics would have the same atherosclerotic changes leading to cystic medial necrosis (the most common lesion in dissection), yet perhaps aortic wall homeostasis is preserved despite the peripheral vascular changes thought to be promulgated by glycosylated proteins.

M. Arnold, MD

Early experience with off-the-shelf endografts using a zone 0 proximal landing site to treat the ascending aorta and arch

Bernardes RC, Navarro TP, Reis FR, et al (Hosp Madre Teresa, Belo Horizonte, Minas Gerais, Brazil; Instituto Panamericano da Circulação, Belo Horizonte, Minas Gerais, Brazil; et al)

J Thorac Cardiovasc Surg 148:105-112, 2014

Objective.—Acute type A aortic syndromes and its chronic complications are fatal diseases traditionally treated by open surgery, with high mortality rates. An endovascular approach to the ascending aorta could reduce the morbidity and mortality associated with open surgery. Our aim was to report our initial experience in treating ascending aortic pathology using commercially available descending thoracic endografts.

Methods.—From 2007 to 2012, 69 patients presented to our center in Belo Horizonte, Brazil, with acute type A aortic syndrome or its chronic complications. Of the 69 patients, 8 high-risk patients had suitable anatomy, and 7 agreed to participate in the present study.

Results.—Of the 7 patients, 4 had penetrating ulcers, 2 had acute dissections, and 1 had chronic dissection with an aneurysm. The technical success rate was 87%, with 1 intraoperative death from acute aortic valve insufficiency. The proximal landing zone was, on average, 21 mm above the aortic valve in all patients. Three patients required intraoperative cervical debranching due to a lesion in the distal third of the ascending aorta, compromising the supra-aortic branches. The distal landing zone was at zone 0 in 4 patients, zone 2 in 1 patient, and in zone 4 in 2 patients. The mean follow-up was 26.3 months. Two repeat dissections developed an average of 2 months after treatment. Both presented with acute dissection that was treated with additional open surgery and both patients survived. Thereafter, no patient had presented again with an acute aortic syndrome or other referable symptoms.

Conclusions.—Endovascular treatment of the ascending aorta is feasible. We had 4 good mid-term results in 7 patients who had presented with penetrating ulcers or aneurysm formation. Acute dissections seem to be more unstable, and additional research is mandatory.

▶ This is an interesting article using currently available thoracic aortic devices to treat ascending aortic pathology. The study is limited given that only 7 patients were included, but it highlights some challenges with the ascending aorta. Zone 0 continues to present challenges for proximal seal because both the proximal and distal seal sites can be compromised. As with any aneurysm, the goal should be to land a device into "normal" aorta. The ascending aorta is often <10 cm, which is why this series is predominantly dissections and penetrating ulcers. It appears of all pathology, penetrating ulcers are the most stable with acute dissection being the least hospitable entity. Certainly this observation has been seen in the descending aorta as well. In this series, 2 patients with acute dissection required additional open surgery because of secondary dissection. This brings up 2 important areas of interest: first, the ascending aorta is a challenging area to image using standard angiography given the immense motion. One must consider that the failure in these 2 patients is secondary to the initial dissection flap not being fully excluded. Second, the devices used for this study are designed for descending aortic work, some of which have active fixation (barbs). Could these devices, when placed in a highly mobile area, induce new intimal tears? What is clear is that the endovascular ascending interventions are coming quickly, and technology is rapidly changing to create better devices that can be deployed with less challenge to the user and less risk for local cardioaortic complications.

B. W. Propper, MD

Editor's Choice – Treatment Decisions for Descending Thoracic Aneurysm: Preferences for Thoracic Endovascular Aneurysm Repair or Surveillance in a Discrete Choice Experiment

Rudarakanchana N, Reeves BC, Bicknell CD, et al (Imperial College Healthcare NHS Trust, London, UK; Univ of Bristol, Bristol, UK; et al)

Eur J Vasc Endovasc Surg 48:13-22, 2014

Objective.—To investigate and rank factors that influence endovascular treatment decisions by specialists for patients with descending thoracic aortic aneurysm (dTAA).

Methods.—Specialists completed a diagrammatic survey describing uncertainty about the benefit of thoracic endovascular aneurysm repair (TEVAR) for dTAA with respect to age, sex, and aneurysm diameter. Subsequently, a detailed discrete choice experiment was designed. Specialists were recruited and asked to indicate treatment of their preference (TEVAR or surveillance) in 25 hypothetical cases of dTAA, with variable patient attributes: age, sex, American Society of Anesthesiologists (ASA) grade, aneurysm diameter, adequate landing zone distal to left subclavian artery (LSA), and length of aortic coverage. Data were analysed using multiple logistic regression.

Results.—The diagrammatic survey, based on 50 respondents, showed that uncertainty about the benefits of TEVAR was greatest for patients aged 80–85 years (up to 47% of respondents were "unsure") and that uncertainty increased with increasing aneurysm diameter (for an 80-year-old man, 7% were unsure at 5.5 cm and 33% were unsure at 7.0 cm). Seventy-one specialists (mainly from Europe and North America, 86% vascular surgeons and 98% working in units offering TEVAR) completed the discrete choice experiment. Preference for TEVAR increased greatly with enlarging diameter: adjusted odds ratios (OR) >5.5–6.0 cm = 15.8 (95% confidence interval [CI] 9.83–25.40); >6.0–6.5 cm = 393.0 (95% CI 202.00–766.00); >6.5–7.0 cm = 1829.0 (95% CI 400.00–4,181.00). TEVAR was less likely to be preferred in patients older than 75 years (>75–80 years OR 0.32, 95% CI 0.21–0.49; >80–85 years = 0.18, 95% CI 0.11–0.28); in women (OR 0.52, 95% CI 0.37–0.74); in patients classified as ASA grade 4 (OR 0.44, 95% CI 0.36–0.57); and in patients with aorta coverage >25 cm (OR 0.48, 95% CI 0.32–0.74). The proximal landing zone did not influence preference.

Conclusion.—Specialists' preferences for endovascular repair of degenerative dTAA vary widely, and demonstrate clinical uncertainty, especially in octogenarians, and a reluctance to offer TEVAR to women. Aneurysm diameter dominates treatment preferences, but patient fitness and length of aortic coverage (>25 cm) also were influential, although the landing zone distal to LSA was not (Fig 1).

▶ Currently there is wide variation and lack of evidence guiding management of descending thoracic aortic aneurysms (dTAA) especially for patients older than 75 years in age. The authors of this study sought to investigate those factors that were most influential concerning decision for thoracic endovascular aneurysm repair (TEVAR) versus surveillance in dTAA. To accomplish this, they used 2 survey modalities. The first asked respondents to chart their uncertainty for repair versus surveillance based on age, sex, and diameter. The results of this survey demonstrated the greatest uncertainty for patients aged 80 to 85 years and that uncertainty increased with increasing aortic diameter (Fig 1).

For me, the weightier part of the study was the second survey, which was a discrete choice experiment. Respondents were given 25 scenarios with variable age, American Society of Anesthesiologist (ASA) grade, sex, aortic diameter, need for left subclavian artery coverage, and length of aortic coverage. They were asked to choose surveillance or TEVAR based on the information. The authors found that aortic diameter had a strong influence on repair: adjusted odds ratio (OR) > 5.5 to 6.0 cm = 15.8, > 6.0 to 6.5 cm = 393.0, > 6.5 to 7.0 cm = 1829.0. TEVAR was less likely to be preferred in patients older than 75 years (OR = 0.32), in women (OR = 0.52), ASA grade 4 (OR = 0.44), and coverage > 25 cm (OR 0.48).

The biggest limitation of the study is that it does not truly reflect reality. Surgeons make treatment decisions based on multiple factors and looking at the

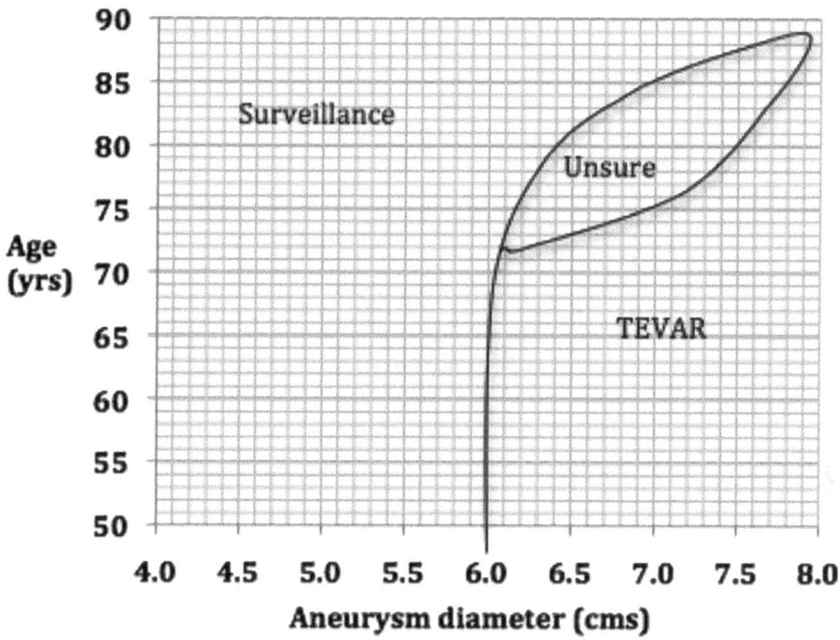

FIGURE 1.—Diagrammatic survey graph. *Note.* TEVAR = thoracic endovascular aortic repair. (Reprinted from the European Journal of Vascular and Endovascular Surgery. Rudarakanchana N, Reeves BC, Bicknell CD, et al. Editor's choice – treatment decisions for descending thoracic aneurysm: preferences for thoracic endovascular aneurysm repair or surveillance in a discrete choice experiment. *Eur J Vasc Endovasc Surg*. 2014;48:13-22, Copyright 2014, with permission from the European Society for Vascular Surgery.)

patient as a "whole." What this study does expose is an inherent ageism and sexism in the treatment of dTAA. It also supports the need for new treatment guidelines based on the natural history of dTAA in the context of the most current medical treatment

M. Arnold, MD

Editor's Choice – Temporary Aneurysm Sac Perfusion as an Adjunct for Prevention of Spinal Cord Ischemia After Branched Endovascular Repair of Thoracoabdominal Aneurysms

Kasprzak PM, Gallis K, Cucuruz B, et al (Univ of Regensburg, Germany)
Eur J Vasc Endovasc Surg 48:258-265, 2014

Objective.—To report experience with the concept of temporary aneurysm sac perfusion (TASP) and second stage side branch completion to prevent severe spinal cord ischemia (SCI) after branched endovascular aortic repair (bEVAR) for thoracoabdominal aortic aneurysm (TAAA).

Methods.—Patients were treated for TAAA with bEVAR between January 2009 and September 2012. TASP was performed by non-completion of side branches to one of the reno-visceral arteries, distal aortic or iliac extensions with secondary side branch completion. Primary endpoints of the study were overall technical success, side branch patency, perioperative mortality, and the rate of severe SCI.

Results.—Eighty-three patients were treated for TAAA with branched aortic stent grafts with ($n = 40$) or without ($n = 43$) TASP. Overall technical success, including aneurysm exclusion, absence of persistent type I or III endoleak, TASP side branch patency, and secondary side branch completion was 35/40 (88%). Secondary TASP side branch completion was performed after a median of 48 days (range 1–370 days). The rate of early reinterventions for reno-visceral side branch complications was 8/283 (3%) and 6/83 (7%) for perioperative mortality, with three patients in both groups. Severe SCI or paraplegia was observed in 11/83 (13%) of the patients and reduced in the TASP group (2/40) compared with the non-TASP group (9/43; $p = .03$), especially in Crawford I–III aneurysms (1/29 vs. 7/24; $p = .01$). However, one TASP patient died 4 months after bEVAR during the TASP interval from suspected aorto-bronchial fistula.

Conclusion.—The concept of TASP after bEVAR for TAAA is feasible and seems to reduce the risk of SCI. Early side TASP branch completion within 4 weeks is recommended to reduce the risk of rupture, although, according to the individual clinical presentation, a longer TASP interval might improve neurological rehabilitation from SCI (Fig 4).

▶ Temporary aneurysm sac perfusion (TASP) to decrease spinal cord ischemia (SCI) is a novel concept, in line with the suggestion from centers of expertise that staged branched endovascular repairs (bEVAR) decrease the incidence of paraplegia. The authors here present an eloquent series of patients undergoing thoracoabdominal aortic aneurysm (TAAA) repair with bEVAR. Although there was a paraplegia rate of 13%, 9 of those 11 patients were in the non-TASP

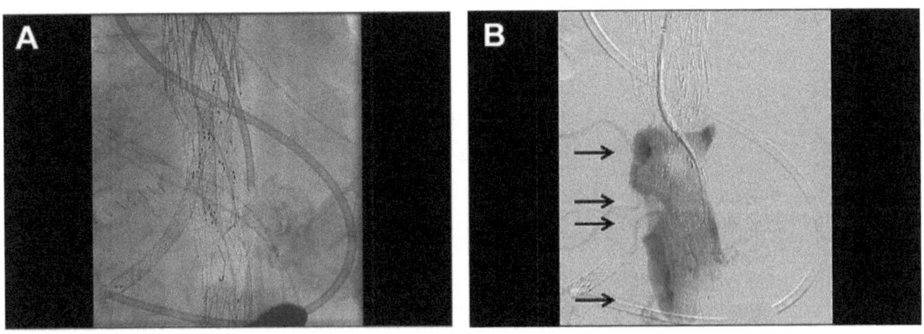

FIGURE 4.—(A) Intraoperative angiogram showing implantation of branched endograft with connecting stent grafts to the celiac trunk and the superior mesenteric artery. (B) Temporary aneurysm sac perfusion via the right renal artery with flow to the aneurysm and at least four lumbar arteries (black arrows). The patient has had left nephrectomy for renal cancer. (Reprinted from the European Journal of Vascular and Endovascular Surgery. Kasprzak PM, Gallis K, Cucuruz B, et al. Editor's choice – temporary aneurysm sac perfusion as an adjunct for prevention of spinal cord ischemia after branched endovascular repair of thoracoabdominal aneurysms. *Eur J Vasc Endovasc Surg*. 2014;48:258-265, Copyright 2014, with permission from the European Society for Vascular Surgery.)

group ($P = .03$). They found that if patients are asymptomatic after their initial procedure, side branch completion should be performed within 4 weeks to decrease the risk of further TAAA degeneration and rupture. However, the staged procedure may be delayed for patients who necessitate recovery from SCI. It would be interesting to note how many patients suffering SCI during the primary procedure will actually return for completion of side branches. Alternatively, the authors do report 1 patient with severe SCI after the secondary side branch completion 2 months later, and appropriately, the question of whether TASP can definitively prevent these delayed serious complications is thus unresolved. One option for these patients is to perform the side branch completion under local and monitored anesthesia so a temporary side branch balloon occlusion can identify neurological deficits early and alternative measures can be taken. These authors preferentially left the celiac trunk noncompleted to perfuse the sac but reflect that it may be more physiological to position an additional patent side branch proximal and distal to the renovisceral aortic segment and in a more dorsal location (presumably to feed the region of the intercostals from T8-T12). Nonetheless, it is clear that cerebrospinal fluid drainage, normal hemoglobin levels, and prevention of hypotension are still the most crucial elements for risk reduction of SCI as a clinical strategy for the practitioner to embrace. As our experience with branched endografts matures, TASP may play an increasing role in the design and fabrication of evolving endovascular devices.

K. C. Orion, MD

Five-year results for endovascular repair of acute complicated type B aortic dissection

Hanna JM, Andersen ND, Ganapathi AM, et al (Duke Univ Med Ctr, Durham, NC)

J Vasc Surg 59:96-106, 2014

Introduction.—Despite a current lack of U.S. Food and Drug Administration approval for the indication, thoracic endovascular aortic repair (TEVAR) has replaced open surgical management for acute complicated type B aortic dissection due to promising short- and midterm data. However, long-term results, with a view toward durability and need for secondary procedures, are limited. As such, the objective of the present study is to report long-term outcomes of TEVAR for acute (≤2 weeks from symptom onset) complicated type B dissection.

Methods.—Between July 2005 and September 2012, 50 consecutive patients underwent TEVAR for management of acute complicated type B dissection at a single referral institution. Patient records were retrospectively reviewed from a prospectively maintained clinical database.

Results.—Indications for intervention included rupture in 10 (20%), malperfusion in 24 (48%), and/or refractory pain/impending rupture in 17 (34%). One patient (2%) had both rupture and malperfusion indications. Ten (20%) patients required one or more adjunctive procedures, in addition to TEVAR, to treat malperfusion syndromes. In-hospital and 30-day rates of death were both 0%; 30-day/in-hospital rates of stroke, permanent paraplegia/paraparesis, and new-onset dialysis were 2% (n = 1), 2% (n = 1), and 4% (n = 2), respectively. Median follow-up was 33.8 months [interquartile range, 12.3-56.6 months]. Overall survival at 5 and 7 years was 84%, with no deaths attributable to aortic pathology. Thirteen (26%) patients required a total of 17 reinterventions over the study period for type I endoleak (n = 5), metachronous aortic pathology (n = 5), persistent false lumen pressurization via distal fenestrations (n = 4), type II endoleak (n = 2), or retrograde acute type A aortic dissection (n = 1). Median time to first reintervention was 4.5 months (range, 0 days-40.3 months). Of the 17 total reinterventions, six (35%) were performed using open techniques and 11 (65%) with endovascular or hybrid methods; there was no difference in survival between patients who did or did not require reintervention.

Conclusions.—This study confirms the excellent short-term outcomes of TEVAR for acute complicated type B dissection and demonstrates the results to be durable and sustained over long-term follow-up. Although aortic reinterventions were required in one-quarter of patients, no aortic-related deaths were observed. These data support the use of TEVAR for acute complicated type B aortic dissection but also highlight the importance of life-long aortic surveillance by an experienced aortic referral center in order to identify and treat complications of the underlying disease process and treatment, as well as new aortic pathologies, as they arise (Table 6).

▶ Since the publication of the IRAD and INSTEAD trials, our treatment of acute type B thoracic aortic dissection (TBAD) continues to evolve. Evidence suggests that there is a patient population in whom thoracic endovascular aortic repair (TEVAR) may be advantageous for uncomplicated acute TBAD. For complicated TBAD, TEVAR has all but replaced open surgery despite the lack of US Food and Drug Administration approval, and short-term outcomes after TEVAR are exceptional compared with conventional open repair. Herein, durable results are reported in long-term follow-up in complicated TBAD. Overall survival at 5 and 7 years was 84%, with no aortic-related deaths. This would compare favorably with the INSTEAD XL follow-up. To this end, the authors comment that these improved outcomes may reflect the fact that they included patients with unrelenting chest or back pain, without organ malperfusion, as complicated type B dissection—17 of the 50 patients. However, we agree that these patients are at high risk for impending rupture, and it is our practice to include them in the group of complicated TBAD. Interestingly, the reintervention rate here (26%) is higher than prior reports, but this is to be expected with longer duration of follow-up (see Table 6). There were also 4 patients with Marfan syndrome. These patients do not do well with endovascular grafts for chronic degenerating dissections but can absolutely benefit in the acute phase, especially in situations of impending rupture. These patients, however, will most certainly require a delayed open conversion for graft explantation and a more

TABLE 6.—Reinterventions

Patient	Reason for Reintervention	Procedure	Time to Reintervention, Months
1	Type II endoleak via the LSCA	Proximal extension TEVAR, LSCA coil embolization	5.0
2	a) Proximal type IA endoleak	Proximal extension TEVAR	1.4
	b) Persistent type IA endoleak	Zone 0 hybrid arch debranching	1.5
	c) Metachronous aortic pathology (AAA)	Open AAA repair	40.3
3	a) Persistent false lumen pressurization via distal fenestrations	Distal extension TEVAR	1.0
	b) Persistent false lumen pressurization via distal fenestrations	Open DTAA repair	5.8
4	Partial proximal endograft collapse and type IA endoleak	Proximal extension TEVAR with LSCA coverage	30.5
5	a) Metachronous aortic pathology (ascending aneurysm)	Ascending aortic and hemi-arch replacement	10.8
	b) Metachronous aortic pathology (DTAA)	Distal extension TEVAR	11.1
6	Metachronous aortic pathology (ascending aneurysm)	Ascending aortic and hemi-arch replacement	1.6
7	Distal type IB endoleak, proximal descending TAA above existing stent graft	Zone 0 hybrid arch debranching with distal extension endograft	13.6
8	Partial endograft collapse and type IA endoleak	Proximal and distal extension TEVAR	0.2
9	Persistent false lumen pressurization via distal fenestrations	a) Distal extension TEVAR b) EVAR of abdominal dissection	4.5
10	Acute retrograde TAAD	Aortic root reconstruction with AV resuspension	0.0
11	Persistent false lumen pressurization via distal fenestrations and type II endoleak via LSCA	a) Distal extension TEVAR b) EVAR of abdominal dissection c) Occlusion of LSCA	5.1
12	Persistent false lumen pressurization via distal fenestrations	Open TAAA repair	2.3
13	Metachronous aortic pathology (DTAA)	Proximal and distal extension TEVAR	8.1

AAA, Abdominal aortic aneurysm; *AV*, aortic valve; *DTAA*, descending thoracic aortic aneurysm; *EVAR*, endovascular abdominal aortic aneurysm repair; *LSCA*, left subclavian artery; *TAA*, thoracic aortic aneurysm; *TAAA*, thoracoabdominal aortic aneurysm; *TAAD*, type A aortic dissection; *TEVAR*, thoracic endovascular aortic repair.

Reprinted from the Journal of Vascular Surgery. Hanna JM, Andersen ND, Ganapathi AM, et al. Five-year results for endovascular repair of acute complicated type B aortic dissection. *J Vasc Surg*. 2014;59:96-106, Copyright 2014, with permission from The Society for Vascular Surgery.

durable repair despite presence of endoleak. If one were to exclude the Marfan patients, which greatly accounted for the 6 of 13 surgical open conversions, the reintervention rate then drops to 18%. This is admirable for patients with such a difficult disease, especially given that reintervention did not worsen long-term survival in this study.

K. C. Orion, MD

Follow-up outcomes of hybrid procedures for thoracoabdominal aortic pathologies with special focus on graft patency and late mortality

Bianchini Massoni C, Geisbüsch P, Gallitto E, et al (Univ of Bologna, Italy; Ruprecht Karls Univ, Heidelberg, Germany)

J Vasc Surg 59:1265-1273, 2014

Objective.—The purpose of this study was to analyze midterm results of bypass patency and overall and aortic-related mortality rates of hybrid aortic procedures for thoracoabdominal aortic pathologies.

Methods.—A retrospective study was performed considering prospectively collected data in two centers. From January 2001 to December 2012, 45 patients (33 men; mean age, 67.8 ± 7.6 years) received hybrid aortic procedures for thoracoabdominal aortic diseases (31 atherosclerotic aneurysms, 7 chronic expanding type B aortic dissections, 2 penetrating aortic ulcers, and 5 pseudoaneurysms), corresponding to 155 revascularized visceral abdominal arteries. Elective/emergency and staged/simultaneous approaches were 31 of 14 and 28 of 17, respectively. Patient demographics, clinical risk factors, and aortic morphological and procedural data were collected. End points were technical success, 30-day morbidity, reintervention and mortality, bypass graft patency, freedom from reintervention, and overall and aortic-related mortality during midterm follow-up. Mean follow-up was 2.2 ± 2.4 years.

Results.—Technical success was achieved in 86.6% (39/45) of patients. Thirty-day morbidity rate was 60% (paraplegia/paraparesis: 13.3%, stroke: 6.7%, renal failure: 31.3%, permanent dialysis: 4.4%). Thirty-day freedom from reintervention rates were 67.1% and 78.5%, respectively. Thirty-day occlusion of revascularized visceral vessels occurred in 11 (7.1%, 11/155) target arteries. In-hospital mortality rate was 24.4%. Primary graft patency after 1, 2, and 4 years was 89.7%, 85.3%, and 79%, respectively. Bypass thrombosis or stenosis developed in nine (6.8%, 9/132) vessels during follow-up. Of these, three patients required reintervention and one died. Freedom from reintervention rates after 1, 2, and 4 years were 45.6%, 45.6%, and 34.2%, respectively. Overall and aortic-related mortality rates after 1, 2, and 4 years were 32.6%, 41.4%, and 45.3% and 9.1%, 13.9%, and 13.9%, respectively.

Conclusions.—A hybrid procedure for thoracoabdominal aortic pathologies in high-risk patient is feasible but carries a significant rate of early and midterm reintervention and death. Long-term surveillance of the visceral bypass is necessary because one-third of the patients will have bypass-related complications.

▶ The thoracoabdominal aneurysm in the elderly patient continues to present challenges as all previous reporting has shown high morbidity and mortality. This study supports those findings and shows similar outcomes to previous work looking at this issue. Of interest is the rate of 10% graft thrombosis at 1 year and close to 20% at 4 years. The article highlights the notion that vigilant surveillance is needed to maintain primary patency when hybrid procedures are used. From the analysis, superior mesenteric artery and celiac thrombosis yielded higher rates of subsequent death, whereas renal thrombosis ended predictably with dialysis. Although almost one-third of patients following hybrid approach had renal failure (which speaks to the initial surgical insult), only 4% went on to dialysis. From these data, we can assume that aggressive surveillance will help find impending graft failure and early intervention is warranted to preserve graft patency. The authors also discuss the important issue of whether such hybrid procedures should be simultaneous versus staged (this reviewer and the Hopkins group strongly favor the latter in every circumstance except free rupture). This series promotes the notion of staging also, with the paraplegia rate of only 6.3% in staged repair versus 17.3% in simultaneous repair. Indeed, in the old and infirmed, an outcome of paraplegia is usually synonymous with death, so the every effort should be directed against it.

B. W. Propper, MD

Global experience with an inner branched arch endograft

Haulon S, Greenberg RK, Spear R, et al (Universitaire de Lille, France; et al)

J Thorac Cardiovasc Surg 148:1709-1716, 2014

Background.—Branched endografts are a new option to treat arch aneurysm in high-risk patients.

Methods and results.—We performed a retrospective multicenter analysis of all patients with arch aneurysms treated with a new branched endograft designed with 2 inner branches to perfuse the supra aortic trunks. Thirty-eight patients were included. The median age was 71 years (range, 64-74 years). An American Society of Anesthesiologists score of 3 or 4 was reported in 89.5% (95% confidence interval [CI], 79.7-99.3) of patients. The 30-day mortality rate was 13.2% (95% CI, 2.2-24.2). Technical success was obtained in 32 patients (84.2% [95% CI, 72.4-95.9]). Early secondary procedures were performed in 4 patients (10.5% [95% CI, 0.7-20.3]). Early cerebrovascular complications were diagnosed in 6 patients (15.8% [95% CI, 4.0-27.6]), including 4 transient ischemic attacks, 1 stroke, and 1 subarachnoid hemorrhage. The median follow-up was 12 months (range, 6-12 months). During follow-up, no aneurysm-related death was detected. Secondary procedures during follow-up were performed in 3 patients (9.1% [95% CI, 0.0-19.1]), including 1 conversion to open surgery. We compared the first 10 patients (early experience group) with the subsequent 28 patients. Intraoperative complications and secondary procedures were significantly higher in the early experience group. Although not statistically significant, the early mortality was higher in the early experience group (30% [95% CI, 0.0-60.0]) versus the remainder (7.1% [95% CI, 0.0-16.9]; $P = .066$). Being part of the early experience group and ascending aortic diameter ≥38 mm were found to be associated to higher rates of combined early mortality and neurologic complications.

Conclusions.—Our preliminary study confirms the feasibility and safety of the endovascular repair of arch aneurysms in selected patients who may not have other conventional options. Clinical trial registration information: Thoracic IDE NCT00583817, FDA IDE# 000101 (Fig 2).

▶ Aortic arch aneurysms require complex and challenging surgical repair. Open repair is associated with a high level of morbidity and mortality. As branched endograft technology has progressed, a totally endovascular approach to repair has been developed. This article looks at the first reported experience with taking the endovascular concept into the arch, a true Zone 0 solution. Multiple centers participated and shared their experience in the work, and their trials and errors across centers to improve outcomes are insightful.

The device is a Cook endograft with 2 inner branches to perfuse the supra-aortic trunks. Deployment requires 3 main steps: (1) left subclavian artery revascularization, (2) deployment of the device in the aortic arch, and (3) cannulation of the inner branches in the innominate artery and left common carotid and bridging these branches with a covered stent (see Fig 2).

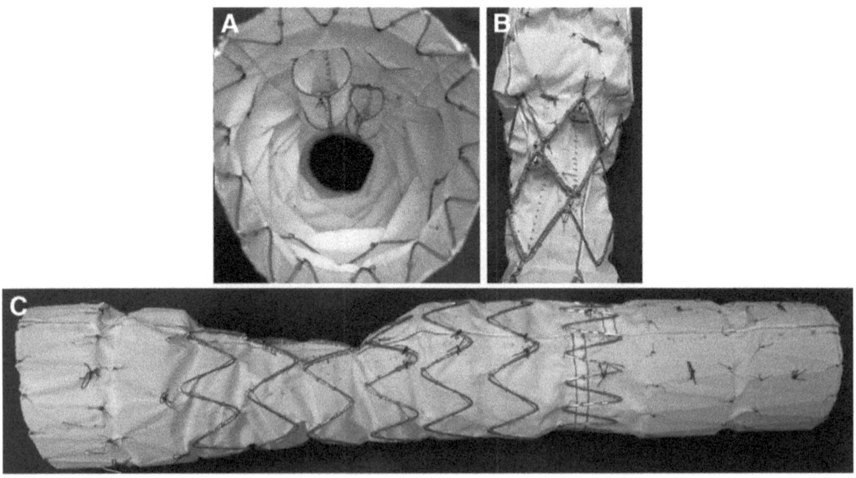

FIGURE 2.—The arch endograft. A, Two internal side branches. B, An enlarged external opening at each distal end. C, The middle of the endograft is narrow to separate the opening of the side branches from the orifices of the supra-aortic trunks to facilitate catheterization and preserve blood flow to the supra-aortic trunks. (Reprinted from the Journal of Thoracic and Cardiovascular Surgery. Haulon S, Greenberg RK, Spear R, et al. Global experience with an inner branched arch endograft. *J Thorac Cardiovasc Surg*. 2014;148:1709-1716, Copyright 2014, with permission from The American Association for Thoracic Surgery.)

Overall 30-day mortality was 13.2%. Technical success was achieved in 84.2% (32 patients). Early cerebrovascular complications were seen in 15.8% of patients. In evaluating their results, the authors noted that there was a significantly higher number of intraoperative complications and secondary procedures in the first 10 patients, designated the early experience group ($P = .04$). This led the authors to conclude that there is a significant learning curve associated with the procedure. The identification of an ascending aorta diameter of 38 mm as predictive of complications is interesting; whether this was a function of atherosclerosis and embolization being the source of problems was not clear. Nonetheless, there will almost certainly evolve a "sweet spot" for this technology, and the article underscores a healthy proximal landing zone (in Zone 0) is key.

Although this study is limited by its small number of patients, it does demonstrate the feasibility for a total endovascular repair for this complicated pathology. Clearly further study and experience is needed with this technology before it becomes mainstream, but this article is a key first step.

M. Arnold, MD

Preoperative percutaneous coronary intervention in patients undergoing open thoracoabdominal and descending thoracic aneurysm repair

Girardi LN, Rabotnikov Y, Avgerinos DV (Weill Cornell Med College, NY)
J Thorac Cardiovasc Surg 147:163-168, 2014

Objective.—Current guidelines have recommended against coronary revascularization before noncardiac surgery in patients with asymptomatic coronary artery disease. However, myocardial infarction after thoracic aneurysm (TA) repair dramatically increases the morbidity and mortality. Revascularization with coronary artery bypass grafting before TA repair minimizes the incidence of perioperative ischemia. However, the recovery can be prolonged, and a percentage of patients will either never return for aneurysm repair or will develop a rupture during convalescence. Percutaneous coronary intervention (PCI) before TA repair might be preferable. Previous studies examining PCI before major vascular surgery included few patients with TAs. We examined the outcomes of patients undergoing PCI before TA repair.

Methods.—From 1997 to 2012, 592 patients underwent TA repair. Patients presenting for elective repair underwent cardiac catheterization before surgery. Those with significant single- or double-vessel coronary artery disease underwent PCI. The perioperative outcomes were examined and compared with those of patients undergoing TA repair without revascularization.

Results.—A total of 44 patients (7.4%) underwent PCI with bare metal stents before surgery. No PCI-related complications occurred. Dual antiplatelet therapy was administered for 4 to 6 weeks. No instances of aneurysm rupture occurred in the interval between PCI and surgery. The incidence of stent thrombosis, myocardial infarction, and mortality for those undergoing PCI was 0. No bleeding complications occurred.

Conclusions.—PCI is safe and efficacious in patients undergoing TA repair. Aneurysm rupture did not occur in the interval before surgery. Antiplatelet therapy did not increase the risk of bleeding complications. Stent thrombosis was not seen. We recommend PCI those with significant single- or double-vessel coronary artery disease before elective TA repair.

▶ The CARP trial revolutionized the preoperative testing for most vascular surgery patients. Indeed, most vascular patients do not require extensive preoperative cardiac evaluation and certainly do not benefit from interventions if they are asymptomatic. The authors herein bring an excellent point that thoracoabdominal and descending thoracic aneurysms (TAA/DTA) are among the most high-risk vascular surgeries and were near excluded from the trials on which the American Heart Association/American College of Cardiology guidelines were developed. The high cross-clamp certainly places significantly more stress on the heart compared with even abdominal aortic aneurysm repairs. The contemporary paper by Wong et al noted that 26.7% of elective TAA had a cardiac complication postoperatively and that these patients had a startling 25.7% mortality rate. Most would agree that it is not unreasonable to pursue cardiac optimization in TAA/DTA patients if they are symptomatic, but most patients are in fact asymptomatic, as shown here. The 2 main concerns addressed are the following: will patients have more bleeding on dual antiplatelet therapy, and will patients rupture their TAA/DTA in the interim between recovering from percutaneous coronary intervention (PCI)/coronary artery bypass grafting (CABG) and aneurysm repair? Although this was a small set of patients, the outcomes were noteworthy. No patients had postoperative bleeding requiring a return to the operative room, and no patients ruptured their aneurysms in the interim, even with the 3-month recovery period after CABG. No patients with preoperative cardiac intervention suffered a myocardial infarction. Only 1 patient suffered spinal cord ischemia, which is also remarkable because 77% of patients underwent a "clamp and sew" method whereas only 23% had extracorporeal circulatory support (there were relatively few type II TAAA in the series). In the reviewer's experience, all Extent type I and II undergo either left-heart bypass or circulatory arrest in an effort to keep such a low percentage of SCI. Furthermore, we routinely perform diagnostic coronary angiogram with full intention for treatment (either PCI or CABG) for all patients planned for circulatory arrest. On some level, this paper is reassuring that when clinical judgment leads to delay in thoracoabdominal aortic aneurysm treatment, such delay is not blatantly unsafe. But moreover, it would be interesting for these authors who have performed 592 thoracic aneurysm repairs to compare the outcomes of asymptomatic patients who underwent coronary revascularization to those who did not to replicate the real question—the true comparative benefit of coronary revascularization that CARP answered.

J. H. Black III, MD, FACS

Severe visceral ischemia and death after multilayer stent deployment for the treatment of a thoracoabdominal aortic aneurysm

Cavalcante RN, Nishinari K, Yazbek G, et al (A.C.Camargo Cancer Ctr, São Paulo, Brazil)

J Vasc Surg:1-4, 2014

The treatment of thoracoabdominal aortic aneurysms, both surgical and endovascular, has always been challenging. In the last years, the multilayer stent has emerged as an alternative device for the treatment of this condition. In this paper, we describe a catastrophic complication of the multilayer stent in a patient with thoracoabdominal aortic aneurysm, a case of massive visceral ischemia and death 3 months after stent deployment.

▶ The Cardiatis multilayer stent has been developed as an alternative to fenestrated or branched endografts for the repair of complex thoracoabdominal aneurysms. This new technology is a multilayered stent that is designed to divert flow from the aneurysm sac leading to sac thrombosis while preserving visceral flow. The fact that aortic pressure continually transmitted to the aortic wall through the multilayer stent is a departure from the traditional aneurysm exclusion is the best outcome. Thus, the ongoing concerns about the device to include continued flow into the aneurysm sac leading to continued sac growth as well as occlusion of critical branches that are fed through the stent has formed a large group of skeptics regarding adoption of the device. The largest published series on outcomes with this device cite 55 treated patients with a 1-year aneurysm-related survival of 93.7%, which would seem favorable on face value.

This article presents a case of severe visceral ischemia 4 months after stent deployment. While the patient was initially placed on clopidogrel and aspirin, clopidogrel was stopped 4 months postoperatively after imaging demonstrated a patent graft with persistent flow into the aneurysm sac. Less than 2 weeks later, the patient was hospitalized and found to have massive and widespread visceral ischemia, leading to death. The authors suggest that, based on this catastrophic outcome, further study on this device is warranted before its widespread use in the treatment of thoracoabdominal aneurysms. New technology is always encumbered by new modes of failure, and the multilayer stent needs to demonstrate efficacy with aneurysm sac stabilization *and* branch vessel patency. This reviewer would hope the surgical community would study the questions separately; why not study its performance in a TAA sac remodeling/growth/rupture before leaping across the visceral segment?

M. Arnold, MD

Use of a novel hybrid vascular graft for sutureless revascularization of the renal arteries during open thoracoabdominal aortic aneurysm repair

Chiesa R, Kahlberg A, Mascia D, et al ("Vita-Salute" Univ School of Medicine, Milan, Italy)

J Vasc Surg 60:622-630, 2014

Objective.—The aim of this study was to assess the safety and short-term effectiveness of a novel hybrid vascular graft used to address renal revascularization during open thoracoabdominal aortic aneurysm (TAAA) repair, performing a sutureless distal anastomosis.

Methods.—Between 2012 and 2013, 25 patients (16 men; mean age, 66 ± 8 years) underwent revascularization of one (24 patients) or both (one patient) renal arteries with the Gore Hybrid Vascular Graft (GHVG; W. L. Gore and Associates, Flagstaff, Ariz) during open TAAA repair. Specific indications included remote location of the ostium of the renal artery, severe atherosclerotic wall degeneration, focal dissection, and stenosis. All surviving patients underwent computed tomography angiography and follow-up visit at 1 month. Preoperative characteristics, intraoperative data, and short-term results were compared with those of 49 concurrent TAAA patients operated on within the same period by standard renal revascularization (SRR) techniques.

Results.—All GHVG target renal vessels (26 of 26) were successfully revascularized without technical concerns. No significant differences were found between GHVG and SRR groups in preoperative and intraoperative data, except for a relative prevalence of aortic dissection (28% vs 6%; $P=.026$) and renal artery stenosis (44% vs 12%; $P=.003$) in the GHVG group and for intraoperative renal bare stenting that was predominantly used in the SRR group (12% vs 28%; $P=.036$). The 30-day mortality was 4% in both groups. Postoperative acute renal failure (doubling of creatinine level and creatinine level >3.0 mg/dL) occurred in two GHVG patients (8%) and seven SRR patients (14%; $P=$NS). Perioperative peak decrease of estimated glomerular filtration rate was lower in the GHVG group (26 ± 18 mL/min/1.73 m^2 vs 37 ± 22 mL/min/1.73 m^2; $P=.034$). At 1-month computed tomography angiography, renal artery patency was 92% for the GHVG vessels, 91% for the contralateral to GHVG renal vessels, and 92% for the SRR group arteries. No GHVG-related complications requiring reintervention or cases of new-onset renal failure requiring dialysis were observed at follow-up.

Conclusions.—Renal revascularization during open TAAA repair by the GHVG with distal sutureless anastomosis is feasible, especially in cases of aortic dissection, remote location of the renal vessel, and severe atherosclerotic disease of the ostium. Short-term results are satisfactory, at least comparable to those of SRR. Larger series and longer follow-up are needed to assess clinical advantages and durability of this new device.

▶ Unfortunately, renal compromise is not an uncommon complication after thoracoabdominal aneurysm (TAA) repair. Many techniques are employed intraoperatively in an attempt to decrease this hit on the kidneys. Here the authors are the first to explore the safety and efficacy of the Gore Hybrid Vascular Graft (GHVG) during open TAA repairs. Results are clearly promising. Renal bypass patency was excellent for both GHVG and the standard renal revascularization group (SRR). There was no significant difference in postoperative complications; specifically no renal complications requiring reintervention in the GHVG group. As one might expect, the actual overall surgical time did not differ between the GHVG group and SRR group. Each renal artery anastomosis on average takes 10 to 15 minutes, but total time for these procedures often exceed 8 to 9 hours. What is notable is the significantly decreased cold renal perfusion time; 28 min versus 34 minutes ($P = .031$). As a result, the perioperative peak decrease glomerular filtration rate was lower in the GHVG group than the SRR. Although we define acute renal failure as doubling of the baseline creatinine or an absolute value above 3.0 mg/dL, it is the vast number of patients who experience a smaller degree of postoperative renal insufficiency where this novel technique may make the most difference. Alternatively, in patients who require individual revascularization of all 4 renovisceral arteries, the time saved using the GHVG can certainly be advantageous. However, many of these patients fall under the category of connective tissue disease, and the question of whether GHVG is better suited than hand-sewn anastomosis in these patients has yet to be answered.

K. C. Orion, MD

Variation in Maximum Diameter Measurements of Descending Thoracic Aortic Aneurysms Using Unformatted Planes versus Images Corrected to Aortic Centerline

Rudarakanchana N, Bicknell CD, Cheshire NJ, et al (Imperial College, London, UK; et al)

Eur J Vasc Endovasc Surg 47:19-26, 2014

Objective.—Evaluation of variation in descending thoracic aortic aneurysm (dTAA) diameters measured on CT scans in different planes and by different observers and the potential impact on treatment decisions.

Methods.—CT angiography of dTAA ($N = 20$) were assessed by three specialists, with measurements repeated after 1 month. Calliper measurements of maximum external diameters were made on unformatted images and perpendicular to the aneurysm centerline after image processing (corrected). Repeatability was assessed using Bland—Altman plots.

Results.—Maximum corrected diameter measurements were smaller than axial measurements (66.3 ± 7.9 mm vs. 74.9 ± 20.9 mm, $p < .001$). Both intraobserver and interobserver variation were less for corrected than for axial measurements (mean intraobserver differences 5.0 ± 3.8 mm vs. 11.8 ± 9.3 mm, $p < .001$; mean interobserver differences 2.8 ± 2.5 mm versus 10.4 ± 14.0 mm, $p < .001$) and interobserver variation increased with aneurysm diameter for maximum axial but not corrected measurements. Using corrected rather than axial measurements could have changed treatment decisions in two patients (10%) using a treatment threshold diameter of 55 mm and 10 patients (50%) using a threshold of 65 mm.

Conclusion.—Corrected diameters were smaller than axial diameters, could be measured with higher repeatability, and were subject to less interobserver variability. Using corrected versus axial measurements would have changed management decisions in up to half of the cases in this study (Fig 1).

▶ Currently, a standardized guideline for obtaining maximum diameter measurements for descending thoracic aortic aneurysms (dTAA) does not exist. Having a standardized protocol in place is essential for comparing data between studies and truly understanding the natural history of dTAA with regard to size and rupture risk. This study sought to define the most reliable and reproducible maximum diameter measurement. The CT scans of 20 patients were presented to 3 expert vascular radiologists, and they were asked to obtain maximal diameter measurements in 3 unformatted planes (axial, coronal, and sagittal) as well

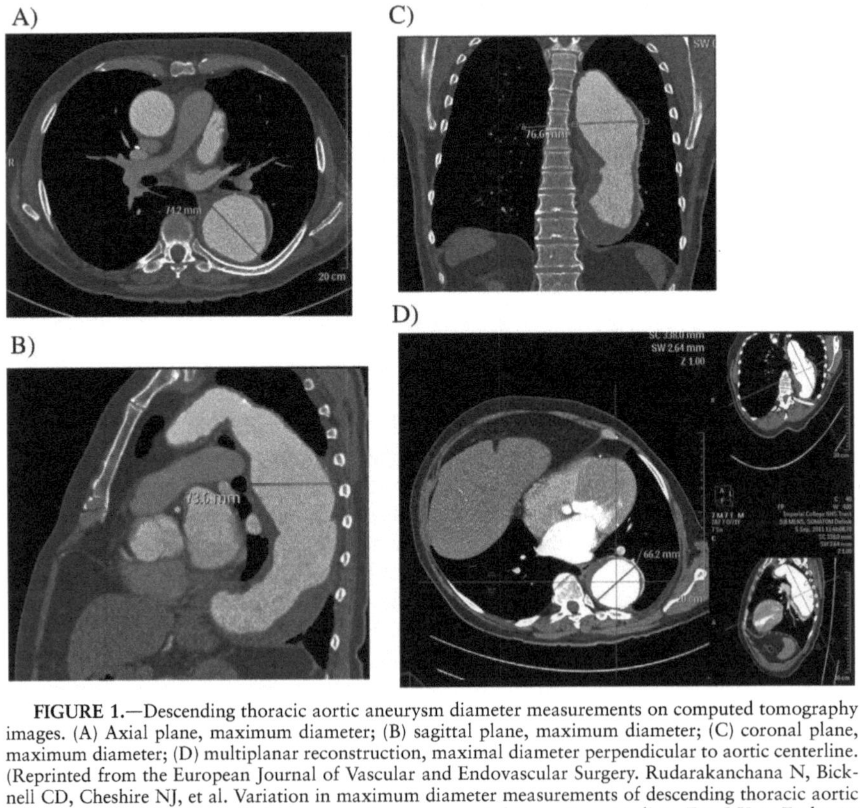

FIGURE 1.—Descending thoracic aortic aneurysm diameter measurements on computed tomography images. (A) Axial plane, maximum diameter; (B) sagittal plane, maximum diameter; (C) coronal plane, maximum diameter; (D) multiplanar reconstruction, maximal diameter perpendicular to aortic centerline. (Reprinted from the European Journal of Vascular and Endovascular Surgery. Rudarakanchana N, Bicknell CD, Cheshire NJ, et al. Variation in maximum diameter measurements of descending thoracic aortic aneurysms using unformatted planes versus images corrected to aortic centerline. *Eur J Vasc Endovasc Surg*. 2014;47:19-26, Copyright 2014, with permission from European Society for Vascular Surgery.)

as after double-oblique multiplanar reconstructions with an aortic centerline (Fig 1).

The average maximal aortic diameter from the axial planes was larger than the maximal corrected diameter (74.9 ± 20.9 mm vs 66.3 ± 7.9 mm, $P < .001$). In addition, both intra- and interobserver variation was less for the corrected images than axial images (mean intraobserver differences 5.0 ± 3.8 mm vs 11.8 ± 9.3 mm, $P < .001$; mean interobserver difference 2.8 ± 2.5 mm vs 10.4 ± 14.0 mm, $P < .001$). Of note, the interobserver variation increased with aneurysm diameter for the axial images but not for the corrected images.

On the basis of these findings, the authors propose that the external corrected diameter become the new reporting standard for dTAA. The biggest limitation of this study is the small number of observers (3). Also, all measurements were done on a single workstation, so this study does not take into account the variability that may come with different processing techniques. Regardless, the establishment of a single measurement method and reporting standard for dTAA is vital for analysis and clinical decision making. Ultimately, some institutions will rely on in-house proprietary workstations that are integrated with their scanner company, and others will pay for additional vendors, but the end effect is to move past axial imaging reporting to centerline corrected methodology.

M. Arnold, MD

Aortic arch debranching and thoracic endovascular repair

De Rango P, Cao P, Ferrer C, et al (Univ of Perugia, Italy; Hosp S. Camillo - Forlanini, Rome)

J Vasc. Surg 59:107-114, 2014

Objective.—Currently, the best approach to the aortic arch remains unsupported by robust evidence. Most of the available data rely on small sample numbers, heterogeneous settings, and limited follow-up. The objective of this study was to evaluate early and midterm results of arch debranching and endovascular procedures.

Methods.—From 2005 through 2013, 104 consecutive patients underwent elective arch treatment with debranching and thoracic endovascular aortic repair. Rates of perioperative (30-day) mortality and neurological complications, and mortality, endoleak, supra-aortic vessel patency, and arch diameter changes at 5 years were analyzed.

Results.—Patients' mean age was 69.8 years, and 90 were males. Twenty arches were repaired for dissection. Nineteen patients required total debranching for diseases extended to zone 0. In 59, debranching and thoracic endovascular aortic repair procedures were staged. At 30 days, death, stroke, and spinal cord ischemia occurred in six, four, and three patients, respectively. Extension to ascending aorta (zone 0 landing) was the only multivariate independent predictor for perioperative mortality (odds ratio, 9.6; 95% confidence interval, 1.54-59.90; $P = .015$), but not for stroke. Four retrograde dissections, two fatal, occurred during the perioperative period. At 1, 3, and 5 years, Kaplan-Meier survival rates were 89.0%, 82.8%, and 70.9%, and freedom from persistent endoleak rates were 96.1%, 92.5%, and 88.3%, respectively. Over 5-year follow-up, 34 aneurysms shrank ≥5 mm, and four grew. Five reinterventions were required. Two supra-aortic vessel occlusions and no late aorta-related mortalities were recorded.

Conclusions.—Despite the perioperative mortality risk, the late outcome of endovascular arch repair presents a low rate of aorta-related deaths and reinterventions and acceptable midterm survival. Furthermore, more than one-third of the aneurysms' diameters decrease over 5 years as a measure of the long-term efficacy of treatment. Retrograde type A dissection remains a major concern in the perioperative period and careful arch approach is required (Figs 1 and 2, Table 2).

▶ I chose this report for this year's Year Book because it represents one of the largest series of combined aortic arch debranching and thoracic endovascular aortic repair procedures with the longest mean follow-up of more than

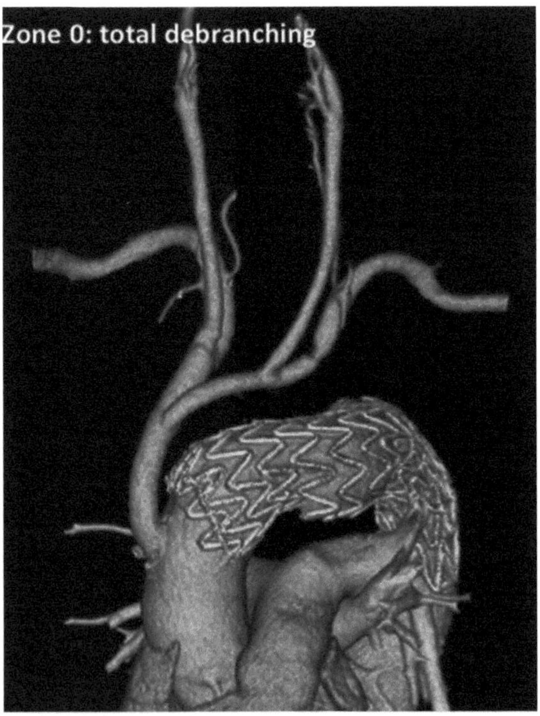

FIGURE 1.—Total debranching (computed tomography angiography [CTA] reconstructions). Bifurcated Dacron bypass from ascending aorta to innominate and left subclavian (LSA) arteries; left common carotid artery attached on the LSA branch associated with thoracic endovascular aortic stent graft. (Reprinted from the Journal of Vascular Surgery. De Rango P, Cao P, Ferrer C, et al. Aortic arch debranching and thoracic endovascular repair. *J Vasc Surg*. 2014;59:107-114, Copyright 2014, with permission from The Society for Vascular Surgery.)

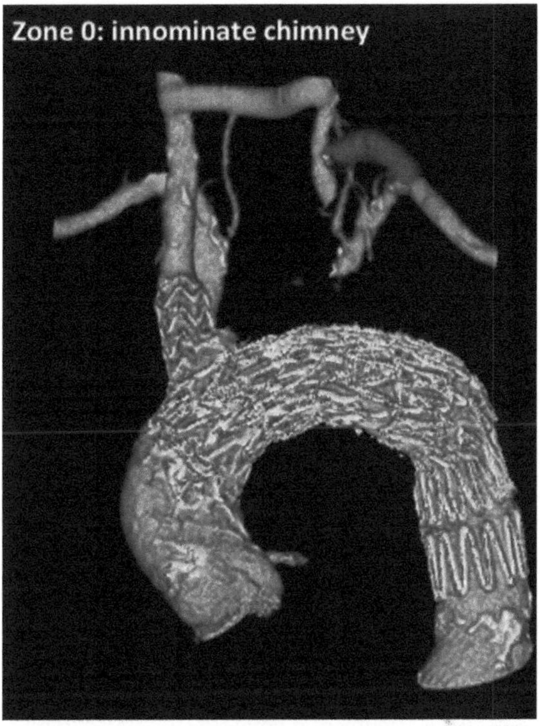

FIGURE 2.—Total debranching (computed tomography angiography [CTA] reconstructions). Innominate chimney and aortic stent graft associated with carotid-carotid-subclavian bypass (in *green* and *red*, respectively) with retropharyngeal tunnel. For interpretation of the references to color in this figure legend, the reader is referred to web version of this article. (Reprinted from the Journal of Vascular Surgery. De Rango P, Cao P, Ferrer C, et al. Aortic arch debranching and thoracic endovascular repair. *J Vasc Surg.* 2014;59:107-114, Copyright 2014, with permission from The Society for Vascular Surgery.)

29 months. A total of 104 consecutive patients with a variety of aortopathies underwent combined or staged treatment for diseased within zones 0 through 2.[1] Technical details of 104 arch debranching procedures are listed in Table 2.

Total debranching (zone 0 landing) accounted for a 30-day mortality risk significantly higher than for the partial debranching group (odds ratio [OR], 11.1; 95% confidence interval [CI], 1.86–65.90; $P = .01$). Thirty-day risk of stroke (OR, 1.5; 95% CI, 0.15–15.45; $P = .56$) and spinal cord ischemia (OR, 2.3; 95% CI, 0.19–26.82; $P = .46$) were not significantly different in the total debranching group.

Technical success was achieved in an impressive 97.1%, and, overall, 4 de novo type A retrograde dissections were recorded at 30 days, 2 being lethal. Zone 0 repair (Figs 1 and 2) was associated with a higher rate of complications.

Despite the relevant perioperative mortality risk, the midterm outcome of endovascular arch repair with different debranching modalities presents a low rate of aorta-related death and reinterventions and acceptable 5-year survival.

TABLE 2.—Technical Details in 104 Arch Debranching Procedures

Technical Details	No. (%)	Procedure Description
Staged procedure	59 (56.7)	16 total surgical debranching
Zone 0	19 (18.3)	1 single (innominate) chimney stent graft + Car-Car-Subcl
		1 single (innominate) branched stent graft + Car-Car-Subcl
		1 triple chimney stent graft
Zone 1	51 (49.0)	Surgical bypass/transposition:
		37 Car-Car-Subcl (20 retropharyngeal; 17 ante-trachea)
		2 Car-Car (ante-trachea)
		6 Car-Subcl (bovine arch)
		6 bilateral Car-Subcl: 4 aberrant Subcl
		2 aberrant Subcl + bovine arch
Zone 2	34 (32.7)	31 Car-Subcl
		3 single (left Subcl) chimney stent graft
Number of aortic stent grafts/repairs[a]	150/103	(1 patient died after 1° stage)
		59 Single stent graft
		39: Two aortic stent grafts
		4: Three aortic stent grafts
		1: Four aortic stent grafts

Car, Carotid; *Car-Car*, right common carotid-left common carotid surgical bypass; *Car-Car-Subcl*, right common carotid-left common carotid-left subclavian surgical bypass/transposition; *Car-Subcl*, common carotid-subclavian surgical bypass/transposition; *Subcl*, subclavian; *TEVAR*, thoracic endovascular aortic repair.

In two patients, left subclavian arteries not revascularized because of urgency or direct vertebral revascularization.

[a]Device models employed in the 103 TEVARs included: 46 Cook Zenith, 22 Gore TAG-C-TAG, 26 Medtronic Talent/Valiant, 9 Bolton Relay.

Furthermore, most of the aneurysm diameters (95.7%) shrank or remained stable over 5 years.

B. W. Starnes, MD

Reference

1. Mitchell RS, Ishimaru S, Ehrlich MP, et al. First international summit on thoracic aortic endografting: round table on thoracic aortic dissection as an indication for endografting. *J Endovasc Ther.* 2002;9:II98-II105.

Aortic arch rupture after multiple multilayer stent treatment of a thoracoabdominal aneurysm

Ferrero E, Gibello L, Ferri M, et al (Mauriziano Umberto I Hosp, Turin, Italy)
J Vasc Surg 60:1348-1352, 2014

Despite the improvement in diagnostic and therapeutic strategies, the treatment of thoracoabdominal aneurysms is still burdened with a high incidence of peri/postoperative morbidity and mortality. The multilayer flow modulator is a new and promising technique for the treatment of such disease; however, some limits are still evident. We report the case of a 76-year-old woman affected by a symptomatic thoracoabdominal aneurysm treated with multiple Cardiatis multilayer flow modulators

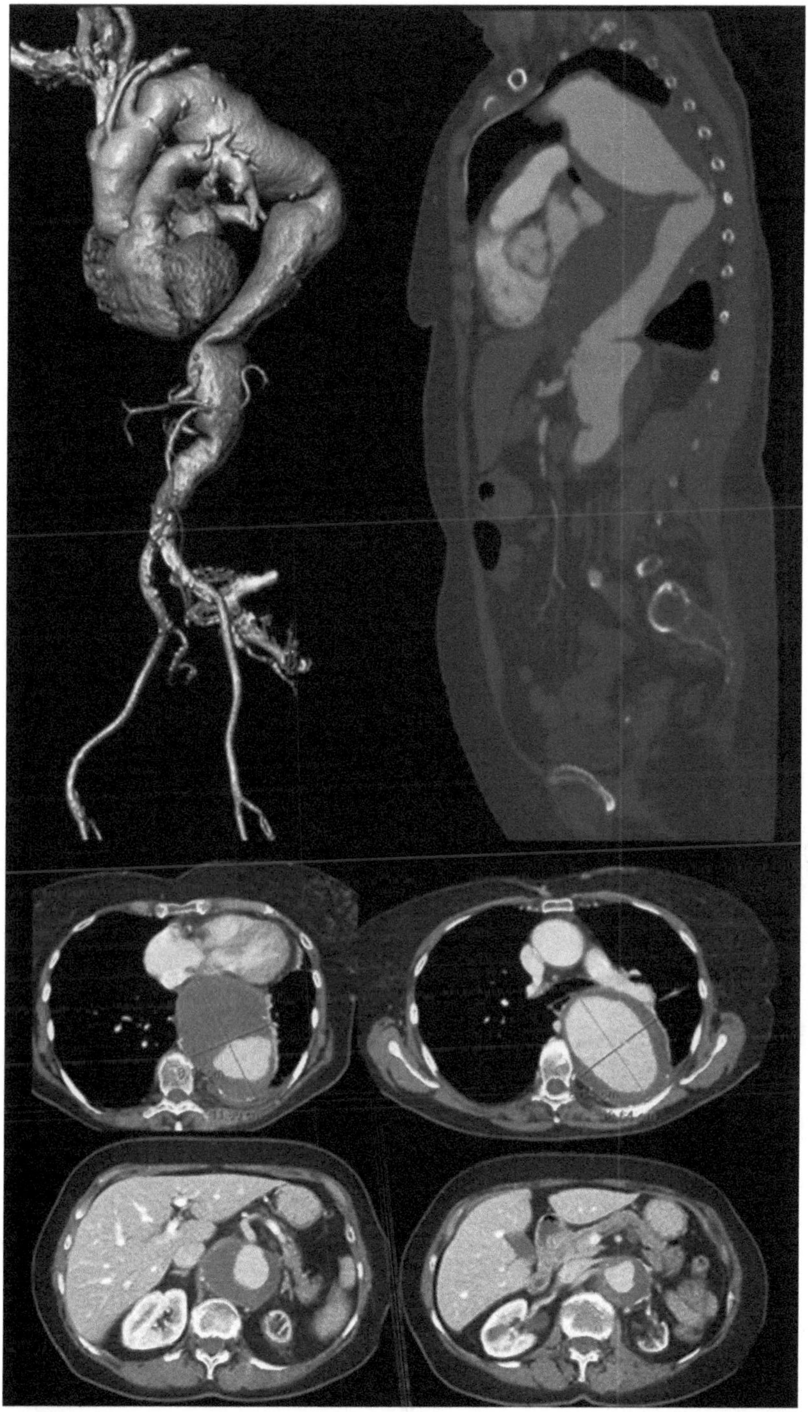

FIGURE 1.—The computed tomography angiography (CTA) showed the maximum increased dilatation of 81 mm at vertebral T4-T6 and a dilatation of infrarenal abdominal aortic aneurysm of 60 mm. The size of the aortic arch at the common carotid artery was 32 mm, at the subclavian artery was 30 mm, and the length between the common carotid artery and the subclavian artery was 15 mm. The distal sealing zone, at the abdominal aortic artery, had a diameter of 26.5 mm and a length of sealing zone of 40 mm. (Reprinted from the Journal of Vascular Surgery. Ferrero E, Gibello L, Ferri M, et al. Aortic arch rupture after multiple multilayer stent treatment of a thoracoabdominal aneurysm. *J Vasc Surg.* 2014;60:1348-1352, Copyright 2014, with permission from The Society for Vascular Surgery.)

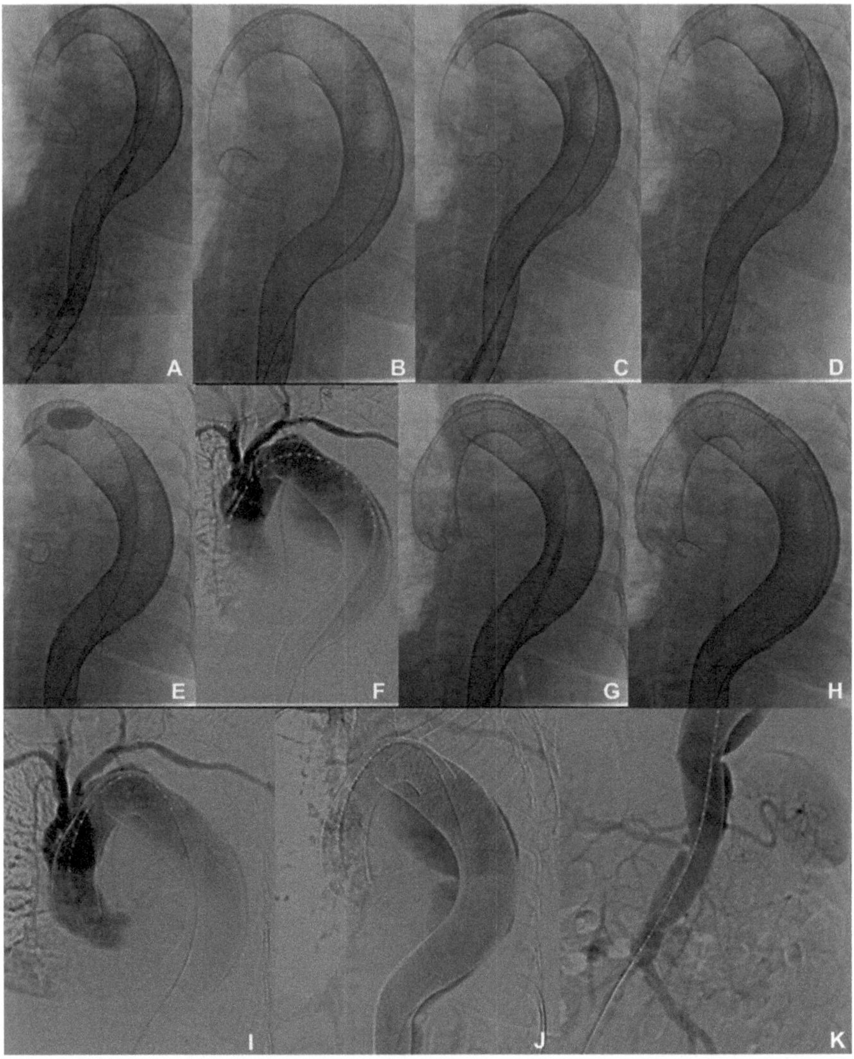

FIGURE 2.—**A,** Fluoroscopic images of Cardiatis multilayer flow modulator (CMFM) deployment. **B,** Modules and the ballooning maneuver showed CMFMs shortening with loss of both central overlapping regions. **C-D,** A fourth CMFM was positioned and ballooned. Presence of an image of infolding in the proximal end point. **E-H,** After the proximal end point ballooning, the CMFM retracted and dislocated, so a fifth CMFM was deployed, covering the whole aortic arch and landing in the ascending aorta. **I-K,** Fluoroscopic images of final control after CMFMs' deployment. (Reprinted from the Journal of Vascular Surgery. Ferrero E, Gibello L, Ferri M, et al. Aortic arch rupture after multiple multilayer stent treatment of a thoracoabdominal aneurysm. *J Vasc Surg.* 2014;60:1348-1352, Copyright 2014, with permission from The Society for Vascular Surgery.)

complicated by aortic arch rupture on the fifth postoperative day, with subsequent patient death (Figs 1-3).

▶ I must admit that I find myself in agreement with many of my colleagues in questioning the validity and reliability of a multilayer uncovered stent approach for treating aortic aneurysmal disease. This case report supports my bias in describing the rapid demise of a patient treated with these techniques. A 76-year-old woman with a symptomatic type II thoracoabdominal aneurysm (Fig 1) was treated with Cardiatis multilayer flow modulator (CMFM; Crossmed, Ines, Belgium) deployment (Fig 2). A total of 5 devices was implanted—mainly because of gross inaccuracy of the deployment process and what appeared to be the unpredictability of where the stents would land. One never wants to have their own postmortem photograph published in a case report (Fig 3).

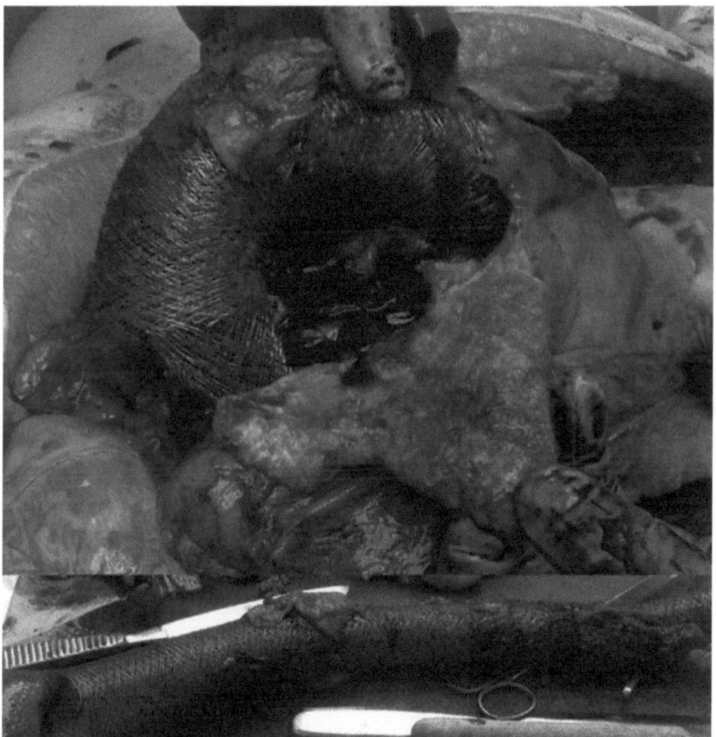

FIGURE 3.—The autopsy images revealed the rupture of the aortic arch in proximity of the descending tract. (Reprinted from the Journal of Vascular Surgery. Ferrero E, Gibello L, Ferri M, et al. Aortic arch rupture after multiple multilayer stent treatment of a thoracoabdominal aneurysm. *J Vasc Surg.* 2014;60:1348-1352, Copyright 2014, with permission from The Society for Vascular Surgery.)

What we do need is more transparent reporting of failures of these unproven techniques or even more robust registries so that we may decide for ourselves if these new strategies actually work.

B. W. Starnes, MD

Assessment of abdominal branch vessel patency after bare-metal stenting of the thoracoabdominal aorta in a human ex vivo model of acute type B aortic dissection

Faure EM, Canaud L, Cathala P, et al (Arnaud de Villeneuve Hosp, Montpellier, France; Lapeyronie Hosp, Montpellier, France; et al)

J Vasc Surg 61:1299-1305, 2015

Objective.—The purpose of this study was to assess the efficiency of bare-metal stenting of the thoracoabdominal aorta in a human ex vivo model of acute type B aortic dissection and the impact of this approach on the patency of the visceral and renal arteries.

Methods.—Fifteen human cadaveric aortas were harvested. Type B aortic dissections were surgically initiated 2 cm below the left subclavian artery. Aortas were thereafter connected to a bench top pulsatile flow to induce propagation of the dissection. A 5-mm 30° lens (Richard Wolf, Vernon Hills, Ill) was introduced successively into the false lumen and the true lumen to monitor the propagation of the dissection. Bare-metal stents were deployed into the true lumen from the primary entry tear to the infrarenal aorta. Measurement of systolic pressure was taken within the abdominal branch vessels before and after stenting. A pressure gradient drop of 15 mm Hg or more after bare-metal stenting was considered hemodynamically relevant.

Results.—Dissection was propagated at least to the renal aorta in 11 cases (73%) and to the infrarenal aorta in 3 cases (20%). Of the 60 abdominal branch vessels studied, 22 (36.7%) were supplied by the false lumen. After extensive aortic bare-metal stenting, complete reattachment of the dissection flap was observed in all cases. Regarding visceral and renal artery patency after bare-metal stenting, a significant pressure gradient drop was reported in 54.5% ($n = 12$) when these arteries were supplied by the false lumen, whereas those originating from the true lumen had a significantly less common pressure gradient drop (7.9% [$n = 3$]; $P < .0001$).

Conclusions.—Bare-metal stenting in this model of acute type B aortic dissection was effective in true lumen reexpansion but induced a high (54.5%) rate of significant pressure drop in the visceral and renal arteries when they were supplied by the false lumen (Figs 1-3).

▶ I chose this article for this year's edition because of the fantastic angioscopic pictures displayed depicting deployment of the bare-metal stent (PETTICOAT) for acute aortic dissection (Figs 1-3). A catheterization attempt of the aortic

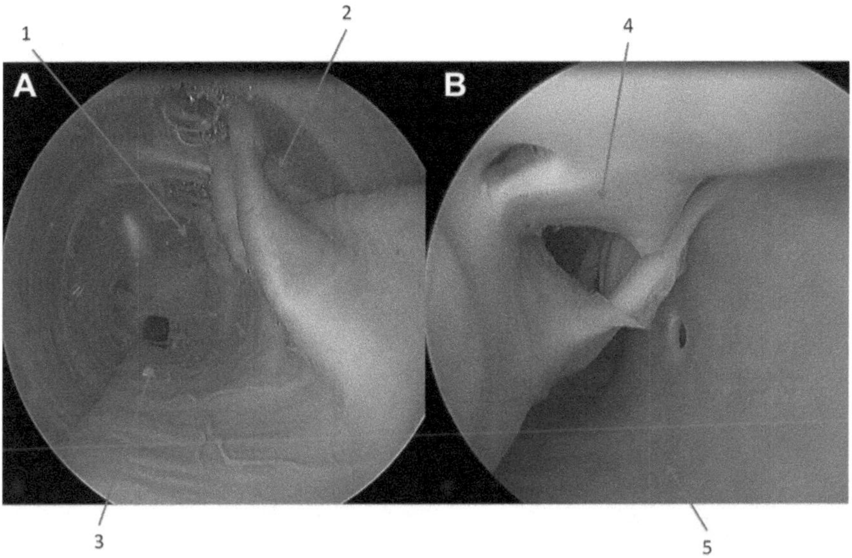

FIGURE 1.—Angioscopy of the false lumen and the true lumen after propagation of the dissection. Views of the false lumen (**A**) and the true lumen (**B**) of a dissected aorta. **A**, False lumen: (*1*) dissected intima of the superior mesenteric artery, (*2*) dissected intima of the celiac trunk, and (*3*) ostium of the left renal artery on the intimal-medial dissected flap. **B**, Dissection flap prolapse within the true lumen: (*4*) ostium of the dissected left renal artery on the flap; (*5*) nondissected aortic wall of the true lumen. (Reprinted from the Journal of Vascular Surgery. Faure EM, Canaud L, Cathala P, et al. Assessment of abdominal branch vessel patency after bare-metal stenting of the thoracoabdominal aorta in a human ex vivo model of acute type B aortic dissection. *J Vasc Surg*. 2015;61:1299-1305, Copyright 2014, with permission from The Society for Vascular Surgery.)

side branches with a significant stenosis and pressure gradient drop through the bare-metal stent was successful in 87% (n = 13 of 15). In the literature, no failure of aortic branch vessel stenting was reported, and stenting of these arteries with a significant pressure gradient drop was a therapeutic choice that appears effective.

Another innovation introduced by this study is the angioscopy performed during the propagation of the dissection (Figs 1 and 2). To the best of my knowledge, it is the first direct and dynamic view of the aortic dissection propagation, the tearing out of its side branches, and the dynamic true lumen collapse during systole due to the false lumen expansion. Angioscopy gave the authors an accurate view of the topography of the branch vessels and the distribution of the intimal-medial tears on the dissected flap.

Extensive bare-metal stenting in this human ex vivo model of Stanford type B aortic dissection is associated with a high rate (54.5%) of significant pressure gradient drop in the visceral and renal arteries when they are supplied by the false lumen. Therefore, according to this experimental model, this therapeutic approach for complicated type B aortic dissection should not be considered as first-line therapy. It could be used with caution as second-line therapy in

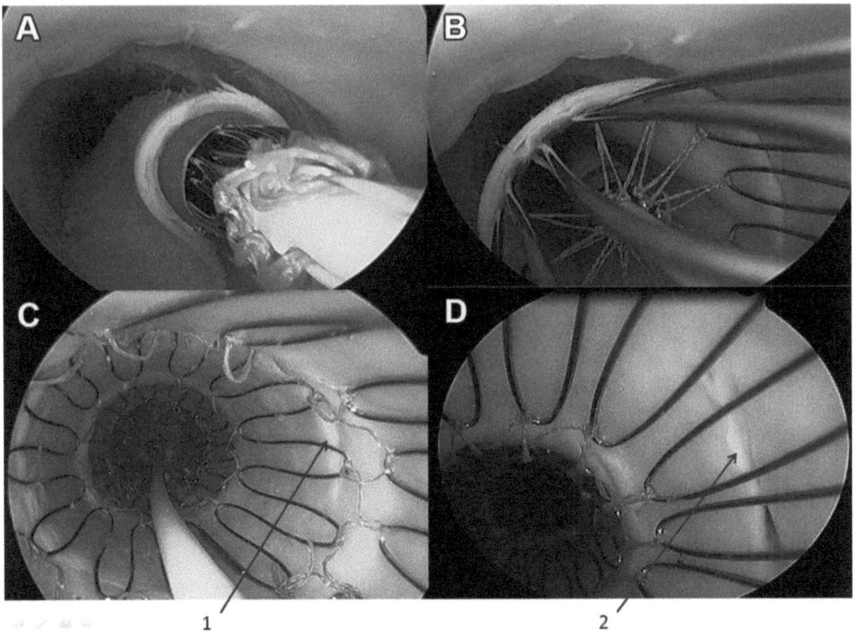

FIGURE 2.—Angioscopy during bare-metal stent deployment within the true lumen of a dissected aorta. **A**, Sheath of the baremetal stent arising from the true lumen, which is collapsed by the false lumen. **B**, Deployment of the stent within the true lumen; the intimal-medial layer is reattached on the aortic wall. **C**, After complete deployment of the bare-metal stent, the intimal-medial flap is completely reattached (*1*). **D**, Right renal artery ostium (*2*) with stenosis after bare-metal stenting. (Reprinted from the Journal of Vascular Surgery. Faure EM, Canaud L, Cathala P, et al. Assessment of abdominal branch vessel patency after bare-metal stenting of the thoracoabdominal aorta in a human ex vivo model of acute type B aortic dissection. *J Vasc Surg*. 2015;61:1299-1305, Copyright 2014, with permission from The Society for Vascular Surgery.)

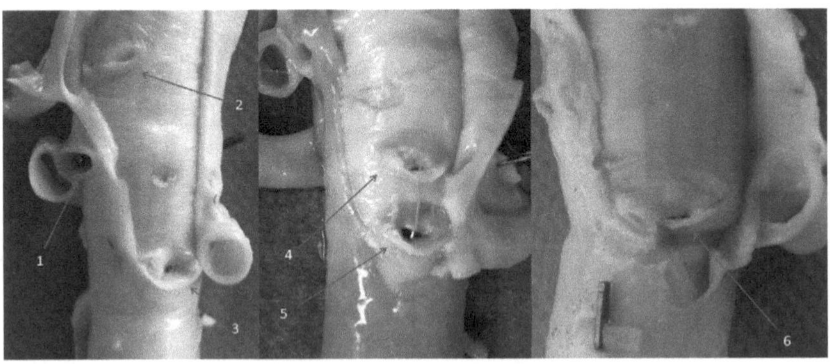

FIGURE 3.—Macroscopic examination of three aortas with visible stenosis of the side branches originating from the false lumen. The dissected part of the aortic wall is open. Bare-metal stent is visible through the intimal-medial flap by transparency. *1*, Ostium of the superior mesenteric artery originating from the true lumen, without stenosis. *2*, Ostium of the celiac trunk within the dissected flap, with stenosis >50%. *3*, Ostium of the left renal artery with stenosis >50%. *4*, Ostium of a supernumerary left renal artery with a stenosis >50%. *5*, Ostium of the left renal artery with stenosis >50%. *6*, Ostium of the right renal artery with stenosis >50%. (Reprinted from the Journal of Vascular Surgery. Faure EM, Canaud L, Cathala P, et al. Assessment of abdominal branch vessel patency after bare-metal stenting of the thoracoabdominal aorta in a human ex vivo model of acute type B aortic dissection. *J Vasc Surg*. 2015;61:1299-1305, Copyright 2014, with permission from The Society for Vascular Surgery.)

the case of persistence of dynamic malperfusion after closure of the primary entry by a thoracic stent-graft.

B. W. Starnes, MD

Contemporary management of symptomatic primary aortic mural thrombus

Verma H, Meda N, Vora S, et al (Narayana Inst of Vascular Sciences, Bangalore, India)

J Vasc Surg 60:1524-1534, 2014

Objective.—Primary aortic mural thrombus (PAMT) is an uncommon condition but an important source of noncardiogenic emboli with a difficult diagnosis and a high rate of complications, including high mortality. We report our experience of thromboembolic disease from PAMT and review its contemporary management.

Methods.—Retrospective analysis of prospectively collected data of all patients who presented with acute occlusion of a limb or visceral vessels between January 2011 and September 2013 was performed.

Results.—A total of 88 patients presented with acute occlusion of the extremities or visceral arteries. All underwent extensive evaluation for the possible source of the embolism. Of these 88 patients, 19 patients (mean age, 41.2 years; male:female ratio, 1:2.1) were found to have aortic mural thrombus as the source of distal embolism. Thrombus was located in the thoracic aorta in 10 patients, in the perivisceral aorta in three patients, and in the infrarenal aorta in six patients. Thrombus in the thoracic aorta was treated with stent grafts in four patients, bare metal stents in three patients, and anticoagulation alone in two patients. In the suprarenal abdominal aorta, all three patients underwent trapdoor aortic thrombectomy. Infrarenal aortic thrombus was managed by aortobifemoral embolectomy in two patients, aortic stenting in two patients, surgical thrombectomy in one patient, and anticoagulation alone in one patient. Successful treatment, defined as freedom from further embolic events or recurrence of thrombus, was achieved in 14 of 19 patients (76.4%) with a mean follow-up period of 16.2 months (range, 2-28 months). There were four (21%) thrombus-related deaths, all due to primary thromboembolic insults. One patient needed a below-knee amputation because of a recurrent thrombotic episode.

Conclusions.—Symptomatic PAMT is an uncommon but important source of noncardiogenic embolus. It appears to occur more frequently in young women. Endovascular coverage of the aortic thrombus, when feasible, appears to be an effective and safe procedure with either stent grafts or closed-cell metal stents. When thrombus is located adjacent to visceral vessels, it should be managed with an open trapdoor thromboembolectomy (Figs 1 and 5).

► Having worked in a high-volume aortic center for nearly 10 years, I have seen many patients with primary aortic mural thrombus (PAMT) in a variety of

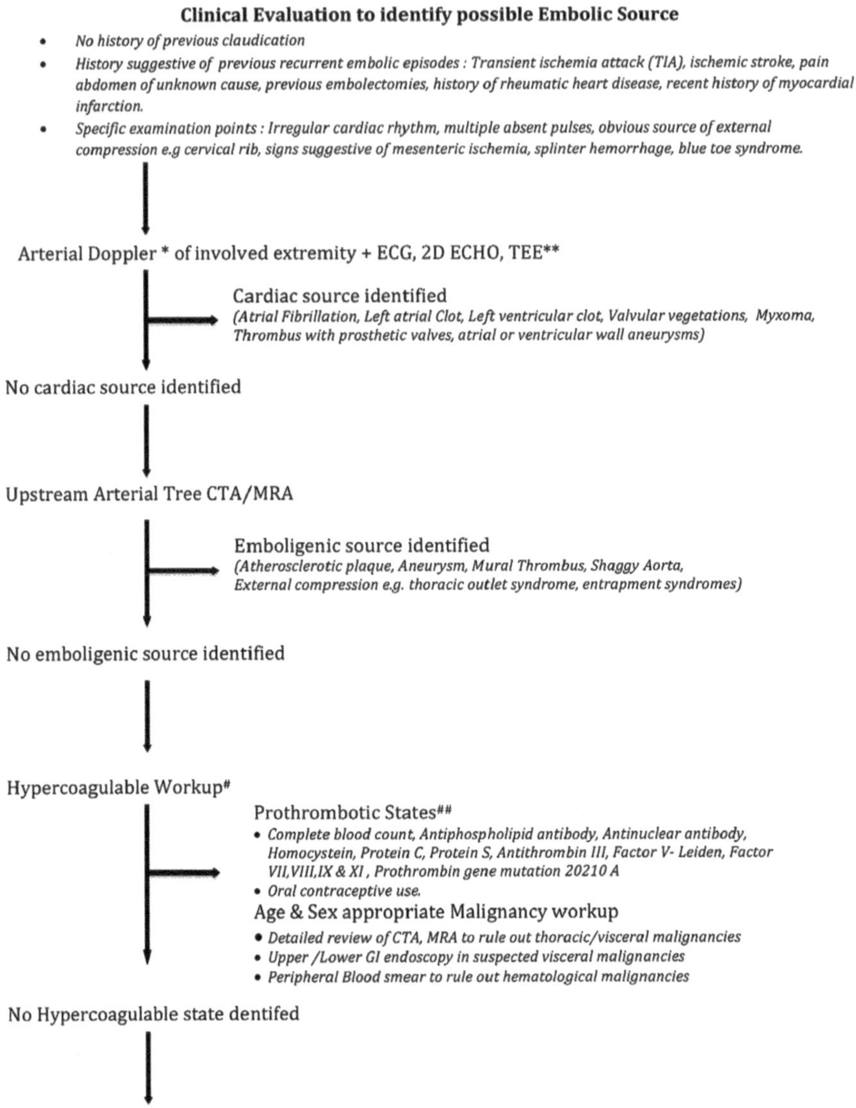

** CECT abdomen & pelvis in suspected visceral ischemia*

*** Transesophageal Echocardiography (TEE) is done in patients with irregular cardiac rhythm with no embolic source identified on Trans thoracic 2D ECHO.*

 # Patients with Aortic mural thrombus also undergo hypercoaguable workup.

##Patients diagnosed with hypercoagulable states were reassessed after completion of a minimum of 6 months of anticoagulation therapy and discontinuation of oral anticoagulation at least for 3 weeks.

FIGURE 1.—Institutional protocol for investigating acute arterial thrombosis. *CTA*, Computed tomography angiography; *ECG*, electrocardiography; *MRA*, magnetic resonance angiography. (Reprinted from the Journal of Vascular Surgery. Verma H, Meda N, Vora S, et al. Contemporary management of symptomatic primary aortic mural thrombus. *J Vasc Surg*. 2014;60:1524-1534, Copyright 2014, with permission from The Society for Vascular Surgery.)

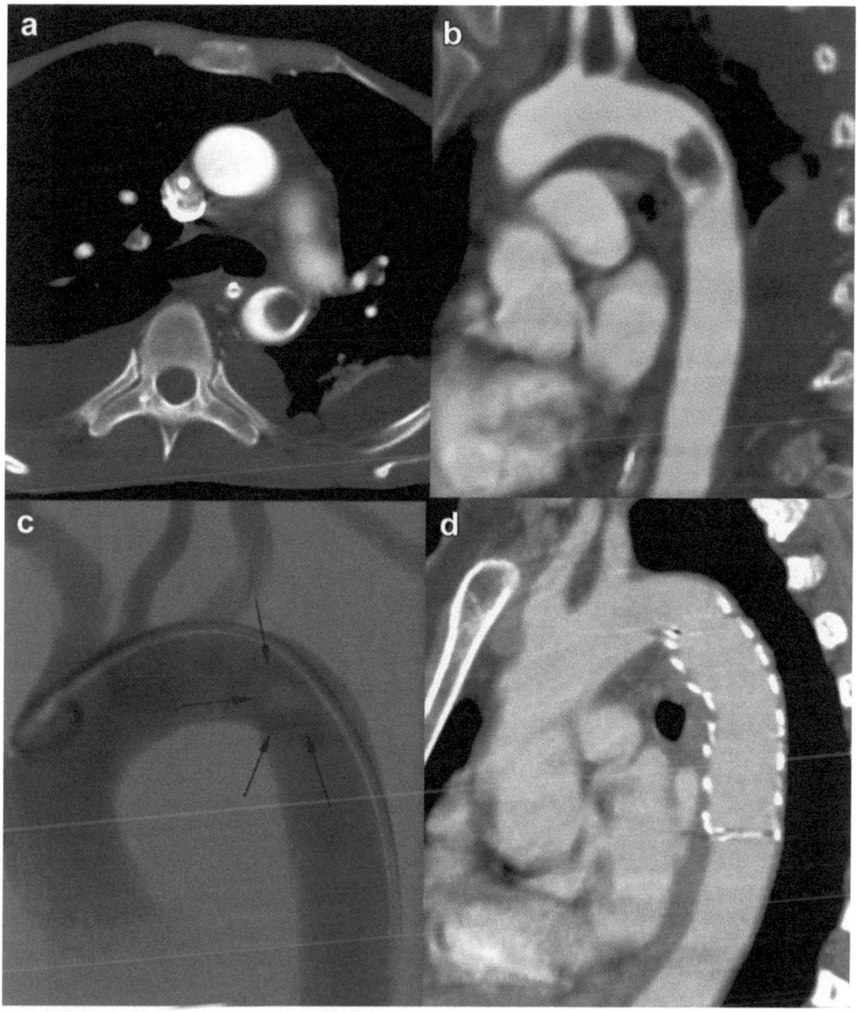

FIGURE 5.—Type IIa primary aortic mural thrombus (PAMT). **a** and **b**, Preoperative computed tomography (CT) scan showing pedunculated thrombus distal to left subclavian artery. **c**, Intraoperative angiogram showing shadow of thrombus (*arrows*). **d**, Six-month follow-up CT scan showing complete exclusion of thrombus. (Reprinted from the Journal of Vascular Surgery. Verma H, Meda N, Vora S, et al. Contemporary management of symptomatic primary aortic mural thrombus. *J Vasc Surg.* 2014;60:1524-1534, Copyright 2014, with permission from The Society for Vascular Surgery.)

different clinical presentations. These authors present a series of 88 patients presenting with some form of acute arterial thromboembolism over a 2.5-year period when 19 were found to have PAMT as the source of the distal embolism. The authors present a nice algorithm for working up these patients (Fig 1) and suggest stent grafts when appropriate and open surgical thrombectomy when the vascular territory becomes pricey (perivisceral segment) (Fig 5). I have 1 criticism of this article, and that is the failure to recognize the rare entity of essential thrombocythemia. Somewhere in this algorithm, a platelet count should be checked before considering any sort of operative therapy. The treatment for a platelet count of >1 million is systemic administration of hydroxylurea compounds, which typically causes the thrombus to completely evaporate on follow-up imaging.

PAMT is a significant problem in young patients and has poor outcomes despite aggressive treatment. Advanced organ ischemia is a poor prognostic sign.

B. W. Starnes, MD

Emergency endovascular stent grafting in acute complicated type B dissection

Wiedemann D, Ehrlich M, Amabile P, et al (Med Univ of Vienna, Austria; Hôpital de la Timone, Marseille, France; et al)
J Vasc Surg 60:1204-1208, 2014

Objective.—The objective of this study was to assess midterm results of emergency endovascular stent grafting for patients with life-threatening complications of acute type B aortic dissection.

Methods.—Between March 1999 and November 2011, 110 patients (86 men, 24 women) with complications of acute type B aortic dissection (mean age, 61 years; range, 19-87 years) were treated with thoracic endovascular aortic repair for malperfusion (55.5%) or aortic rupture (53.6%) in five major European referral centers and one U.S. referral center. Additional comorbidities included hypertension in 90 patients (82%), diabetes in 14 patients (13%), and chronic obstructive pulmonary disease in six patients (6%). Eleven patients (10%) had undergone previous aortic surgery.

Results.—Overall hospital mortality was 12% (n = 13), with 14 late deaths after hospital discharge. In-hospital complications occurred in 32 patients (36%); 10 patients developed postoperative renal failure, five patients experienced new permanent neurologic symptoms, and six patients (5.4%) experienced retrograde type A aortic dissection. Furthermore, nine patients (8%) developed an early type I endoleak. Actuarial survival at 1 and 5 years was 85% and 73%, respectively. Postprocedural computed tomography angiography showed complete or partial thrombosis of the false lumen at the stent graft level in 61% and 23% of all patients, respectively. Freedom from treatment failure according to the Stanford classification was 82%, 75%, and 59% at 1, 3, and 5 years.

Conclusions.—Endovascular repair of complicated acute type B aortic dissection is proven to be a technically feasible and effective treatment modality in this relatively difficult patient cohort. Short-term and midterm results are persuasive; however, the long-term efficacy needs to be further evaluated.

► My impression after reading this article was that is was at least a decade old, but not so. Recently published in the *Journal of Vascular Surgery*. I am shocked that the authors stated that there existed ongoing debate as to how to manage acute type B aortic dissection with either malperfusion or frank rupture! How about Class I, Level A recommendations (the highest evidence available) published 5 years ago in 2010?[1]

I think we all know the standard of care for the management of these sick patients in transthoracic endovascular aortic repair (TEVAR) with intention to reperfuse the true lumen and promote false lumen thrombosis. There are some valuable points from this article, however. First, the incidence of retrograde type A dissection in this series of 110 patients was 5.4% (6 patients). In all 6 cases, overstenting of the left subclavian artery was performed. In this small subset of patients, device type did not matter because there were 2 Talent, 3 Gore, and 1 Valiant stent grafts.

Retrograde type A dissection is the most feared complication of this treatment strategy because it can rapidly be fatal. The European experience with TEVAR for acute uncomplicated type B aortic dissection suggests that the incidence of retrograde type A associated with TEVAR is 8% (personal communication, Matthew Thompson, MD), and as such a strategy of treatment delay of 4 to 8 weeks is encouraged. In patients with malperfusion or rupture, treatment delay is not feasible.

Another interesting piece of data would be to know where the entry tear was located, in the convexity (outer curvature) or concavity (inner curvature) of the genu of the arch. There are data to suggest that entry tears located along the concavity have a higher rate of retrograde extension and dissection with TEVAR.

B. W. Starnes, MD

Reference

1. Hiratzka LF, Bakris GL, Beckman JA, et al. 2010 ACCF/AHA/AATS/ACR/ASA/SCA/SCAI/SIR/STS/SVM guidelines for the diagnosis and management of patients with thoracic aortic disease: executive summary. A report of the American College of Cardiology Foundation/American Heart Association Task Force on Practice Guidelines, American Association for Thoracic Surgery, American College of Radiology, American Stroke Association, Society of Cardiovascular Anesthesiologists, Society for Cardiovascular Angiography and Interventions, Society of Interventional Radiology, Society of Thoracic Surgeons, and Society for Vascular Medicine. *Catheter Cardiovasc Interv.* 2010;76:E43-E86.

Endovascular longitudinal fenestration and stent graft placement for treatment of aneurysms developing after chronic type B aortic dissection

Barshes NR, Gravereaux EC, Semel M, et al (Baylor College of Medicine, Houston, TX; Brigham and Women's Hosp, Boston, MA)

J Vasc Surg 61:1366-1369, 2015

The thickened intimal flap present in cases of chronic aortic dissection can present a challenge to attempts at endovascular stent graft treatment performed for subsequent aneurysmal degeneration by precluding adequate landing zones for the endograft and by constraining the endograft from full expansion. In this report we describe our technique and outcome for longitudinal endovascular fenestration of chronic aortic dissection flaps to facilitate endovascular stent graft treatment for thoracic aortic aneurysms developing after aortic dissection (Figs 3 and 5).

▶ The endovascular technique of longitudinal disruption of a chronic aortic dissection flap described in this report may allow for the effective endovascular

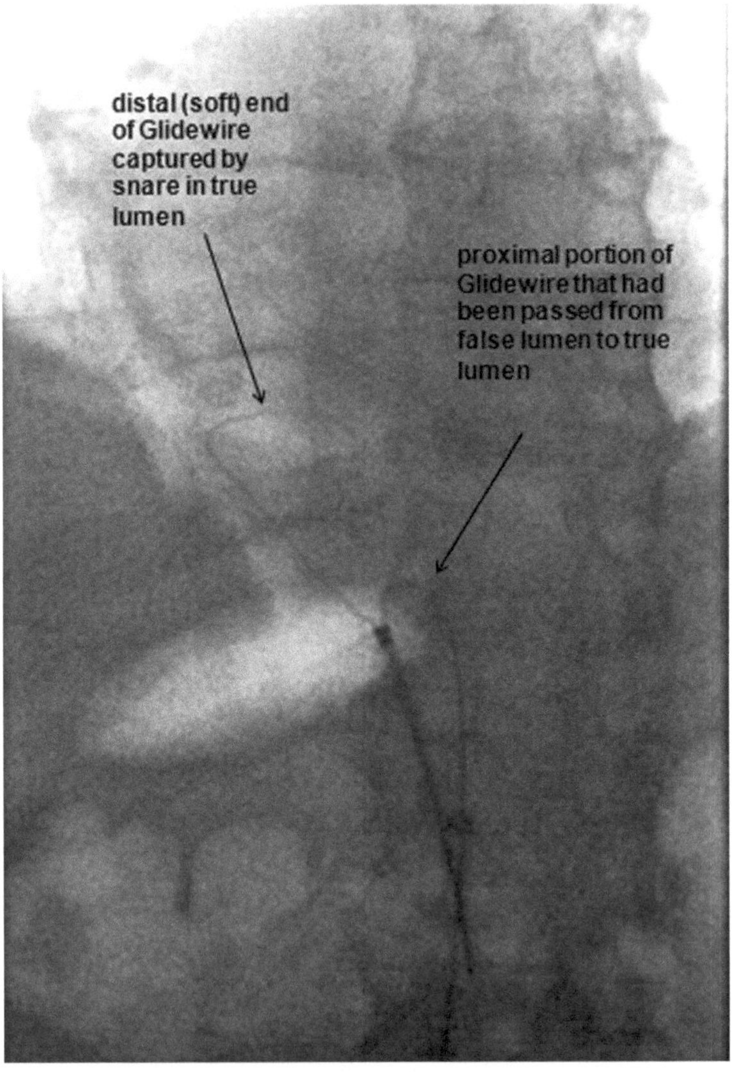

FIGURE 3.—Obliteration of the chronic aortic dissection flap (ie, reestablishment of a single lumen) was achieved by traction on a stiff guidewire "lassoed" around the false membrane. (Reprinted from the Journal of Vascular Surgery. Barshes NR, Gravereaux EC, Semel M, et al. Endovascular longitudinal fenestration and stent graft placement for treatment of aneurysms developing after chronic type B aortic dissection. *J Vasc Surg*. 2015;61:1366-1369, Copyright 2014, with permission from The Society for Vascular Surgery.)

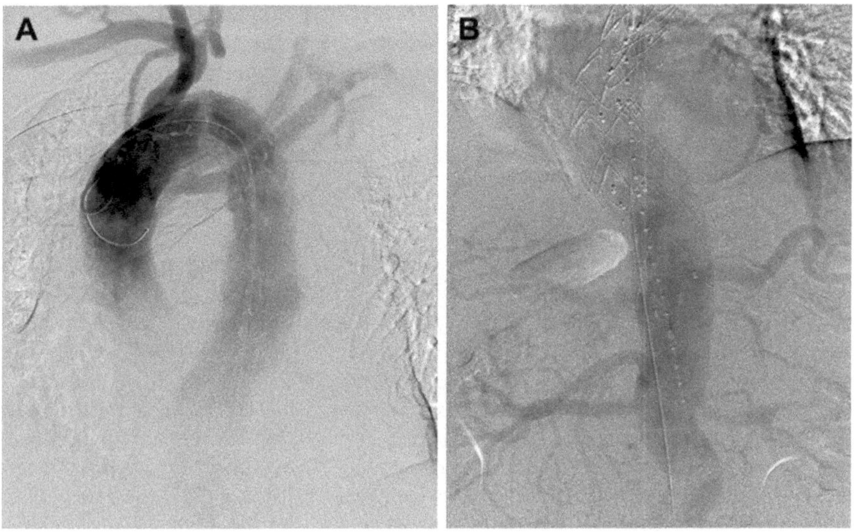

FIGURE 5.—A, Completion thoracic angiogram and (B) abdominal aortogram demonstrate absence of filling of the aneurysmal segment of aorta and filling of all the aortic arch branches, renal arteries, and visceral branches. (Reprinted from the Journal of Vascular Surgery. Barshes NR, Gravereaux EC, Semel M, et al. Endovascular longitudinal fenestration and stent graft placement for treatment of aneurysms developing after chronic type B aortic dissection. *J Vasc Surg*. 2015;61:1366-1369, Copyright 2014, with permission from The Society for Vascular Surgery.)

stent graft treatment of descending thoracic aortic aneurysms that might otherwise not be amenable to endovascular therapy because of the proximity of the intimal flap to important branch vessels (Figs 3 and 5). The authors recommend that this technique be included among the "array of strategies and tactics" surgeons use in the contemporary management of thoracic aneurysms with chronic dissection.

A few lessons were learned and highlighted in the text from this preliminary experience. In 1 patient, the authors were able to take advantage of preexisting tears in the aorta to gain false lumen access. Access to the false lumen can be challenging using reentry devices in these thick, chronic septa. The distal reentry points can often be identified using intravascular ultrasound (IVUS) imaging and by carefully studying the preoperative CT scan. I personally cannot emphasize enough how important IVUS is in the management of these dissection patients!

Second, the authors recommend that true lumen access be maintained from both femoral access sheaths because, as in cases of acute dissection and malperfusion, the fenestrated dissection membrane may pull down into the infrarenal aorta and obstruct iliac flow. I have personally seen this happen. Surgeons should be prepared to reestablish distal perfusion with endovascular or surgical techniques if the septum occludes the distal aorta, a potential hazard of this technique.

B. W. Starnes, MD

Hybrid endovascular repair of a dissecting thoracoabdominal aortic aneurysm with stent graft implantation through the false lumen

Watanabe Y, Kuratani T, Shirakawa Y, et al (Osaka Univ Graduate School of Medicine, Japan)

J Vasc Surg 59:264-267, 2014

We report the first successful hybrid endovascular technique for treating a residual dissecting thoracoabdominal aortic aneurysm with a compressed true lumen in a 48-year-old man in whom multiple stent grafts were deployed through the false lumen. The first stage of the procedure involved debranching of the visceral vessels from the right external iliac artery. In the second stage, a Gore excluder iliac extender (W. L. Gore and Associates, Flagstaff, Ariz) was deployed through the false lumen of the left common iliac artery; then, a Powerlink bifurcated stent graft (Endologix, Irvine, Calif) was positioned at the false lumen of the abdominal aorta. Overlapping with this stent graft, three Gore TAG stent grafts were deployed upward toward the Dacron (DuPont, Wilmington, Del) graft implanted during a previous operation on the descending aorta. Subsequently, the patient had an uneventful postoperative course, with no complications at the 3-year follow-up. The successful results of our new hybrid endovascular technique suggest the feasibility and efficacy of stent graft implantation through the false lumen (Fig 2).

▶ We see these sorts of case reports emerge more in the literature, and they should caution us to pause and await for more case experience before wide adoption takes place. I first saw a case of this sort presented by Mark Fillinger a few years ago, and I thought that his approach was innovative. The premise is that in many of these cases of chronic aortic dissection with subsequent aneurysmal degeneration, treating the aneurysm to prevent death from rupture should be the main goal, regardless of which lumen is preserved.

Surgeons who have played in this space have published on small case series of endoluminal stent grafting into the true lumen with the intent of obliterating false lumen flow. We all know that sometimes this is impossible because of anatomic features. This case is illustrative of successful treatment of a patient harboring a large thoraco-abdominal aneurysm by stent grafting into the larger false lumen after visceral artery debranching to successfully obliterate the aneurysm (Fig 2). This is thought provoking but we need more data.

B. W. Starnes, MD

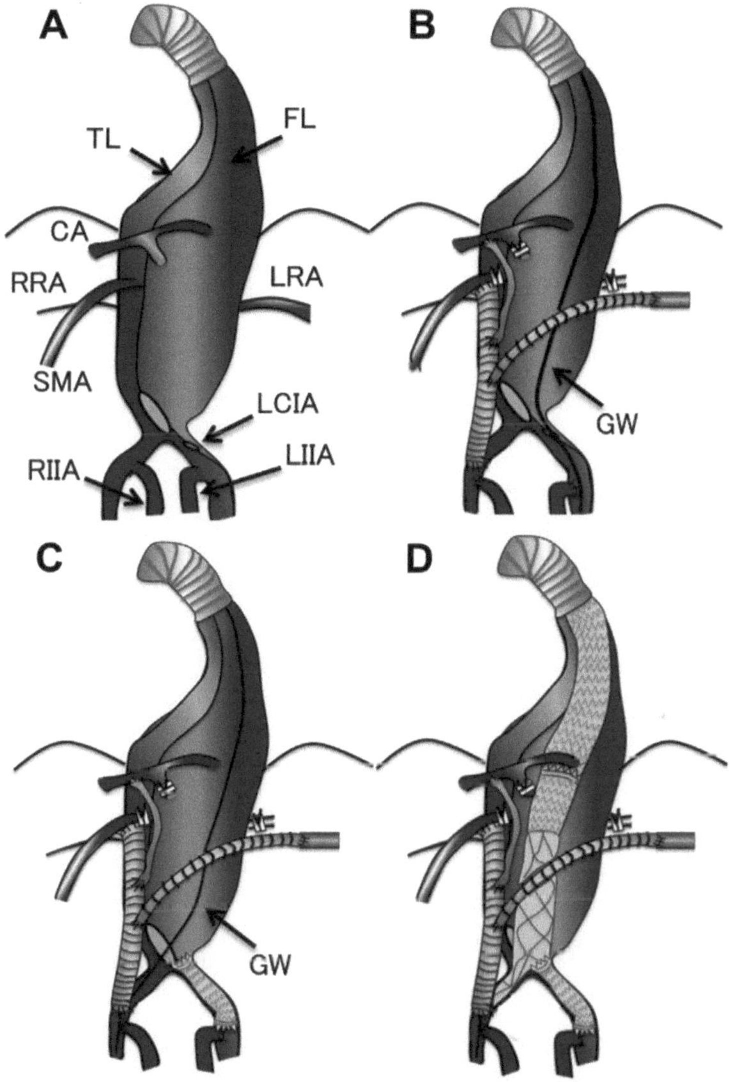

FIGURE 2.—Diagrammatic representation of the procedure. A, A dissecting aortic aneurysm extended from the double-barrel anastomosis of the previous surgery to the left common iliac artery (*LCIA*). Distal tears existed immediately proximal to the aortoiliac bifurcation and the LCIA. B, After the right (*RIIA*) and left internal iliac arteries (*LIIA*) were interposed onto a more distal portion of the external iliac arteries (*EIAs*), debranching of the visceral vessels from the right CIA was performed. A guidewire (*GW*) was advanced into the false lumen (*FL*) of the dissecting aorta through the distal tear of the LCIA. C, A Gore Excluder iliac extender component was deployed into the left iliac artery, and a GW was advanced through the distal tear immediately proximal to the aortoiliac bifurcation. D, A Powerlink bifurcated stent graft and three Gore TAG stent grafts were placed at the FL of the dissecting aortic aneurysm. *CA*, Celiac artery; *LRA*, left renal artery; *RRA*, right renal artery; *SMA*, superior mesenteric artery; *TL*, true lumen. (Reprinted from the Journal of Vascular Surgery. Watanabe Y, Kuratani T, Shirakawa Y, et al. Hybrid endovascular repair of a dissecting thoracoabdominal aortic aneurysm with stent graft implantation through the false lumen. *J Vasc Surg*. 2014;59:264-267, Copyright 2014,with permission from The Society for Vascular Surgery.)

Mid-term Outcomes and Aortic Remodelling After Thoracic Endovascular Repair for Acute, Subacute, and Chronic Aortic Dissection: The VIRTUE Registry

The VIRTUE Registry Investigators (St. Antonius Ziekenhuis, Nieuwegein, Netherlands; Ospedale Sant'Orsola Malpighi, Bologna, Italy; St George's Vascular Inst, London, UK; et al)

Eur J Vasc Endovasc Surg 48:363-371, 2014

Objective.—The VIRTUE Registry describes the mid-term clinical and morphological results of thoracic endovascular repair (TEVR) in patients with type B aortic dissection.

Methods.—This was a prospective cohort study. The VIRTUE Registry is a prospective, multicentre clinical trial that enrolled patients with complicated acute (<15 days), subacute (15–92 days), and chronic (>92 days) type B aortic dissections treated with the Valiant endograft. One hundred patients were enrolled and the clinical outcomes described at the 3-year follow-up. Analysis of the aortic area and false lumen thrombosis rates defined the morphological response to TEVR in the three clinical groups.

Results.—Three-year all-cause mortality (18%, 4%, and 24%), dissection related mortality (12%, 4%, and 9%), aortic rupture (2%, 0%, and 4%), retrograde type A dissection (5%, 0%, and 0%), and aortic reintervention rates (20%, 22%, and 39%) were, respectively, defined for patients with acute ($n = 50$), subacute ($n = 24$), and chronic ($n = 26$) dissections. Analysis of aortic morphology observed that patients with subacute dissection demonstrated a similar degree of aortic remodelling to patients with acute dissection. Patients with acute and subacute dissection exhibited greater aortic plasticity than patients with chronic dissection.

Conclusions.—The principle clinical findings suggest that TEVR is able to provide good protection from aorticrelated death in the mid-term, but with a high rate of aortic reintervention. Analysis of aortic morphology suggested that aortic remodelling in subacute patients is similar to the acute group. Retention of aortic plasticity in the subacute group lengthens the therapeutic window for the treatment of uncomplicated type B dissection (Fig 1).

▶ The traditional 2-week distinction between the acute and chronic phases of aortic dissection relate to the timing of death in the era of open surgery[1] and is probably not as useful in describing the aortic response to endovascular repair. There has been some suggestion that defining the response to aortic surgery in a subacute phase (15-92 days) of dissection might be useful to investigate when the aorta becomes less plastic in its ability to remodel and whether this has any implications on clinical outcomes. This study describes the midterm results of the VIRTUE Registry. The registry enrolled patients with acute, subacute, and chronic type B aortic dissections treated with the Valiant thoracic endograft (Medtronic, Santa Rosa, CA, USA). The current report details the later outcomes with reference to clinical results and aortic remodeling (Fig 1).

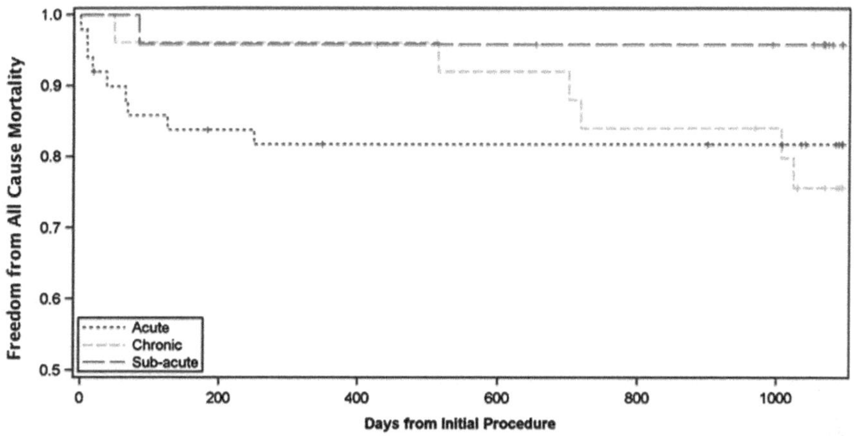

	Post TEVR	30	90	180	270	365	730	1095
Acute	49	45	42	41	39	38	38	37
Chronic	26	26	25	25	25	25	21	18
Sub-acute	24	24	23	23	23	23	21	19

FIGURE 1.—Freedom from all-cause mortality by clinical group. There was no overall difference in survival between the three groups ($p = .200$). Numbers at risk at each time point (days) are tabulated below the figure. *Note.* TEVR = thoracic endovascular repair; Post TEVR = number of patients at risk immediately after TEVR. (Reprinted from the European Journal of Vascular and Endovascular Surgery. The VIRTUE Registry Investigators. Mid-term outcomes and aortic remodelling after thoracic endovascular repair for acute, subacute, and chronic aortic dissection: the VIRTUE Registry. *Eur J Vasc Endovasc Surg*. 2014;48:363-371, Copyright 2014, with permission from European Society for Vascular Surgery.)

The VIRTUE study has provided detailed clinical and morphological data regarding endovascular treatment of type B aortic dissection. The principle clinical findings suggest that thoracic endovascular repair (TEVAR) is able to provide good protection from aortic related death in the midterm, but with a high rate of aortic reintervention. This study has identified that technical refinements to the operative procedure might be able to reduce the rate of reintervention in the chronic groups with greater aortic coverage in the primary procedure. Analysis of aortic morphology has suggested that aortic remodeling in the subacute patients is similar to the acute group. Retention of aortic plasticity in the subacute group lengthens the therapeutic window for the treatment of uncomplicated type B dissection.

Ladies and gentleman, the treatment of most uncomplicated type B dissections with TEVAR is coming, and the Europeans are leading the way in this endeavor. It appears that the safe window for intervening is within 4 to 6 weeks (subacute) to lessen the risk of retrograde type A dissection in the acute phase (Matthew Thompson, personal communication, April 2015).

B. W. Starnes, MD

Reference

1. Hirst AE Jr, Johns VJ Jr, Kime SW Jr. Dissecting aneurysm of the aorta: a review of 505 cases. *Medicine (Baltimore)*. 1958;37:217-279.

Outcomes after false lumen embolization with covered stent devices in chronic dissection

Idrees J, Roselli EE, Shafii S, et al (Cleveland Clinic, OH)
J Vasc Surg 60:1507-1513, 2014

Objective.—Persistent retrograde false lumen perfusion is a common mode of failure after thoracic endovascular aortic repair (TEVAR) for chronic dissection. Objectives were to describe a novel endovascular approach for false lumen occlusion and assess outcomes.

Methods.—From 2009 to 2013, 21 patients (mean age, 64 ± 11 years) with chronic thoracoabdominal dissection underwent adjunctive false lumen embolization using covered stent devices for persistent retrograde perfusion. Eight patients had type B dissection, 13 had residual dissection after prior type A repair, and all were deemed high risk for open operation. False lumen embolization in 17 patients was an adjunct at the initial TEVAR or extension, including two as elephant trunk completion. In the other four, this was done as an isolated procedure, and three had previously undergone TEVAR sparing the celiac artery. Covered stent devices included iliac plugs in 18, nitinol embolization plugs in two, and occluded stent graft in one. More than one device was used in 15 patients.

Results.—There was one hospital death due to left subclavian artery aneurysm rupture but no patient had stroke, paraplegia, myocardial infarction, or renal failure. Mean follow-up was 25 ± 19 months. During surveillance computed tomography imaging, false lumen thrombosis was noted in all patients, but four required further embolization because the thrombosis was incomplete. Mean maximum aortic diameter decreased from 64 ± 14 to 59 ± 15 mm. There was one late death from intracranial hemorrhage and no aortic ruptures.

Conclusions.—Adjunctive false lumen embolization with a covered stent device promotes thrombosis and remodeling after stent grafting the true lumen for chronic dissection. Further study of this strategy is warranted (Figs 3 and 4).

▶ For those surgeons who manage thoracic aortic aneurysm in association with chronic aortic dissection, the main purpose of thoracic endovascular aortic repair is to prevent death from aneurysm rupture, not to treat the underlying dissection. That said, paramount to the success of any endovascular method in this subset of patients is complete false lumen thrombosis. Unfortunately, this is not achievable in a certain percentage of patients. What are desperately needed are better false lumen obliteration strategies. Coils and plugs are typically too small for the job.

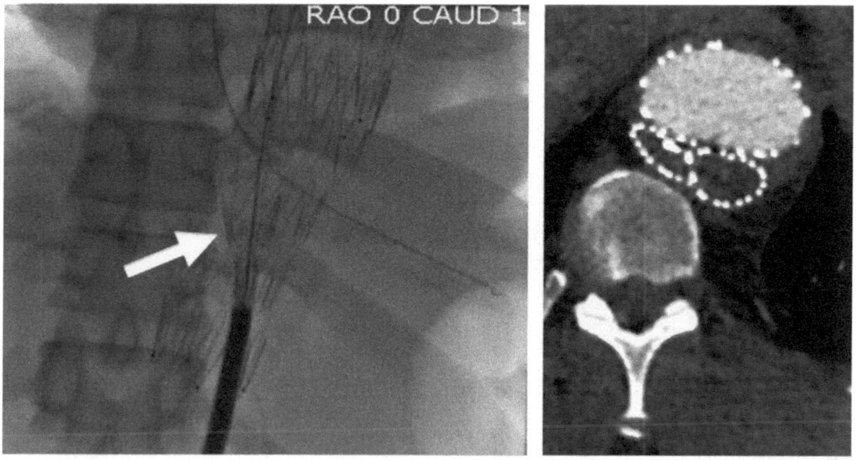

FIGURE 3.—**Left**, Intraoperative fluoroscopic image shows deployment of the iliac occluder devices into the false lumen (*arrow*). **Right**, Postoperative computed tomography (CT) image shows iliac occluder devices in the false lumen, with complete thrombosis. (Reprinted from the Journal of Vascular Surgery. Idrees J, Roselli EE, Shafii S, et al. Outcomes after false lumen embolization with covered stent devices in chronic dissection. *J Vasc Surg*. 2014;60:1507-1513, Copyright 2014, with permission from The Society for Vascular Surgery.)

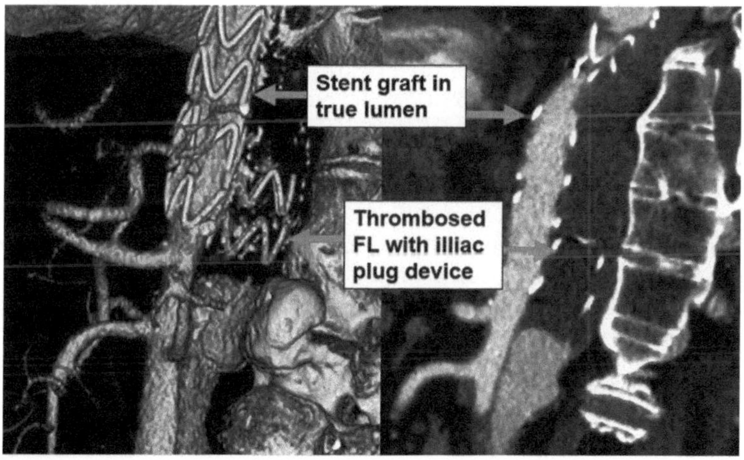

FIGURE 4.—False lumen embolization using covered stent device in chronic dissection. **Left**, Volume-rendered computed tomography (CT) image at the 2-year follow-up shows the stent graft in the true lumen and an iliac plug device adjacent in the false lumen. **Right**, Complete thrombosis of the false lumen in the area of the iliac plug device and intact flow through the true lumen with the stent graft are shown. (Reprinted from the Journal of Vascular Surgery. Idrees J, Roselli EE, Shafii S, et al. Outcomes after false lumen embolization with covered stent devices in chronic dissection. *J Vasc Surg*. 2014;60:1507-1513, Copyright 2014, with permission from The Society for Vascular Surgery.)

These authors at a high-volume institution describe their early experience using stent graft occluders (iliac occlude devices) to obliterate false lumen flow (Figs 3 and 4). Hopefully, we will see more unique devices on the horizon for this type of therapy.

B. W. Starnes, MD

Short-term Outcome of Spinal Cord Ischemia after Endovascular Repair of Thoracoabdominal Aortic Aneurysms

Dias NV, Sonesson B, Kristmundsson T, et al (Skåne Univ Hosp, Malmö, Sweden)

Eur J Vasc Endovasc Surg 49:403-409, 2015

Objective.—To analyze the incidence and short-term outcome of SCI after endovascular repair of thoracoabdominal aneurysms (eTAAA).

Methods.—All patients undergoing eTAAA with branched and fenestrated stent grafts between 2008 and 2014 were retrospectively reviewed concerning pre-, intra- and post-operative clinical data and imaging.

Results.—Seventy-two patients (53 males, 68 [64–73] years old) underwent eTAAA (51 elective, 21 acute including 7 ruptures). Patients were classified anatomically according to Crawford: type I ($n = 11$), type II ($n = 26$), type III ($n = 18$), and type IV ($n = 17$). Thirty-day mortality was 6.9% (3.9% for elective, 7.1% for symptomatic and 28.6% for ruptures, including one intra-operative death). Twenty-two of the 71 patients who survived the operation (31.0%) developed SCI: type I ($n = 2$, 20.0%), type II ($n = 13$, 50.0%), type III ($n = 3$, 16.7%), type IV ($n = 4$, 23.5%). SCI incidence decreased in the latter part of the experience (23.7% vs. 39.4%, $p = .201$). SCI development was independently associated with Crawford type II TAAA (OR 4.497 (1.331–15.195), $p = .016$) and higher contrast volume (OR 3.736 [1.054–13.242], $p = .041$). Fifteen of these 22 patients with SCI showed some improvement of their deficits before hospital discharge. The introduction of a standardized protocol in the last 38 patients aiming at the early diagnosis and treatment of SCI led to more frequent regression of SCI symptoms (100% vs. 46.2%, $p = .017$) and a higher rate of regaining ambulatory capacity (55.6% vs. 15.4%, $p = .027$). After the introduction of this protocol, the residual SCI rate at hospital discharge was 13.2% as opposed to 33.3% in the initial group.

Conclusion.—eTAAA has low peri-operative mortality, but SCI incidence is high albeit that it decreased with increasing experience. More extensive repair and use of larger volumes of contrast were associated with higher risk of SCI. Acute repair does not significantly increase SCI risk. A standardized protocol for early diagnosis and treatment of SCI leads to a higher recovery rate with a greater likelihood of regaining ambulatory capacity (Tables 4 and 5).

▶ This article analyses spinal cord ischemia (SCI) after thoracoabdominal endovascular aneurysm repair in 71 patients. It suggests that SCI development

TABLE 4.—Spinal Cord Ischemia

	SCI	No SCI	*p*
Previous aortic surgery	11 (26.8)	30 (73.2)	.441
Crawford			.068
I	2 (20.0)	8 (80.0)	
II	13 (50.0)	13 (50.0)	.015
III	3 (16.7)	15 (83.3)	
IV	4 (23.5)	13 (76.5)	
Hypogastric occlusion			
Pre-operative	5 (22.7)	5 (10.2)	.161
Post-operative	6 (27.3)	8 (16.3)	.339
Elective/acute repair	15 (29.4)/7 (35.0)	36 (70.6)/13 (65.0)	.776
Operation time, min	470 (404–547)	392 (308–461)	.009
Intra-operative bleeding, mL	2,050 (1,075–4,425)	1000 (525–1700)	.004
Contrast volume, mL	322 (279–389)	244 (180–298)	.001
Iodine dose, g	53 (39–62)	39 (25–50)	.008
Fluoroscopy time, min	122 (102–172)	120 (88–142)	.263
Radiation, μGym^2	71,257 (45,643–93,738)	50,646 (34,526–76,247)	.039
CO_2 use intra-operatively	20 (33.9)	39 (66.1)	.319
Primary technical success	20 (29.9)	47 (70.1)	.583
Post-operative			
Absolute GFR increase, %[a]	45 (33–84)	22 (1–42)	.001
Atrial fibrillation	7 (63.6)	4 (36.4)	.031
Lower limb fasciotomy	3 (100)	0 (0)	.028
Standardized SCI observation			
Yes	9 (23.7)	29 (76.3)	.201
No	13 (39.4)	20 (60.6)	

[a]Percent in relation to the pre-operative absolute GFR.

Reprinted from the European Journal of Vascular and Endovascular Surgery. Dias NV, Sonesson B, Kristmundsson T, et al. Short-term outcome of spinal cord ischemia after endovascular repair of thoracoabdominal aortic aneurysms. *Eur J Vasc Endovasc Surg*. 2015;49:403-409, Copyright 2014, with permission from the European Society for Vascular Surgery.

TABLE 5.—Effect of a Standardized Protocol for Early Diagnosis of SCI

	Standardized Protocol for Early SCI Diagnosis	
	Yes $n = 9/38$	No $n = 13/33$
Degree of SCI symptoms regression[a]		
Complete	4	2
Partial	5	4
None	0	7
Residual symptoms[b]		
Ambulatory	5[c]	2
Non-ambulatory	4	11
Crawford		
All	5 (13.2)	11 (33.3)
I	1 (14.3)	1 (33.3)
II	3 (30.0)	8 (50.0)
III	1 (9.1)	1 (14.3)
IV	0 (0.0)[d]	1 (14.3)

[a]$p = .027$.
[b]$p = .074$.
[c]One patient needing minimal assistance.
[d]Out of 10 patients.

Reprinted from the European Journal of Vascular and Endovascular Surgery. Dias NV, Sonesson B, Kristmundsson T, et al. Short-term outcome of spinal cord ischemia after endovascular repair of thoracoabdominal aortic aneurysms. *Eur J Vasc Endovasc Surg*. 2015;49:403-409, Copyright 2014, with permission from the European Society for Vascular Surgery.

is associated with more extensive repairs but not with the acuteness of the operation. Moreover, it shows the positive impact of the use of standardized postoperative protocols for the early detection and treatment of spinal cord ischemia, reinforcing the need of finding more strategies for preventing this serious complication.

A whopping 22 (31.0%) of the 71 patients surviving the operation developed postoperative SCI. SCI was more common after repair of Crawford type II aneurysms ($n = 13$, 50%) than the other types of thoracoabdominal aneurysms (TAAA; $P = .015$, Table 4). Another preoperative anatomic feature associated with the development of SCI was hypogastric occlusion, although this did not reach statistical significance ($P = .266$). Intraoperative variables associated with the subsequent development of SCI were the operating time ($P = .009$), intraoperative bleeding (which was probably directly related to hypotension; $P = .004$), contrast volume use ($P = .001$), iodine dose ($P = .008$), and radiation dose ($P = .039$). Occlusion of the hypogastric arteries after endovascular TAAA (eTAAA) was not significantly associated with SCI development ($P = .339$).

Of note, the incidence of SCI was lower after the introduction of a formal perioperative standardized SCI protocol, was decreasing in the latter part of the study, but this did not reach to any statistical significance (23.7% vs 39.4%, $p = .201$, Table 4). Patients undergoing eTAAA in the last part of the study received less contrast volume, iodine dose, and radiation, probably related to operator experience.

This study reiterates the low perioperative mortality of eTAAA and the importance of SCI as the major complication. It suggests that increasing experience leads to a decrease in the incidence of SCI and, more importantly, shows that standardized protocols for the early diagnosis and treatment of SCI increase the chances of symptom regression.

The introduction of a standardized protocol for early diagnosis of SCI (last 38 patients) led to universal improvement of the neurological deficits of the 9 patients experiencing SCI during this period. In the early period, SCI deficits remained unchanged in 7 (53.8%) patients, and only 6 (46.2%) showed some improvement ($P = .017$). Moreover, the protocol for early diagnosis of SCI was also associated with a higher level of symptom regression, with more patients regaining their ambulatory capacity ($P = .027$, Table 5).

B. W. Starnes, MD

Thoracic endovascular aortic repair in management of aortoesophageal fistulas

Canaud L, Ozdemir BA, Bee WW, et al (St George's Vascular Inst, London, UK)
J Vasc Surg 59:248-254, 2014

Objective.—To provide a systematic review of the outcomes of thoracic endovascular aortic repair (TEVAR) for aortoesophageal fistula (AEF) and to identify prognostic factors associated with poor outcomes.

Methods.—Literature searches of the Embase, Medline, and Cochrane databases identified relevant articles reporting results of TEVAR for AEF. The main outcome measure was the composite of aortic mortality, recurrence of the AEF, and stent graft explantation. The secondary outcome measure was aortic-related mortality.

Results.—Fifty-five articles were integrated after a literature search identified 72 patients treated by TEVAR for AEFs. The technical success rate of TEVAR was 87.3%. The overall 30-day mortality was 19.4%. Prolonged antibiotics (>4 weeks) were administered in 80% of patients. Concomitant or staged resection or repair of the esophagus was performed in 44.4% of patients. Stent graft explantation was performed within the first month after TEVAR as a planned treatment in 11.1%. After a mean follow-up of 7.4 months (range, 1-33 months), the all-cause mortality was 40.2%, and the aortic-related mortality was 33.3. Prolonged antibiotic treatment ($P = .001$) and repair of AEFs due to a foreign body ($P = .038$) were associated with a significant lower aortic mortality. On univariate analysis, TEVAR and concomitant or staged adjunctive procedures (resection, repair of the esophagus, or a planned stent graft explantation) were associated with a significantly lower incidence of aortic-related mortality ($P = .0121$). When entered into a binary logistic regression analysis, prolonged antibiotic treatment was the only factor associated with a significant lower incidence of the endpoint ($P = .003$).

Conclusions.—Late infection or recurrence of the AEF and associated mortality rates are high when TEVAR is used as a sole therapeutic strategy. Prolonged antibiotic treatment has a strong negative association with mortality. A strategy of a temporizing endovascular procedure to stabilize the patient in extremis, and upon recovery, an open surgical esophageal repair with or without stent graft explantation is advocated (Table 4).

▶ Finally! Some sensible recommendations for managing vascular disease with implantable stent grafts when it involves any sort of contamination. We should all realize that many of these case series reported in the literature do not include

TABLE 4.—Logistic Regression Model

Variable	OR	95% CI	*P* value
Outcome composite end point			
Combined procedure: TEVAR and surgery	1.03	0.19-5.40	.96784
Antibiotic therapy >4 weeks	0.03	0.001-0.21	.00389
Foreign body	0.22	0.005-2.57	.31503
Outcome aortic-related mortality			
Combined procedure: TEVAR and surgery	0.63	0.077-3.79	.62
Antibiotic therapy >4 weeks	<0.001	<0.001->100	.994
Foreign body	<0.001	<0.001->100	.993

CI, Confidence interval; *OR*, odds ratio; *TEVAR*, thoracic endovascular aortic repair.

Reprinted from the Journal of Vascular Surgery. Canaud L, Ozdemir BA, Bee WW, et al. Thoracic endovascular aortic repair in management of aortoesophageal fistulas. *J Vasc Surg*. 2014;59:248-254, Copyright 2014, with permission from The Society for Vascular Surgery.

the disasters because clinicians are least likely to publish their bad outcomes. That means that the complication rates are likely even higher than reported.

Thoracic endovascular aortic repair (TEVAR) recently gained popularity as an emergent treatment for aorto-enteric fistulas (AEFs), despite the high risk of infection. Reports often feature favorable short-term outcomes. Although endovascular stent grafting is faster and safer than surgery in unstable patients, the major concern is the durability of this approach. TEVAR does nothing to address the issue of the defect in the digestive tract, leaving the patients at risk of AEF recurrence and/or stent graft infection.

The aim of this article is to define the outcomes of TEVAR for AEFs with a particular focus on midterm results and to determine the prognostic factors associated with poor outcomes.

The main conclusions of this article were that TEVAR for AEFs often achieves the primary goal of therapy (i.e., control of bleeding, preventing fatal exsanguination). The high rate of secondary stent graft infection or recurrence of the AEF clearly proves that even combined with broad-spectrum antibiotics, TEVAR cannot replace surgical debridement and/or drainage of the infected mediastinum. Whether this is best achieved by drainage and primary repair/resection of the esophagus alone with or without removal of the stent graft remains to be proven. However, prolonged antibiotic treatment has a strong negative association with mortality (Table 4).

Message: Get the job done surgically instead of trying to buy more time with herbs and spices!

B. W. Starnes, MD

9 Aortoiliac Disease and Leg Ischemia

Retrograde pedal access for patients with critical limb ischemia

Bazan HA, Le L, Donovan M, et al (Ochsner Clinic, New Orleans, LA)

J Vasc Surg 60:375-382, 2014

Objective.—Retrograde pedal access may allow the treatment of tibial occlusive lesions when standard endovascular techniques fail. We aimed to analyze the outcomes in patients with chronic limb ischemia (Rutherford class IV and V) who were not surgical candidates for a tibial bypass and had undergone an unsuccessful attempt at revascularization through an antegrade access.

Methods.—During a 3-year period, a retrograde pedal access was selectively chosen when a popliteal or tibial lesion could not be crossed through an antegrade approach. Retrograde pedal access was performed under ultrasound guidance using a 4F micropuncture coaxial sheath. All interventions were performed in a sheathless fashion using a 0.014- or 0.018-inch "bareback" wire as support for a 2- or 2.5-mm balloon angioplasty catheter to cross and treat tibial chronic total occlusions that could not be treated through an antegrade approach. Routine anticoagulation and dual-antiplatelet therapy were used periprocedurally. Antegrade access was used to treat any lesion that required a stent placement after the retrograde wire was snared and brought through the antegrade guide-catheter. Patient indications and comorbidities were recorded. Outcomes analyzed were limb salvage rate, periprocedural complications, and mortality. Mean and standard deviations were calculated. The Kaplan-Meier method was used to calculate limb salvage rates.

Results.—A review of the 681 lower extremity angiograms in which a patient had an intervention from July 2010 through December 2013 identified 13 patients (nine men) in whom a retrograde pedal access was performed (mean age, 71.4 ± 12.4 years). Among these, diabetes was present in 10 of 13 (77%) and chronic renal insufficiency (stages II-V) in nine (69%). Five (38%) had undergone contralateral amputation. Indications for a retrograde pedal revascularization were Rutherford chronic limb ischemia class IV in two (15%) and class V in 11 (85%). Technical success rate was 69% (nine of 13). A variety of popliteal (two of 13) and tibial (13 of 13) vessels were treated with angioplasty alone (10 of 13) or angioplasty/stent placement (three of 13) through a retrograde approach. The technical failures were due to inability to cross the occlusion(s). Periprocedurally, there was one myocardial infarction but no local complications, worsening renal insufficiency, or deaths. At a mean follow-up of 17.1 ± 10.3 months, the limb salvage rate was 77% (10 of 13). There was a high mortality rate of 23% (three of 13) on follow-up in this cohort, occurring at median 6 ± 4 months.

Conclusions.—Retrograde pedal access for limb salvage in high-risk patients is feasible and safe, with acceptable limb salvage rates at intermediate follow-up. Appropriate candidates are those who have failed an antegrade intervention and are poor candidates for a tibial bypass. Future studies should test whether this mode of revascularization has favorable limb salvage rates in larger patient populations and seek to identify specific patient populations who will benefit from this technique.

▶ The 69% technical success rate for retrograde pedal access reported in this study underscores the challenging nature of this technique. Although retrograde access is a demanding procedure associated with a significant failure rate, these odds nonetheless may be acceptable to patients and providers without alternative revascularization options seeking to avoid amputation. This report provides a useful technical description for providers who lack experience with this approach. Several technical details included are distinct from more proximal access approaches, including application of gentle pressure with the ultrasound probe during access to compress the pedal veins while revealing pedal artery pulsation (if present), "bareback" (ie, sheathless) advancement of a low profile balloon following removal of the microcatheter sheath, adjunctive use of vasodilator flush solution (including their recipe), and approaches to establish hemostasis.

The implications of technical failure with attempted retrograde pedal access are important to consider, particularly if the procedure may eliminate pedal bypass as an alternative treatment option owing to access-related thrombosis of the recipient vessel. Providers who perform lower extremity endovascular intervention but not lower extremity bypass might be predisposed to plan revascularization from the perspective of exhausting endovascular options, sometimes at the expense of remaining surgical options. Consistent with this concern, the surgeon investigators who conducted this study concluded that patients who are poor candidates for a tibial bypass are appropriate to consider for retrograde pedal access. Given this conclusion, however, it is somewhat ironic that one patient in this series underwent a popliteal-tibial bypass after technical failure of attempted retrograde pedal access, showing that availability of new techniques sometimes impacts providers' perceptions of what can be achieved with old ones.

M. A. Corriere, MD, MS

Risk factors for readmission after lower extremity bypass in the American College of Surgeons National Surgery Quality Improvement Program

Zhang JQ, Curran T, McCallum JC, et al (Beth Israel Deaconess Med Ctr, Boston, MA)

J Vasc Surg 59:1331-1339, 2014

Objective.—Readmission is associated with high mortality, morbidity, and cost. We used the American College of Surgeons National Surgery Quality Improvement Program (ACS-NSQIP) to determine risk factors for readmission after lower extremity bypass (LEB).

Methods.—We identified all patients who received LEB in the 2011 ACS-NSQIP database. Multivariable logistic regression was used to assess independent predictors of 30-day readmission. We also identified our institutional contribution of LEB patients to the ACS-NSQIP from 2005 to 2011 to determine our institution's rate of readmission and readmission indications.

Results.—Among 5018 patients undergoing LEB, ACS-NSQIP readmission analysis was performed on 4512, excluding those whose readmission data were unavailable, who suffered a death on index admission, or who remained in the hospital at 30 days. Overall readmission rate was 18%, and readmission rate of those with NSQIP-captured complications was 8%. Multivariable predictors of readmission were dependent on functional status (odds ratio [OR], 1.40; 95% confidence interval [CI], 1.08-1.79), dyspnea (OR, 1.28; 95% CI, 1.02-1.60), cardiac comorbidity (OR, 1.46; 95% CI, 1.16-1.84), dialysis dependence (OR, 1.44; 95% CI, 1.05-1.97), obesity (OR, 1.28; 95% CI, 1.07-1.53), malnutrition (OR, 1.42; 95% CI, 1.12-1.79), critical limb ischemia operative indication (OR, 1.40; 95% CI, 1.10-1.79), and return to the operating room on index admission (OR, 8.0; 95% CI, 6.68-9.60). The most common postdischarge complications occurring in readmitted patients included wound complications (55%), multiple complications (22%), and graft failure (5%). Our institutional data contributed 465 LEB patients to the ACS-NSQIP from 2005 to 2012, with an overall readmission rate of 14%. Unplanned readmissions related to the original LEB (related unplanned) made up 75% of cases. The remainder 25% included readmissions that were planned staged procedures related to the original LEB (related planned, 11%) and admissions for a completely unrelated reason (unrelated unplanned, 14%). The most common readmission indications included wound infection (37%) and graft failure (10%). Readmissions were attributable to NSQIP-captured postdischarge complications in 44% of cases, an additional 44% had a non-NSQIP-defined reason for readmission, and the remainder (12%) included patients admitted for complications described in NSQIP but not meeting strict NSQIP criteria.

Conclusions.—Readmissions are common after LEB. Optimization of select chronic conditions, closer follow-up of patients in poor health and those who required return to the operating room, and early detection of surgical site infections may improve readmission rates. Our finding that

25% of readmissions after LEB are not procedure related informs the broader discussion of how a readmission penalty affects vascular surgery in particular.

▶ The finding that surgery for peripheral arterial disease is among the top 3 diagnoses associated with highest readmission rates should not be a shock to anyone who performs lower extremity bypass, particularly for patients with critical limb ischemia who present with ulcers, gangrene, or infection requiring debridement in addition to the revascuarlization.[1] Readmission is a phenomenon that probably cannot (although "should not" might be a better choice of words) be eliminated among patients undergoing lower extremity bypass. High rates of readmission may be more reflective of the diagnosis under consideration than an a priori indicator of globally flawed care, and the notion that conditions with highest readmission rates will benefit or respond predictably to reimbursement penalties may be inherently flawed. Punitive action based on readmission may, in fact, have several negative consequences that ultimately inflate rather than control costs. If cost-driven quality initiatives incentivize providers to prioritize minimizing risk of readmission over maximizing rates of limb salvage, adoption of a more aggressive approach toward primary amputation among patients with tissue loss (who are among those at greatest risk for readmission) might avoid readmissions related to wound-related issues but would trade this improvement for the higher costs (both societal and financial) associated with amputation. The importance of avoiding readmission therefore depends on whether we assume the perspective of the payer (Medicare, in the case of this analysis), the provider, or the patient. Each of these parties might prioritize cost control, readmission, or limb salvage, respectively, as the most important objective depending on the circumstances, incentives, and contingencies in place.

Reducing readmissions therefore may come at the expense of other outcomes and may place short-term and long-term perspectives at odds with one another. It is interesting to note that the majority of surgical site infections (SSIs) identified in this study were diagnosed postdischarge. A provider interpreting the results therefore might correctly conclude that some readmissions might have been related to premature discharges, which potentially eliminate the opportunity to manage an SSI during the same hospital stay. Within this framework, providers seeking to minimize readmissions might adopt a more conservative attitude toward timing of discharge and/or implementation of intravenous antibiotics for superficial SSIs, which might lead to an inflated length of stay. Deciding which outcomes deserve priority is therefore critically important when attempting to operationalize initiatives to reduce readmission. As we observe the consequences (both intended and unintended) of policy measures focused on short-term costs and outcomes, it will be interesting to see whether the pendulum eventually swings in the other direction.

M. A. Corriere, MD, MS

Reference

1. Jencks SF, Williams MV, Coleman EA. Rehospitalizations among patients in the Medicare fee-for-service program. *N Engl J Med.* 2009;360:1418-1428.

Objective measurement of lower extremity function and quality of life after surgical revascularization for critical lower extremity ischemia

Landry GJ, Esmonde NO, Lewis JR, et al (Oregon Health & Science Univ, Portland)

J Vasc Surg 60:136-142, 2014

Background.—Outcomes of revascularization for critical limb ischemia (CLI) have historically been patency, limb salvage, and survival. Functional status and quality of life have not been well described. This study used functional and quality of life assessments to measure patient-centered outcomes after revascularization for CLI.

Methods.—The study observed 18 patients (age, 65 ± 11 years) prospectively before and after lower extremity bypass for CLI. Patients completed the Short Physical Performance Battery, which measures walking speed, leg strength, and balance, as well as performed a 6-minute walk, and calorie expenditure was measured by an accelerometer. Isometric muscle strength was assessed with the Muscle Function Evaluation chair (Metitur, Helsinki, Finland). Quality of life instruments included the 36-Item Short Form Health Survey and the Vascular Quality of Life questionnaire. Patients' preoperative status was compared with 4-month postoperative status.

Results.—Muscle Function Evaluation chair measurements of ipsilateral leg strength demonstrated a significant increase in knee flexion from 64 ± 62 N to 135 ± 133 N ($P = .038$) and nearly significant increase in knee extension from 120 ± 110 N to 186 ± 85 N ($P = .062$) and ankle plantar flexion from 178 ± 126 N to 267 ± 252 N ($P = .078$). In the contralateral leg, knee flexion increased from 71 ± 96 N to 149 ± 162 N ($P = .028$) and knee extension from 162 ± 112 N to 239 ± 158 N ($P = .036$). Absolute improvements were noted in 6-minute walk distance, daily calorie expenditure, and individual domains and overall Short Physical Performance Battery scores, and upper extremity strength decreased, although none were significant. The Vascular Quality of Life questionnaire captured significant improvement in all individual domains and overall score ($P < .015$). Significant improvement was noted only for bodily pain ($P = .011$) on the 36-Item Short Form Health Survey.

Conclusions.—Despite lack of statistical improvement in most functional test results, revascularization for CLI results in improved patient-perceived leg function. Significant improvements in isometric muscle

strength may explain the measured improvement in quality of life after revascularization for CLI.

▶ This study explores novel parameters beyond those conventionally used to assess peripheral arterial disease (PAD) outcomes in clinical research, and the authors are to be commended for attempting to establish a more holistic and patient-centered perspective than the status quo. The authors identified improvements in several outcomes after surgical revascularization, including all domains of the Vascular Quality of Life Questionnaire, the bodily pain domain of the SF-36 questionnaire, and muscle strength. No significant changes, however, were observed in several outcomes that could generally be categorized as assessments of walking or physical activity: the 6-minute walk test, accelerometer-based calorie expenditure (used as a surrogate measure of overall physical activity), or the short physical performance battery. The results therefore seem to indicate that walking impairment may be less relevant to quality of life than other issues, such as pain or wound healing, for patients with critical limb ischemia. Along those lines, it would be worthwhile to perform a similar evaluation among patients with intermittent claudication; walking impairment may be more directly relevant to quality of life in these patients, who might also be expected to have more potential for postrevascularization improvement in some of these measures. It is also important to remember that this study (which was limited to patients with critical limb ischemia) did not include any controls (such as patients undergoing endovascular intervention, amputation, or medical treatment without a procedure) for comparison. The natural history of critical limb ischemia without revascularization is poorly understood but important to consider; it is possible that revascularization may halt or alter a trajectory of progressive functional decline, resulting in benefits that would not be apparent when assessed based on improvement (vs lack of further deterioration).

PAD affects an elderly patient population with a significant prevalence of other comorbidities (including chronic obstructive pulmonary disease, coronary artery disease, and osteoarthritis) that may affect physical function, activities of daily living, and quality of life. The elements of the Summary Performance Score (including the timed 4-meter walk, Tinetti balance test, and sit-stand test) potentially provide insight into how diagnoses other than PAD may independently contribute to both walking and global functional impairment. Objective assessment of these other variables may be useful for providers attempting to predict which benefits are likely to be gained through revascularization.

Although the authors observed postrevascularization improvement in leg strength (assessed based on leg flexion and extension), this variable has not been traditionally included in assessment of PAD symptoms or treatment responses. Curiously, significant postoperative improvements in both knee flexion and extension were identified in the contralateral leg, whereas only knee flexion was significantly improved in the bypassed leg. Perhaps these results indicate either an indirect effect resulting from bypass or a practice effect unmasked by repeat testing. The description of the approach to isometric muscle strength measurement (performed with the Muscle Function Evaluation Chair) suggests that it is cumbersome and may be challenging to link directly to daily physical activities; this outcome therefore will likely require further validation to establish its relevance to quality of life and/or walking impairment in PAD before wider use.

M. A. Corriere, MD, MS

Race and gender affect outcomes of lower extremity bypass

Jain AK, Kalbaugh CA, Farber MA, et al (Univ of North Carolina, Chapel Hill)

J Vasc Surg 60:1275-1281, 2014

Background.—Race and gender have individually been associated with affecting outcomes in vascular interventions. We hypothesized that race and gender stratification would identify variations in outcomes of lower extremity bypass (LEB) procedures.

Methods.—LEB procedures were identified using Current Procedural Terminology (American Medical Association, Chicago, Ill) codes from the 2011 American College of Surgeons National Surgical Quality Improvement Program database. Individuals of races other than black or white were excluded because of small sample size. Preoperative variables, such as age, demographics, medical comorbidities, and laboratory values, were evaluated across race and gender groups using χ^2, the Student t-test, and least square means testing. Significant predictors were entered into a multivariate logistic regression model. Six primary outcomes were evaluated: major complications, minor complications, 30-day mortality, early graft failure, readmission, and length of stay (LOS).

Results.—There were 4518 LEB procedures performed on black (n = 839; male [BM], 56.5%; female [BF], 43.5%) or white (n = 3679; male [WM], 66.4%; female [WF], 33.6%) patients. Black patients were more likely to be younger, diabetic, smokers, functionally dependent, dialysis dependent, and have hypertension, critical limb ischemia, higher creatinine, lower hematocrits, and higher platelet counts. Multivariate analysis revealed no statistically significant gender differences within the white cohort with respect to complications, death, graft failure, or readmission rates. WF and BM had longer LOS than WM (reference group; 4.7 ± 1.9 days and 5.4 ± 2.0 days vs 4.3 ± 2.0 days, respectively; $P < .006$ and $P < .0001$) after LEB procedures, but outcomes among these groups did not differ significantly. BF had a longer LOS than WM (5.8 ± 2.0 days vs 4.3 ± 2.0 days; $P < .0001$) and trended toward higher readmission rates (odds ratio, 1.28; 95% confidence interval, 0.97-1.70; $P = .08$). BF had a higher risk of early graft failure than WM (odds ratio, 2.90; 95% confidence interval, 1.52-5.49; $P = .001$).

Conclusions.—BF had higher early graft failure and LOS compared with WM. WF and BM also had increased LOS compared with WM. Race-gender stratification may predict outcomes in patients undergoing LEB procedures that may not be predicted by gender or race alone. Further

studies using this stratification methodology may provide better insight into optimal therapeutic strategies and preventative measures for these patient subgroups. Investigation into causes of increased LOS in black patients and increased graft failure in BF may help improve outcomes.

▶ This analysis of the American College of Surgeons National Quality Improvement Project (ACS-NSQIP) Participant Use Datafile further validates race- and gender-based disparities associated with lower extremity bypass outcomes that have been previously identified by others using this and other datasets. Female gender and black race are factors that have been identified by others as predictors of adverse outcomes associated with lower extremity bypass, although the authors do provide some novel and specific observations by providing gender-specific outcomes stratified by black versus white race. It is interesting to note that they did not evaluate Hispanic ethnicity as part of their analysis, which has also been suggested as a risk factor for adverse outcomes; a query into this additional potential source of disparities might have provided additional insight relevant to a growing proportion of the US population. The analysis is victim to many of the limitations common to NSQIP-based studies; the endpoints are limited to perioperative events and do not include highly relevant long-term outcomes such as amputation-free survival, quality of life, or limb salvage. The authors were also unable to adjust for medical therapy, physiologic data (such as ankle brachial index), or anatomic factors.

These limitations aside, this study provides further validation that race- and gender-based outcome disparities exist for lower extremity bypass. Given that the existence of these disparities is no longer controversial, the key questions that remain are (1) what are the contributing etiologic factors? and (2) how can they be modified or eliminated? Biological factors (such as vessel diameter or distinct pathophysiology) might be responsible for some of the observed disparities and might require development of tailored approaches to pharmacotherapy or distinct intervention criteria. Alternatively, these disparities may instead be the result of differences in how these patients interact with the health care system. Given that race and gender disparities are also being identified across an ever-increasing array of outcomes other than lower extremity bypass (including coronary disease, aortic aneurysm, and hemodialysis access, to name a few), this latter explanation seems plausible. Differences in disease severity at presentation, which have been seen among women with peripheral arterial disease but are poorly understood,[1] may indicate barriers to screening, timely diagnosis, or appropriate provider access. Cultural factors may also influence health risk behaviors and provider trust. The race- and gender-based differences in length of stay identified in this analysis may also reflect challenges with accessing important postdischarge outpatient resources (such as rehabilitation, home health, and wound care) that impact outcomes. Sorting out which of these factors contribute most to disparities will likely be challenging and extend beyond the scope of secondary data analysis but is nonetheless essential if we hope to identify actionable opportunities. The time has come to move on from observing disparities to addressing them.

M. A. Corriere, MD, MS

Reference

1. Hirsch AT, Allison MA, Gomes AS, et al. A call to action: women and peripheral artery disease: a scientific statement from the American Heart Association. *Circulation.* 2012;125:1449-1472.

Open bypass and endovascular procedures among diabetic foot ulcer cases in the United States from 2001 to 2010

Skrepnek GH, Armstrong DG, Mills JL (Univ of Arizona College of Medicine, Tucson)

J Vasc Surg 60:1255-1265, 2014

Objective.—The objective of this study was to evaluate trends in outcomes of inpatient mortality, surgical complications, charges, and length of stay stratified according to open vs endovascular revascularization and amputation status in patients admitted to the hospital with diabetic foot ulcers (DFUs).

Methods.—Inpatient discharge records from the Agency for Healthcare Research and Quality Healthcare Cost and Utilization Project were used in this retrospective cohort study spanning 2001 to 2010. Multivariate regression analyses were used to simultaneously control for patient demographic and socioeconomic attributes, hospital characteristics, and comorbid case-mix disease severity.

Results.—During the study period, 2.5 million inpatient DFU cases were observed, of which 412,051 (16.5%) involved amputation (34.8% major, 61.2% minor). Overall, 211,534 (8.5%) of DFU cases underwent revascularization (43.5% open, 51.1% endovascular treatment [EVT], 5.4% both). From 2001 vs 2010, the volume of open procedures decreased 34.9%, and EVT volume increased 197.1%. The percentage of amputations for DFUs remained relatively unchanged, and a major:minor ratio of 0.534 was observed among all cases. Across specific procedure type and amputation status, multivariate analyses indicated equal or decreased inpatient mortality and lengths of stay since 2001, and inflation adjusted charges generally increased. The presence of a surgical complication, however, was observed to increase by >50% for open procedures involving minor amputations and >30% for open procedures involving no amputations. Because of many potential factors, surgical complications were noted to exceed approximately 900% among cases of EVT involving major amputations beginning in 2007 relative to 2001.

Conclusions.—This nationally-representative investigation found that DFU admissions are common, long, and costly (often >$100,000 per case), with a marked shift having occurred from open bypass to EVT. Although hospital mortality and length of stay either remained the same

or have decreased significantly, an increase in procedure-specific surgical complications was observed across several intervention categories.

▶ The relationship between diabetic foot ulcer (DFU) and peripheral arterial disease (PAD) is a complex one, particularly when explored within the realm of administrative data. Providers caring for patients with both of these diagnoses often face treatment decision-making challenges, especially when PAD is mild and uncertainty exists regarding whether revascularization is necessary to achieve wound healing. A trial of outpatient wound therapy may fail without a revascularization, but preemptive revascularization subjects the patient to procedure-related risks and isn't always absolutely necessary. This analysis of the Nationwide Inpatient Sample Dataset provides an assessment of resource utilization and outcomes associated with DFU care over a decade (2001-2012), focusing specifically on patients who received a revascularization during their inpatient hospitalization. The authors describe what they perceive as a paradigm shift in inpatient DFU management characterized by increasing utilization of endovascular versus open surgical techniques. Trends over the study period included decreases in periprocedural mortality but increases in both patient complexity (assessed based on the Deyo-Charleson Comorbidity index) and surgical complications, whereas amputation rates remained relatively stable.

Although the authors conclude that their findings characterize the prevalence, clinical significance, and economic effects of the DFU, it would be more correct to say that this study characterizes these factors as they relate to inpatient hospitalization for DFU, and the results should be interpreted accordingly. Over the 10-year period during which this study was conducted, an increasing number of outpatient environments emerged and established increasing roles in DFU care in the United States, including outpatient wound care centers, endovascular suites, home health agencies, and podiatric surgery centers. The increasing case mix severity and lack of decline in amputation rates observed by these investigators, therefore, may reflect the growing share of lower-acuity DFU care that has been taken over by outpatient centers, with a corresponding shift to more selective use of inpatient care for increasingly complex cases. Unfortunately, it is not possible to ascertain what treatment(s), if any, preceded inpatient hospitalization for DFU in this study or other specific details related to the scenario that preceded revascularization. Resources dedicated to outpatient treatment environments are likely substantial and probably account for a significant proportion of the overall costs associated with DFU but were not accounted for in this study; costs related to inpatient care, therefore, may only reflect the tip of the proverbial iceberg. Efficient care for DFU requires effective interaction between these inpatient and outpatient centers (which often involve separate providers or health systems). Many patients may require a combination of inpatient and outpatient treatment, and data from both of these settings are necessary to develop evidence-based approaches to directing care delivery into the resource-appropriate environment providing the greatest value.

M. A. Corriere, MD, MS

Patients carrying *CYP2C19* loss of function alleles have a reduced response to clopidogrel therapy and a greater risk of in-stent restenosis after endovascular treatment of lower extremity peripheral arterial disease

Guo B, Tan Q, Guo D, et al (Fudan Univ, Shanghai, China)

J Vasc Surg 60:993-1001, 2014

Objective.—This study evaluated the relationship between the cytochrome P450 (*CYP*) *2C19* genotype and the antiplatelet effect of clopidogrel therapy and investigated whether genotyping can predict the risk of ischemic events after endovascular treatment (ET) of lower extremity peripheral arterial disease.

Methods.—From January 2011 to July 2012, 120 consecutive patients with arteriosclerosis obliterans (TransAtlantic Inter-Society Consensus for the Management of Peripheral Arterial Disease [TASC II] A-C) in the superficial femoral artery were included in a prospectively maintained database. Patients received 75 mg clopidogrel and 100 mg aspirin daily for at least 5 days before TaqMan (Life Technologies, Grand Island, NY) of *CYP2C19* single-nucleotide polymorphisms and thromboelastography of the clopidogrel response. ET was subsequently performed, and follow-up evaluations, including duplex ultrasound imaging and ankle-brachial index assessment, were performed at 1, 3, 6, and 12 months after ET. During the follow-up, stent patency was assessed by ultrasound imaging, computed tomography angiography, or digital subtraction angiography.

Results.—A total of 74 ET procedures were performed. Fifty of the enrolled patients (41.7%) completed the follow-up examinations and were included in the analysis. The mean duration of follow up was 9.8 6 2.1 months (range, 1-30 months). Carriers of at least one *CYP2C19* loss-of-function (LOF) allele had a diminished pharmacodynamic response to clopidogrel (51.6 6 20.1 vs 39.8 6 15.2 for patients without and with LOF alleles, respectively; $P = .022$). Carriers of one LOF allele had an increased incidence of ischemic events compared with patients without any LOF alleles (59.0% vs 20.8%, respectively; $P = .008$). This trend was even more evident in patients with two LOF alleles compared with patients with no LOF alleles (100% vs 20.8% ischemic events; $P = .002$). The cumulative primary patency rate at 12 months was 56.0%, with significant differences between groups (73.1% vs 34.6% in patients without and with LOF alleles, respectively; $P = .0.006$). *CYP2C19* LOF carrier status was associated with an increased rate of primary end points ($P = .007$). On the basis of their adenosine diphosphate-induced platelet aggregation, patients with high platelet reactivity had a significantly higher risk of ischemic events ($P = .012$). *CYP2C19* genotypic classification (adjusted hazard ratio, 2.688; 95% confidence interval, 1.366-5.288; $P = .004$) and history of smoking (adjusted hazard ratio, 2.430; 95% confidence interval, 1.024-5.765; $P = .044$) were independent risk factors for ischemic events.

Conclusions.—*CYP2C19* LOF alleles were associated with a diminished platelet response to clopidogrel treatment. Patients carrying *CYP2C19*

LOF alleles who are treated with clopidogrel may trend toward a poor prognosis after ET (Figs 2 and 3).

▶ The results of this study show that single nucleotide polymorphisms involving the cytochrome P450 2C19 (CYP2C19) resulting in loss of function (LOF) can have profound impact on the outcomes of endovascular treatment of lower extremity peripheral arterial disease (PAD). Although the study has several limitations (the greatest of which being exclusion of nearly 60% of the cohort because of lack of follow-up and lack of investigator blinding), the large magnitude of effect that CYP2C19 LOF had on platelet function (measured using thromboelastography) and risk of ischemic events resulted in several highly significant observations that should command the attention of anyone who treats PAD. Participants with CYP2C19 LOF had increased risk of ischemic events and significantly diminished pharmacologic responses to clopidogrel (Figs 2 and 3, respectively), with even greater risk among those with 2 versus 1 LOF allele (with 100% vs 21%, respectively, experiencing ischemic events during follow-up). Smoking was the only other independent risk factor for ischemic events identified, and active smoking was associated with a risk nearly equivalent to 2 LOF alleles.

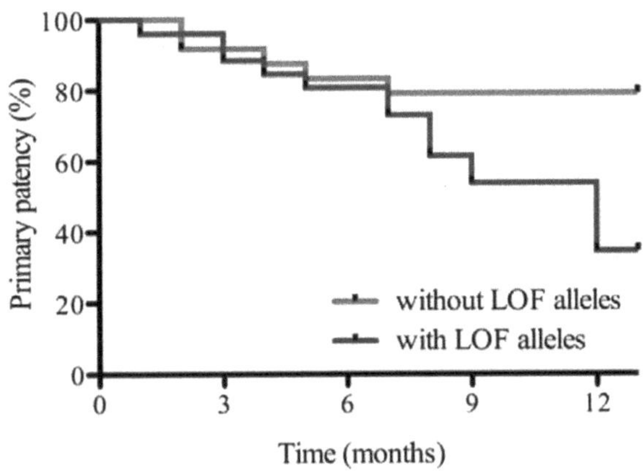

Without LOF alleles					
Numbers at risk	24	22	20	19	19
Standard error	0.00	0.05	0.08	0.08	0.08
With LOF alleles					
Numbers at risk	26	23	21	14	9
Standard error	0.00	0.06	0.07	0.09	0.09

FIGURE 2.—Kaplan-Meier curve shows primary vessel patency during follow-up in patients with and without the cytochrome P450 *(CYP) 2C19* loss-of-function (*LOF*) allele (n = 50). *P* = .006 by log-rank test. (Reprinted from the Journal of Vascular Surgery. Guo B, Tan Q, Guo D, et al. Patients carrying *CYP2C19* loss of function alleles have a reduced response to clopidogrel therapy and a greater risk of in-stent restenosis after endovascular treatment of lower extremity peripheral arterial disease. *J Vasc Surg*. 2014;60:993-1001, Copyright 2014, with permission from the Society for Vascular Surgery.)

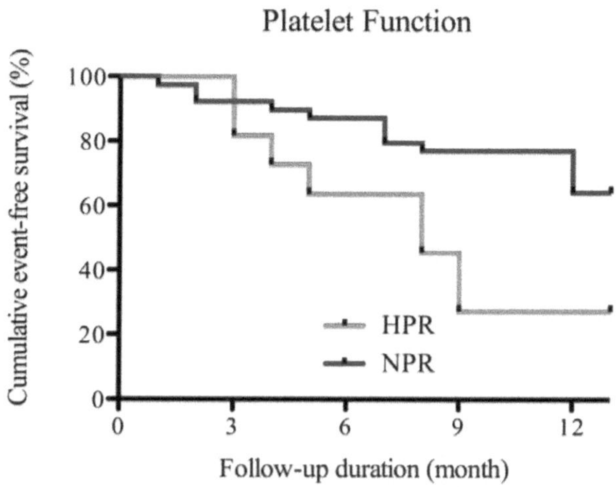

HPR					
Numbers at risk	11	9	7	3	3
Standard error	0.00	**0.11**	**0.14**	**0.13**	**0.13**
NPR					
Numbers at risk	39	36	34	30	25
Standard error	0.00	0.04	0.05	0.06	0.07

FIGURE 3.—Estimated rates of primary end points are shown according to platelet reactivity characteristics (n = 50). $P = .012$ by log-rank test. *HPR*, High platelet reactivity; *NPR*, normal platelet reactivity. (Reprinted from the Journal of Vascular Surgery. Guo B, Tan Q, Guo D, et al. Patients carrying *CYP2C19* loss of function alleles have a reduced response to clopidogrel therapy and a greater risk of in-stent restenosis after endovascular treatment of lower extremity peripheral arterial disease. *J Vasc Surg.* 2014;60:993-1001, Copyright 2014, with permission from the Society for Vascular Surgery.)

Although these results are certainly noteworthy, several challenges exist to applying the findings to clinical practice. Ideally, providers could screen all patients being considered for the CYP2C19 LOF mutation and then apply a specific management strategy to those testing positive to decrease their risk for adverse outcomes. The authors identified at least one CYP2C19 LOF allele in 52% of the study population, suggesting that the polymorphisms are common among patients with symptomatic PAD and, therefore, might warrant the cost of screening. From an epidemiologic perspective, however, readers should be mindful that this study was conducted in Shanghai, China and, therefore, may have issues related to external validity; the prevalence of CYP2C19 LOF might not be the same in other more racially heterogeneous populations (potentially reducing the yield and value of screening). Additionally, exactly how identification of the CYP2C19 LOF allele should affect clinical management or decision making is unclear. Although the authors did not provide stratified outcomes based on rates of dual antiplatelet therapy use, their clinical protocol mentioned use of dual antiplatelet treatment among all participants without contraindications. Presumably, then, the high rates of ischemic events occurred in the setting of dual antiplatelet therapy for many participants. Providers considering intervention in the setting of a known CYP2C19 LOF polymorphism are, therefore, left without an evidence-based modification of medical therapy to invoke if they hope to improve outcomes, apart from perhaps deciding to withhold intervention (a strategy that would certainly be acceptable in this study population, which was dominated by patients with intermittent claudication). The results additionally suggest that claudicants with the CYP2C19 LOF who are actively smoking should expect especially poor outcomes with endovascular treatment. Interestingly, participants with the CYP2C19 LOF had a smoking prevalence nearly double of those without (35% vs 17%). While we await additional evidence to support specific screening and management approaches related to CYP2C19 LOF, the best and simplest approach may be to focus on risk reduction and noninterventional treatment strategies in claudicants, particularly those who smoke.

M. A. Corriere, MD, MS

An early validation of the Society for Vascular Surgery Lower Extremity Threatened Limb Classification System

Cull DL, Manos G, Hartley MC, et al (Univ of South Carolina School of Medicine-Greenville)

J Vasc Surg 60:1535-1542, 2014

Objective.—The Society for Vascular Surgery (SVS) recently established the Lower Extremity Threatened Limb Classification System, a staging system using Wound characteristic, Ischemia, and foot Infection (WIfI) to stratify the risk for limb amputation at 1 year. Although intuitive in nature, this new system has not been validated. The purpose of the following study was to determine whether the WIfI system is predictive of limb amputation and wound healing.

Methods.—Between 2007 and 2010, we prospectively obtained data related to wound characteristics, extent of infection, and degree of postrevascularization ischemia in 139 patients with foot wounds who presented for lower extremity revascularization (158 revascularization procedures). After adapting those data to the WIfI classifications, we analyzed the influence of wound characteristics, extent of infection, and degree of ischemia on time to wound healing; empirical Kaplan-Meier survival curves were compared with theoretical outcomes predicted by WIfI expert consensus opinion.

Results.—Of the 158 foot wounds, 125 (79%) healed. The median time to wound healing was 2.7 months (range, 1-18 months). Factors associated with wound healing included presence of diabetes mellitus ($P = .013$), wound location ($P = .049$), wound size ($P = .007$), wound depth ($P = .004$), and degree of ischemia ($P < .001$). The WIfI clinical stage was predictive of 1-year limb amputation (stage 1, 3%; stage 2, 10%; stage 3, 23%; stage 4, 40%) and wound nonhealing (stage 1, 8%; stage 2, 10%; stage 3, 23%; stage 4, 40%) and correlated with the theoretical outcome estimated by the SVS expert panel.

Conclusions.—The theoretical framework for risk stratification among patients with critical limb ischemia provided by the SVS expert panel appears valid. Further validation of the WIfI classification system with multicenter data is justified (Table 1).

► Patients with a foot wound in the setting of critical limb ischemia (CLI) present a high-stakes challenge that requires dedicated and resource-intensive management. Wound healing and limb salvage are major accomplishments in this patient population, even at specialized centers with focused interest in CLI outcomes (including the center where this study was performed). This analysis provides a valuable assessment of the recently proposed Society for Vascular Surgery Lower Extremity Threatened Limb Classification System that uses wound, ischemia, and infection (WIFI) criteria to categorize amputation risk. The WIFI system was developed based on expert consensus without directly supporting data out of necessity because preceding evidence has tended to consider its components separately and few applicable natural history studies exist.[1] Although proposing a classification system without direct evidence validating its predictive value is a somewhat unorthodox approach that seems to put the proverbial cart before the horse, this represents an attempt by the WIFI experts to address a long-standing disconnect among diabetes, neuropathy, and peripheral artery disease as important factors that have an impact on amputation outcomes and often coexist.

In this study, Cull et al retrospectively adapted their own institutional dataset to the WIFI classification system to evaluate its predictive accuracy. Although their system has many similarities with WIFI, there were also several important differences: the former has more ischemia grade strata, whereas the latter provides greater detail related to wound characteristics (Table 1). The authors system also omits the neuropathy assessment recommended by the WIFI authors. Given that WIFI's stated intent was to merge separate CLI and diabetic foot classification systems, it is also curious to note that neither WIFI nor the authors' system includes diabetes as a component. As the authors mention, they applied the WIFI spectrum score (designed for grading before a revascularization procedure) to patients with CLI who were postrevascularization. Although their justification for this approach (that ischemia grade affects likelihood of wound healing/amputation regardless of whether a revascularization has been performed) seems reasonable, this distinction should be considered when interpreting the results. Use of photographs rather than clinical examinations for wound classification may also have resulted in misclassification (particularly for depth and tissue involvement) within this retrospective study. The retrospective design may have also introduced potential for bias among unblinded observers assigning scores because all 1-year endpoints (including amputation) in the study cohort had occurred before publication of the WIFI classification system.

These limitations aside, this study leverages a high-quality data set to provide a preliminary validation of the WIFI classification system. As ongoing investigations continue to evaluate the predictive accuracy of WIFI, it will be of interest to evaluate the potential contributions of other patient-level factors

TABLE 1.—Comparison of Study Data Categories With the Wound Characteristic, Ischemia, and Foot Infection (*WIfI*) Grades

Study Data Categories		WIfI
Wound characteristics[a]		Wound grade[b]
Wound size		0 No rest pain
1	<1 cm^2	1 Small, shallow ulcer
2	1-3 cm^2	No exposed bone, unless limited to distal phalanx
3	>3 cm^2	No gangrene
Wound depth		2 Deeper ulcer with exposed bone joint, or tendon, not involving the tissue heel
1	Ulcer not extending to SQ	Shallow heel ulcer without calcaneal involvement
2	Ulcer extending to SQ tissue	Gangrenous changes limited to digits
3	Ulcer extending to bone or joint space	3 Extensive, deep ulcer involving forefoot/midfoot
Wound type		Deep, full thickness heel ulcer + calcaneal involvement
1	Ulcer	Extensive gangrene involving forefoot/midfoot
2	Gangrene	Full thickness heel necrosis + calcaneal involvement
Location		Infection grade
1	Forefoot	0 No symptoms or signs of infection
2	Midfoot	1 Local infection involving only skin, SQ tissue
3	Heel	2 Local infection with erythema >2 cm, or involving structures deeper than skin, SQ (eg, abscess, osteomyelitis)
Infection categories		3 Local infection with signs of SIRS
1	None	Ischemia grade
2	Erythema	0 TP >60 mm Hg
3	Purulence	ABI >0.8
4	Systemic evidence of infection	AP >100 mm Hg
Ischemia categories[c]		1 TP 40-59 mm Hg
1	TP >60 mm Hg	ABI 0.6-0.79
	ABI >0.9	AP 70-100 mm Hg
	Palpable pulse	2 TP 30-39 mm Hg
	AP >80 mm Hg	ABI 0.4-0.59
2	TP 30-60 mm Hg	AP 50-70 mm Hg
	ABI 0.5-0.9	3 TP <30 mm Hg
	AP 50-79 mm Hg	ABI <0.39
3	TP <30 mm Hg	AP <30 mm Hg
	ABI <0.5	
	AP <50 mm Hg	

ABI, Ankle-brachial index; *AP*, systolic ankle pressure; *SIRS*, systemic inflammatory response syndrome; *SQ*, subcutaneous tissue; *TP*, toe pressure.

[a]Study only included patients with foot wounds.

[b]WIfI classification dictates that wound depth take priority over wound size.

[c]If ABI and TP resulted in different grades in patients with diabetes mellitus, TP was used to determine grade.

(such as diabetes, neuropathy, age, and smoking) to overall predictive accuracy. Given the relative complexity of WIFI, it also remains to be seen whether this system is widely adopted for routine clinical decision making, research, or both.

M. A. Corriere, MD, MS

Reference

1. Mills JL Sr, Conte MS, Armstrong DG, et al. The society for vascular surgery lower extremity threatened limb classification system: risk stratification based on wound, ischemia, and foot infection (WIfI). *J Vasc Surg*. 2014;59:220-234.e1-2.

Lower extremity autologous vein bypass for critical limb ischemia is not adversely affected by prior endovascular procedure

Santo VJ, Dargon P, Azarbal AF, et al (Oregon Health and Science Univ, Portland)

J Vasc Surg 60:129-135, 2014

Objective.—It has been reported that a failed endovascular intervention adversely affects results of lower extremity bypass (LEB). We reviewed rates of prior endovascular intervention (PEI) in patients undergoing LEB with autologous vein for critical limb ischemia (CLI) to determine effects on graft patency, limb salvage, and amputation-free survival.

Methods.—Retrospective review was conducted of consecutive autologous vein LEBs performed for CLI between 2005 and 2012 at a tertiary care academic medical center.

Results.—Overall, 314 autologous vein LEBs were performed for CLI, 71% for tissue loss. TransAtlantic Inter-Society Consensus II type D or type C lesions were present in 62% and 25%, respectively. The great saphenous vein was used as a conduit in 83%, and the distal target was infrapopliteal in 60%. The 30-day mortality rate was 3.5%. Primary patency rates at 1 year and 5 years were 61% and 45%. Secondary patency rates at 1 year and 5 years were 88% and 64%, with 23% requiring an intervention to maintain patency. The 5-year limb salvage rate was 89%, and the 5-year amputation-free survival was 49%. There were 61 patients (19%) who had undergone a PEI and 253 (81%) who underwent bypass with no prior endovascular intervention (NPEI). There were 19 iliac stents, 29 femoral interventions, 13 popliteal interventions, 9 crural interventions, 9 infrainguinal thrombectomies, and 13 infrainguinal thrombolyses. PEI and NPEI patients had similar demographics and prevalence of atherosclerotic risk factors. The 1-year primary patency rate was 62% for NPEI patients vs 59% for PEI patients ($P=.759$). The 1-year and 2-year secondary patency rates were 87% and 79% for NPEI patients vs 89% and 78% for PEI patients ($P=.947$). The 3-year limb salvage rate was 89% for NPEI patients vs 92% for PEI patients ($P=.445$). The 3-year amputation-free survival was 59% for NPEI patients vs 52% for

PEI patients (P=.399). Median follow-up time was 323 days for NPEI patients (interquartile range, 83-918) vs 463 days for PEI patients (interquartile range, 145-946; P=.275).

Conclusions.—Overall operative mortality, patency rates, and limb salvage for autologous vein LEB in CLI patients continue to be excellent in the endovascular era and are not necessarily affected by a prior ipsilateral endovascular procedure. Long-term survival remains poor in CLI patients requiring LEB (Tables 1-4).

▶ The results of this retrospective analysis from a single center—that prior endovascular procedures do not adversely impact outcomes of subsequent autologous vein bypasses for patients with critical limb ischemia (CLI)—are inconsistent with observations from several prominent multicenter studies and trials.[1-4] Because this analysis did not include an assessment of statistical power, it is possible that an effect related to prior endovascular procedures was present but not detected (a type II statistical error). The authors performed extensive comparisons, however, between groups stratified by prior endovascular intervention status. Tables 2-4 contain 48 statistical tests, but the authors identified only one between-group difference (higher prevalence of hypertension within the group without prior endovascular intervention); at an alpha level of 0.05, more between-group differences would be expected owing to random chance. Because data collection for this study was performed using an electronic health record from a single center, it is also possible that adverse events or re-interventions that were managed elsewhere were not accounted for.

Statistical considerations aside, there may be other potential explanations for the reported results and their lack of consistency with other multicenter studies. One variable of potential interest that was not analyzed (and would be challenging to include within a retrospective study) is whether the previous

TABLE 1.—Prior Endovascular Interventions (*PEIs*)

	No. (%)
Pelvic stent	19 (31.1)
Femoral stent	8 (13.1)
Femoral angioplasty	14 (23.0)
Femoral atherectomy	7 (11.4)
Popliteal stent	5 (8.2)
Popliteal angioplasty	5 (8.2)
Popliteal atherectomy	3 (4.9)
Crural stent	1 (1.6)
Crural angioplasty	5 (8.2)
Crural atherectomy	3 (4.9)
Infrainguinal thrombectomy	9 (14.8)
Infrainguinal thrombolysis	13 (21.3)

There were 92 PEIs performed in 61 patients.

TABLE 2.—Baseline Patient Characteristics and Comorbidities

	NPEI (n = 253)	PEI (n = 61)	*P* Value
Male/female[a]	163/90 (64.4/35.6)	34/27 (55.7/44.3)	.208
Age,[b] years	67.2 ± 12.5	66.9 ± 12.7	.883
BMI,[c] kg/m^2	26.7 (23-32.2)	25.9 (23.6-30.0)	.280
HTN	208 (82.2)	40 (65.6)	.004
HLD	113 (44.7)	23 (37.7)	.325
DM			.578
None	125 (49.4)	28 (45.9)	
NIDDM	59 (23.3)	18 (29.5)	
IDDM	69 (27.3)	15 (24.6)	
CAD	109 (43.1)	27 (44.3)	.867
Prior CVA	48 (19.0)	9 (14.8)	.443
CKD	60 (23.7)	11 (18.0)	.341
Creatinine,[b] mg/dL	1.5 ± 1.3	1.5 ± 1.6	.871
Dialysis	28 (11.1)	7 (11.5)	.928
COPD	33 (13.0)	4 (6.6)	.158
Tobacco use			.445
None	52 (20.6)	17 (27.9)	
Prior	103 (40.7)	25 (41.0)	
Current	98 (38.7)	19 (31.1)	
Normal pulses			
Femoral	168 (69.8)	43 (75.4)	.642
Popliteal	27 (11.1)	8 (14.0)	.619
Pedal	2 (0.8)	0 (0)	.121
Antiplatelet	162 (64.0)	45 (73.8)	.150
Aspirin	145 (57.3)	38 (62.3)	.479
Clopidogrel	40 (15.8)	20 (32.8)	.002
Dipyridamole	4 (1.6)	1 (1.6)	1.000
Beta-blocker	130 (51.4)	33 (54.1)	.703
Statin	117 (46.2)	30 (49.2)	.680
Anticoagulation	41 (16.2)	9 (14.8)	.781

BMI, Body mass index; *CAD*, coronary artery disease; *CKD*, chronic kidney disease (serum creatinine concentration >1.5); *COPD*, chronic obstructive pulmonary disease; *CVA*, cerebrovascular accident; *DM*, diabetes mellitus; *HLD*, hyperlipidemia; *HTN*, hypertension; *IDDM*, insulin-dependent diabetes mellitus; *NIDDM*, noninsulin-dependent diabetes mellitus; *NPEI*, no prior endovascular intervention; *PEI*, prior endovascular intervention.

[a]Categorical variables are presented as number (%), χ^2 analysis.

[b]Mean ± standard deviation, unpaired Student *t*-test, two-tailed analysis.

[c]Median (interquartile range), Mann-Whitney analysis.

Reprinted from the Journal of Vascular Surgery. Santo VJ, Dargon P, Azarbal AF, et al. Lower extremity autologous vein bypass for critical limb ischemia is not adversely affected by prior endovascular procedure. *J Vasc Surg*. 2014;60:129-135, Copyright 2014, with permission from The Society for Vascular Surgery.

endovascular procedure impacted the conduct of the subsequent bypass in terms of the site of proximal anastomosis, the recipient vessel, and the number of patent runoff vessels. Given the authors' admittedly conservative approach toward endovascular treatment for CLI (all patients with TransAtlantic Inter-Society Consensus II C or D disease within this series were preferentially treated with vein bypass provided that they had vein conduit available and were deemed appropriate candidates), the absence of an adverse impact related to previous endovascular intervention may in part be related to a conscious effort to preserve available bypass options during these interventions. Approximately 30% of the previous endovascular interventions consisted of iliac angioplasty (Table 1), an intervention expected to have a positive impact (if any) on the patency of subsequent infrainguinal bypass; it is, therefore, possible that the

TABLE 3.—Preoperative Lesion Characteristics: TransAtlantic Inter-Society Consensus (*TASC*) II

	NPEI (n = 253)	PEI (n = 61)	*P* Value
TASC II classification			.127
Unknown	27 (10.8)	7 (11.7)	
B	4 (1.6)	3 (5.0)	
C	59 (23.5)	20 (33.3)	
D	163 (64.4)	31 (50.8)	

NPEI, No prior endovascular intervention; *PEI*, prior endovascular intervention.
Data are presented as number (%), χ^2 analysis.
Reprinted from the Journal of Vascular Surgery. Santo VJ, Dargon P, Azarbal AF, et al. Lower extremity autologous vein bypass for critical limb ischemia is not adversely affected by prior endovascular procedure. *J Vasc Surg*. 2014;60:129-135,

TABLE 4.—Arterial Inflow and Outflow

	NPEI (n = 253)	PEI (n = 61)	*P* Value
Inflow vessel			
External iliac	4 (1.6)	1 (1.6)	1.000
Common femoral	100 (39.5)	23 (37.7)	.794
Profunda femoris	39 (15.4)	9 (14.8)	.898
Superficial femoral	63 (24.9)	18 (29.5)	.460
Above-knee popliteal	8 (3.2)	2 (3.3)	1.000
Below-knee popliteal	23 (9.1)	6 (9.8)	.857
Aortofemoral graft	3 (1.2)	1 (1.6)	.580
Iliofemoral graft	2 (0.8)	1 (1.6)	.478
Popliteal graft	2 (0.8)	0 (0)	1.000
Axillary-femoral graft	4 (1.6)	0 (0)	1.000
Femoral-femoral graft	5 (2.0)	0 (0)	.587
Outflow vessel			
Above-knee popliteal	25 (9.9)	5 (8.2)	.688
Below-knee popliteal	73 (28.9)	23 (37.7)	.178
Tibioperoneal trunk	4 (1.6)	1 (1.6)	1.000
Posterior tibial	53 (20.9)	12 (19.7)	.825
Anterior tibial	39 (15.4)	8 (13.1)	.651
Peroneal	47 (18.6)	8 (13.1)	.314
Pedal	12 (4.8)	4 (6.6)	.289

NPEI, No prior endovascular intervention; *PEI*, prior endovascular intervention.
Data are presented as number (%), χ^2 analysis.
Reprinted from the Journal of Vascular Surgery. Santo VJ, Dargon P, Azarbal AF, et al. Lower extremity autologous vein bypass for critical limb ischemia is not adversely affected by prior endovascular procedure. *J Vasc Surg*. 2014;60:129-135,

results might have been different if the analysis had limited previous endovascular interventions to procedures distal to the common femoral artery. Finally, as pointed out by the authors in their discussion, this study was limited to patients who underwent a lower extremity bypass; patients who underwent primary endovascular intervention for CLI but subsequently were not candidates for bypass when the initial treatment failed, therefore, are excluded. These results, therefore, should be interpreted within the context of the authors' treatment algorithm and may not be generalizable to environments with relatively aggressive attitudes toward endovascular treatment (or conservative use of bypass) for CLI.

M. A. Corriere, MD, MS

References

1. Bradbury AW, Adam DJ, Bell J, et al. Bypass versus angioplasty in severe ischaemia of the leg (BASIL) trial: analysis of amputation free and overall survival by treatment received. *J Vasc Surg*. 2010;51:18S-31S.
2. Blaurock P, Mansmann U, Schwarzbach M, et al. Early surgical outcome after failed primary stenting for lower limb occlusive disease. *J Endovasc Ther*. 2005; 12:13-21.
3. Joels CS, York JW, Kalbaugh CA, Cull DL, Langan EM 3rd, Taylor SM. Surgical implications of early failed endovascular intervention of the superficial femoral artery. *J Vasc Surg*. 2008;47:562-565.
4. Nolan BW, De Martino RR, Stone DH, et al. Prior failed ipsilateral percutaneous endovascular intervention in patients with critical limb ischemia predicts poor outcome after lower extremity bypass. *J Vasc Surg*. 2011;54:730-735.

Bayesian network meta-analysis of nitinol stents, covered stents, drug-eluting stents, and drug-coated balloons in the femoropopliteal artery

Katsanos K, Spiliopoulos S, Karunanithy N, et al (Guy's and St. Thomas' Hosps, London, UK; Patras Univ Hosp, Rion, Greece; et al)

J Vasc Surg 59:1123-1133.e8, 2014

Objective.—Several randomized controlled trials (RCTs) have shown the superiority of some of these technologies over balloon angioplasty, but direct comparisons between these treatment options are lacking. The authors conducted a network meta-analysis of RCTs comparing bare nitinol stents, covered nitinol stents, paclitaxel- or sirolimus-eluting stents (PES or SES), and paclitaxel-coated balloons (PCB) with plain balloon angioplasty or with each other in the femoropopliteal artery (PROSPERO registry: CRD42013004845).

Methods.—Sixteen RCTs comprising 2532 patients with 4227 person-years of follow-up were analyzed on an intention-totreat basis. Bayesian random effects Poisson and binomial models were used for mixed treatment comparisons (Win- BUGS). Clinical heterogeneity was accounted for by incorporating a meta-regression model on trial-specific baseline risk. End points included technical success, vascular restenosis, target lesion revascularization, and major amputations. Pairwise odds ratios and rate ratios (ORs and RRs) of absolute treatment effects were calculated, and the probabilities of each treatment being best are reported. Summary estimates are reported as the posterior median and associated credible intervals (CrIs) that serve the same purpose as confidence intervals in the context of the Bayesian framework. Extensive sensitivity, meta-regression, and network consistency analyses were performed to evaluate heterogeneity.

Results.—Technical success was highest with covered stents (pooled OR, 13.6; 95% CrI, 3.3-31.1, probability best 82%) followed by uncovered stents (pooled OR, 7.0; 95% CrI, 2.6-129, probability best 18%) when compared with balloon angioplasty (reference treatment). Vascular restenosis was lowest with PES (RR, 0.43; 95% CrI, 0.16-1.18, probability best 45%) followed by PCB (RR, 0.43; 95% CrI, 0.26-0.67, probability best 42%). Target lesion revascularization was lowest with PCB (RR, 0.36; 95% CrI, 0.23-0.55, probability best 56%) followed by PES (RR, 0.42; 95% CrI, 0.16-1.06, probability best 33%). Major amputations were rare in all treatment and control groups (pooled amputation rate of 0.7 events per 100 person-years).

Conclusions.—Immediate technical success is better with the use of covered stents, whereas paclitaxel-eluting stents and paclitaxel-coated balloons offer the best long-term results in the femoropopliteal artery (Fig 3, Supplementary Table 2).

▶ The devil is often in the details when it comes to interpreting meta-analysis results. Although the authors assert that a randomized, controlled trial network (Fig 3) allows indirect comparisons between treatments that were not evaluated with direct head-to-head comparisons within the same trial, several confounding influences may affect these comparisons and warrant consideration when attempting to draw conclusions from the findings. Different inclusion/exclusion criteria (including factors such as previous intentions, lesion characteristics, or anatomic factors such as runoff) and medical management protocols between trials may have led to comparisons within this meta-analysis that the investigators in the original studies never intended (and indeed may have wished to avoid). Although the analysis used advanced modeling methods intended to mitigate bias resulting from differences in study design and inclusion/exclusion criteria, it is difficult to ignore the possibility that some of these details may have set the stage for comparisons between interventions performed under different circumstances and contingencies. Beyond differences in trial design, comparison of the participant characteristics between studies (Supplementary Table 2) shows that percentages of participants with claudication versus critical limb ischemia among included trials were highly variable (if mentioned at all). Antiplatelet therapy was also highly inconsistent between trials, and several covariates that would be anticipated to be influential (including clinical diagnosis, smoking, and comorbidities such as renal disease) were missing for multiple studies or completely absent from individual studies. It is also important to remember that many of the included trials were industry sponsored (some even named after a proprietary device) with protocols that did not include blinding; these factors may have predisposed them to significant bias, particularly for outcomes such as technical success and target lesion revascularization.

Several variables can factor into the choice between endovascular techniques, including patency, cost, risk, and technical success (among others). Although this meta-analysis observed a significant technical success advantage for covered and uncovered stents, concluding that primary stenting should be

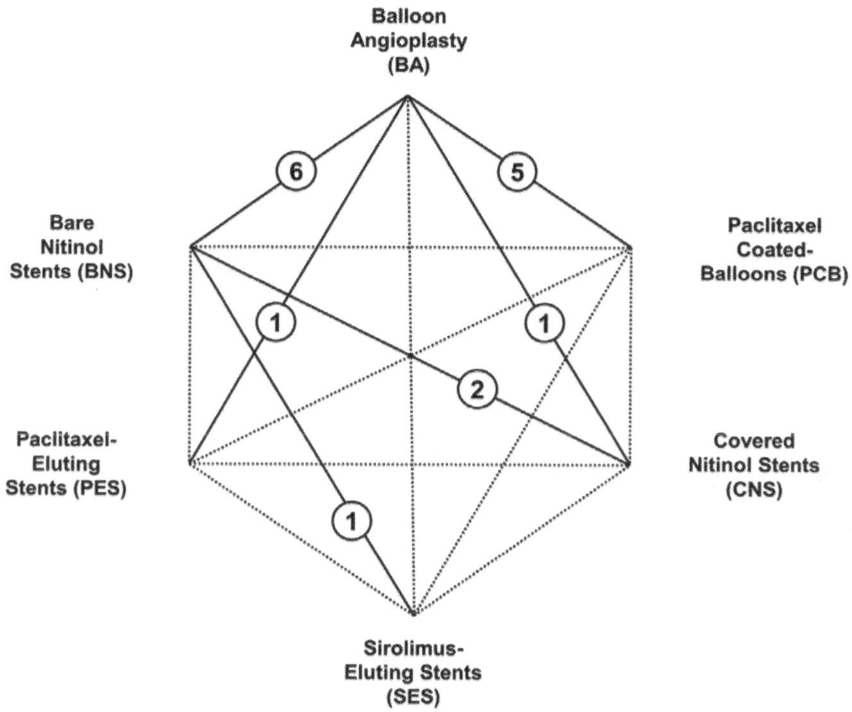

FIGURE 3.—Mixed treatment comparison (MTC) network of evidence. The *straight* lines denote direct head-to-head comparisons and the *dotted lines* denote indirect comparisons in which direct comparison data are missing. The numbers next to the *solid lines* refer to the number of randomized controlled trials (RCTs), with direct comparisons available for each link. (Reprinted from the Journal of Vascular Surgery. Katsanos K, Spiliopoulos S, Karunanithy N, et al. Bayesian network meta-analysis of nitinol stents, covered stents, drug-eluting stents, and drug-coated balloons in the femoropopliteal artery. *J Vasc Surg*. 2014;59:1123-1133.e8, with permission from the Society for Vascular Surgery.)

favored for all femoropopliteal interventions would be an extreme (and expensive) interpretation of the results. Crossovers to other treatment arms were considered technical failures within this study; in clinical practice, however, starting with a treatment that is relatively basic and inexpensive (such as balloon angioplasty) and progressing to more advanced intervention if unsatisfactory results are obtained is a common approach. Starting with the treatment that is simplest and least invasive (ie, requires the smallest sheath access diameter) potentially avoids overtreatment with more complicated, invasive, or expensive options that may be unnecessary. The disadvantage to adopting a "one-size-fits-all" mentality and applying the same algorithm to all patients, however, is that cases requiring more aggressive treatment potentially waste time and equipment through a series of failed interventions performed before the one that eventually succeeds. The ideal approach may, therefore, be the middle ground, where providers selectively utilize more advanced or invasive treatments when they identify factors that predict failure of simpler strategies. If endovascular treatment options are considered from a hierarchical perspective, providers

SUPPLEMENTARY TABLE 2.—Baseline Variables of Randomized Controlled Trials (RCTs) Included in the Network Meta-Analysis

Trial	INTRACOIL Active	INTRACOIL Control	ABSOLUTE Active	ABSOLUTE Control	FAST Active	FAST Control	ASTRON Active	ASTRON Control	RESILIENT Active	RESILIENT Control	SUPER Active	SUPER Control	VIABAHN Active	VIABAHN Control
Study arms	n = 135	n = 131	n = 51	n = 53	n = 123	n = 121	n = 34	n = 39	n = 134	n = 72	n = 74	n = 76	n = 97	n = 100
Age, years	67 ± 11	68 ± 10	65 ± 10	68 ± 10	67 ± 9	66 ± 10	69 ± 9	69 ± 10	68 ± 10	66 ± 9	66 ± 9	70 ± 9	67 ± 10	67 ± 10
Male sex	67%	63%	59%	47%	63%	75%	74%	64%	71%	67%	78%	86%	70%	82%
Smoking	82%	80%	53%	36%	68%	73%	35%	44%	72%	83%	24%	26%	51%	46%
Hypertension	n/a	n/a	92%	87%	83%	83%	82%	80%	84%	94%	66%	67%	68%	65%
Hyperlipidemia	n/a	n/a	92%	87%	60%	61%	91%	92%	80%	76%	n/a	n/a	59%	60%
Diabetes	38%	37%	43%	32%	36%	31%	29%	31%	38%	39%	31%	38%	34%	37%
Renal insufficiency	n/a	n/a	n/a	n/a	15%	6%	n/a	n/a	n/a	n/a	15%	8%	10%	6%
Claudication	n/a	n/a	88%	87%	97%	96%	91%	97%	100%	100%	85%	79%	88%	91%
Critical leg ischemia	n/a	n/a	12%	13%	3%	4%	9%	3%	n/a	n/a	15%	21%	12%	9%
Lesions treated	n = 177	n = 175	n = 51	n = 53	n = 123	n = 121	n = 34	n = 39	n = 134	n = 72	n = 74	n = 76	n = 97	n = 100
Occlusions (CTOs)	23%	17%	37%	32%	37%	25%	38%	39%	n/a	n/a	96%	91%	20%	30%
Lesion length (cm)	3.5 ± 3.0	3.3 ± 3.0	10.1 ± 7.5	9.2 ± 6.4	4.5 ± 2.8	4.5 ± 2.8	8.2 ± 6.7	6.5 ± 4.6	7.1 ± 4.4	6.4 ± 4.1	12.3 ± 5.4	11.7 ± 5.2	7.0 ± 4.0	7.0 ± 4.0
Recommended antiplatelet therapy	Aspirin and ticlopidine for 1 month		Aspirin + clopidogrel for 3 months		Aspirin + clopidogrel for 1 month		Aspirin + clopidogrel for 3 months		Aspirin + clopidogrel for 3 months		Aspirin + clopidogrel for 1 month (or LMWH)		Aspirin (or occasionally ticlopidine)	

Trial	VIBRANT Active	VIBRANT Control	VIASTAR Active	VIASTAR Control	SIROCCO Active	SIROCCO Control	ZILVER-PTX Active	ZILVER-PTX Control	THUNDER Active	THUNDER Control	FEMPAC Active	FEMPAC Control	PACIFIER Active	PACIFIER Control
Study arms	n = 72	n = 76	n = 72	n = 69	n = 47	n = 46	n = 238	n = 241	n = 48	n = 54	n = 45	n = 42	n = 44	n = 47
Age, years	69	63	68	69	66	69	666	11	68	6	10	68	6	11
Male sex	63%	64%	67%	75%	66%	78%	66%	64%	65%	63%	60%	60%	59%	64%
Smoking	n/a	n/a	69%	70%	47%	30%	86%	84%	23%	22%	47%	36%	49%	60%
Hypertension	n/a	n/a	83%	84%	68%	70%	89%	82%	79%	83%	78%	81%	66%	66%
Hyperlipidemia	n/a	n/a	68%	68%	64%	63%	76%	70%	69%	63%	58%	59%	50%	47%
Diabetes	n/a	n/a	35%	36%	43%	35%	49%	42%	50%	46%	40%	55%	43%	28%
Renal insufficiency	n/a	n/a	n/a	n/a	n/a	n/a	10%	11%	n/a	n/a	n/a	n/a	n/a	n/a
Claudication	n/a	n/a	86%	91%	n/a	n/a	90%	91%	n/a	n/a	96%	93%	95%	96%
Critical leg ischemia	n/a	n/a	14%	19%	n/a	n/a	10%	9%	n/a	n/a	4%	7%	5%	4%
Lesions treated (n)	n = 72	n = 76	n = 72	n = 69	n = 47	n = 46	n = 247	n = 251	n = 86	n = 86	n = 100	n = 101	n = 86	n = 47
Occlusions (CTOs)	n/a	n/a	79%	70%	69%	57%	30%	25%	27%	26%	13%	19%	23%	38%

Lesion length (cm)	n/a	n/a	17.3	18.9	8.5 ± 4.4	3.1 ± 5.2	5.4 ± 4.1	5.3 ± 4.0	7.5 ± 6.2	4.4 ± 6.7	4.0	4.7	7.0 ± 5.3	6.6 ± 5.5
Recommended antiplatelet therapy	n/a		Aspirin + clopidogrel for 6 months		Aspirin + clopidogrel/ ticlopidine for 1 month		Aspirin + clopidogrel for 2 months		Aspirin + clopidogrel for 1 month		Aspirin + clopidogrel long-term		Aspirin + clopidogrel for >2 months	

Trial	DEBELLUM Active	DEBELLUM Control	LEVANT 1 Active	LEVANT 1 Control
Study arms	n = 25	n = 25	n = 49	n = 52
Age, years	66 ± 6	67 ± 6	n/a	n/a
Male sex	76%	72%	n/a	n/a
Smoking	68%	56%	n/a	n/a
Hypertension	76%	60%	96%	87%
Hyperlipidemia	48%	68%	59%	69%
Diabetes	52%	36%	45%	50%
Renal insufficiency	n/a	n/a	n/a	n/a
Claudication	64%	60%	94%	93%
Critical leg ischemia	36%	40%	6%	7%
Lesions treated	n = 44	n = 48	n = 49	n = 52
Occlusions (CTOs)	21%	22%	41%	42%
Lesion length (mm)	7.6 ± 0.6	7.8 ± 0.7	8.1 ± 3.7	8.0 ± 3.8
Recommended antiplatelet therapy	Aspirin + clopidogrel for 1 month		n/a	

would therefore be able to maximize efficiency while simultaneously controlling costs if they could predict when option A is likely to succeed or, if technical failure is probable, when starting with option B or C instead is the better choice.

M. A. Corriere, MD, MS

Cilostazol is associated with improved outcomes after peripheral endovascular interventions

Warner CJ, Greaves SW, Larson RJ, et al (Dartmouth-Hitchcock Med Ctr, Lebanon, NH; The Dartmouth Inst for Health Policy and Clinical Practice, Lebanon, NH)

J Vasc Surg 59:1607-1614, 2014

Objective.—Although cilostazol is commonly used as an adjunct after peripheral vascular interventions, its efficacy remains uncertain. We assessed the effect of cilostazol on outcomes after peripheral vascular interventions using meta-analytic techniques.

Methods.—We searched MEDLINE (1946-2012), Cochrane CENTRAL (1996-2012), and trial registries for studies comparing cilostazol in combination with antiplatelet therapy to antiplatelet therapy alone after peripheral vascular interventions. Treatment effects were reported as pooled risk/hazard ratio (HR) with random-effects models.

Results.—Two randomized trials and four retrospective cohorts involving 1522 patients met inclusion criteria. Across studies, mean age ranged from 65 to 76 years, and the majority of patients were male (64%-83%); mean follow-up ranged from 18 to 37 months. Most interventions were in the femoropopliteal segment, and overall, 68% of patients had stents placed. Pooled estimates demonstrated that the addition of cilostazol was associated with decreased restenosis (relative risk [RR], 0.71; 95% confidence interval [CI], 0.60-0.84; $P < .001$), improved amputation-free survival (HR, 0.63; 95% CI, 0.47-0.85; $P = .002$), improved limb salvage (HR, 0.42; 95% CI, 0.27-0.66; $P < .001$), and improved freedom from target lesion revascularization (RR, 1.36; 95% CI, 1.14-1.61; $P < .001$). There was no significant reduction in mortality among those receiving cilostazol (RR, 0.73; 95% CI, 0.45-1.19; $P = .21$).

Conclusions.—The addition of cilostazol to antiplatelet therapy after peripheral vascular interventions is associated with a reduced risk of restenosis, amputation, and target lesion revascularization in our meta-analysis of six studies. Consideration of cilostazol as a medical adjunct after peripheral vascular interventions is warranted, presuming these findings are broadly generalizable (Fig 5, Table 1).

▶ This meta-analysis suggests beneficial pleiotropic effects associated with cilostazol use among patients treated with peripheral endovascular intervention on a variety of outcomes, including restenosis, amputation-free survival, limb salvage, and freedom from target lesion revascularization (Fig 5). Although cilostazol was evaluated as an adjunctive treatment used in combination with

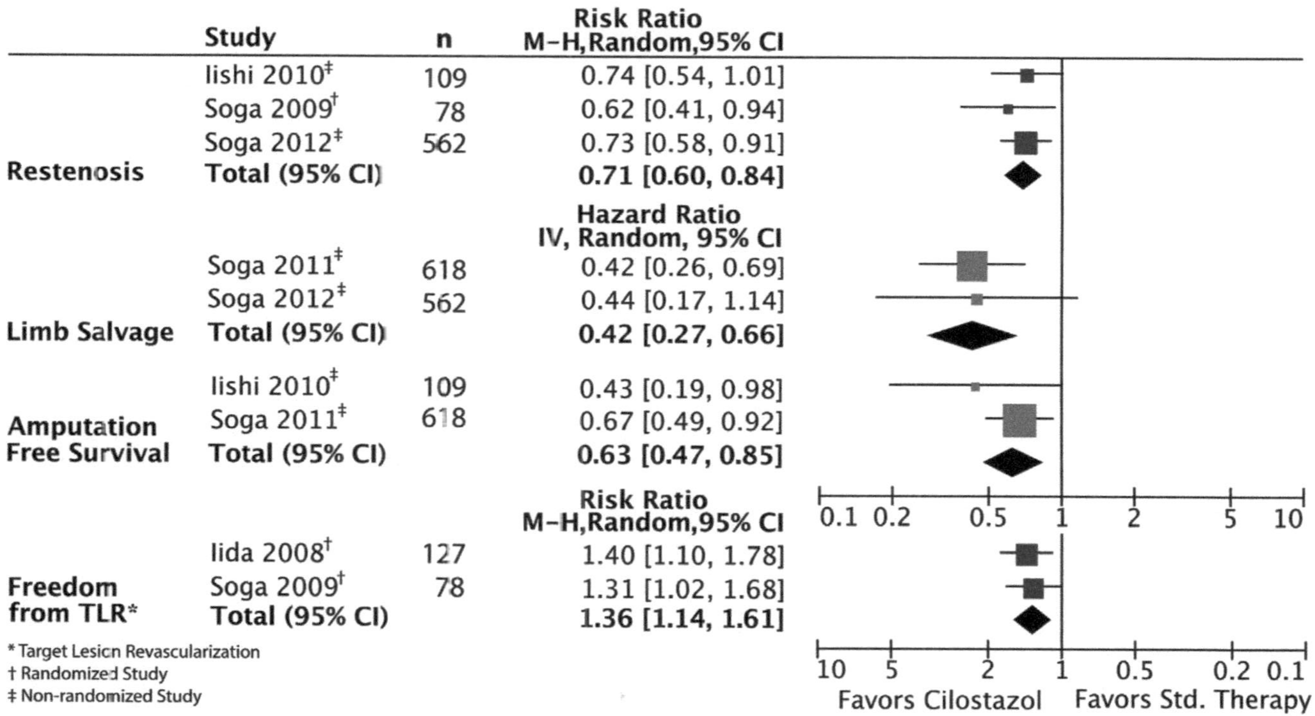

FIGURE 5.—Forest plot of main outcomes. *CI*, Confidence interval. (Reprinted from the Journal of Vascular Surgery. Warner CJ, Greaves SW, Larson RJ, et al. Cilostazol is associated with improved outcomes after peripheral endovascular interventions. *J Vasc Surg*. 2014;59:1607-1614, Copyright 2014, with permission from The Society for Vascular Surgery.)

TABLE 1.—Characteristics of Included Studies

Author	Year	Design	No.	Age, Years	Male, %	Indication, % CLI[a]	Lesion Location, % Femoropopliteal[b]	Intervention, % Stent[c]	Comparison[d]	Cointervention[d]	Mean Follow-up, Months
Soga	2011	Retrospective cohort	618	72 ± 11	69%	100%	35%	37%	No cilostazol	Aspirin, clopidogrel	21
Soga	2012	Retrospective cohort	562	73 ± 9	76%	26%	100%	100%	No cilostazol	Aspirin, clopidogrel	25
Ikushima	2011	Retrospective cohort	28	76 ± 7	82%	36%	100%	100%	Ticlopidine	Aspirin	18
Iishi	2010	Retrospective cohort	109	65 ± 11	64%	21%	100%	65%	No cilostazol	Aspirin	37
Soga	2009	RCT	78	71 ± 8	83%	0%	100%	46%	No cilostazol	Aspirin, ticlopidine	24
Iida	2008	RCT	127	70 ± 8	72%	25%	100%	87%	Ticlopidine	Aspirin	36

CLI, Critical limb ischemia; *RCT*, randomized controlled trial.
[a]Indications included critical limb ischemia vs claudication.
[b]Lesion locations include femoropopliteal and infrapopliteal.
[c]Interventions include stenting (with or without angioplasty) and angioplasty alone.
[d]Aspirin dose, 81-200 mg/day; ticlopidine dose, 200 mg/day; clopidogrel dose, 75 mg/day.

peripheral endovascular intervention for either intermittent claudication (IC) or critical limb ischemia (CLI) within this meta-analysis (Table 1), it is important to bear in mind that this medication can be used not only as an adjunct but as a stand-alone treatment for symptomatic management of IC. Given the relative safety of this medication and the growing body of clinical evidence supporting its benefits beyond IC symptoms, cilostazol pharmacotherapy should probably be considered for all patients with symptomatic peripheral arterial disease (PAD) without contraindications regardless of whether they have IC, CLI, or near-term plans for a revascularization procedure. Along those lines, it may be time to reconsider our approach to PAD treatment selection, particularly for IC. Although the clinical practice guidelines advise a hierarchical approach in which either exercise therapy or cilostazol is implemented initially and the next option is only tried if the first fails,[1] this algorithm potentially delays identification of satisfactory treatment(s) while prolonging morbidity. A more practical approach may be simultaneous (rather than staged) implementation of cilostazol with exercise therapy, with continuation of pharmacotherapy through procedural intervention if an inadequate symptomatic response is obtained.

The primary downside for widespread implementation of cilostazol therapy is cost. Patient adherence can also be an issue because of intolerance related to gastrointestinal or palpitation symptoms, which are relatively common, leading to real-world compliance that unfortunately is often lower than the 90% to 100% rates reported in 3 of the studies included in this analysis. Providers in the United States may also encounter opposition from insurance formulary regulators when prescribing cilostazol for CLI without claudication symptoms, as IC is the only indication for this medication approved by the US Food and Drug Administration. Current practice appears to have outpaced regulation, however, as indicated by the heterogeneity in rates of CLI as the treatment indication (0%–100%) among included studies (Table 1).

M. A. Corriere, MD, MS

Reference

1. Norgren L, Hiatt WR, Dormandy JA, Nehler MR, Harris KA, Fowkes FG. Inter-society consensus for the management of peripheral arterial disease (TASC II). *J Vasc Surg*. 2007;45:S5-S67.

Outcomes of covered versus bare-metal balloon-expandable stents for aortoiliac occlusive disease

Humphries MD, Armstrong E, Laird J, et al (Univ of California Davis Med Ctr, Sacramento; Univ of Colorado, Denver)
J Vasc Surg 60:337-343, 2014

Objective.—Randomized trials and retrospective data suggest that covered balloon-expandable (CBE) stents have better short-term patency compared with balloon-expandable bare-metal stents (BMSs) in the treatment of iliac artery disease. This study evaluated midterm outcomes of BMSs vs

CBE stents placed in the common iliac artery (CIA) for aortoiliac occlusive disease.

Methods.—All endovascular interventions for symptomatic peripheral arterial occlusive disease performed at a single institution from 2006 to 2012 were reviewed. Patients undergoing stent placement in the CIA segment were included in the analysis. Demographic data, TransAtlantic Inter-Society Consensus (TASC) classification, stent type, patency, and limb reinterventions were compared.

Results.—For treatment of de novo distal aorta or CIA stenosis, 254 procedures were performed in 162 patients. BMSs were used in 190 arteries; CBE stents were used in 64 arteries. There was no difference in age, gender, or TASC classification between the two groups. Mean follow-up was 22 ± 16 months. Primary patency, assisted patency, and secondary patency were significantly better in the BMS group. CIAs treated with covered stents were more likely at 1 year or longer to require repeated intervention (hazard ratio, 2.5; 95% confidence interval, 1.2-5.3; $P = .009$). TASC classification did not predict need for reintervention in either group. Multivariate analysis revealed dual antiplatelet therapy to be the only other factor to affect patency during long-term follow-up.

Conclusions.—In this study, BMSs had significantly better patency compared with CBE stents for treatment of aortoiliac occlusive disease. A randomized trial comparing patency as well as restenosis rates with long-term follow-up is needed to determine if there is any benefit from use of covered stents in the aortoiliac segment (Figs 1 and 2 and Table 1).

▶ The authors of this retrospective study tantalize the reader by stating that the selection of covered balloon-expandable (CBE) stents versus bare-metal stents (BMS) was performed on a case-by-case basis at the discretion of the treating physician without providing any insight into what considerations or criteria actually factored into the choice. A standardized approach consistent among the operators is certainly not implied, raising the possibility that selection bias (either generalized or provider-specific) might have contributed to some of the differences observed between groups. It is certainly plausible that lesion-specific factors might have affected stent selection in some situations. In the setting of circumferentially or densely calcified lesions, for example, CBE might be favored because of concerns about the potential for cracking and rupturing the arterial wall during balloon inflation. Alternatively, BMS might instead be favored when access is challenging due to comparatively smaller sheath diameters or for lesions in which tracking and deliverability are concerns (such as long-segment critical stenoses, where friction may have more of a tendency to dislodge a CBE from its balloon delivery system).

One might hypothesize that critical limb ischemia (CLI) patients would have iliac stent patency outcomes worse than claudicants due to relatively poor distal runoff. It is therefore interesting that the results demonstrated superior patency for BMS despite a higher rate of CLI as the procedure indication (34% vs 14% of CBE) (Figs 1 and 2). Another interesting contrast between the patient groups was related to the proportion of participants with acute limb ischemia as their

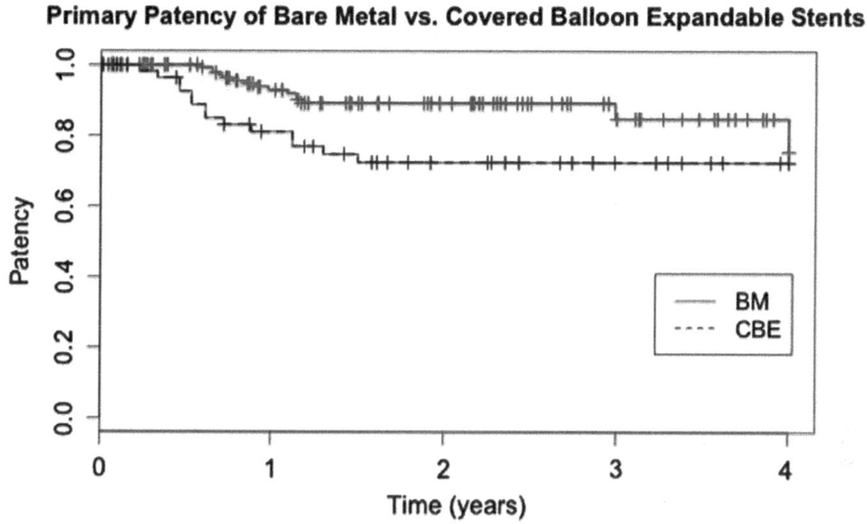

Bare Metal	190	96	65	37
Covered	64	29	19	10

FIGURE 1.—Primary patency of bare-metal (BM) stents (89% ± 3%) compared with covered balloon-expandable (CBE) stents (72% ± 6%) in the common iliac artery (CIA) ($P = .008$). (Reprinted from the Journal of Vascular Surgery. Humphries MD, Armstrong E, Laird J, et al. Outcomes of covered versus bare-metal balloon-expandable stents for aortoiliac occlusive disease. *J Vasc Surg.* 2014;60:337-343, Copyright 2014, with permission from The Society for Vascular Surgery.)

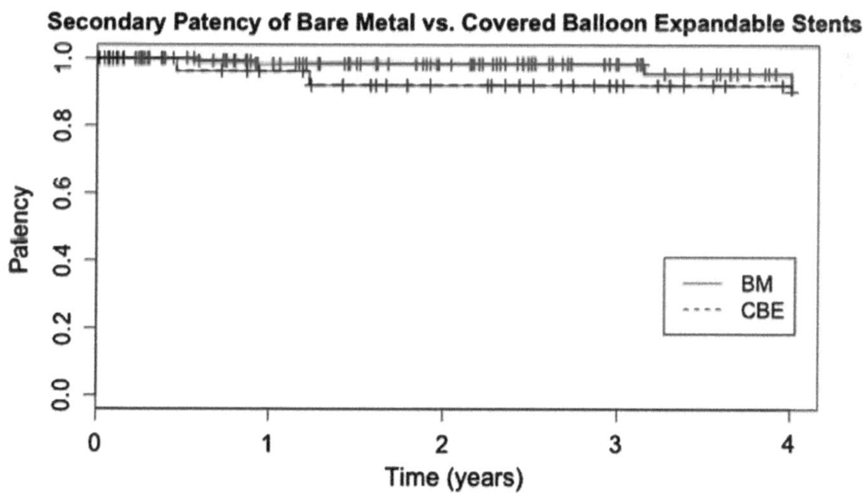

Bare Metal	190	104	68	38
Covered	64	34	23	10

FIGURE 2.—Secondary patency of bare-metal (BM) stents (98% ± 1% compared with covered balloon-expandable (CBE) stents (92% ± 3%) in the common iliac artery (CIA) by limb ($P = .03$). (Reprinted from the Journal of Vascular Surgery. Humphries MD, Armstrong E, Laird J, et al. Outcomes of covered versus bare-metal balloon-expandable stents for aortoiliac occlusive disease. *J Vasc Surg.* 2014;60:337-343, Copyright 2014, with permission from The Society for Vascular Surgery.)

TABLE 1.—Patient Demographic Characteristics by Stent Type

Variable	BMS (n = 125), No. (%)	CBE stent (n = 37), No. (%)	*P* Value
Mean age ± SD, years	65 ± 11	64 ± 11	.69
Male gender	58 (46)	19 (51)	.73
Hypertension	97 (77)	32 (86)	.34
Dyslipidemia	88 (70)	27 (73)	.92
Coronary artery disease	66 (53)	17 (46)	.56
Congestive heart failure	28 (22)	2 (5)	.04
End-stage renal disease	14 (11)	0	.07
Diabetes mellitus	50 (40)	9 (24)	.12
Stoke	25 (20)	7 (19)	1.00
Statin	86 (69)	22 (60)	.39
Smoking status			
Current	55 (44)	13 (35)	.44
Prior	57 (46)	20 (54)	.47
Never	13 (10)	4 (10)	1.00
Anticoagulation	11 (9)	1 (5)	.34
Antiplatelet therapy			
Aspirin	49 (39)	19 (51)	.26
Clopidogrel	6 (5)	2 (5)	1.00
Aspirin + clopidogrel	37 (30)	7 (19)	.28
None	33 (26)	9 (24)	.96
Clinical indication			
Claudication	72 (58)	27 (73)	.13
Critical limb ischemia	44 (35)	5 (14)	.02
Acute limb ischemia	4 (3)	4 (10)	.15

BMS, Bare-metal stent; *CBE*, covered balloon-expandable; *SD*, standard deviation.

procedural indication (3% for BMS vs 10% of CBE) (Table 1). Although this difference was not statistically significant, inferior outcomes associated with acute limb ischemia would be expected for a variety of reasons that would justify exclusion of this group of patients from a randomized trial comparing these treatments. As mentioned in the conclusion, additional randomized comparisons may be available in the near future that will hopefully allow evidence-based approaches to defining the circumstances, if any, where CBE may offer advantages over BMS for aortoiliac occlusive disease.

M. A. Corriere, MD, MS

Routine use of completion imaging after infrainguinal bypass is not associated with higher bypass graft patency

Tan T-W, on behalf of the Vascular Study Group of New England (Louisiana State Univ Health Shreveport, Shreveport, LA; Boston Univ Med Ctr, Boston, NH; et al)

J Vasc Surg 60:678-685.e2, 2014

Background.—Significant variability exists in completion imaging (CIM) after infrainguinal lower extremity bypass (LEB). We evaluated the use of CIM and compared graft patency in patients treated by surgeons who performed routine CIM vs those who performed selective CIM.

Methods.—We reviewed the Vascular Study Group of New England database (2003-2010) and assessed the use of CIM (angiography or duplex ultrasound) among patients undergoing LEB. The surgeon-specific CIM strategy was categorized as routine (≥80% of LEBs) vs selective (<80% of LEBs). Exclusion criteria included acute limb ischemia, bilateral procedures, and surgeon volume <10 cases per study period. Primary graft patency at discharge and at 1 year was analyzed on the basis of CIM use and surgeon-specific CIM strategy. Multivariable analyses were performed using Poisson regression.

Results.—Among 2032 LEB procedures performed by 48 surgeons, CIM was used in 1368 cases (67.3%). CIM was performed in 72% of autogenous LEBs and 52% of prosthetic grafts. Dialysis (odds ratio [OR], 1.7; 95% confidence interval [CI], 1.1-2.6; $P = .01$), elective LEB (OR, 2.6; 95% CI, 1.4-4.8; $P = .002$), great saphenous vein conduit (OR, 2.0; 95% CI, 1.6-2.5; $P < .001$), and tibial or pedal target artery (OR, 1.8; 95% CI, 1.4-2.3; $P < .001$) were associated with CIM use. In multivariate models, CIM was not associated with improved primary graft patency at discharge (OR, 1.1; 95% CI, 0.7-1.7; $P = .64$) or at 1 year (OR, 0.9; 95% CI, 0.7-1.2; $P = .47$). Sixteen surgeons (33%) were routine users and 32 (67%) were selective users of CIM. Among patients of routine vs selective CIM users, primary graft patency at discharge and at 1 year was 96% vs 94% ($P = .21$) and 68% vs 72% ($P = .09$), respectively. In multivariate analysis, routine or selective CIM strategy was not associated with improved discharge (rate ratio, 0.8; 95% CI, 0.6-1.1; $P = .31$) or 1-year (rate ratio, 1.1; 95% CI, 0.9-1.2; $P = .56$) graft patency.

Conclusions.—In our observational cohort, CIM does not improve short-term and 1-year bypass graft patency in infrainguinal LEB. The surgeon-specific strategy of selective CIM after LEB has outcomes comparable to those of routine CIM (Fig 2, Tables 1 and 2).

▶ Perioperative graft failure following lower extremity bypass is a challenging complication that often has negative impact on long-term outcomes, even when patency is reestablished. Apart from the clinical implications for the individual patient, rates of readmission and reoperation are the subject of increasing focus from quality and insurance organizations, sometimes with financial or other punitive consequences. Although it is unreasonable to expect that rates of perioperative graft thrombosis can be reduced to zero, providers performing leg bypass are under increasing scrutiny to produce results that minimize both clinical and financial jeopardy. Within this context, it is, therefore, easy to understand surgeons adopting an aggressive attitude toward completion imaging (CIM) to improve outcomes. Although CIM is perhaps inconvenient from a time and logistical perspective, it does provide the surgeon with either confirmation of a technically satisfactory result (and the peace of mind that accompanies this information) or an opportunity to resolve a technical issue

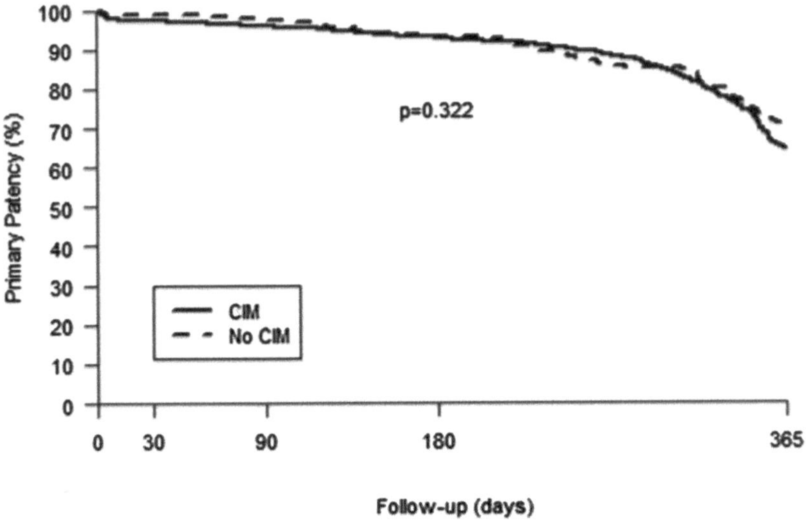

Sample					
CIM :	872	817	778	711	264
No CIM:	389	371	351	310	116

FIGURE 2.—Kaplan-Meier curves of primary bypass graft patency among patients treated with lower extremity bypass (LEB) performed with or without completion imaging (CIM). (Reprinted from the Journal of Vascular Surgery. Tan T-W, on behalf of the Vascular Study Group of New England. Routine use of completion imaging after infrainguinal bypass is not associated with higher bypass graft patency. *J Vasc Surg*. 2014;60:678-685, Copyright 2014, with permission from The Society for Vascular Surgery.)

without the need for a return to the operating room under more adverse circumstances.

When comparing outcomes from surgeons who use CIM following infrainguinal bypass routinely versus selectively (defined based on a cut-point of ≥80% among surgeons performing a minimum of 10 cases during the 7-year study period), this analysis observed no patency advantage associated with routine CIM. Several interesting contrasts between the patients who had CIM versus those who did not are evident and perhaps provide insight into the rationale behind the decision making. Patients who underwent CIM had higher rates of rest pain, tissue loss, and distal (tibial or pedal) versus popliteal graft recipient vessels (Table 1). These variables were associated with graft patency (Table 2), although routine use of CIM was not (Fig 2). Providers performing a greater proportion of their bypasses with saphenous or arm vein and using distal targets more frequently also might be more inclined to push the envelope with borderline vein conduit (although vein diameter was not included as covariate in this study), which might further predispose them toward routine CIM in these relatively extenuating circumstances. Routine CIM, therefore, may have a confounding relationship with many factors associated with increased risk for loss of patency, potentially justifying the desire for increased sensitivity in detecting technical problems when several adverse factors exist despite lack of

TABLE 1.—Demographic, Patient, and Operative Characteristics of Patients Who Did and Did Not Undergo Completion Imaging (*CIM*) During Lower Extremity Bypass (LEB)

Characteristic	Overall (N = 2032)	CIM (n = 1368)	No CIM (n = 664)	*P* value
Demographic				
Age, years	68.2 ± 11.9	68.5 ± 12	67.5 ± 11.8	.08
Male gender	1386 (68.2)	936 (68.4)	450 (67.8)	.80
White race	1999 (99.1)	1347 (99.3)	652 (98.6)	.13
Smoking				
Never	378 (18.6)	264 (19.3)	114 (17.2)	.02
Prior	890 (43.9)	619 (45.3)	271 (40.9)	
Current	761 (37.5)	483 (35.4)	278 (41.9)	
Medical comorbidity				
Hypertension	1748 (86)	1186 (86.7)	562 (84.6)	.22
Diabetes mellitus	1064 (52.4)	742 (54.2)	322 (48.5)	.02
Coronary artery disease	768 (37.8)	527 (38.5)	241 (36.4)	.38
Congestive heart failure	331 (16.3)	214 (15.6)	117 (17.6)	.28
Chronic pulmonary disease	525 (25.9)	349 (25.5)	176 (26.5)	.63
ESRD	157 (7.7)	121 (8.8)	36 (5.4)	.01
Aspirin	1436 (70.7)	961 (70.2)	475 (71.5)	.57
Clopidogrel	171 (8.4)	114 (8.3)	57 (8.6)	.87
Statin	1251 (61.6)	831 (60.8)	420 (63.3)	.28
Previous bypass	657 (32.3)	445 (32.5)	212 (31.9)	.80
Creatinine, mg/dL	1.5 ± 1.5	1.5 ± 1.6	1.5 ± 1.3	.28
Procedure detail				
Indication				
Claudication	544 (26.8)	340 (24.9)	204 (30.7)	.001
Rest pain	515 (25.3)	336 (24.6)	179 (27)	
Tissue loss	973 (47.9)	692 (50.6)	281 (42.3)	
Urgency				
Elective	1673 (82.3)	1150 (84.1)	523 (78.8)	.002
Urgent	345 (17)	213 (15.6)	132 (19.9)	
Emergent	14 (0.7)	5 (0.4)	9 (1.4)	
Anesthesia				
Spinal	330 (16.2)	231 (16.9)	99 (14.9)	.49
Epidural	138 (6.8)	90 (6.6)	48 (7.2)	
General	1563 (77)	1047 (76.5)	516 (77.8)	
Graft origin				
CFA, profunda, or SFA	1767 (88.8)	1209 (89.6)	558 (87.2)	.11
Above- and below-knee PA	222 (11.2)	140 (10.4)	82 (12.8)	
Graft recipient				
Above- and below-knee PA	1132 (55.8)	688 (50.3)	444 (67.1)	<.001
Tibioperoneal trunk, tibial or pedal artery	898 (44.2)	680 (49.7)	218 (32.9)	
Conduit type				
GSV	1364 (67.1)	979 (71.6)	385 (58)	<.001
Single segment	1329 (65.4)	950 (69.4)	379 (57.2)	
Multiple segments	34 (1.7)	29 (2.1)	5 (0.8)	
Arm vein	161 (7.9)	125 (9.1)	36 (5.4)	
Prosthetic	507 (25)	264 (19.3)	243 (36.6)	<.001

CFA, Common femoral artery; *ESRD*, end-stage renal disease; *GSV*, great saphenous vein; *PA*, popliteal artery; *SD*, standard deviation; *SFA*, superficial femoral artery.

Continuous data are presented as mean ± standard deviation and categorical data as number (%).

TABLE 2.—Multivariable Analysis of the Association Between Completion Imaging (CIM) and Primary Bypass Graft Patency During Lower Extremity Bypass (LEB)

	Adjusted Estimate[a]	95% Lower Confidence Limit	95% Upper Confidence Limit	P Value
Discharge patency				
CIM	1.11	0.72	1.70	.64
Age	1.01	0.99	1.03	.17
Hypertension	1.59	0.95	2.66	.08
Indication for surgery: claudication vs critical limb ischemia	1.54	0.89	2.66	.12
Graft recipient: popliteal vs tibial or pedal artery	2.86	1.79	4.53	<.001
Conduit type				
GSV vs prosthetic	1.43	0.86	2.38	.17
Arm vein vs prosthetic	0.83	0.41	1.69	.61
Autologous vs prosthetic	1.09	0.64	1.88	.75
One-year patency				
CIM	0.90	.68	1.20	.47
Age	1.01	1.0	1.02	.06
Indication for surgery: claudication vs critical limb ischemia	1.52	1.11	2.07	.01
Graft recipient: popliteal vs tibial or pedal artery	2.12	1.59	2.81	<.001
Conduit type				
GSV vs prosthetic	1.21	0.88	1.66	.24
Arm vein vs prosthetic	0.78	0.48	1.31	.36
Autologous vs prosthetic	0.98	0.68	1.40	.90
Patency loss hazard				
CIM	0.97	0.74	1.28	.83
Hypertension	0.72	0.52	1.01	.06
Graft recipient: popliteal vs tibial or pedal artery	0.48	0.36	0.64	<.001
Conduit type				
GSV vs prosthetic	0.69	0.51	0.94	.02
Arm vein vs prosthetic	0.97	0.62	1.52	.89
Autologous vs prosthetic	0.82	0.58	1.15	.24

AOR, Adjusted odds ratio; *GSV*, great saphenous vein; *HR*, hazard ratio.
[a]AOR for initial patency and 1-year patency and adjusted HR for patency loss.
Reprinted from the Journal of Vascular Surgery. Tan T-W, on behalf of the Vascular Study Group of New England. Routine use of completion imaging after infrainguinal bypass is not associated with higher bypass graft patency. *J Vasc Surg.* 2014;60:678-685, Copyright 2014, with permission from The Society for Vascular Surgery.

independent association with patency. The take-home message, therefore, may be that although indication, graft conduit, and bypass anatomic configuration affect patency, these associations aren't necessarily attributable to technical problems that left the operating room unrecognized and uncorrected.

It would be interesting to know whether the surgeons using routine CIM who participated in this study would be willing to change this practice based on the results. A consideration relevant to the utility of routine CIM that was not reported was the percentage of studies with findings that led to a bypass revision prior to leaving the operating room. If this occurred with significant frequency, one might assume that outcomes might suffer if routine CIM were abandoned. Given that CIM adds little risk or morbidity to the procedure, it would not be surprising to discover that some surgeons prioritize the peace of mind generated by a negative completion study over the time and logistical issues associated with obtaining one.

M. A. Corriere, MD, MS

Endovascular treatment of lesions in the below-knee popliteal artery

Siracuse JJ, Gill HL, Cassidy SP, et al (Columbia Univ, NY)
J Vasc Surg 60:356-361, 2014

Background.—Endovascular interventions are increasing; however, there are little data regarding outcomes of complex interventions involving the below-knee popliteal/P3 artery. This study evaluated the short-term and long-term results and predictors of success of below-knee popliteal artery endovascular interventions.

Methods.—This was a retrospective review of a prospectively maintained endovascular lower extremity database of all patients with below-knee popliteal interventions from 2004 to 2012. Patient demographics, angiographic findings, interventions, primary and secondary patency, limb loss, and mortality were recorded. Analysis was performed using Kaplan-Meier life-table and multivariate analysis, with $P < .05$ indicating significance.

Results.—There were 221 patients (56% male) with below-knee popliteal/P3 artery lesions. Mean age was 73 ± 11.2 years. Claudication was present in 22% and critical limb ischemia (CLI) in 78%. Mean lesion length was 10 ± 8.5 cm, with 45% having total occlusions. Treatment included percutaneous transluminal angioplasty (PTA) with or without a stent (47%), atherectomy (ATH) with or without PTA/stent (52%), and stenting with PTA and ATH (3%). Complications included embolization (0.4%), hematoma (2.7%), pseudoaneurysm (1.3%), and dissection (7%). Freedom from restenosis (peak systolic velocity ratio >2.4) was 65% at 1 year. Independent predictors of restenosis were CLI (hazard risk [HR], 4.4; 95% confidence interval [CI], 1.9-9.9) and stenting combined with PTA and ATH (HR, 2.7; 95% CI, 1.01-7.4). Primary assisted and secondary patencies were 95% and 85% at 1 year. ATH with PTA had lower short-term restenosis in diabetic patients compared with nondiabetic patients (95% vs 78% at 4 months). Limb loss was 18% at 4 years. Mortality was 24% at 4 years. Statin use was protective against primary restenosis (HR, 0.39; 95% CI, 0.23-0.67) and death (HR, 0.5; 95% CI, 0.28-1.0).

Conclusions.—Endovascular intervention for lesions involving the below-knee popliteal artery is a safe and effective therapy for claudication and CLI. Diabetic patients benefit most from ATH with PTA. Statin use is protective against restenosis and mortality and should be the standard of care in patients undergoing peripheral endovascular interventions (Tables 1-3).

▶ The title of this article is somewhat misleading, as only 9% of lesions involved only the below-knee popliteal artery, whereas 78% of patients underwent treatment of multiple levels (including the femoral or tibial vessels; Table 2). The below-knee popliteal artery, therefore, was often included within the treated arterial segment but seldom defined it completely. Three different treatments (atherectomy, percutaneous transluminal angioplasty, and stenting) were used either alone or in combination in this study, and use of all 3 treatments within the same procedure was associated with increased risk of restenosis (Table 3). It is unclear whether patients with all 3 of these techniques had this approach used by design or instead out of necessity in the setting of technically poor results from the interventions that were performed first. If the latter explanation is correct, the increased risk of restenosis associated with the use of all 3 interventions in combination would certainly be expected.

Critical limb ischemia was also associated with restenosis in the multivariable model; this diagnosis was prevalent among 78% of patients in this cohort (with tissue loss being more common than rest pain), whereas 22% had intermittent claudication (Table 1). Because intermittent claudication and critical limb ischemia have natural histories distinguished by differences in amputation-free and overall survival, interpretation of these outcomes is challenging when the results are not stratified by diagnosis. Because claudicants whose interventions fail may not progress to critical limb ischemia, their inclusion in analyses of limb salvage (or, conversely, amputation-free survival) has

TABLE 1.—Demographic and Comorbidities

Variables	Mean ± SD or No. (%)
Demographics	
Age, years	73 ± 11.2
Males	124 (56)
Comorbidities	
Claudication	48 (22)
Rest pain	17 (37)
Tissue Loss	136 (61)
Diabetes	151 (68)
Coronary artery disease	131 (59)
Congestive heart failure	57 (26)
CRI	79 (36)
End-stage renal disease	38 (17)
Hypertension	190 (86)
Tobacco history	107 (48)
Obesity	33 (15)
COPD	25 (11)
Previous intervention	108 (49)
Previous bypass	10 (5)

COPD, Chronic obstructive pulmonary disease; CRI, chronic renal insufficiency; SD, standard deviation.

Reprinted from the Journal of Vascular Surgery. Siracuse JJ, Gill HL, Cassidy SP, et al. Endovascular treatment of lesions in the below-knee popliteal artery. *J Vasc Surg*. 2014;60:356-361, Copyright 2014, with permission from The Society for Vascular Surgery.

TABLE 2.—Lesion and Intervention Details

Variables	No. (%)
TASC	
A	20 (9)
B	75 (34)
C	76 (34)
D	50 (23)
Artery treated	
Femoral	108 (49)
Above-knee popliteal	102 (46)
Retrogeniculate popliteal	129 (58)
Tibial	129 (58)
Multiple levels treated	172 (78)
Below-knee popliteal artery	
PTA	95 (43)
PTA+stent	9 (4)
ATH	48 (22)
ATH+PTA	38 (17)
ATH+stent	24 (11)
ATH+PTA+stent	7 (3)
Complications	
Contrast-induced nephropathy	0 (0)
Embolization	1 (0.4)
Pseudoaneurysm	3 (1.4)
Hematoma	6 (3)
Dissection	16 (7)

ATH, Atherectomy; *PTA*, percutaneous transluminal angioplasty; *TASC*, TransAtlantic Inter-Society Consensus.

Reprinted from the Journal of Vascular Surgery. Siracuse JJ, Gill HL, Cassidy SP, et al. Endovascular treatment of lesions in the below-knee popliteal artery. *J Vasc Surg*. 2014;60:356-361, Copyright 2014, with permission from The Society for Vascular Surgery.

TABLE 3.—Multivariate Predictors of Primary Restenosis of the Below-Knee Popliteal Artery

Covariate	HR (95% CI)	*P*
CLI	4.4 (1.9-9.9)	<.001
ATH+PTA+stent	2.7 (1.01-7.4)	<.001
Statin use	0.39 (0.23-0.67)	<.001

ATH, Atherectomy; *CI*, confidence interval; *CLI*, critical limb ischemia; *HR*, hazard risk; *PTA*, percutaneous transluminal angioplasty.

Reprinted from the Journal of Vascular Surgery. Siracuse JJ, Gill HL, Cassidy SP, et al. Endovascular treatment of lesions in the below-knee popliteal artery. *J Vasc Surg*. 2014;60:356-361, Copyright 2014, with permission from The Society for Vascular Surgery.

significant potential to impact results. The reported outcomes, therefore, should be interpreted with this limitation in mind. It is also conceivable that differences in anatomic disease severity (including both inflow disease and patent runoff vessels) between participants with claudication versus critical limb ischemia may have affected patency results.

Although the authors concluded that many patients with femoropopliteal occlusive disease "are high surgical risk and can benefit from a minimally invasive approach," it is important to note that no surgical group was provided as a control. Without a direct comparison, these results, therefore, do not show an implicit advantage (or disadvantage) versus surgical therapy. Some patients (5%) in this cohort actually had a previous bypass procedure (Table 1), however, showing that less-invasive approaches occasionally provide options for patients whose surgical options may have been exhausted or whose risk for repeat surgical intervention is prohibitive.

M. A. Corriere, MD, MS

Determinants of invasive treatment in lower extremity peripheral arterial disease

van Zitteren M, Vriens PW, Burger DH, et al (Tilburg Univ, Kansas City, MO; St. Elisabeth Hosp, Kansas City, MO)

J Vasc Surg 59:400-408.e2, 2014

Objective.—Since it is unknown what factors are weighed in a clinician's decision to refer patients with symptomatic lower extremity peripheral arterial disease (PAD) for invasive treatment, we examined the relationship between health status, lesion location, and site variations and invasive treatment referral ≤1 year following diagnosis in patients with PAD.

Methods.—This was a prospective observational cohort study on ambulatory patients that presented themselves at two vascular surgery outpatient clinics. A total of 970 patients with new symptoms of PAD or with an exacerbation of existing PAD symptoms that required clinical evaluation and treatment (Rutherford Grade I) were eligible, 884 consented and were included between March 2006 and November 2010. We report on 505 patients in the current study. Prior to patients' initial PAD evaluation, the Short Form-12, Physical Component Scale (PCS) was administered to measure health status. Anatomical lesion location (proximal vs distal) was derived from duplex ultrasounds. PCS scores, lesion location, and site were evaluated as determinants of receiving invasive (endovascular, surgery) vs noninvasive treatment ≤1 year following diagnosis in Poisson regression analyses, adjusting for demographics, ankle-brachial index, and risk factors.

Results.—Invasive treatment as a first-choice was offered to 167 (33%) patients. While an association between poorer health status and invasive therapy was found in unadjusted analyses (relative risk [RR], 0.98; 95% confidence interval [CI], 0.97-1.00; $P = .011$), proximal lesion location (RR, 3.66; 95% CI, 2.70-4.96; $P < .0001$) and site (RR, 1.69; 95% CI, 1.11-2.58; $P = .014$) were independent predictors of invasive treatment referral in the final model.

Conclusions.—One-third of patients were treated invasively following PAD diagnosis. Patients' health status was considered in providers' decision to refer patients for invasive treatment, but having a proximal lesion was the strongest predictor. This study also found some important first indications of site variations in offering invasive treatment among patients with PAD. Future work is needed to further document these variations in care (Table 1).

▶ This study from the Netherlands engages an important issue that some providers may find uncomfortable discussing: provider biases affecting treatment selection for peripheral arterial disease (PAD). In addition to the presence of a proximal (aortoiliac) lesion, the authors identified the clinic site as a factor predicting selection of an invasive versus noninvasive initial treatment option. These results imply that the process of treatment selection is not solely guided by clinical guidelines and patient-specific factors in a "sterile" environment, and that provider biases (some of which may be unrelated to either evidence or patient welfare) may drive choices. These findings might prompt negative publication bias because of their sensitive nature, and the authors are to be commended for sharing the results. Treatment selection heterogeneity resulting from provider bias and potential secondary gain has been brought to public attention for coronary artery disease care and, more recently, has entered the public consciousness for PAD through media coverage of regulatory audits by insurance providers (including Medicare) targeting inexplicably aggressive peripheral interventionalists.

The participant cohort for this study was identified based on patients who presented themselves to 2 outpatient vascular surgery clinics with new onset or exacerbation of PAD symptoms. Self-referral to a specialist is not a route that all patients with PAD take to arrive at their first treatment choice, however, particularly in health care environments where initial evaluation by a primary care provider may be required and direct self-referral to specialists may not be allowed. Given that one-third of the participants in this study were managed with invasive treatment as the first choice despite mild (Rutherford class I) symptoms, a 50% smoking prevalence (Table 1), and availability of a supervised exercise program (a luxury that is not accessible to many patients); however, it may be that placing a gatekeeper between interventionalists and patients is sometimes for the best. Although a recent randomized trial demonstrated that an aggressive approach toward revascularization has potential advantages for patients with intermittent claudication (IC),[1] it is important to bear in mind that PAD is a chronic disease in which failure of an intervention may be accompanied by progression of symptom severity. A long-term perspective is therefore appropriate, and patients may benefit in the long run if the provider considering a choice between options a, b, and c is also thinking about how early choices will potentially affect long-term amputation-free survival and options x, y, and z. Several studies have demonstrated that failed endovascular procedures can have significant negative impact on the outcomes of subsequent interventions.[2-5] For patients who are amputation-free, the so-called final treatment (a term the authors used to define the last treatment used during the 1-year study period) always looms in the future, a consideration that may not be central to the decision-making process for some providers who do not continue to manage patients toward the "end of the line" when endovascular options have been exhausted.

TABLE 1.—Baseline Characteristics of the Total Sample and Stratified by First-Choice Treatment Strategy

	Total Sample (N = 505)	First-Choice Treatment Strategy Invasive (n = 167)	Noninvasive (n = 338)	P Value
Demographics				
Mean age (range), years	64.7 ± 9.7 (37-92)	**62.6 ± 9.8**	**65.8 ± 9.5**	**<.0001**
Male gender	324 (64.2)	105 (62.9)	219 (64.8)	.67
Socioeconomic factors				
No partner	123 (24.5)	35 (21.2)	88 (26.0)	.24
Less than high school education	127 (25.5)	46 (28.0)	81 (24.2)	.35
Working full- or part-time	135 (27.6)	**54 (33.3)**	**81 (24.8)**	.046
Cardiovascular history				
Angina pectoris	69 (13.7)	17 (10.2)	52 (15.4)	.11
Myocardial infarction	85 (16.8)	23 (13.8)	62 (18.3)	.20
Coronary artery bypass graft surgery	60 (11.9)	15 (9.0)	45 (13.3)	.16
Percutaneous coronary intervention	45 (8.9)	12 (7.2)	33 (9.8)	.34
Congestive heart failure	20 (4.0)	3 (1.8)	17 (5.0)	.08
Stroke	38 (7.5)	14 (8.4)	24 (7.1)	.61
Transient ischemic attack	43 (8.5)	10 (6.0)	33 (9.8)	.15
Clinical factors				
Smoking	250 (49.5)	93 (55.7)	157 (46.4)	.05[b]
Diabetes mellitus	121 (24.0)	38 (22.8)	83 (24.6)	.66
Hypercholesterolemia	342 (67.7)	111 (66.5)	231 (68.3)	.67
Hypertension	308 (61.0)	95 (56.9)	213 (63.0)	.18
Mean BMI	26.7 ± 4.6	**25.9 ± 3.6**	**27.1 ± 5.0**	**.001**
Chronic obstructive pulmonary disease	79 (15.6)	23 (13.8)	56 (16.6)	.42
Renal dysfunction	38 (7.5)	10 (6.0)	28 (8.3)	.36
Back pain	75 (14.9)	31 (18.6)	44 (13.0)	.10
Hip or knee pain	105 (20.8)	39 (23.4)	66 (19.5)	.32
Medication use				
Overall anticoagulants	447 (88.5)	**138 (82.6)**	**309 (91.4)**	**.004**
Aspirin	406 (80.4)	**124 (74.3)**	**282 (83.4)**	**.014**
Anticoagulants	82 (16.2)	28 (16.8)	54 (16.0)	.82
Statins	416 (82.4)	130 (77.8)	286 (84.6)	.06
Beta blocker	210 (41.6)	60 (35.9)	150 (44.4)	.07
Diuretics	116 (23.0)	32 (19.2)	84 (24.9)	.15
ACE inhibitor	159 (31.5)	54 (32.3)	105 (31.1)	.77
Calcium antagonist	106 (21.0)	29 (17.4)	77 (22.8)	.16
Nitroglycerine	44 (8.7)	9 (5.4)	35 (10.4)	.06
Digoxin	9 (1.8)	2 (1.2)	7 (2.1)	.49
Antiarrhythmics	15 (3.0)	5 (3.0)	10 (3.0)	.98
Antidepressives	29 (5.7)	13 (7.8)	16 (4.7)	.17
Anxiolytics	20 (4.0)	3 (1.8)	17 (5.0)	.08
Hypnotics	27 (5.3)	10 (6.0)	17 (5.0)	.65
Vascular laboratory assessment				
Median pain-free walking distance, m	80.0 ± 128.9	70.0 ± 131.3	80.0 ± 127.6	.14
Mean resting ABI[a]	0.66 ± 0.17	**0.63 ± 0.17**	**0.67 ± 0.16**	**.011**
Prior lower extremity revascularization				
Endovascular	54 (10.7)	24 (14.4)	30 (8.9)	.06
Endarterectomy	9 (1.8)	1 (0.6)	8 (2.4)	.16
Psychological factors				
Depression	143 (28.5)	47 (28.3)	96 (28.7)	.94
Anxiety	126 (25.1)	45 (27.1)	81 (24.2)	.48
Type D personality	111 (22.1)	42 (25.1)	69 (20.5)	.24

ABI, Ankle-brachial index; *ACE*, angiotensin-converting-enzyme; *BMI*, body mass index; *SD*, standard deviation.

Boldface entries indicate statistical significance. Continuous data are shown as mean or median ± standard deviation and categoric data as number (%).

[a]Lowest ABI measured.

[b]Not significant.

Treatment selection for PAD is a complex decision process in which some treatment options (like revascularization) are relatively passive, and others (like exercise therapy) require more buy-in and active participation from the patient, which sometimes can be challenging to assess. Patients may be unable to participate in exercise therapy due to inflow disease or comorbidities or may reject it based on their own expectations and values. To make matters more complicated, patients unlikely to adhere to an exercise plan that may not disclose this to their provider at the time of treatment selection due to a desire to avoid what they perceive as a negative response to a recommended treatment. Patients may therefore leave the clinic with a treatment plan that is unlikely to succeed and end up either returning for a follow-up appointment unimproved (and frustrated by wasted time) to consider the next option or instead seeking treatment elsewhere. On the other end of the spectrum, as demonstrated in this study, patients may also encounter providers with aggressive attitudes toward revascularization leading to potential overtreatment of some patients who would have responded to exercise and/or pharmacotherapy if given the chance. The "best" approach, if one exists, is likely a middle ground where both patient and provider contribute to treatment selection. Emerging evidence suggests that patients are interested in contributing to PAD treatment selection,[6] but providers need to identify efficient ways to get them involved and must be willing to embrace their input.

M. A. Corriere, MD, MS

References

1. Nordanstig J, Taft C, Hensäter M, Perlander A, Osterberg K, Jivegård L. Improved quality of life after 1 year with an invasive versus a noninvasive treatment strategy in claudicants: one-year results of the Invasive Revascularization or Not in Intermittent Claudication (IRONIC) Trial. *Circulation.* 2014;130:939-947.
2. Bradbury AW, Adam DJ, Bell J, et al. Bypass versus Angioplasty in Severe Ischaemia of the Leg (BASIL) trial: analysis of amputation free and overall survival by treatment received. *J Vasc Surg.* 2010;51:18S-31S.
3. Blaurock P, Mansmann U, Schwarzbach M, et al. Early surgical outcome after failed primary stenting for lower limb occlusive disease. *J Endovasc Ther.* 2005; 12:13-21.
4. Joels CS, York JW, Kalbaugh CA, Cull DL, Langan EM 3rd, Taylor SM. Surgical implications of early failed endovascular intervention of the superficial femoral artery. *J Vasc Surg.* 2008;47:562-565.
5. Nolan BW, De Martino RR, Stone DH, et al. Prior failed ipsilateral percutaneous endovascular intervention in patients with critical limb ischemia predicts poor outcome after lower extremity bypass. *J Vasc Surg.* 2011;54:730-735.
6. Corriere MA, Avise JA, Peterson LA, et al. Exploring patient involvement in decision making for vascular procedures. *J Vasc Surg.* 2015; http://dx.doi.org/10.1016/j.jvs.2015.04.443.

Percutaneous transluminal angioplasty versus primary stenting in infrapopliteal arterial disease: A meta-analysis of randomized trials

Wu R, Yao C, Wang S, et al (The First Affiliated Hosp of Sun Yat-sen Univ, Guangzhou, China)
J Vasc Surg 59:1711-1720, 2014

Background.—Percutaneous transluminal angioplasty (PTA) and primary stenting are commonly used endovascular therapeutic procedures for the treatment of infrapopliteal arterial occlusive disease. However, which procedure is more beneficial for patients with infrapopliteal arterial occlusive disease is unknown.

Methods and Results.—We performed a meta-analysis, searching PubMed, EMBASE, the Cochrane Central Register of Controlled Trials, ISI Web of Knowledge, and relevant websites without language or publication date restrictions for randomized trials that compared primary stenting with PTA in patients with infrapopliteal arterial occlusive disease. The keywords were "stents," "angioplasty," "infrapopliteal," "tibial arteries," and "below knee." We selected immediate technical success, primary and secondary patency, limb salvage, and patient survival as the outcomes of this meta-analysis. On the basis of the inclusion criteria, we identified six prospective randomized trials. One-year outcomes did not show any significant differences between the PTA and primary stenting groups, respectively: technical success (93.3% vs 96.2%; odds ratio [OR], 0.59; 95% confidence interval [CI], 0.24-1.47; P=.25), primary patency (57.1% vs 65.7%; OR, 0.95; 95% CI, 0.35-2.58; P=.92), secondary patency (73.5% vs 57.6%; OR, 2.08; 95% CI, 0.81-5.34; P=.13), limb salvage (82.2% vs 87.5%; OR, 0.64; 95% CI, 0.29-1.41; P=.27), and patient survival (84.0% vs 87.5%; OR, 0.79; 95% CI, 0.40-1.55; P=.49).

Conclusions.—For infrapopliteal arterial occlusive disease, primary stenting has the same 1-year benefits as PTA. There is insufficient evidence to support the superiority of either method. Primary stenting is associated with a trend toward higher primary patency and lower secondary patency. Further large-scale prospective randomized trials should produce more reliable results (Figs 3 and 5; Table 2).

▶ Comparing the results between clinical studies evaluating lower extremity revascularization is often problematic due to heterogeneity of inclusion/exclusion criteria, medical management, primary outcomes, and duration of follow-up. This meta-analysis includes 6 randomized controlled trials that included a combined total of 548 participants with critical limb ischemia (rest pain and/or tissue loss); although not incorporated into the analytic approach by design, this factor greatly facilitates interpretation of the results by avoiding inclusion of claudicants, whose distinct disease severity and anticipated amputation-free survival would potentially confound the results. Table 2 provides some insight into the challenges of comparing studies and then attempting to extrapolate a conclusion reflected by the results when considered in combination, even when limiting studies to randomized controlled trials

A

Study or Subgroup	PTA Events	PTA Total	Stent Events	Stent Total	Weight	Odds Ratio M-H, Fixed, 95% CI	Year
Rand 2006	12	20	14	17	33.9%	0.32 [0.07, 1.49]	2006
Bosiers 2009	35	40	30	37	21.8%	1.63 [0.47, 5.68]	2009
Randon 2010	17	22	13	16	19.1%	0.78 [0.16, 3.90]	2010
Rand 2011	16	27	9	17	25.2%	1.29 [0.38, 4.39]	2011
Total (95% CI)		**109**		**87**	**100.0%**	**0.94 [0.48, 1.83]**	
Total events	80		66				

Heterogeneity: Chi² = 2.94, df = 3 (P = 0.40); I² = 0%
Test for overall effect: Z = 0.18 (P = 0.86)

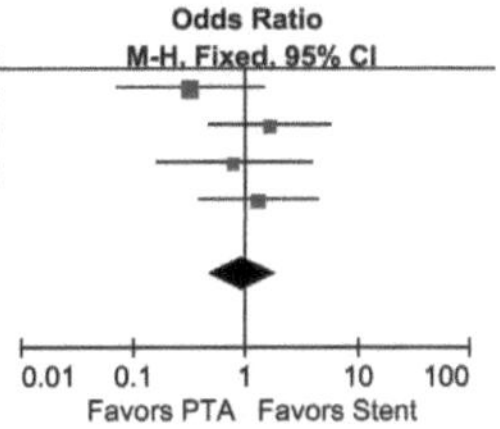

B

Study or Subgroup	PTA Events	PTA Total	Stent Events	Stent Total	Weight	Odds Ratio M-H, Fixed, 95% CI	Year
Randon 2010	17	22	13	16	11.0%	0.78 [0.16, 3.90]	2010
Brodmann 2011	13	27	6	17	12.3%	1.70 [0.49, 5.93]	2011
Scheinert 2012	44	77	54	72	76.8%	0.44 [0.22, 0.89]	2012
Total (95% CI)		**126**		**105**	**100.0%**	**0.64 [0.36, 1.11]**	
Total events	74		73				

Heterogeneity: Chi² = 3.46, df = 2 (P = 0.18); I² = 42%
Test for overall effect: Z = 1.59 (P = 0.11)

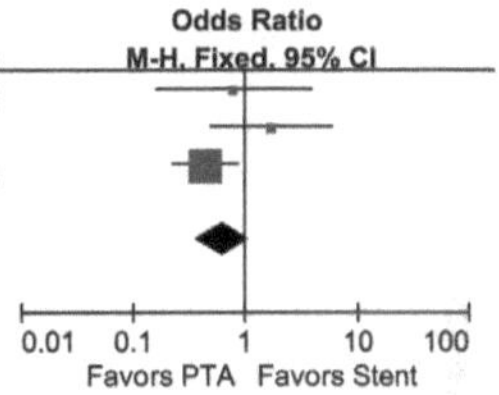

FIGURE 3.—Forest plots of the estimated individual and overall effect of the primary patency between percutaneous transluminal angioplasty (*PTA*) and primary stenting groups at 6 months (**A**) and 12 months (**B**). *CI*, Confidence interval; *M-H*, Mantel-Haenszel. (Reprinted from the Journal of Vascular Surgery. Wu R, Yao C, Wang S, et al. Percutaneous transluminal angioplasty versus primary stenting in infrapopliteal arterial disease: a meta-analysis of randomized trials. *J Vasc Surg*. 2014;59:1711-1720, Copyright 2014, with permission from The Society for Vascular Surgery.)

A

Study or Subgroup	PTA Events	PTA Total	Stent Events	Stent Total	Weight	Odds Ratio M-H, Fixed, 95% CI	Year
Rand 2006	20	21	17	19	14.0%	2.35 [0.20, 28.27]	2006
Bosiers 2009	53	57	53	60	59.9%	1.75 [0.48, 6.33]	2009
Randon 2010	20	22	15	16	26.1%	0.67 [0.06, 8.06]	2010
Total (95% CI)		**100**		**95**	**100.0%**	**1.55 [0.56, 4.29]**	
Total events	93		85				

Heterogeneity: Chi² = 0.58, df = 2 (P = 0.75); I² = 0%
Test for overall effect: Z = 0.85 (P = 0.40)

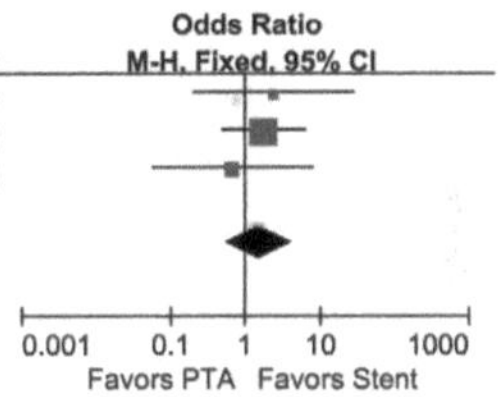

B

Study or Subgroup	PTA Events	PTA Total	Stent Events	Stent Total	Weight	Odds Ratio M-H, Fixed, 95% CI
Randon 2010	20	22	15	16	10.0%	0.67 [0.06, 0.00]
Scheinert 2012	68	85	69	80	90.0%	0.64 [0.28, 1.46]
Total (95% CI)		**107**		**96**	**100.0%**	**0.64 [0.29, 1.41]**
Total events	88		84			

Heterogeneity: Chi² = 0.00, df = 1 (P = 0.97); I² = 0%
Test for overall effect: Z = 1.11 (P = 0.27)

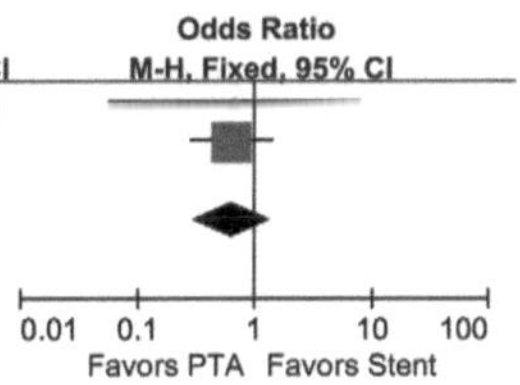

FIGURE 5.—Forest plots of the estimated individual and overall effect of the limb salvage between percutaneous transluminal angioplasty (*PTA*) and primary stenting groups at 6 months (*A*) and 12 months (*B*). *CI*, Confidence interval; *M-H*, Mantel-Haenszel. (Reprinted from the Journal of Vascular Surgery. Wu R, Yao C, Wang S, et al. Percutaneous transluminal angioplasty versus primary stenting in infrapopliteal arterial disease: a meta-analysis of randomized trials. *J Vasc Surg*. 2014;59:1711-1720, Copyright 2014, with permission from The Society for Vascular Surgery.)

comparing two specific treatment interventions (primary angioplasty vs stenting) within a defined anatomic location (infrapopliteal disease). Anatomic inclusion criteria varied considerably between trials, incorporating combinations of percent stenosis, vessel diameter, presence of inflow or outflow disease,

TABLE 2.—Main Features of Included Trials

	Rand 2006		Bosiers 2009		Randon 2010	
	PTA (n = 27)	Stent (n = 24)	PTA (n = 57)	Stent (n = 60)	PTA (n = 22)	Stent (n = 16)
Age, years	72	72	73.1 ± 8.5	74.7 ± 7.8	72 ± 10	72 ± 9
Male gender	NA	NA	41 (71.9%)	31 (51.7%)	14 (63.6%)	6 (37.5%)
DM	19 (70%)	16 (67%)	39 (68.4%)	43 (71.7%)	12 (55%)	10 (63%)
CAD	11 (41%)	9 (38%)	NA	NA	18 (82%)	12 (75%)
CKD	3 (11%)	5 (21%)	NA	NA	12 (55%)	5 (31%)
Smoking	17 (63%)	14 (58%)	26 (45.6%)	24 (40%)	4 (18%)	1 (6%)
Hypertension	NA	NA	51 (89%)	51 (85%)	22 (100%)	16 (100%)
Dyslipidemia	NA	NA	35 (61.4%)	32 (53.3%)	9 (41%)	7 (44%)
Type of balloon/stent	Non-drug eluting	Carbofilm coated	Non-drug eluting	Absorbable metal	Non-drug eluting	Bare metal
Lesion length, mm	24.0		12.0 ± 5.0	10.6 ± 4.9	NA	NA
Inclusion criteria	Fontaine III and IV; stenosis >70% or occlusion; lesions ≤3, lesion length ≤3 cm; cumulative lesion length ≤9 cm		Rutherford 4 and 5; stenosis >50% or occlusion; life expectancy >6 months; vessel diameter 3-3.5 mm		Fontaine III and IV; Rutherford 4 to 6; stenosis >70% or occlusion	
Exclusion criteria	Inflow or outflow obstruction; coagulopathy; peptic ulcer; inflammatory vascular disease		Inflow obstruction; previous treatment; allergy to antiplatelet or anticoagulant; participation in another clinical trial; pregnant; mentally ill or retarded		Inflow obstruction; acute limb ischemia; myocardial infarction; blue toe syndrome; inability to ambulate	
Angiographic follow-up/time	Yes/6 months		Yes/6 months		Yes/3, 6, 12, 18, 24 months	

CAD, Coronary artery disease; *CKD*, chronic kidney disease; *DM*, diabetes mellitus; *DVT*, deep venous thrombosis; *NA*, not reported; *PTA*, percutaneous transluminal angioplasty.

Reprinted from the Journal of Vascular Surgery. Wu R, Yao C, Wang S, et al. Percutaneous transluminal angioplasty versus primary stenting in infrapopliteal arterial disease: a meta-analysis of randomized trials. *J Vasc Surg*. 2014;59:1711-1720, Copyright 2014, with permission from The Society for Vascular Surgery.

and lesion length and/or number. Exclusion criteria were also quite variable, with only some studies specifically mentioning exclusion of acute limb ischemia (which affects a different patient population and management considerations) or patients with renal disease (who would be expected to have inferior outcomes across most clinical endpoints). As noted by the authors, the 6 trials included also used 6 different types of stents (including bare-metal, drug-eluting, and carbon-coating technologies). Periprocedural adverse events were not analyzed but might have been anticipated to differ between groups due to stenting's greater technical difficulty and larger minimum sheath diameter; the impact of these factors is evident from the inferior technical success observed with primary stenting. Amputation-free survival has also been previously suggested as an efficacy endpoint for trials evaluating catheter-based intervention for critical limb ischemia (CLI) but was not analyzed in this study[1]; physiologic outcomes (such as toe pressures or toe-brachial index), quality of life, and cost are among other variables of potential interest that were not evaluated. These limitations aside, the combined results suggest that primary stenting offers no obvious advantage over angioplasty in terms of technical success, short-term patency (Fig 3), or limb salvage (Fig 5).

When interpreting these results, it is important to remember the contingencies implied by inclusion in a randomized clinical trial, the most important of which is perhaps anatomic suitability for either treatment. These results therefore may not carry immense practical impact within clinical practice outside a randomized trial scenario, where the operator faced with a choice between options would presumably select the safest, lowest risk, and/or lowest cost option (primary angioplasty being the choice for all 3 of these criteria). In clinical practice, endovascular treatment of CLI often involves proceeding from cheaper and simpler to more expensive and technically demanding treatment options unless factors are identified that favor the latter (such as dense calcification) are identified. In the setting of challenging anatomy or lesion characteristics, providers may increasingly resort to combinations of treatments (including angioplasty, stenting, and atherectomy with the use of adjunctive tools such as crossing devices and retrograde access). In these situations, providers often consider the suitability of bypass as an alternative option (based on factors such as operative risk and availability of single segment vein conduit) when deciding how far to push the envelope to accomplish endovascular treatment. These contingencies are frequently encountered in clinical practice and often result in situations bearing little resemblance to randomized trial protocols, resulting in challenges to direct application of available evidence to specific treatment decisions for individual patients.

M. A. Corriere, MD, MS

Reference

1. Conte MS, Geraghty PJ, Bradbury AW, et al. Suggested objective performance goals and clinical trial design for evaluating catheter-based treatment of critical limb ischemia. *J Vasc Surg*. 2009;50:1462-1473.e1-3.

Surgical vein graft preparation promotes cellular dysfunction, oxidative stress, and intimal hyperplasia in human saphenous vein

Osgood MJ, Hocking KM, Voskresensky IV, et al (Vanderbilt Univ Med Ctr, Nashville, TN; et al)

J Vasc Surg 60:202-211, 2014

Introduction.—Human saphenous vein (HSV) is the most widely used bypass conduit for peripheral and coronary vascular reconstructions. However, outcomes are limited by a high rate of intimal hyperplasia (IH). HSV undergoes a series of ex vivo surgical manipulations prior to implantation, including hydrostatic distension, marking, and warm ischemia in solution. We investigated the impact of surgical preparation on HSV cellular function and development of IH in organ culture. We hypothesized that oxidative stress is a mediator of HSV dysfunction.

Methods.—HSV was collected from patients undergoing vascular bypass before and after surgical preparation. Smooth muscle and endothelial function were measured using a muscle bath. Endothelial preservation was assessed with immunohistochemical staining. An organ culture model was used to investigate the influence of surgical preparation injury on the development of IH. Superoxide levels were measured using a high-performance liquid chromatography-based assay. The influence of oxidative stress on HSV physiologic responses was investigated by exposing HSV to hydrogen peroxide (H_2O_2).

Results.—Surgical vein graft preparation resulted in smooth muscle and endothelial dysfunction, endothelial denudation, diminished endothelial nitric oxide synthase staining, development of increased IH, and increased levels of reactive oxygen species. Experimental induction of oxidative stress in unmanipulated HSV by treatment with H_2O_2 promoted endothelial dysfunction. Duration of storage time in solution did not contribute to smooth muscle or endothelial dysfunction.

Conclusions.—Surgical vein graft preparation causes dysfunction of the smooth muscle and endothelium, endothelial denudation, reduced endothelial nitric oxide synthase expression, and promotes IH in organ culture. Moreover, increased levels of reactive oxygen species are produced and may promote further vein graft dysfunction. These results argue for less injurious means of preparing HSV prior to autologous transplantation into the arterial circulation.

▶ Reducing the trauma to precious saphenous conduit has been taught for years at institutions with robust open surgical bypass practices. Using several distinct sophisticated metrics, the authors show that "standard" surgical manipulation makes the harvested saphenous vein more dysfunctional at a cellular level, including alterations in the smooth muscle and endothelial cell function. The implications are 2-fold: (1) there is likely cellular-mediated injury that is brought on by surgical trauma, and (2) this injury may promote intimal hyperplasia. The next step in a study such as this should ideally include quantification of level of cellular injury and attempting to find a correlation with clinical outcomes. Even without the advanced biological testing, the act of saphenous vein harvest should be approached with appropriate reverence. Physical, thermal, and mechanical injury to conduit is likely to decrease its long-term success.

R. J. Feezor, MD, FACS

Clinical significance of embolic events in patients undergoing endovascular femoropopliteal interventions with or without embolic protection devices

Mendes BC, Oderich GS, Fleming MD, et al (Mayo Clinic, Rochester, MN)
J Vasc Surg 59:359-367.e1, 2014

Objective.—The purpose of this study was to evaluate the incidence and clinical significance of embolic events in patients undergoing endovascular femoropopliteal interventions with or without embolic protection devices (EPDs).

Methods.—We reviewed the clinical data of 566 patients treated by 836 endovascular femoropopliteal interventions for lower extremity claudication (46%) or critical limb ischemia (54%) from 2002 to 2012. Outcomes were analyzed in 74 patients/87 interventions performed with EPDs (Spider Rx; Covidien, Plymouth, Minn) and 513 patients/749 interventions performed without EPDs. TransAtlantic Inter-Society Consensus (TASC) II classification, runoff scores, and embolic events were analyzed. End points were morbidity, mortality, reintervention, patency, and major amputation rates.

Results.—Both groups had similar demographics, indications, cardiovascular risk factors, and runoff scores, but patients treated with EPDs had significantly ($P < .05$) longer lesions (109 ± 94 mm vs 85 ± 76 mm) and more often had occlusions (64% vs 30%) and TASC C/D lesions (56% vs 30%). Embolic events occurred in 35 of 836 interventions (4%), including two (2%) performed with EPD and 33 (4%) without EPD ($P = .35$). Macroscopic debris was noted in 59 (68%) filter baskets. Embolic events were not associated with lesion length, TASC classification, runoff scores, treatment type, or indication but were independently associated with occlusion. Patients who had embolization required more reinterventions (20% vs 3%; $P < .001$) and major amputations at 30 days (11% vs 3%; $P = .02$). There was no difference in hospital stay (2.4 ± 4 days vs 1.6 ± 2 days; $P = .08$), reintervention (2% vs 4%), and major amputation (1% vs 4%) among patients treated with or without EPD, respectively. The two patients who developed embolization with EPDs had no clinical sequela and required no reintervention. Most emboli were successfully treated by catheter aspiration or thrombolysis, but eight patients (24%) treated without EPD required prolonged hospital stay, seven (21%) had multiple reinterventions, one (3%) had unanticipated major amputation, and one (3%) died from hemorrhagic complications of thrombolysis. Median follow-up was 20 months. At 2 years, primary patency and freedom from reintervention was similar for TASC A/B and TASC C/D lesions treated with or without EPDs.

Conclusions.—Rates of embolization are low in patients undergoing endovascular femoropopliteal interventions with (4%) or without (2%) EPD. Embolization is more frequent in patients with occlusions. While emboli in patients with EPD had no clinical sequel, those treated without EPD required multiple reinterventions in 21% or resulted in major amputation or death in 3%. Late outcomes were similar in patients treated with or without EPDs.

▶ The use of embolic protection devices during peripheral endovascular interventions remains debated. This report documents a single-center, retrospective analysis of 836 femoropopliteal interventions performed over a decade, and specifically compares the outcomes and embolic complication rates between 87 interventions performed with embolic protection devices (EPD) and 749 interventions without EPD. Clearly there is selection bias, and in fact 74% of the EPD interventions were performed by 1 interventionalist. Overall, embolic events were noted more frequently in patients treated with arterial occlusions, but lesion length, TransAtlantic Inter-Society Consensus classification, indication for intervention, and runoff score did not bear out as predictive of embolism. As expected, the patients who had embolic events required more early reinterventions and had more early major amputations. Importantly, although the numbers are low, there may have been a protective effect of the use of EPD in that the clinical sequelae noted were less catastrophic compared with patients who had embolic events and had an EPD used. The overall rate of embolic events was not affected by the use of EPD, but this clearly may have been influenced by the selection bias inherent to a retrospective review. Additionally, the authors treated only 5% of lesions with atherectomy, and a higher prevalence of this treatment modality is potentially associated with increased embolic sequelae. As alluded to in the discussion, much like carotid interventions, there is radiographic proof of embolic events at a much higher frequency than clinical sequelae, so the question remains as to the value of EPD overall. In this report, there appears to be few complications attributable to EPD, and likely there are some lesions and runoff anatomies that justify their use. The challenge of identifying these lesions and/or anatomic characteristics remains.

R. J. Feezor, MD, FACS

Impact of severe chronic kidney disease on outcomes of infrainguinal peripheral arterial intervention

Patel VI, Mukhopadhyay S, Guest JM, et al (Massachusetts General Hosp, Boston)

J Vasc Surg 59:368-375, 2014

Objective.—Patients with severe chronic kidney disease (CKD) and peripheral vascular disease are at increased risk of major adverse limb events (MALEs) and death; however, patients with end-stage renal disease have been excluded in current objective performance goals. We evaluated the effect of severe (class 4 and 5) CKD on outcomes after infrainguinal endovascular arterial interventions.

Methods.—All primary peripheral vascular interventions (PVIs) performed at a single institution (January 2002 through December 2009) were included. End points were defined by Society for Vascular Surgery objective performance goals for critical limb ischemia (CLI), which include all-cause mortality, reintervention, and composite end points of death or amputation and MALEs (reintervention or amputation). Univariate and multivariable analysis was used to examine the effect of severe CKD on study end points.

Results.—A total of 879 PVIs were performed, with severe CKD in 125 (14%). Severe CKD patients were significantly ($P < .05$) more likely to have diabetes (64% vs 46%), CLI (72% vs 11%), and need a multilevel PVI (34% vs 19%) or tibial intervention (35% vs 20%) compared with the remainder of the cohort. Distribution of TransAtlantic Inter-Society Consensus C and D lesions were similar (19% severe CKD vs 15%; $P = .2$). Severe CKD predicted perioperative (30-day) reintervention (odds ratio [OR], 2.3; 95% confidence interval [CI], 1.5-4; $P = .05$), amputation or death (OR, 3.1; 95% CI, 1.1-9; $P = .04$), and MALEs (OR, 2.8; 95% CI, 1.3-6.1; $P = .04$), which was independent of CLI in multivariable regression analysis. On Kaplan-Meier analysis, severe CKD was significantly (log-rank $P < .05$) associated with death (31% ± 4% vs 7% ± 1%), amputation (14% ± 3% vs 3% ± 1%), and MALEs (40% ± 5% vs 26% ± 2%) at 1 year. Freedom from reintervention was similar at 1 year (70% 6 5% severe CKD vs 75% ± 2%; $P = .23$). Risk-adjusted (age, CLI, diabetes, coronary artery disease) Cox proportional hazards regression showed that severe CKD increased the risk of late mortality (hazard ratio [HR], 2.4; 95% CI, 1.8-3.2; $P < .01$), amputation (HR, 2.1; 95% CI, 1.1-3.9; $P = .02$), and death or amputation (HR, 1.8; 95% CI, 1.3-2.4; $P = .04$), without increasing the risk of late reinterventions or MALEs.

Conclusions.—CKD independently predicts early and late adverse events after a PVI, in particular, excessive mortality. CKD should figure prominently in clinical decision making for patients with peripheral vascular disease.

► Lower extremity revascularization outcomes are typically measured by statistics such as amputation rate, need for reintervention, and the recently debated target-lesion revascularization. Clinical vascular surgeons have known for years that restoration of limb perfusion is only half the battle in the typical patient with peripheral arterial disease (PAD). Patients' systemic risk factors and comorbidities are, for some, likely to overwhelm the beneficial effects of any elegantly performed revascularization by whatever means. The authors report that patients with severe renal insufficiency (glomerular filtration rate ≤30 mL/min/1.73 m^2) have depressingly poor overall survival as well as increased amputation rates, and this discrimination held true even when adjusting for age, indication of intervention (critical limb ischemia), diabetes, and coronary artery disease. In essence, and perhaps over simplistically, there are some patients for whom revascularization is not likely to be "worth it." Consideration of a patient's overall survival must factor into clinical decisions to treat (or not) any part of the vascular system, and this balance will be more important as health care resources continue to be limited, either because of economics or availability.

R. J. Feezor, MD, FACS

Surgical vein graft preparation promotes cellular dysfunction, oxidative stress, and intimal hyperplasia in human saphenous vein

Osgood MJ, Hocking KM, Voskresensky IV, et al (Vanderbilt Univ Med Ctr, Nashville, TN; et al)

J Vasc Surg 60:202-211, 2014

Introduction.—Human saphenous vein (HSV) is the most widely used bypass conduit for peripheral and coronary vascular reconstructions. However, outcomes are limited by a high rate of intimal hyperplasia (IH). HSV undergoes a series of ex vivo surgical manipulations prior to implantation, including hydrostatic distension, marking, and warm ischemia in solution. We investigated the impact of surgical preparation on HSV cellular function and development of IH in organ culture. We hypothesized that oxidative stress is a mediator of HSV dysfunction.

Methods.—HSV was collected from patients undergoing vascular bypass before and after surgical preparation. Smooth muscle and endothelial function were measured using a muscle bath. Endothelial preservation was assessed with immunohistochemical staining. An organ culture model was used to investigate the influence of surgical preparation injury on the development of IH. Superoxide levels were measured using a high-performance liquid chromatography based assay. The influence of oxidative stress on HSV physiologic responses was investigated by exposing HSV to hydrogen peroxide (H_2O_2).

Results.—Surgical vein graft preparation resulted in smooth muscle and endothelial dysfunction, endothelial denudation, diminished endothelial nitric oxide synthase staining, development of increased IH, and increased levels of reactive oxygen species. Experimental induction of oxidative stress in unmanipulated HSV by treatment with H_2O_2 promoted endothelial dysfunction. Duration of storage time in solution did not contribute to smooth muscle or endothelial dysfunction.

Conclusions.—Surgical vein graft preparation causes dysfunction of the smooth muscle and endothelium, endothelial denudation, reduced endothelial nitric oxide synthase expression, and promotes IH in organ culture. Moreover, increased levels of reactive oxygen species are produced and may promote further vein graft dysfunction. These results argue for less injurious means of preparing HSV prior to autologous transplantation into the arterial circulation.

► Reducing the trauma to precious saphenous conduit has been taught for years at institutions with robust open surgical bypass practices. Using several distinct sophisticated metrics, the authors show that "standard" surgical manipulation makes the harvested saphenous vein more dysfunctional at a cellular level, including alterations in the smooth muscle and endothelial cell function. The implications are 2-fold: (1) there is likely cellular-mediated injury that is brought on by surgical trauma, and (2) this injury may promote intimal hyperplasia. The next step in a study such as this ideally should include quantification of level of cellular injury and attempting to find a correlation with clinical outcomes. Even without the advanced biological testing, the act of saphenous vein harvest should be approached with appropriate reverence. Physical, thermal, and mechanical injury to conduit is likely to decrease its long-term success.

R. J. Feezor, MD, FACS

Safety and feasibility of adjunctive dexamethasone infusion into the adventitia of the femoropopliteal artery following endovascular revascularization

Owens CD, Gasper WJ, Walker JP, et al (Univ of California San Francisco Med Ctr)

J Vasc Surg 59:1016-1024, 2014

Objective.—Restenosis following endovascular treatment of the femoropopliteal segment is associated with the inflammatory response produced in the artery wall at the time of the procedure. Although local drug delivery to the superficial femoral and popliteal arteries promises improved patency, data are currently limited. We hypothesized that improved percutaneous delivery of an anti-inflammatory compound into the adventitia of the femoropopliteal at the time of endovascular treatment would be safe, feasible, and decrease the inflammatory response.

Methods.—This was a prospective, investigator-initiated, phase I, first-in-man study testing the safety and feasibility of percutaneous adventitial delivery of dexamethasone. Following successful intervention, an adventitial microinfusion catheter was advanced over a 0.014-inch wire to the treated segment. Its microneedle (0.9 mm long × 140-μm diameter) was deployed into the adventitia to deliver dexamethasone (4 mg/mL) mixed with contrast agent (80:20 ratio), providing fluoroscopic visualization. The primary safety outcome measure was freedom from vessel dissection, thrombosis, or extravasation while the primary efficacy outcome was duplex-determined binary restenosis defined as a peak systolic velocity ratio >2.5.

Results.—Twenty patients with Rutherford clinical category 2-5 enrolled in this study. The mean age was 66, and 55% had diabetes mellitus. Treated lesion length was 8.9 ± 5.3 cm, and 50% were chronic total occlusions. Eighty percent of treated lesions were in the distal superficial femoral or popliteal arteries. All lesions were treated by balloon angioplasty with provisional stenting (n = 6) for suboptimal result. Three patients were treated with atherectomy as well. A mean of 1.6 ± 1.1 mg (0.5 ± 0.3 mL) of dexamethasone sodium phosphate was injected per centimeter of lesion length. In total, a mean of 12.1 ± 6.1 mg of dexamethasone was injected per patient. The mean number of injections required per lesion was 3.0 ± 1.3 cm, minimum one and maximum six injections. There was 100% technical success of drug delivery and no procedural or drug-related adverse events. The mean Rutherford score decreased from 3.1 ± .7 (median, 3.0) preoperatively to .5 ± .7 at 6 months (median, 0.0; $P < .00001$). Over this same time interval, the index leg ankle-brachial index increased from .68 ± .15 to .89 ± .19 ($P = .0003$). The preoperative C-reactive protein in this study was 6.9 ± 8.5 indicating severe baseline inflammation, which increased to 14.0 ± 23.1 mg/L (103% increase) at 24 hours following the procedure. However, this increase did not reach statistical significance of $P = .14$. Two patients met the primary efficacy end point of loss of primary patency by reoccluding their treated segment of the index lesion during the follow-up period.

Conclusions.—Adventitial drug delivery via a microinfusion catheter is a safe and feasible alternative to intimal-based methods for adjunctive treatment in the femoropopliteal segment. The 6-month preliminary results suggest perivascular dexamethasone treatment may improve outcomes following angioplasty to the femoral and popliteal arteries, and support further clinical investigation of this approach.

▶ The vast majority of published studies investigating the treatment of symptomatic lower extremity peripheral artery disease has focused on the anatomic repair: in other words, fixing the anatomy. There is growing evidence that despite improved initial technical success, the durability of such interventions remains disappointing, and the mechanism of failure likely is mediated at least in part by inflammatory actors. In other vascular territories, systemic modulation of the immune response has been associated with a significant number of untoward side effects. This 20-patient report focused on the safety of a first-in-man administration of glucocorticoid into the adventitia surrounding atherosclerotic lesions that have been treated with standard endovascular means. The authors used a proprietary Bullfrog microinfusion catheter (Mercator Medsystems, San Leandro, CA) to infiltrate a mixture of dexamethasone and contrast from the lumen into the adventitia. They had intraprocedural radiographic confirmation that the injections, spaced every 3 cm based on cadaveric data, were able to longitudinally deliver the drug to the entire length of the lesion with a mean of 3.0 ± 1.3 injections per lesion (range, 1-6). Attributable to the primary intervention of angioplasty, angioplasty and stent, or atherectomy the postprocedure ankle-brachial indices increased. Notably, there were no dissections pseudoaneurysms, or 30-day thrombosis, suggesting that the mechanism of delivery of the drug was safe. There was a modest but not statistically significant increase in serum inflammatory markers. Two of the 20 patients had ultrasonographically detected restenosis at 6 months. The study provides early evidence that transluminal delivery of a drug into the arterial adventitia can be accomplished safely but provides no data into the efficacy of achieving the ultimate goal of increasing durability of endovascular intervention. The principle in concept is at the least intriguing enough to warrant subsequent investigation.

R. J. Feezor, MD, FACS

Walking disability in patients with peripheral artery disease is associated with arterial endothelial function

Grenon SM, Chong K, Alley H, et al (Univ of California San Francisco)
J Vasc Surg 59:1025-1034, 2014

Objective.—Patients with peripheral artery disease (PAD) have varying degrees of walking disability that do not completely correlate with ankle-brachial index (ABI) or angiographic anatomy. We hypothesized that endothelial function (EF) is an independent predictor of symptom severity in PAD patients.

Methods.—This was a cross-sectional study of 100 PAD patients presenting to a vascular surgery clinic. All patients received ABI testing and brachial artery flow-mediated, endothelium-dependent vasodilation (FMD) to assess arterial EF. Symptom severity and walking disability reported by Rutherford category was based on the patient's self-report during the clinic visit and recorded by the investigator-vascular surgeons. Demographic, biochemical, and physiologic parameters were entered into regression equations to determine association with symptom severity.

Results.—Patients were a mean age of 66 ± 8 years, and 43% had diabetes. Mean FMD was 7.4%, indicating impaired EF. EF progressively declined as Rutherford category increased ($P = .01$). Brachial artery FMD, ABI, systolic blood pressure, C-reactive protein, low-density lipoprotein, high-density lipoprotein, β-blocker use, and a history of diabetes or coronary artery disease were all associated with Rutherford category (all $P < .05$). Multivariable regression showed EF ($P < .02$) and ABI ($P < .0001$) were independently associated with walking disability. When the cohort was restricted to claudicant patients ($n = 73$), EF remained associated with walking disability after adjustment for other covariates ($P = .0001$).

Conclusions.—Symptom severity in PAD is multifactorial, reflecting impaired hemodynamics and vascular dysfunction. This is the first report demonstrating that walking disability in PAD is associated with arterial EF. The mechanistic link underlying these observations remains to be defined.

▶ The prevalence of walking dysfunction among patients with peripheral artery disease (PAD) has been well documented, but the exact pathophysiology has yet to be ascertained because it is a complex process involving more than restriction of blood flow in large vessels. There has been recent emphasis on systemic markers of inflammation in addition to well-studied atherosclerosis-associated factors such as serum cholesterol. The ankle-brachial index (ABI) is perhaps a crude test of the degree of diminution of blood flow to the lower extremity. The authors tested 100 male subjects from a single VA Medical Center, the majority of whom had PAD. They found, predictably, that patients with PAD severe enough to manifest as limb-threatening ischemia had higher systolic blood pressure and a higher incidence of diabetes mellitus. Worsening clinical severity of PAD was also associated with increasing low-density lipoprotein, total cholesterol, and C-reactive protein. Naturally, worse PAD was associated with lower ABI as well. Most interestingly, the authors tested brachial artery flow-mediated vasodilation (FMD), which is a well-established test of endothelial function, and found that higher Rutherford classification was associated with a decline in FMD. In subgroup analysis, among the 73 patients with claudication, the discrimination between mild (> 3 blocks), moderate (> 1 and ≤3 blocks), or severe (≤1 block) was not possible with ABI measurement but was possible with FMD. This suggests that the dynamic FMD test was more sensitive than the static ABI. The natural extension of this type of observational study is to investigate whether some intervention can halt the progression or even induce regression of FMD dysfunction.

R. J. Feezor, MD, FACS

Pedal bypass surgery after crural endovascular intervention

Uhl C, Hock C, Betz T, et al (Krankenhaus Barmherzige Brüder Regensburg, Germany)

J Vasc Surg 59:1583-1587, 2014

Background.—Many centers choose endovascular intervention as their first-line treatment for crural occlusions in patients with critical limb ischemia (Rutherford 4-6). However, unsuccessful interventions often result in major amputation. Therefore, pedal bypass surgery should be considered as an alternative first-line treatment. We reviewed the impact of a prior endovascular intervention on the outcome of our patients' pedal bypass procedures.

Methods.—A retrospective analysis was conducted for all patients who had undergone pedal bypass surgery in our department from February 2008 to October 2012. We performed 75 pedal bypass operations in 71 patients (male, 54; female, 17; median age, 72 years; range, 29-90 years). In 36 of those cases, patients had undergone a prior infrapopliteal endovascular intervention (PEI group). In 39 cases, patients underwent bypass surgery as first-line treatment because their prior angiography had resulted in either unsuccessful endovascular intervention, or intervention had been deemed 'not feasible' (BSF group). Only autologous vein grafts were used, and no retrograde intervention was done via the pedal arteries. Endpoints of the analysis were primary and secondary patency rates, mortality, and limb salvage at 1 year postoperatively.

Results.—Overall primary patency at 1 year was 58.3%, and secondary patency was 61.3%. Limb salvage was 76.8% and survival was 80.4%. Graft occlusion within 30 days was 18.7%. Revision in those cases was futile and 78.6% of patients had to undergo major amputation. Primary patency at 1 year was 67.0% in PEI group vs 48.3% in BSF group (P =.409) and secondary patency was 73.5% vs 48.6% (P =.100). Prior endovascular intervention had no significant impact on either limb salvage (82.3% vs 71.6% at 1 year; P =.515) or graft occlusions within 30 days (19.4% vs 17.9%; P =.547). Survival rate at 1 year was 79.5% in PEI group and 81.3% in BSF group (P =.765). Risk factors and indications were similar in both groups.

Conclusions.—Crural endovascular intervention does not seem to have a negative impact on the outcome of subsequent pedal bypass surgery. Requirements are avoiding a destruction of the target vessel and opting for timely bypass surgery whenever endovascular treatment does not achieve a sufficient perfusion for wounds to heal. Early graft occlusions are associated with a higher risk for major amputation.

▶ The limb-salvage impact of failed endovascular interventions is one of the most important issues facing treating physicians in the coming years, and this has been made more vital by the impressively increasing numbers of interventionalists capable of performing such interventions, the appropriate emphasis on cost-effective quality care delivery, and the inevitable increase in the "typical" patient's systemic comorbidities. The authors reviewed the outcomes of 75 pedal bypass procedures (75% of which had the dorsalis pedis as the target outflow vessel) and compared the subsets of patients with prior crural endovascular interventions (n = 36, 48%) with those without prior intervention (n = 39, 52%). The 4% reported mortality, 19% 30-day graft failure, and 16% 30-day major amputation rate are simultaneously laudable, sobering, and consistent with real-world outcomes of centers of expertise. Among the endovascular interventions, there were no crural stents placed and only 1 tibial atherectomy. All bypasses were done with autologous conduit. There was no difference in primary patency, secondary patency, limb salvage, or graft occlusion between patients with prior endovascular intervention and those without. The deliverable message, therefore, is that patients can safely undergo attempts at endovascular therapy for infrageniculate lesions contributing to critical limb ischemia without compromising future distal bypass options. The clear caveat to this message is that an aura of conservatism should dictate the aggressiveness of the endovascular therapy. Extensive atherectomy, tibial stenting, and the inherent trauma of retrograde pedal/crural access to achieve early technical endovascular success were not tested. It is likely that these maneuvers, despite helping to gain early technical success, may be associated with loss of anatomic outflow and hence worse bypass and potentially limb-salvage outcomes in an arena where the results are already disheartening.

R. J. Feezor, MD, FACS

Endovascular recanalization of infrapopliteal occlusions in patients with critical limb ischemia

Singh GD, Armstrong EJ, Yeo K-K, et al (Univ of California, Sacramento; et al)
J Vasc Surg 59:1300-1307, 2014

Background.—Endovascular therapies are increasingly used for treatment of critical limb ischemia (CLI). Infrapopliteal (IP) occlusions are common in CLI, and successful limb salvage may require restoration of arterial flow in the distribution of a chronically occluded vessel. We sought to describe the procedural characteristics and outcomes of patients with IP occlusions who underwent endovascular intervention for treatment of CLI.

Methods.—All patients with IP interventions for treatment of CLI from 2006 to 2012 were included. Angiographic and procedural data were compared between patients who underwent intervention for IP occlusions vs IP stenosis. Restenosis was determined by Doppler ultrasound imaging. Limb salvage was the primary end point of the study. Additional end points included primary patency, primary assisted patency, secondary patency, occlusion crossing success, procedural success, and amputation-free survival.

Results.—A total of 187 patients with CLI underwent interventions for 356 IP lesions, and 77 patients (41%) had interventions for an IP occlusion. Patients with an intervention for IP occlusion were more likely to have zero to one vessel runoff (83% vs 56%; $P < .001$) compared with interventions for stenosis. Compared with IP stenoses, IP occlusions were longer (118 ± 86 vs 73 ± 67 mm; $P < .001$) and had a smaller vessel diameter (2.5 ± 0.8 vs 2.7 ± 0.5 mm; $P = .02$). Wire crossing was achieved in 83% of IP occlusions, and the overall procedural success for IP occlusions was 79%. The overall 1-year limb salvage rate was 84%. Limb salvage was highest in the stenosis group, slightly lower in the successful occlusion group, and lowest in the failed occlusion group (92% vs 75% vs 58%, respectively; $P = .02$). Unsuccessfully treated IP occlusions were associated with a significantly higher likelihood of major amputation (hazard ratio, 5.79; 95% confidence interval, 1.89-17.7) and major amputation or death (hazard ratio, 2.69; 95% confidence interval, 1.09-6.63).

Conclusions.—Successful endovascular recanalization of IP occlusions can be achieved with guidewire and support catheter techniques in most patients. In patients selected for an endovascular-first approach for IP occlusions in CLI, this strategy can be successfully implemented with favorable rates of limb salvage.

► The techniques, familiarity, and expertise among practitioners performing endovascular procedures to treat limb-threatening ischemia continue to increase and progress. Patients with Rutherford classification 4 through 6 often have infrapopliteal disease. Despite the relative certainty that surgical revascularization remains the gold standard, this report gives results with an anatomically challenging cohort of patients, namely, infrapopliteal occlusions. With a mean length of infrapopliteal occlusion of nearly 12 cm, the authors achieved a 79% procedural success, usually with a standard contralateral femoral approach, and only a modest number of retrograde (pedal) access techniques. Despite early technical success, however, occlusions tended to recur at a frequency greater than in lesions that presented as mere stenoses. Similarly, the early technical achievements were associated with a sobering rate of 12-month primary patency, primary assisted patency, and secondary patency, all of which were lower than that seen in stenotic lesions. The limb salvage rate of 75% for tibial occlusions successfully treated was lower than the 92% seen in patients who had tibial stenoses successfully treated. Interestingly, tibial occlusions that were not successfully treated were seen to have a 12-month limb salvage rate of 58%. Although these results after nonintervention almost seem too good to be true, the authors are to be commended on their initial technical successes and their overall limb salvage rates. Clearly, "success" in the infrapopliteal space has to be a relative measure.

R. J. Feezor, MD, FACS

Utility of direct angiosome revascularization and runoff scores in predicting outcomes in patients undergoing revascularization for critical limb ischemia

Kret MR, Cheng D, Azarbal AF, et al (Oregon Health and Science Univ, Portland; Northwest Permanente Physicians and Surgeons, Clackamas, OR)
J Vasc Surg 59:121-128, 2014

Objective.—Both runoff scores and direct (DR) vs indirect revascularization (IR) according to pedal angiosomes have unclear impact on outcome for patients with critical limb ischemia (CLI). We compared DR vs IR and runoff scores in CLI patients undergoing infrapopliteal bypass for foot wounds.

Methods.—Patients who had tibial/pedal bypass for a foot/ankle wound from 2005-2011 were identified and operations classified as DR or IR based on wound location and bypass target. A blinded observer reviewed angiograms for an intact pedal arch and calculated standard Society for Vascular Surgery (single tibial) and modified (composite tibial) runoff scores. Comorbidities, wound characteristics, wound healing, major amputation, and overall survival were determined.

Results.—A total of 106 limbs were revascularized in 97 patients; 54 limbs had DR and 52 had IR, although only 36% of wounds corresponded to a single, distinct angiosome. Wound characteristics and comorbidities were similar between groups. Mean standard (7.9 vs 7.2; $P=.001$) and modified (22.2 vs 20.0; $P=.02$) runoff scores were worse (higher number indicates worse runoff) in the IR vs DR groups; 33% had a complete pedal arch. Complete wound healing (78% vs 46%; $P=.001$) and time to complete healing (99 vs 195 days; $P=.002$) were superior with DR vs IR but were not influenced by runoff score, modified runoff score or presence of complete plantar arch. In multivariate models controlling for runoff score, DR remained a significant predictor for wound healing (odds ratio, 2.9; 95% confidence interval, 1.1-7.4; $P = .028$) and reduced healing time (hazard ratio, 2.1; 95% confidence interval, 1.2-3.7; $P = .012$). Mean amputation-free survival (75 vs 71 months for DR vs IR; $P = .82$) and median survival (36 vs 33 months DR vs IR; $P = .22$) were not different for DR vs IR.

Conclusions.—DR according to pedal angiosomes provides more efficient wound healing, but is possible in only one-half of the patients and does not affect amputation-free or overall survival. DR is associated with improved runoff scores, but current runoff scores have little clinical utility in predicting outcomes in CLI patients.

▶ Very often, surgeons do not have a choice in target tibial vessel for revascularization efforts for ischemic tissue loss. The concept of the angiosome, although not new, has recently resurfaced, ironically perhaps largely within the endovascular realm. Clinicians are using the concept to target therapy based on the blood supply to a foot wound. When that is indeed possible with open surgical bypass, the authors show that wounds heal more often and significantly more quickly. However, wound healing is still possible, albeit less likely, with indirect revascularization or performing a bypass to a distal target that does not correspond to the offending angiosome. Interestingly, the runoff score and presence of a patent pedal arch did not have any bearing on wound healing at all. This well-done analysis supports the notion that surgeons should bypass to the best blood vessel possible and additionally pay attention to the angiosome concept for tissue loss. However, indirect revascularization, associated with less effective wound healing, is not associated with any elevation in amputation rate. The bottom line—bypass to the best blood vessel possible, and do it well with autologous vein; if there are 2 (or more) equivalent targets, remember the angiosome.

R. J. Feezor, MD, FACS

The effect of graft configuration on 30-day failure of infrapopliteal bypasses

Nguyen B-N, Neville RF, Abugideiri M, et al (George Washington Univ, DC; et al)

J Vasc Surg 59:1003-1008, 2014

Background.—Despite advances in endovascular techniques, infrapopliteal bypasses are still required for limb salvage. Short-term graft patency is an important outcome parameter reflecting technical considerations and acute graft thrombosis. Both are important prerequisites for long-term patency. In this analysis, we compared the 30-day patency of all conduit configurations for infrapopliteal bypasses.

Methods.—All primary infrapopliteal bypasses from the American College of Surgeons-National Surgical Quality Improvement Program database between 2005 and 2010 were divided into six groups: (1) great saphenous vein (GSV); (2) prosthetic conduit (prosthetic); (3) prosthetic conduit with a distal anastomotic venous adjunct (ADJ), such as a cuff or patch (prosthetic + ADJ); (4) composite graft of prosthetic and a vein segment (composite); (5) spliced autogenous vein (spliced vein); and (6) arm vein. Thirty-day graft failure, patient demographics, and operative details were compared among groups. A multivariate model was used for statistical analysis.

Results.—A total of 5375 infrapopliteal bypasses were analyzed by conduit: GSV, 3983 (75%); prosthetic, 898 (17%); spliced vein, 160 (3%); prosthetic + ADJ, 112 (2%); arm vein, 93 (2%); and composite, 91 (2%). The difference among groups in demographics and comorbidities was not statistically significant. Perioperative mortality rates were similar among different conduits. After adjusting for sex, age, weight, race, and previous cardiac surgery, the bypass conduit had a significant independent association with 30-day graft patency ($P = .006$). The GSV failure rate was 7.5%. Composite had a significantly higher 30-day failure rate (15.4%, $P = .006$). There was no significant difference in 30-day failure rate of spliced vein (5.6%, $P = .37$) or arm vein (4.3%, $P = .24$) conduits compared with GSV. Prosthetic had significantly higher 30-day failure rate than GSV (10.5%, $P = .004$). The addition of adjuvant venous tissue at the distal anastomosis of prosthetic bypasses did not significantly improve their 30-day patency (failure rate of 9.8% for prosthetic + ADJ and 10.5% for prosthetic). There was no significant difference in graft patency between alternative venous conduits (arm vein/spliced vein) and prosthetic + ADJ.

Conclusions.—Venous conduits (GSV, spliced vein, arm vein) deliver the best 30-day patency for infrapopliteal bypasses, and GSV remains the most commonly used graft. Prosthetic grafts had a higher 30-day failure rate. Composite grafts should be abandoned because their early patency is not better than pure prosthetic conduits. The addition of a distal venous adjunct did not seem to improve acute prosthetic graft patency, which may reflect lack of effect on thrombogenicity rather than the myointimal hyperplastic response that effects long-term failure of infrapopliteal bypass.

▶ The availability and choice of conduit clearly influences the success of a bypass. For patients whose anatomic occlusions warrant a bypass from the femoral artery to an infrapopliteal artery, the great saphenous vein (GSV) should always be used preferentially. The dilemma starts in the 30% (at least) of patients without suitable GSV to perform the bypass. This report mines the National Surgical Quality Improvement Program database based on Current Procedural Terminology codes to determine the early failure rates as a function of conduit configuration. The authors show that prosthetic conduit has a significantly higher early failure rate (10.5%) than GSV, arm vein, or spliced vein

(7.5%, 4.3%, and 5.6%, respectively). The puzzling conclusions lie within the realm of the bypasses done with prosthetic and an adjuvant technique such as a cuff or a patch. The 30-day failure rate is 9.8%, which is not statistically different from the autologous, non-GSV conduit. Based on that conclusion, there is a suggestion that the 2 conduit choices are equivalent. This result should be interpreted with caution, as the study was likely underpowered given the small sample size. Certainly, the choice of conduit has to balance the likelihood of success with morbidity of the surgery.

R. J. Feezor, MD, FACS

Open versus endoscopic great saphenous vein harvest for lower extremity revascularization of critical limb ischemia

Santo VJ, Dargon PT, Azarbal AF, et al (Oregon Health and Science Univ, Portland)

J Vasc Surg 59:427-434, 2014

Objective.—This study determined wound complication rates, intervention rates, failure mechanisms, patency, limb salvage, and overall survival after lower extremity revascularization using open vein harvest (OVH) vs endoscopic vein harvest (EVH) for critical limb ischemia.

Methods.—A single-institution review was conducted of consecutive patients who underwent infrainguinal bypass with a single-segment reversed great saphenous vein between 2005 and 2012.

Results.—A total of 251 patients with critical limb ischemia underwent revascularization, comprising 153 with OVH and 98 with EVH. The OVH group had a lower mean body mass index (26.7 vs 29.9 kg/m^2; $P = .001$). There were no other differences in demographics, comorbidities, medications, smoking, or in the proximal or distal anastomotic site. Median operative times were 249 minutes (OVH) vs 316 minutes (EVH; $P < .001$). Median postoperative hospital length of stay was 7 days (OVH) vs 5 days (EVH; $P < .001$). Median follow-up was 295 days (OVH) vs 313 days (EVH; $P = .416$). During follow-up, 21 OVH grafts (14%) and 27 EVH grafts (28%) underwent an intervention ($P = .048$). There were a similar number of surgical interventions: 50% (OVH) vs 61% (EVH; $P = .449$). Failed grafts had a mean of 1.2 stenoses per graft, regardless of harvest method. Median stenosis length was 2.1 cm (OVH) vs 2.5 cm (EVH; $P = .402$). At 1 and 3 years, the primary patency was 71% and 52% (OVH) vs 58% and 41% (EVH; $P = .010$), and secondary patency was 88% and 71% (OVH) vs 88% and 64% (EVH; $P = .266$). A secondary patency Cox proportional hazard model showed EVH had a hazard ratio of 2.93 (95% confidence interval, 1.03-8.33; $P = .044$). Overall and harvest-related wound complications were 44% and 29% (OVH) vs 37% and 12% (EVH; $P = .226$ and $P = .002$). At 5 years, amputation-free survival was 48% (OVH) vs 54% (EVH; $P = .305$), and limb salvage was 89% (OVH) and 91% (EVH; $P = .615$).

Conclusions.—OVH and EVH have similar failure mechanisms, limb salvage, amputation-free survival, and overall survival. EVH is associated with impaired patency, increased need for intervention, longer operative times, shorter hospital stays, and decreased vein harvest site wound complications. OVH of the great saphenous vein may provide optimal patency but was not necessarily associated with better patient-centered outcomes. Similar limb salvage rates and amputation-free survival may justify the use of EVH, despite inferior patency, to capture shorter hospital stays and decreased wound complications.

▶ For open surgical revascularization, wound complications remain a great challenge. The advent of endoscopic vein harvest for coronary bypass has led some peripheral vascular surgeons to attempt to adapt the technique to saphenectomy for lower extremity bypasses, with predominantly disappointing results. The authors show that endoscopic vein harvest (EVH) is associated with longer operating times compared with open vein harvest (OVH) but a significantly lower in-hospital length of stay and lower incidence of saphenous wound complications. As with prior studies, there is a lower primary patency at 1 and 3 years with EVH and twice the incidence of secondary interventions, but these factors led to no increase in amputation rates. As surgeons, our goal of "do no harm" really means in the long run, acknowledging short-term disability for long-term improvement. Do we do a less morbid but less durable operation (EVH) or do we do a more invasive procedure first (OVH)? Clearly, the debate is not cut and dried. Both sides—open and endoscopic saphenectomy—should work to improve their results. Open saphenectomy harvest can be performed with smaller, more directed "skip" incisions, with attention to tissue handling and wound closure; endoscopic saphenectomy can continue to be practiced in an effort to decrease operating times and accidental vein injury. There likely is a role for both in the right hands.

R. J. Feezor, MD, FACS

Presentation, treatment, and outcome differences between men and women undergoing revascularization or amputation for lower extremity peripheral arterial disease

Lo RC, Bensley RP, Dahlberg SE, et al (Beth Israel Deaconess Med Ctr and Harvard Med School, Boston, MA)

J Vasc Surg 59:409-418, 2014

Objective.—Prior studies have suggested treatment and outcome disparities between men and women for lower extremity peripheral arterial disease after surgical bypass. Given the recent shift toward endovascular therapy, which has increasingly been used to treat claudication, we sought to analyze sex disparities in presentation, revascularization, amputation, and inpatient mortality.

Methods.—We identified individuals with intermittent claudication and critical limb ischemia (CLI) using International Classification of Diseases, Ninth Revision codes in the Nationwide Inpatient Sample from 1998 to 2009. We compared presentation at time of intervention (intermittent claudication vs CLI), procedure (open surgery vs percutaneous transluminal angioplasty or stenting vs major amputation), and in-hospital mortality for men and women. Regional and ambulatory trends were evaluated by performing a separate analysis of the State Inpatient and Ambulatory Surgery Databases from four geographically diverse states: California, Florida, Maryland, and New Jersey.

Results.—From the Nationwide Inpatient Sample, we identified 1,797,885 patients (56% male) with intermittent claudication (26%) and CLI (74%), who underwent 1,865,999 procedures (41% open surgery, 20% percutaneous transluminal angioplasty or stenting, and 24% amputation). Women were older at the time of intervention by 3.5 years on average and more likely to present with CLI (75.9% vs 72.3%; odds ratio [OR], 1.21; 95% confidence interval [CI], 1.21-1.23; $P < .01$). Women were more likely to undergo endovascular procedures for both intermittent claudication (47% vs 41%; OR, 1.27; 95% CI, 1.25-1.28; $P < .01$) and CLI (21% vs 19%; OR, 1.14; 95% CI, 1.13-1.15; $P < .01$). From 1998 to 2009, major amputations declined from 18 to 11 per 100,000 in men and 16 to 7 per 100,000 in women, predating an increase in total CLI revascularization procedures that was seen starting in 2005 for both men and women. In-hospital mortality was higher in women regardless of disease severity or procedure performed even after adjusting for age and baseline comorbidities (.5% vs .2% after percutaneous transluminal angioplasty or stenting for intermittent claudication; 1.0% vs .7% after open surgery for intermittent claudication; 2.3% vs 1.6% after percutaneous transluminal angioplasty or stenting for CLI; 2.7% vs 2.2% after open surgery for CLI; $P < .01$ for all comparisons).

Conclusions.—There appears to be a preference to perform endovascular over surgical revascularization among women, who are older and have more advanced disease at presentation. Percutaneous transluminal angioplasty or stenting continues to be popular and is increasingly being performed in the outpatient setting. Amputation and in-hospital mortality rates have been declining, and women now have lower amputation but higher mortality rates than men. Recent improvements in outcomes are likely the result of a combination of improved medical management and risk factor reduction.

▶ Disparities in health care delivery and outcomes are historically tough to investigate. The most frequent means of doing so involve retrospective reviews of large administrative databases such as those used here. The authors show that despite presenting with more significant disease burden at a later chronologic age, there is a trend for women to be treated more often with endovascular techniques. One potential conclusion is that the health care system at large should continue to strive to identify women with symptomatic peripheral arterial disease and refer them to treating specialists sooner. Alternatively, there could be inherent differences in biology or anatomy that make options either limited or less successful. What is definitely seen is that women have higher mortality rates after overall less-invasive procedures, likely because of the higher cardiovascular comorbidities seen and known preoperatively. Beyond that conclusion lies a danger in this type of analysis. It may be an overstatement to assume that the treatment decisions are directly reflective of physician bias based on gender as opposed to sound clinical judgment based on the presenting state of the patient and known comorbidities. To claim that there is a preference for one therapy over another may be an inaccurate interpretation. It may come down to the timing of disease presentation, detection, and treatment as well as the biology of the pathologic state and patient overall.

R. J. Feezor, MD, FACS

Primary stenting of femoropopliteal atherosclerotic lesions using new helical interwoven nitinol stents

Chan YC, Cheng SW, Ting AC, et al (Univ of Hong Kong Med Ctr)

J Vasc Surg 59:384-391, 2014

Background.—The Supera helical interwoven nitinol stent has enhanced flexibility in counteracting fractures when placed in the femoropopliteal arteries and may improve patency. The aim of this study is to assess the early results of the Supera stent in symptomatic patients with femoropopliteal atherosclerotic lesions.

Methods.—From October 2011 to April 2013, patients with symptomatic femoropopliteal lesions were treated with angioplasty and primary stenting using the Supera stent. They were followed up at 1, 3, 6, and 12 months with clinical, duplex, and radiographic assessments. Failure was defined as >50% restenosis of the target lesion on duplex ultrasound imaging or stent fracture on X rays.

Results.—A total of 78 consecutive patients (46 males, 32 females) with 82 legs, mean age of 78.5 years (range, 57-97 years) were included. Symptoms of claudication, rest pain, and tissue loss were 48 (59%), 8 (10.1%), and 30 (37%), respectively. Ninety-six Supera stents were inserted in total. In 44 (53.7%) of the legs, stents were extended to the popliteal segments. The mean stented length was 12.6 cm (range, 4.0-38.0 cm). The primary patency rates at 6 and 12 months were 83.5% and 78.6%, respectively. The ankle brachial index increased from 0.58 ± 0.16 preoperative to 0.87 ± 0.14 postoperative. There were no stent fractures. Patency rate was not affected by severity of symptoms, stent lengths, femoro/popliteal stents (log-rank test, $P = .50, .13, .52$). All the patients reported symptomatic improvement. There was no procedural- or device-related morbidity or mortality, no major amputation after revascularization, and 10 patients died of unrelated cardiopulmonary/renal causes on follow-up.

Conclusions.—Our early experience shows that the Supera stents are effective in our cohort of elderly patients, with acceptable patency rates. There were no stent fractures so far even with stenting of the popliteal segments.

▶ The authors report a single-center series of 78 consecutive patients with femoropopliteal occlusive disease treated with primary stenting using the novel Supera stent (IDEV Technologies, Inc, Houston, TX). The results are consistent with those of other published stent trials, with a 78.6% 12-month primary patency rate, appropriate improvement in ankle-brachial index (0.58 to 0.87), and no major amputations. The patient cohort studied, however, tended to be older (mean age, 78.5 years), and 35 patients (45%) presented with limb-threatening ischemia (rest pain or tissue loss), which may make the results slightly more laudable. The stent that was tested is a novel design of interwoven nitinol wires arranged in a helical pattern and is reported to resist fracture. Consistent with manufacturer's instructions, as opposed to standard practice, Supera stents are 1 mm smaller than the prestent angioplasty balloon used in the diseased arterial segment. The helical geometry is touted to tolerate flexion better than standard self-expanding nitinol stents. To support that tenet, 54% of the patients had disease treated in the above-knee popliteal artery and 12% in the below-knee popliteal artery. None of the 96 implanted stents had stent fracture. Six patients had significant in-stent stenosis and 3 had stent occlusions during the follow-up period. The new stent design seems to have tested well in a relatively challenging anatomic location and in older, potentially more significantly diseased vessels, but widespread application and results will determine its ultimate role in the armamentarium against peripheral arterial disease.

R. J. Feezor, MD, FACS

Comparison of surgical bypass with angioplasty and stenting of superficial femoral artery disease

Malas MB, Enwerem N, Qazi U, et al (Johns Hopkins Hosp, Baltimore, MD)
J Vasc Surg 59:129-135, 2014

Objective.—To evaluate the contemporary outcome of femoral-popliteal bypass compared with angioplasty and stenting in patients with symptomatic peripheral arterial disease (PAD) in terms of patency and reintervention rates.

Methods.—We identified all patients evaluated at the Johns Hopkins Bayview Medical Center with the presumptive diagnosis of PAD from September 2005 to September 2010. In this group, we selected all symptomatic patients after failing medical management who received percutaneous transluminal angioplasty/stenting of the superficial femoral artery or femoral-popliteal bypass. We compared the overall patency and reintervention rates between the two groups as well as patency within TransAtlantic Inter-Society Consensus (TASC) II subgroups. Descriptive analyses were performed using χ^2 and two-sided *t*-tests. The Mann-Whitney *U* test was used to compare distributions of continuous variables and the Fisher exact test for categorical variables. Cox proportional hazard model was used to examine the treatment effect within each lesion type, using bypass as the reference group.

Results.—Out of 1237 patients evaluated at Johns Hopkins Bayview Medical Center for PAD from September 2005 to September 2010, we identified 104 symptomatic patients who received percutaneous transluminal angioplasty/stenting of the superficial femoral artery or femoral-popliteal bypass after failing medical management. There were 61 male patients (56%), and the mean age was 68 years in both groups. Both treatment groups had similar risk factors. Overall, 77% of patients with TASC II A and B lesions underwent angioplasty and stenting, whereas 73% of patients with TASC C and D lesions underwent bypass ($P < .01$). The primary patency at 24 months was better for the stent group 67% (95% confidence interval [CI], 0.52-0.78) vs bypass group 49% (95% CI, 0.32-0.64; $P = .05$). The rate of reintervention within the 2-year period was higher in the bypass group compared with the stent group (54% vs 31%; $P = .02$). TASC A and B lesions combined demonstrated a reduced hazard of patency failure compared with TASC C or D lesions combined (hazard ratio, 2.42; 95% CI, 1.26, 4.65; $P < .01$).

Conclusions.—This is the first study that documents higher reintervention rates for femoral-popliteal bypass compared with angioplasty and stenting. We believe that the main reason for this finding is the fact that the bypass patients had significantly more advanced disease. This, emphasizes that one must consider the patient population undergoing intervention when comparing revascularization procedures. A prospective randomized trial is needed to determine the overall better treatment option.

▶ The debate goes on over endovascular and open surgical bypass. This type of retrospective analysis is fraught with selection bias, mostly, as the authors point out, resulting from the anatomy. TransAtlantic Inter-Society Consensus (TASC) A and B lesions are treated endovascularly and TASC C and D are treated with open surgery. It is difficult to make any meaningful comparative statements between the 2 treatment modalities because the success and failure are driven primarily by the anatomy and not the method of revascularization. Indeed the improvements in endovascular technology and resultant patient selection bias may change the current experience with open surgery; those patients historically most likely to have a successful distal bypass (TASC A/B) are now being offered endovascular revascularization. The planned upcoming randomized trials will be focused on the patients squarely in the middle of the decision spectrum. Patients with TASC A disease will likely be offered endovascular treatment first, whereas those with TASC D lesions and robust conduit are likely (or at least should be) to be offered open surgical bypass.

R. J. Feezor, MD, FACS

Independence and mobility after infrainguinal lower limb bypass surgery for critical limb ischemia

Ambler GK, Dapaah A, Al Zuhir N, et al (Cambridge Univ Hosps NHS Foundation Trust, UK)
J Vasc Surg 59:983-987, 2014

Background.—Critical limb ischemia (CLI) is a common condition associated with high levels of morbidity and mortality. Most work to date has focused on surgeon-oriented outcomes such as patency, but there is increasing interest in patient-oriented outcomes such as mobility and independence.

Objective.—This study was conducted to determine the effect of infrainguinal lower limb bypass surgery (LLBS) on postoperative mobility in a United Kingdom tertiary vascular surgery unit and to investigate causes and consequences of poor postoperative mobility.

Methods.—We collected data on all patients undergoing LLBS for CLI at our institution during a 3-year period and analyzed potential factors that correlated with poor postoperative mobility.

Results.—During the study period, 93 index LLBS procedures were performed for patients with CLI. Median length of stay was 11 days (interquartile range, 11 days). The 12-month rates of graft patency, major amputation, and mortality were 75%, 9%, and 6%, respectively. Rates of dependence increased fourfold during the first postoperative year, from 5% preoperatively to 21% at 12 months. Predictors of poor postoperative mobility were female sex ($P = .04$) and poor postoperative mobility ($P < .001$), initially and at the 12-month follow-up. Patients with poor postoperative mobility had significantly prolonged hospital length of stay (15 vs 8 days; $P < .001$).

Conclusions.—Patients undergoing LLBS for CLI suffer significantly impaired postoperative mobility, and this is associated with prolonged hospital stay, irrespective of successful revascularization. Further work is needed to better predict patients who will benefit from revascularization and in whom a nonoperative strategy is optimal.

► Most of the reported outcomes after lower extremity bypasses performed for critical limb ischemia are with surgery-specific (primary, primary-assisted, secondary patency) or crudely patient-specific (limb salvage, mortality). However, perhaps a more important metric to examine is the actual benefit that a patient might receive from such a major surgery on a patient with well-defined comorbidities. In this report, patients are classified as independent, aided, or dependent based on an assessment of their mobility. Although one could argue about the specific inclusions for each category, the definitions were consistently applied to a group of 93 patients who underwent distal bypasses. Patients were assessed preoperatively, upon discharge (mean, 11 days postoperatively), and at 12 months postoperatively. Among the 68 patients deemed independent preoperatively, only 39 retained independence at a year. Equally valuable, no patient who was preoperatively determined to be aided or dependent ever became independent at any time point postoperatively. The message is clear: patients who cannot ambulate independently preoperatively will almost assuredly not gain ambulatory independence despite the best effort of surgical teams. This knowledge should be useful when clinicians have the discussion with patients and their families balancing the risks and benefits of a distal bypass. Moreover, because these patients all have limited life expectancy, it would be prudent to inquire of a patient's specific goals for any surgery before embarking on it. Dependent patients who aspire to heal their wounds and begin walking should be counseled specifically preoperatively.

R. J. Feezor, MD, FACS

Mortality rates and mortality predictors in patients with symptomatic peripheral artery disease stratified according to age and diabetes

Mueller T, Hinterreiter F, Luft C, et al (Konventhospital Barmherzige Brueder, Linz, Austria)

J Vasc Surg 59:1291-1299, 2014

Objective.—Atherosclerotic peripheral arterial disease (PAD) is one of the most prevalent, morbid, and mortal diseases. The aim of this study was to evaluate mortality rates of patients with atherosclerotic PAD stratified according to age and diabetes and to determine predictors of death.

Methods.—We studied 487 patients with symptomatic PAD consecutively admitted to the hospital. This cohort included the following four patient subgroups: (1) 216 patients with PAD <75 years of age without diabetes mellitus; (2) 115 patients with PAD <75 years of age with diabetes mellitus; (3) 102 patients with PAD ≥75 years of age without diabetes mellitus; and (4) 54 patients with PAD ≥75 years of age with diabetes mellitus. Control subjects without atherosclerotic disease were matched to the patients with PAD in a 1:1 design by sex, age (±2 years), and diabetes mellitus status. Outcome measure was all-cause mortality at 5 years.

Results.—Mortality rates at 5 years were 10% in nondiabetic patients with PAD <75 years of age (vs 5% in control subjects; risk ratio [RR], 2.15; 95% confidence interval [CI], 1.60-4.34); 23% in diabetic patients with PAD <75 years of age (vs 7% in control subjects; RR, 3.53; 95% CI, 1.80-6.91); 38% in nondiabetic patients with PAD ≥75 years of age (vs 22% in control subjects; RR, 2.08; 95% CI, 1.26-3.44); and 52% in diabetic patients with PAD ≥75 years of age. Applying multivariate Cox proportional hazards regression analyses (with cardiovascular risk factors, coexisting atherosclerotic disease, clinical stage of PAD, and several biochemical markers as predictor variables), we found the following independent predictors of outcome: in the 216 nondiabetic patients with PAD <75 years of age, high-sensitivity C-reactive protein (hs-CRP) (RR, 3.04; 95% CI, 1.48-6.26); in the 115 diabetic patients with PAD <75 years of age, amino-terminal proe—B-type natriuretic peptide

(NT-proBNP) (RR, 2.63; 95% CI, 1.65-4.19); in the 102 nondiabetic patients with PAD ≥75 years of age, critical limb ischemia (RR, 3.70; 95% CI, 1.82-7.52) and NT-proBNP (RR, 1.93; 95% CI, 1.32-2.82); and in the 54 diabetic patients with PAD ≥75 years of age, hs-CRP (RR, 2.61; 95% CI, 1.45-4.67) and NT-proBNP (RR, 3.31; 95% CI, 1.96-5.60).

Conclusions.—Mortality rates at 5 years varied considerably among patients with PAD stratified according to age and diabetes. Predictors of death differed among the four patient subgroups in this study and included critical limb ischemia, hs-CRP, and NT-proBNP. Our results might help to develop future strategies for optimized treatment of hospitalized patients with symptomatic PAD.

▶ Treating clinicians are all versed in the overall mortality statistics of patients with peripheral arterial disease (PAD), and the worse the PAD, the higher the mortality, but not necessarily because of the limb that precipitated the patient's presentation. PAD is an overwhelming marker for systemic disease, and any therapy aimed at treating the limb dysfunction must include an overall assessment of the patient comorbidities, including cardiac and cerebrovascular disease. As with other disease states, there are degrees of severity: not all patients with PAD are the same. The 4 major categories studied in this well-done 5-year observational trial, namely patients with PAD who are older and those who are younger than 75 years and those with and without diabetes, stratified their respective 5-year mortality rates as expected: 10% for nondiabetics younger than 75 years, 23% for diabetics younger than 75, 38% for nondiabetics older than 75, and 52% for diabetics older than 75. Each of these rates was 2- to 3-fold greater than matched control patients without PAD. In each of the cohorts, there was an identifiable systemic marker that independently predicted mortality. This type of observational case-control study presents valuable natural history data and confirms the clinical suspicion that all PAD is not equal. Treatment strategies and the respective intensity with which they are applied should be altered based on the intrinsic risk for each subgroup. Risk reduction strategies should be more aggressive for higher-risk subgroups.

R. J. Feezor, MD, FACS

Endoscopic versus open saphenous vein graft harvest for lower extremity bypass in critical limb ischemia

Eid RE, Wang L, Kuzman M, et al (Univ of Pittsburgh Med Ctr, PA; Univ of Pittsburgh, PA)

J Vasc Surg 59:136-144, 2014

Objective.—Endoscopic vein harvest (EVH) has been demonstrated to improve early morbidity when compared with conventional open vein harvest (OVH) technique for infrainguinal bypass surgery. However, recent literature suggests conflicting results regarding mid- and long-term patency with EVH. The purpose of this study is to compare graft patency between harvest techniques specifically in patients with critical limb ischemia.

Methods.—This retrospective study compared two groups of patients (EVH = 39 and OVH = 49) undergoing lower extremity revascularization from January 2009 to December 2011. Outcome measures included patency rates, postoperative complications, and wound infection. Graft patency was assessed using Kaplan-Meier curves.

Results.—Both groups were matched for demographics and indications for bypass (critical limb ischemia). Median follow-up was 22 months. There was a significant reduction in the incidence of wound infection at the vein harvest site in the EVH group (OVH = 20%; EVH = 0%; $P < .001$), nevertheless, the difference was not significant when only the anastomotic sites were included (OVH = 12.2%; EVH = 15.4%; $P = .43$). The hospital length of stay was comparable between the two groups (EVH = 8.73 ± 9.69; OVH = 6.35 ± 3.28; $P = .26$) with no significant difference in the recovery time. Primary graft patency rate was 43.2% in the EVH group and 69.4% in the OVH group ($P = .007$) at 3 years. The most common reason for loss of primary patency was graft occlusion (61.5%) in the OVH group and vein graft stenosis (54.5%) in the EVH group. The average number of vascular reinterventions per bypass graft was significantly lower in the OVH group compared with the EVH group (OVH = 0.37; EVH = 1.28; $P < .001$).

Conclusions.—Our findings demonstrate inferior primary patency when using the technique of EVH. Additionally, we identified a significantly higher rate of reintervention in the EVH cohort as well as a higher rate of vein graft body stenosis. However, EVH was associated with a decreased rate of wound complications with similar limb salvage and secondary patency rates when compared to OVH. EVH should therefore be selectively utilized in patients at high risk for wound complications.

▶ Among the many systemic and local complications of open infrainguinal bypass surgery, wound infections and breakdown remain among the most prevalent. In an era of monitoring of in-patient length of stay and readmission rates, wound complications have the potential to have impact beyond the obvious patient disadvantage. Endoscopic vein harvest has gained popularity among cardiac surgeons and some vascular surgeons, but the initial short-term benefit of a decrease in wound infection rates has been offset by suggestions of a decline in long-term graft patency. Eid et al follow up with their series of 78 patients who underwent infrainguinal bypass for critical limb ischemia using saphenous vein conduit harvested by endoscopic methods (endoscopic vein harvest [EVH]) or traditional open vein harvest (OVH). Despite having EVH performed by an experienced surgeon, the operating times were nearly twice as long (392 vs 195 minutes; $P < .001$) and didn't reduce estimated blood loss. The postoperative length of stay was similar. The overall wound complication rate was similar between EVH and OVH, but the saphenectomy-specific wound complication rate was dramatically lower with EVH. Most notably, the bypass primary patency at 30 months was considerably better for OVH compared with EVH (69% vs 43%, $P = -.007$). The implication is that the perioperative trauma caused by EVH has deleterious long-term effects on the bypass graft. In interpreting these results, it should be noted that the operative technique used for Occupational Safety and Health was a single long incision. Perhaps the most prudent management is a middle ground: open surgical exposure with judicious use of "skip incisions" and paying close attention to saphenectomy dissection techniques, such as the avoidance of undermining skin flaps and meticulous attention to closure. This way, one can maintain the positive effects of OVH but minimize the wound complications.

R. J. Feezor, MD, FACS

Incidence, predictors, and prognosis of in-stent occlusion after endovascular treatment with nitinol stents for femoropopliteal lesions

Dohi T, Iida O, Soga Y, et al (Osaka Univ Graduate School of Medicine, Suita, Japan; Kansai Rosai Hosp Cardiovascular Ctr, Amagasaki, Japan; Kokura Memorial Hosp, Kitakyusyu, Japan; et al)

J Vasc Surg 59:1009-1015.e1, 2014

Objective.—Widespread use of self-expanding nitinol stent-based endovascular treatment (EVT) for femoropopliteal (FP) lesions has been fueled by its less-invasive nature and modest durability; however, prevalence, predictors and prognosis of in-stent occlusion are undefined and were investigated here.

Methods.—This study entailed a multicenter, retrospective analysis of a prospectively maintained database. Between January 2004 and December 2011, 2447 de novo FP lesions (mean length, 143 ± 87 mm; 52% chronic total occlusions) from 2008 patients (mean age, 73.0 ± 9.2 years; 71% male; 61% diabetics; 32% critical limb ischemia; and 24% on hemodialysis) were treated with nitinol stent-based EVT. Study outcome was in-stent occlusion: rates (1, 3, and 5 years), predictors and association with limb prognosis.

Results.—In-stent occlusion rate was 5.2%, 11.2%, and 16.4% at 1, 3, and 5 years, respectively (mean follow-up, 2.3 ± 1.7 years). Female sex, critical limb ischemia, and Transatlantic Inter-Society Consensus II class C/D (multivariate Cox proportional hazard ratio [HR], 1.75, 1.49, and 3.34, respectively) were independent predictors of in-stent occlusion after FP stenting, which was associated with poor limb prognosis (major amputation, HR 6.35; major adverse limb event, major adverse limb event, HR, 21.1).

Conclusions.—Moderate in-stent occlusion rates were observed after nitinol stent-based EVT. Closer attention is warranted with high-risk cases because of poorer limb prognosis.

► Registry data often are more insightful than initial clinical trials because of the inclusion of what is typically felt to be "real world" scenarios and patients.

This 13-center registry examined the outcomes of 3623 limbs treated for de novo femoropopliteal occlusive disease, of which, 2447 (70%) were stented. More than three-fourths of these procedures were performed using a single commercially available stent. The authors reported an in-stent occlusion rate of 8.2% at over 2 years, but the patient follow-up dramatically declined after 1 year. The clinical factors predictive of in-stent occlusion were predictable: women had more severe presenting symptoms and worse anatomic disease. Although 87% of stent occlusions were successfully treated with remedial endovascular therapy, stent occlusion remained a major risk for amputation. Taken together, the conclusions are not novel but still worthwhile: stents in the femoropopliteal artery are effective and associated with acceptable patency. By virtue of the registry itself, there remain several unanswered questions, including (1) what lesion(s) truly deserve stenting as opposed to, for example, angioplasty or atherectomy; (2) are there differences in the outcomes of different stents; and perhaps most important, (3) do stents serve any detrimental role for future revascularization compared with angioplasty alone?

R. J. Feezor, MD, FACS

Outcomes of endovascular lower extremity interventions depend more on indication than physician specialty

Wallace JR, Yuo T, Marone L, et al (Univ of Pittsburgh Med Ctr, PA)
J Vasc Surg 59:376-383.e3, 2014

Objective.—Outcomes of endovascular lower extremity interventions (eLEIs) have been recently linked to provider specialty; however, the indication for intervention was not examined. We sought to compare outcomes between specialties performing eLEI for different indications, in a recent statewide inpatient discharge dataset.

Methods.—The Florida hospital discharge data from 2005 to 2009 were reviewed for patients with LEI during hospitalization. We assigned provider specialty as interventional radiology (IR), interventional cardiology (IC), or vascular surgery (VS) based on provider-associated procedures. Clinical indication was claudication or critical limb ischemia (CLI). We limited our analysis to patients without concomitant open surgery during hospitalization. We compared mortality, length of stay (LOS), major use of intensive care unit (ICU), discharge disposition, and total charges between specialties with regression models, both unadjusted and adjusted for demographic and clinical characteristics.

Results.—A total of 15,398 patients (47% with CLI) had an eLEI. Clinical indication was significantly associated with provider type ($P < .001$) and outcomes. VS and IR were more likely than IC to treat CLI patients (VS 59%, IR 65%, IC 26%; $P < .001$). IC performed the majority of procedures on claudicants (VS 30%, IC 57%, IR 13%; $P < .001$), while VS performed the majority of procedures on CLI patients (VS 50%, IC

23%, IR 27%; $P < .001$). Adjusted analyses demonstrated no difference in mortality rates between the three specialties (odds ratio [OR] VS: reference, IR: 1.24, IC: 0.79; $P = \text{NS}$ for both). However, compared with VS, IR-treated patients were less likely to be discharged home (OR, 0.74; $P < .001$), LOS was longer (β, 1.16 days; $P < .001$), major ICU use was more common (OR, 1.49; $P < .001$), and total charges were higher (β, $341; $P = .001$). CLI predicted poorer results for all outcomes: death (OR, 4.19; $P < .001$), discharge home (OR, 0.50; $P < .001$), increased LOS (β, 3.26 days; $P < .001$), major ICU use (OR, 1.95; $P < .001$), and total charges (β, $18,730; $P < .001$).

Conclusions.—The majority of eLEI done by VS are for CLI, whereas the majority of patients treated by IC are claudicants. Although provider specialty does correlate with several clinical results, the clinical indication for eLEI is a stronger predictor of adverse outcomes. Future analyses of eLEI should adjust for clinical indication.

▶ A recently much-maligned article published in a specialty journal indicted vascular surgeons as having inferior outcomes after endovascular interventions to treat peripheral arterial disease. Naturally, the societal response was appropriate outrage, as the publication did not account for procedural indications in its analysis, among other methodologic flaws. In contrast, this state hospital discharge data review reveals 2 relevant findings: the portion of "market share" formerly controlled by interventional radiologists is being transitioned to vascular surgeons while that under control by interventional cardiology remains stable and, more clinically relevant, interventional cardiologists overwhelmingly treat less-severe peripheral arterial disease than radiology/vascular surgeons. Hence, despite the effort to show specialty-specific outcome data, the outcomes will continue to be dictated by the patients treated. In all reality, there are varying levels of skill and judgment in any specialty, and hopefully all continue to strive for improvement.

R. J. Feezor, MD, FACS

Endovascular-first approach is not associated with worse amputation-free survival in appropriately selected patients with critical limb ischemia

Garg K, Kaszubski PA, Moridzadeh R, et al (New York Univ School of Medicine)

J Vasc Surg 59:392-399, 2014

Objective.—Endovascular interventions for critical limb ischemia are associated with inferior limb salvage (LS) rates in most randomized trials and large series. This study examined the long-term outcomes of selective use of endovascular-first (endo-first) and open-first strategies in 302 patients from March 2007 to December 2010.

Methods.—Endo-first was selected if (1) the patient had short (5-cm to 7-cm occlusions or stenoses in crural vessels); (2) the disease in the superficial femoral artery was limited to TransAtlantic Inter-Society Consensus II A, B, or C; and (3) no impending limb loss. Endo-first was performed in 187 (62%), open-first in 105 (35%), and 10 (3%) had hybrid procedures.

Results.—The endo-first group was older, with more diabetes and tissue loss. Bypass was used more to infrapopliteal targets (70% vs 50%, $P=.031$). The 5-year mortality was similar (open, 48%; endo, 42%; $P=.107$). Secondary procedures (endo or open) were more common after open-first (open, 71 of 105 [68%] vs endo, 102 of 187 [55%]; $P=.029$). Compared with open-first, the 5-year LS rate for endo-first was 85% vs 83% ($P=.586$), and amputation-free survival (AFS) was 45% vs 50% ($P=.785$). Predictors of death were age >75 years (hazard ratio [HR], 3.3; 95% confidence interval [CI], 1.7-6.6; $P=.0007$), end-stage renal disease (ESRD) (HR, 3.4; 95% CI, 2.1-5.6; $P<.0001$), and prior stroke (HR, 1.6; 95% CI, 1.03-2.3; $P=.036$). Predictors of limb loss were ESRD (HR, 2.5; 95% CI, 1.2-5.4; $P=.015$) and below-the-knee intervention ($P=.041$). Predictors of worse AFS were older age (HR, 2.03; 95% CI, 1.13-3.7; $P=.018$), ESRD (HR, 3.2; 95% CI, 2.1-5.11; $P<.0001$), prior stroke ($P=.0054$), and gangrene ($P=.024$).

Conclusions.—At 5 years, endo-first and open-first revascularization strategies had equivalent LS rates and AFS in patients with critical limb ischemia when properly selected. A patient-centered approach with close surveillance improves long-term outcomes for both open and endo approaches.

▶ Defining the exact role for endovascular attempts at revascularization will be one of the greatest unanswered challenges in the treatment of peripheral arterial disease. Clearly, if there were equivalent clinical results, the minimally invasive nature of endovascular revascularization would support its unanimous adoption. As the techniques become more disruptive of the native vessel with barotrauma (angioplasty), permanent intimal disruption (stent) or intimomedial excision (atherectomy), the immediate visual results may indeed improve; however, the long-term results are still debated. Most alarming, there is longstanding concern that future open surgical revascularization options are made more challenging or potentially impossible because of prior endovascular interventions. The authors report no decline in limb salvage or amputation-free survival among patients with an "endo first" approach. However, what they actually show is that their clinical selection criteria are reasonable and likely appropriate. Patients with nonimminent limb threat who have anything short of TransAtlantic Inter-Society Consensus II D lesions can safely undergo endovascular attempts at revascularization as a first-line approach. An interesting follow-up study would be the fate of patients who did not respond to endovascular interventions and a comparison with patients with similar clinical presentations who were treated with open surgery first. The true test, clearly, would be a randomized study between endovascular revascularization first (and maybe second, third, and so on) and open surgical bypass.

R. J. Feezor, MD, FACS

Atherectomy offers no benefits over balloon angioplasty in tibial interventions for critical limb ischemia

Todd KE Jr, Ahanchi SS, Maurer CA, et al (Eastern Virginia Med School, Norfolk, VA)

J Vasc Surg 58:941-948, 2013

Background.—Endovascular adjuncts, like atherectomy, were developed to improve outcomes of endovascular arterial interventions. The true impact of atherectomy on endovascular outcomes remains to be determined, and little data exist on the influence of atherectomy on tibial interventions. Our study compares early and late outcomes of tibial intervention with angioplasty vs atherectomy-assisted interventions.

Methods.—We completed a retrospective review of all tibial interventions between 2008 and 2010. Outcomes were analyzed using single and multivariate analysis, Cox regression, and Kaplan-Meier curves. Primary outcomes were primary, primary assisted, and secondary patency rates, as well as limb salvage and survival rates.

Results.—Over a 2-year period, 480 tibial interventions were completed for 421 patients. Eighty-seven percent (n = 418) of interventions were performed for critical limb ischemia (CLI) and 13% (n = 62) for claudication. The CLI cohort of 418 interventions was analyzed. These patients had a mean age of 71 years with a mean follow-up time of 16 ± 15 months (range, 0-59 months). Of the 418 interventions, 339 underwent percutaneous transluminal angioplasty (PTA): 333 PTA alone, six PTA + stent. The remaining 79 interventions received atherectomy: 33 laser, 13 directional, and 33 orbital either alone or in conjunction with PTA (11 atherectomy only, 68 atherectomy + PTA). The groups did not differ significantly in terms of demographics, risk factors, or technical success. The atherectomy group had more TASC B lesions (54% vs 38%; $P = .013$), while the PTA-alone group had more TASC D lesions (25% vs 13%; $P = .004$). TASC A and C lesions did not differ significantly between the groups. No significant differences existed with respect to the early (30-day) outcomes of loss of patency (11% vs 13%; $P = .699$), complications (8% vs 13%; $P = .292$), or major amputation (17% vs 13%; $P = .344$) in the PTA-alone group vs the atherectomy-assisted group. Kaplan-Meier analysis revealed no difference for all primary outcomes of PTA alone vs the atherectomy-assisted group at 12 and 36 months: primary patency (69%, 55% vs 61%, 46%; $P = .158$), primary assisted patency (83%, 71% vs 85%, 67%; $P = .801$), secondary patency (94%, 89% vs 95%, 89%; $P = .892$), limb salvage (79%, 70% vs 81%, 77%; $P = .485$), or survival (77%, 56% vs 80%, 50%; $P = .944$).

Conclusions.—The adjunctive use of atherectomy offered no improvement in primary outcomes over PTA alone in either early or late outcomes in CLI patients who underwent endovascular tibial interventions.

Considering the additional cost and increased procedural time, these findings put into question the routine use of adjunctive atherectomy.

▶ Tibial artery interventions, open or endovascular, are the most challenging interventions performed for the treatment of lower-extremity atherosclerosis, with patency rates most vascular surgeons would like to improve. The desire to find adjunctive technologies that would improve simple angioplasty is, therefore, understandable. This retrospective review, however, clearly shows that atherectomy does not provide the answer to the problem. Certainly the authors concede that the definitive answer can only be provided by a large, randomized, prospective trial, but they offer compelling evidence that the extra costs of atherectomy in money and time are not currently justified.

P. W. White, MD, FACS

Vascular Quality of Life Questionnaire-6 facilitates health-related quality of life assessment in peripheral arterial disease

Nordanstig J, Wann-Hansson C, Karlsson J, et al (Sahlgrenska Univ Hosp and Academy, Gothenburg, Sweden; Malmö Univ, Sweden; Örebro Univ Hosp, Sweden; et al)

J Vasc Surg 59:700-707.e1, 2014

Background.—Most commonly used outcome measures in peripheral arterial disease (PAD) provide scarce information about achieved patient benefit. Therefore, patient-reported outcome measures have become increasingly important as complementary outcome measures. The abundance of items in most health-related quality of life instruments makes everyday clinical use difficult. This study aimed to develop a short version of the 25-item Vascular Quality of Life Questionnaire (VascuQoL-25), a PAD-specific health-related quality of life instrument.

Methods.—The study recruited 129 individuals with intermittent claudication and 71 with critical limb ischemia from two university hospitals. Participants were a mean age of 70 ± 9 years, and 57% were men. All patients completed the original VascuQoL when evaluated for treatment, and 127 also completed the questionnaire 6 months after a vascular procedure. The VascuQoL-25 was reduced based on cognitive interviews and psychometric testing. The short instrument, the VascuQoL-6, was tested using item-response theory, exploring structure, precision, item fit, and targeting. A subgroup of 21 individuals with intermittent claudication was also tested correlating the results of VascuQoL-6 to the actual walking capacity, as measured using global positioning system technology.

Results.—On the basis of structured psychometric testing, the six most informative items were selected (VascuQoL-6) and tested vs the original VascuQoL-25. The correlation between VascuQoL-25 and VascuQoL-6 was $r = 0.88$ before intervention, $r = 0.96$ after intervention, and the difference was $r = 0.91$ ($P < .001$). The Cronbach α for the VascuQoL-6 was .85 before and .94 after intervention. Cognitive interviews indicated that the responders considered all six items to be relevant and comprehensible. Rasch analysis was used to reduce response options from seven (VascuQoL-25) to four (VascuQoL-6). VascuQol-6 was shown to have high precision and discriminative properties. Item fit was excellent, with both "infit" and "outfit" between 0.7 and 1.3 for all six items. The standardized response mean after intervention was 1.15, indicating good responsiveness to clinical change. VascuQoL-6 results correlated strongly ($r = 0.72$; $P < .001$) with the actual measured walking ability ($n = 21$).

Conclusions.—VascuQoL-6 is a valid and responsive instrument for the assessment of health-related quality of life in PAD. The main advantage is the compact format that offers a possibility for routine use in busy clinical settings.

▶ Not having a doctorate in statistics, I was somewhat intimidated by the analysis of the results in this study. Nevertheless, the authors present and validate an excellent, easy-to-use and easy-to-complete quality-of-life questionnaire designed specifically for patients with peripheral artery disease.

Although amputation-free survival and noninvasive vascular testing are commonly used to assess outcomes in peripheral artery disease patients, these outcomes do not address the patient's own perception of their disease. The previously validated Vascular Quality of Life (VascuQoL) questionnaire[1] included 25 questions with 7 potential answers to each. Here, the authors consolidate their VascuQoL-6 questionnaire to 6 questions with 4 choices to each question. The questions assess each of the domains of the previous questionnaire: pain, symptoms, activities, social, and emotional, and, importantly, the mean time taken to complete the VascuQoL-6 was significantly less than that of the VascuQoL-25 (1.4 vs 9.6 minutes; $P < .001$).

This validated, abbreviated questionnaire is an excellent, concise tool for assessing a patient's perception of his or her disease and can be used to assess the effectiveness of intervention. The questionnaire is included in the article Appendix, and permission for its use can be obtained by contacting Dr Morgan.

B. Peterson, MD, FACS

Reference

1. Morgan MB, Crayford T, Murrin B, Fraser SC. Developing the Vascular Quality of Life Questionnaire: a new disease-specific quality of life measure for use in lower limb ischemia. *J Vasc Surg*. 2001;33:679-687.

Early graft failure after infrainguinal arterial bypass

Soma G, Greenblatt DY, Nelson MT, et al (Univ of Wisconsin School of Medicine & Public Health, Madison)

Surgery 155:300-310, 2014

Introduction.—Early graft failure (EGF), defined as failure within 30 days of an index procedure, is a serious complication after infrainguinal arterial bypass. EGF has not been examined by the use of national data since the widespread adoption of percutaneous treatments for arterial occlusive disease.

Methods.—We used data from the American College of Surgeons National Surgical Quality Improvement Program. Patients who underwent infrainguinal arterial bypass from 2005 to 2011 were selected from the American College of Surgeons National Surgical Quality Improvement Program database. The frequency of 30-day EGF was determined. Univariate and multivariate analyses evaluated risk factors for EGF.

Results.—Of 23,468 patients who underwent open infrainguinal arterial bypass, 1,065 (4.5%) had EGF. Patients who had EGF were more likely to have a prolonged duration of stay (34.8% vs 12.0%, $P < .001$), greater rates of reoperation (82.1% vs 14.3%, $P < .001$) and increased 30-day mortality (5.1% vs 2.1%, $P < .001$). The rate of additional complications in patients who experienced EGF was 42.0%, compared with 25.4% in those who did not have EGF ($P < .001$). Patients who experienced complications in addition to EGF were more likely to have complications after graft failure (69.5% vs 31.3%). In multivariable analysis, EGF was associated with younger age, female sex, black race, obesity, thrombocytosis, increased international normalized ratio, femoral-to-tibial bypass, prosthetic graft, and emergent operation.

Conclusion.—The incidence of EGF after open lower extremity arterial bypass has not increased in an era of increased use of percutaneous techniques. Nevertheless, EGF occurs in almost 5% of patients and is strongly associated with additional complications and mortality. Identifying patients at risk for EGF may facilitate modification of contributing factors. Diminishing the incidence of graft occlusion will lead to decreased morbidity and mortality in this cohort of patients.

► In this detailed American College of Surgeon National Surgical Quality Improvement Program study, Soma et al soberly remind us of the consequences of early graft failure after infrainguinal bypass. Two novel findings are the identification that prosthetic grafts carry an almost 30% association with early graft failure and that duration of operation greater than 6 hours is also associated with a greater likelihood of early graft failure.

The finding that diabetes mellitus was not associated with early graft failure but rather had a marginally inverse association fit well with my own evidence-based bias. Indeed, an increased graft patency in diabetics was also identified by Pomposelli et al[1] in their landmark series involving more than a thousand dorsalis pedis bypasses in a primarily diabetic population.

The authors' expert demonstration that early graft failure leads to additional postoperative complications—most commonly infectious but also including myocardial infarction and cardiac arrest—is a timely reminder to practicing vascular surgeons that careful patient selection remains paramount for infrainguinal bypass. Furthermore, consideration of endovascular intervention and perhaps even primary amputation should be explored for the candidate presenting with severe claudication or critical limb ischemia. In this deliberation, I would argue that routine relegation of diabetes mellitus as a negative risk factor is no longer justifiable.[2]

K. Hughes, MD, FACS

References

1. Pomposelli FB, Kansal N, Hamdan AD, et al. A decade of experience with dorsalis pedis artery bypass: analysis of outcome in more than 1000 cases. *J Vasc Surg.* 2003;37:307-315.
2. Hughes K, Padilla L, Al-Zubeidy B, et al. Diabetes is not associated with an increased peri-operative mortality or non-infectious morbidity following lower extremity arterial reconstruction. *Am J Surg.* 2014;207:573-577.

Determinants of Outcome after Endovascular Therapy for Critical Limb Ischemia with Tissue Loss

Meltzer AJ, Evangelisti G, Graham AR, et al (New York–Presbyterian Hosp)
Ann Vasc Surg 28:144-151, 2014

Background.—In this study we examine outcomes of endovascular therapy for critical limb ischemia with tissue loss and identify risk factors for failure of endovascular therapy across a panel of outcome metrics.

Methods.—A retrospective review (2006–2010) of patients undergoing endovascular therapy for critical limb ischemia with tissue loss provided data for multivariate models of overall survival, amputation-free survival, limb salvage (LS), and wound healing.

Results.—One hundred six patients underwent endovascular therapy for Rutherford class 5 (88%) or class 6 (12%) ischemia with ulceration and/or gangrene of the heel (15%), forefoot (16%), toe(s) (43%), calf/ankle (11%), or multiple locations (15%). Sustained limb salvage at 1 year was 87%. One-year overall survival and amputation-free survival were 65% and 49%, respectively. Multivariate regression models identified independent risk factors for reduced primary patency: Rutherford 6 ischemia ($P = 0.008$; HR 4.7 [95% confidence interval 1.5–14.8]) and infrapopliteal intervention ($P = 0.03$; HR 2.58 [95% CI 1.08–6.14]). Rutherford class 6 ischemia was independently associated with reduced assisted patency ($P = 0.004$; HR 5.39 [95% CI 1.74–16.73]). Wound healing was adversely affected by diabetes ($P = 0.02$; HR 7.0 [95% CI 1.4–36.2]), continued smoking ($P = 0.04$; HR 5.3 [95% CI 1.1–26.3]), and patency loss ($P = 0.04$; HR 4.8 [95% CI 1.1–22.30]). Rutherford class 6 ischemia was independently associated with reduced limb salvage

($P < 0.0001$; HR 35.1 [95% CI 5.4–231.2]) and amputation-free survival ($P = 0.007$; HR 3.61 [95% CI 1.4–9.18]), in addition to COPD ($P = 0.01$; 3.58 [95% 1.28–9.55]). Independent predictors of poor overall survival included end-stage renal disease ($P = 0.03$; HR 2.99 [95% CI 1.1–8.05]), history of angina ($P = 0.02$; HR 5.08 [95% CI 1.28–20.29]), and COPD ($P = 0.001$; HR 3.77 [95% CI 1.76–8.34]).

Conclusions.—Both increasing severity of tissue loss as well as the presence of severe medical comorbidities are associated with poorer outcomes of endovascular therapy in these patients. Although sustained limb salvage in patients with tissue loss may be achieved with endovascular therapy, this is due to poor overall survival and a competing mortality hazard.

▶ This report focuses on the dilemma that continually faces vascular/endovascular surgeons: the fact that patients who need an operation the most are often the least able to tolerate that specific operation. Meltzer et al soberly draw our attention to another rather troubling conundrum: the fact that many of the same comorbidities associated with adverse outcomes after surgical bypass are also associated with failure of endovascular therapy. The authors show that the seemingly encouraging limb salvage rate of 87% at 1 year after endovascular therapy for critical limb ischemia is achieved only because one-third of the patients are dead in 1 year—with a 1-year amputation-free survival rate of only 49%.

It is most appropriate that this study should come from this particular group of authors, as a previous report from the same institution (and several of the same authors) strongly advocated the endovascular-first approach for limb salvage revascularization.[1] Those of us who use the endovascular-first approach (author included) should take appropriate caution: this philosophy may not always lead to ultimate limb salvage, particularly for patients with severe tissue loss as well as those with severe medical comorbidities. But are these same patients with severe medical comorbidities not the very ones for whom surgical bypass often pose prohibitive risks? Thus, the vascular conundrum continues.

K. Hughes, MD, FACS

Reference

1. DeRubertis BG. Shifting paradigms in the treatment of lower extremity vascular disease. *Ann Surg*. 2007;246:415-424.

Correlation of Patient-reported Symptom Outcomes and Treadmill Test Outcomes after Treatment for Aortoiliac Claudication

Murphy TP, Reynolds MR, Cohen DJ, et al (Rhode Island Hosp, Providence, RI; Beth Israel Deaconess Med Ctr, Boston, MA; Univ of Missouri-Kansas City, MO; et al)

J Vasc Interv Radiol 24:1427-1435, 2013

Purpose.—To examine the relationship between objective treadmill test outcomes and subjective symptom outcomes among patients with claudication treated with stent revascularization (ST) compared with supervised exercise (SE).

Materials and Methods.—Five scales of the Peripheral Artery Questionnaire and Walking Impairment Questionnaire were correlated with peak walking time and treadmill claudication onset time.

Results.—The correlation between change in disease-specific quality of life (QOL) and change in peak walking time differed according to treatment group, with statistically significant correlations for all five scales for the ST group and weaker trends for the SE group, only one of which was statistically significant. In contrast, improvements in disease-specific QOL correlated well with increases in claudication onset time, with no significant interaction with treatment group for any of the five scales.

Conclusions.—Disease-specific QOL results at 6 months in the Claudication: Exercise Vs. Endoluminal Revascularization (CLEVER) study show that improved maximal treadmill walking in patients with claudication treated with SE correlated poorly with self-reported symptom relief. Conversely, patients treated with ST showed good correlation between improved maximal treadmill walking and self-reported symptom improvement. The correlation between claudication onset time and self-reported symptom relief was good across treatment groups. This finding indicates that traditional objective treadmill test outcomes may not correlate well with symptom relief in patients with claudication. Future studies should investigate these data and improve understanding of patient relevance of traditional objective treadmill-based treatment outcomes.

► This post hoc analysis probes the still-unexplained findings of the CLEVER (Claudication: Exercise vs Endoluminal Revascularization) Study[1]: that although both supervised exercise and stenting for aortoiliac claudicants led to significant benefits in treadmill walking and symptoms, stenting achieved superior symptom-related outcomes, whereas exercise led to greater improvement in peak walking times (PWT). Murphy et al bring increased clarification by showing that although there is a correlation between patient-perceived symptom-related outcomes and PWT for the individual stent patient (as well as the stenting cohort in the study), a specific correlation between PWT and symptom improvement for the patient undergoing supervised exercise actually does not exist (although a correlation exists for the supervised exercise cohort). In addition to serving as a reminder that the mechanisms by which exercise therapy leads to symptomatic improvement for claudication remain to be fully elucidated, the report also calls into question whether PWT should be regarded as the gold standard endpoint in claudication studies.[2] In this report, claudication onset time was much more reliably correlated with symptom relief.

An interesting suggestion by the authors is that careful elicitation of patient preferences for functional versus symptomatic benefit could help individualize decision making for patients with claudication. I, for one, am not quite sure if practicing vascular surgeons/specialists are ready to begin recommending stenting for patients primarily interested in symptom relief and supervised exercise for those primarily interested in functional benefit. But then, of course, time will tell.

K. Hughes, MD, FACS

References

1. Murphy TP, Cutlip DE, Regensteiner JG, et al. Supervised exercise versus primary stenting for claudication resulting from aortoiliac peripheral artery disease: six-month outcomes from the claudication: exercise versus endoluminal revascularization (CLEVER) study. *Circulation.* 2012;125:130-139.
2. Hiatt WR, Hirsch AT, Regensteiner JG, Brass EP. Clinical trials for claudication. Assessment of exercise performance, functional status, and clinical end points. Vascular clinical trialists. *Circulation.* 1995;92:614-621.

Outcomes of endovascular lower extremity interventions depend more on indication than physician specialty

Wallace JR, Yuo T, Marone L, et al (Univ of Pittsburgh Med Ctr, PA)
J Vasc Surg 59:376-383.e3, 2014

Objective.—Outcomes of endovascular lower extremity interventions (eLEIs) have been recently linked to provider specialty; however, the indication for intervention was not examined. We sought to compare outcomes between specialties performing eLEI for different indications, in a recent statewide inpatient discharge dataset.

Methods.—The Florida hospital discharge data from 2005 to 2009 were reviewed for patients with LEI during hospitalization. We assigned provider specialty as interventional radiology (IR), interventional cardiology (IC), or vascular surgery (VS) based on provider-associated procedures. Clinical indication was claudication or critical limb ischemia (CLI). We limited our analysis to patients without concomitant open surgery during hospitalization. We compared mortality, length of stay (LOS), major use of intensive care unit (ICU), discharge disposition, and total charges between specialties with regression models, both unadjusted and adjusted for demographic and clinical characteristics.

Results.—A total of 15,398 patients (47% with CLI) had an eLEI. Clinical indication was significantly associated with provider type ($P < .001$) and outcomes. VS and IR were more likely than IC to treat CLI patients (VS 59%, IR 65%, IC 26%; $P < .001$). IC performed the majority of procedures on claudicants (VS 30%, IC 57%, IR 13%; $P < .001$), while VS performed the majority of procedures on CLI patients (VS 50%, IC 23%, IR 27%; $P < .001$). Adjusted analyses demonstrated no difference in mortality rates between the three specialties (odds ratio [OR] VS: reference, IR: 1.24, IC: 0.79; $P =$ NS for both). However, compared with VS, IR-treated patients were less likely to be discharged home (OR, 0.74;

$P < .001$), LOS was longer (β, 1.16 days; $P < .001$), major ICU use was more common (OR, 1.49; $P < .001$), and total charges were higher (β, $341; $P = .001$). CLI predicted poorer results for all outcomes: death (OR, 4.19; $P < .001$), discharge home (OR, 0.50; $P < .001$), increased LOS (b, 3.26 days; $P < .001$), major ICU use (OR, 1.95; $P < .001$), and total charges (β, $18,730; $P < .001$).

Conclusions.—The majority of eLEI done by VS are for CLI, whereas the majority of patients treated by IC are claudicants. Although provider specialty does correlate with several clinical results, the clinical indication for eLEI is a stronger predictor of adverse outcomes. Future analyses of eLEI should adjust for clinical indication.

▶ This study is seemingly largely conducted as a response to an article previously published by Zafar et al, suggesting that vascular surgeons have poorer outcomes than interventional radiologists and interventional cardiologists when performing endovascular lower extremity interventions (eLEIs).[1] In this study, the authors clearly show that outcomes after eLEIs are more closely related to the clinical indications for intervention rather than physician specialty.

Analyzing the Florida Agency for Health Care Administration hospital inpatient data from 2005 to 2009, a cohort of 15 398 patients undergoing eLEIs was studied. Univariate analysis found that critical limb ischemia (CLI), as opposed to claudication, significantly led to poorer outcomes in all endpoints: in-hospital mortality, length of stay, discharge disposition (home vs not home), major intensive care use, and total hospital charges—independent of provider specialty. Clearly, clinical indication is a confounder that the prior study ignored and justifies the use of a multivariable regression model to evaluate outcomes after eLEIs, as is done in this article.

Vascular surgeons treated as many patients with CLI as the other 2 groups combined, whereas interventional cardiologists performed most eLEIs in claudicants (57%). Using multivariable regression to control for the confounding of clinical indication, outcomes were clearly more closely related to clinical indication for intervention rather than physician specialty. This study invalidates the results of the prior study by showing that analyzing outcomes by provider specialty without adjusting for clinical indication (patients with CLI are naturally going to have poorer outcomes than patients with claudication) leads to bias and suggests that future eLEI studies need to control for clinical indication.

B. Peterson, MD, FACS

Reference

1. Zafar AM, Dhangana R, Murphy TP, et al. Lower-extremity endovascular interventions for Medicare beneficiaries: comparative effectiveness as a function of provider specialty. *J Vasc Interv Radiol.* 2012;23:3-9.e1–14.

Effect of Progenitor Cell Mobilization With Granulocyte-Macrophage Colony-Stimulating Factor in Patients With Peripheral Artery Disease: A Randomized Clinical Trial

Poole J, Mavromatis K, Binongo JN, et al (Emory Univ School of Medicine, Atlanta, GA; Atlanta Veterans Affairs Med Ctr, Decatur, GA; Emory Univ, Atlanta, GA; et al)

JAMA 310:2631-2639, 2013

Importance.—Many patients with peripheral artery disease (PAD) have walking impairment despite therapy. Experimental studies in animals demonstrate improved perfusion in ischemic hind limb after mobilization of bone marrow progenitor cells (PCs), but whether this is effective in patients with PAD is unknown.

Objective.—To investigate whether therapy with granulocyte-macrophage colony-stimulating factor (GM-CSF) improves exercise capacity in patients with intermittent claudication.

Design, Setting, and Participants.—In a phase 2 double-blind, placebo-controlled study, 159 patients (median [SD] age, 64 [8] years; 87% male, 37% with diabetes) with intermittent claudication were enrolled at medical centers affiliated with Emory University in Atlanta, Georgia, between January 2010 and July 2012.

Interventions.—Participants were randomized (1:1) to received 4 weeks of subcutaneous injections of GM-CSF (leukine), 500 μg/day 3 times a week, or placebo. Both groups were encouraged to walk to claudication daily.

Main Outcomes and Measures.—The primary outcome was peak treadmill walking time (PWT) at 3 months. Secondary outcomes were PWT at 6 months and changes in circulating PC levels, ankle brachial index (ABI), and walking impairment questionnaire (WIQ) and 36-item Short-Form Health Survey (SF-36) scores.

Results.—Of the 159 patients randomized, 80 were assigned to the GM-CSF group. The mean (SD) PWT at 3 months increased in the GM-CSF group from 296 (151) seconds to 405 (248) seconds (mean change, 109 seconds [95% CI, 67 to 151]) and in the placebo group from 308 (161) seconds to 376 (182) seconds (change of 56 seconds [95% CI, 14 to 98]), but this difference was not significant (mean difference in change in PWT, 53 seconds [95% CI, −6 to 112], P =.08). At 3 months, compared with placebo, GM-CSF improved the physical functioning subscore of the SF-36 questionnaire by 11.4 (95% CI, 6.7 to 16.1) vs 4.8 (95% CI, −0.1 to 9.6), with a mean difference in change for GM-CSF vs placebo of 7.5 (95% CI, 1.0 to 14.0; P =.03). Similarly, the distance score of the WIQ improved by 12.5 (95% CI, 6.4 to 18.7) vs 4.8 (95% CI, −0.2 to 9.8) with GM-CSF compared with placebo (mean difference in change, 7.9 [95% CI, 0.2 to 15.7], P =.047). There were no significant differences in the ABI, WIQ distance and speed scores, claudication onset time, or mental or physical component scores of the SF-36 between the groups.

Conclusions and Relevance.—Therapy with GM-CSF 3 times a week did not improve treadmill walking performance at the 3-month follow-up. The improvements in some secondary outcomes with GM-CSF suggest that it may warrant further study in patients with claudication.

Trial Registration.—clinicaltrials.gov Identifier: NCT01041417.

▶ Progenitor cell (PC) therapy, for the promotion of angiogenesis, in the treatment of peripheral arterial disease is an active area of ongoing investigation that carries considerable promise. The outcomes from clinical trials, however, are equivocal. Unfortunately, this well-conducted trial was unable to show a clear benefit, at least in peak walking times at 3 months for patients with moderate to severe angiographically proven claudication. Claudication onset time, considered by some to be more reliably correlated with symptom relief,[1] was also not significantly improved when the PC group was compared with the placebo group.

The CLEVER (Claudication: Exercise vs Endoluminal Revascularization) Trial suggested that revascularization may lead to improved subjective patient-perceived symptom improvement, whereas supervised exercise therapy may lead to improvement in objective treadmill peak walking times.[2] In light of this finding, the fact that PC therapy led to the improvement of some subjective parameters (ie, the distance score of the Walking Impairment Questionnaire and the physical functioning subscore of the Short Form—36) is quite encouraging.

I agree with the authors that additional studies are clearly needed in this area. My hope is that future claudication trials will also compare PC therapy with supervised exercise therapy and standard revascularization techniques.

K. Hughes, MD, FACS

References

1. Murphy TP, Reynolds MR, Cohen DJ, et al. Correlation of patient-reported symptom outcomes and treadmill test outcomes after treatment for aortoiliac claudication. *J Vasc Interv Radiol.* 2013;24:1427-1435.
2. Murphy TP, Cutlip DE, Regensteiner JG, et al. Supervised exercise versus primary stenting for claudication resulting from aortoiliac peripheral artery disease: six-month outcomes from the claudication: exercise versus endoluminal revascularization (CLEVER) study. *Circulation.* 2012;125:130-139.

10 Upper Extremity Ischemia/Dialysis Access

Percutaneous Angioplasty Using a Paclitaxel-Coated Balloon Improves Target Lesion Restenosis on Inflow Lesions of Autogenous Radiocephalic Fistulas: A Pilot Study

Lai C-C, Fang H-C, Tseng C-J, et al (Kaohsiung Veterans General Hosp, Taiwan; Natl Yang-Ming Univ, Taipei; et al)

J Vasc Interv Radiol 25:535-541, 2014

Purpose.—To determine whether the use of a paclitaxel-coated balloon (PCB) improves patency in patients undergoing percutaneous transluminal angioplasty (PTA) for recurrent juxtaanastomotic stenosis of radiocephalic arteriovenous fistulas (RCAVFs).

Material and Methods.—This prospective study recruited hemodialysis patients with two short (<2 cm) and separated inflow RCAVF lesions. After dilation of lesions using a 4-mm plain balloon (PB), half of the lesions were randomly selected for treatment with PTA using PCB (size, 4 mm; length, 2 cm) and PB (size, 5-mm or 6-mm) (group 1), and the other half were treated with PTA using PB alone (group 2). After the index PTA, dysfunction-driven angiography was performed to confirm target lesion restenosis (TLR). TLR and lesion patency were compared in the two groups by χ^2 test, *t* test, and Kaplan-Meier analysis.

Results.—The analysis of 20 lesions in 10 patients revealed that the TLR-free duration in group 1 was significantly longer than the TLR-free duration in group 2 (251.2 d vs 103.2 d; $P < .01$). The patency rate of the target lesion was significantly higher in group 1 than in group 2 at 6 months (70% vs 0%; $P < .01$) but not at 12 months (20% vs 0%; $P > .05$).

Conclusions.—This early study suggests that, for improving short-term patency, PTA with PCB and PB is more effective than PTA with PB alone, warranting further study.

► Arteriovenous fistulas (AVFs) are regarded as the vascular access of choice for hemodialysis. Juxta-anastomotic venous stenosis is a frequent complication of radiocephalic AVF (RCAVF) dysfunction or nonmaturation, which is commonly treated by balloon percutaneous transluminal angioplasty (PTA). Target lesion restenosis (TLR) after PTA is mainly caused by neointimal hyperplasia, particularly in lesions treated by repeated PTA using an uncoated plain balloon (PB). Studies have found that paclitaxel-coated balloons (PCBs) safely and effectively reduce in-stent restenosis in percutaneous coronary intervention and reduce in-stent restenosis or de novo stenosis in peripheral artery intervention. However, few studies address the use of PCB for endovascular management of hemodialysis access vascular stenosis. In this study, the authors compared PTA performed with PCB plus PB versus PTA performed with conventional PB alone in patients with RCAVF and recurrent inflow lesions. Their results established that for treating artery-anastomosed venous lesions, the use of PCB plus PB is safe (ie, no added complications compared with PB) and effective (100% technical success rate). In addition, PCB plus PB use delays short-term TLR and prolongs the TLR-free duration compared with conventional PB, and this beneficial effect of PCB plus PB was observed at 6 months but declined in subsequent months. Together, the results of this study indicate that drug-coated balloons improve short-term patency and possibly inhibit neointimal hyperplasia in the artery-anastomosed vein, similar to the results described earlier in the coronary artery and in the peripheral artery. These results may be of importance as a potential intervention for the endovascular management of hemodialysis access vascular stenosis; however, there are some limitations in this study that need to be addressed. Primarily, this study was performed at a single center with a small sample of only 20 patients. In addition, after PTA-PCB, the use of PB may alter the effectiveness of drug delivery to the vessel wall and may diffuse the release of paclitaxel to the adjacent segment. Therefore, further studies with a larger number of cases are needed to confirm these findings.

J. P. Cullen, PhD

Vascular remodeling and intimal hyperplasia in a novel murine model of arteriovenous fistula failure

Wong C-Y, de Vries MR, Wang Y, et al (Univ Med Ctr, Leiden, The Netherlands; Univ of Cincinnati, OH)
J Vasc Surg 59:192-201, 2014

Objective.—The arteriovenous fistula (AVF) still suffers from a high number of failures caused by insufficient outward remodeling and intimal hyperplasia (IH) formation from which the exact mechanism is largely unknown. A suitable animal model is of vital importance in the unraveling of the underlying pathophysiology. However, current murine models of AVF failure do not incorporate the surgical configuration that is commonly used in humans. Because the hemodynamic profile is one of the key determinants that play a role in vascular remodeling in the AVF, it is preferable to use this same configuration in an animal model. Here we describe a novel murine model of AVF failure in which the configuration (end-to-side) is similar to what is most frequently performed in humans.

Methods.—An AVF was created in 45 C57BL/6 mice by anastomosing the end of a branch of the external jugular vein to the side of the common carotid artery with interrupted sutures. The AVFs were harvested and analyzed histologically at days 7, 14, and 28. Identical veins of unoperated-on mice served as controls. Intravenous near-infrared fluorescent fluorophores were used to assess the patency of the fistula.

Results.—The patency rates at days 7, 14, and 28 days were 88%, 90%, and 50%, respectively. The mean circumference increased up to day 14, with a maximum 1.4-fold increase at day 7 compared with the control group (1.82 ± 0.7 vs 1.33 ± 0.3 mm; $P = .443$). Between days 14 and 28, the circumference remained constant (2.36 ± 0.2 vs 2.45 ± 0.2 mm; $P = .996$). At 7 days after surgery, the intimal area consisted mainly of an acellular layer that was structurally analogous to a focal adherent thrombus. Starting at 14 days after surgery, venous IH increased significantly compared with the unoperated-on group (14 days: 115,090 ± 22,594 μm^2, 28 days: 234,619 ± 47,828 μm^2, unoperated group: 2368 ± 1056 μm^2; $P = .001$ and $P < .001$, respectively) and was mainly composed of cells positive for α-smooth muscle actin. We observed leukocytes in the adventitial side of the vein at all time points.

Conclusions.—Our novel murine AVF model, which incorporates a clinically relevant configuration of the anastomosis, displays similar features that are characteristic of failing human AVFs. Moreover, our findings suggest that coagulation and inflammation could both potentially play an important role in the formation of IH and subsequent AVF failure. Near-infrared fluoroscopy was a suitable alternative for conventional imaging techniques. This murine AVF-model is a valuable addition to the AVF animal model arsenal.

▶ The consensus among dialysis experts is that the safest and longest lasting of the access types is the arteriovenous fistula (AVF). Hemodialysis vascular access dysfunction remains a huge clinical problem, and despite their superior patency rates, the utility of AVFs is hampered by 2 distinct causes of failure: (1) an initial failure to mature and (2) the later development of stenotic lesions in the outflow tract. To date, numerous animal models have been designed to study AVF failure. Large animals, such as pigs, are more suitable for intervention studies, but murine models have the greatest potential to gain more insight in the molecular mechanisms underlying this pathologic process because of the availability of transgenic mice. Previous studies have described a murine AVF model in which the fistula was constructed in an end-to-end manner. However, AVFs in hemodialysis patients are usually constructed by anastomosing the end of a vein to the side of an artery. Therefore, incorporating an AVF configuration resembling the human AVF is preferable, as the configuration is an important contributor to endothelial dysfunction and subsequent development of intimal hyperplasia (IH). In this study, the authors developed a novel murine model with an identical anatomic configuration as that used in humans. Using C57BL/6 mice, they created AVFs by anastomosing the end of a branch of the external jugular vein to the side of the common carotid artery with interrupted sutures. In their analysis, they focused on outward remodeling (OR) as well as the formation of IH in the venous outflow tract. Their results show that the venous outflow tract of AVFs is characterized by OR in the first 14 days. Furthermore, the authors hypothesize that focal adherent thrombi appear to serve as fertile soil for the formation of progressive intimal lesions positive for α–smooth muscle actin, ultimately leading to a 50% loss of patency 28 days after surgery. Anticoagulant therapy was necessary for creating a patent AVF, and finding the correct balance between acute thrombosis and hemorrhage proved to be of crucial importance. Using their protocol with heparin, they observed early thrombosis in 3% of the mice and bleeding complications in 7%. This end-to-side configuration, while providing a more accurate reflection of human AVF pathophysiology, can also yield novel insight into this process by being effectively applied in myriad transgenic animals. This is an interesting preclinical model that should yield important results in the study of AVF failure.

J. P. Cullen, PhD

Comparison of Surgical and Endovascular Salvage Procedures for Juxta-anastomotic Stenosis in Autogenous Wrist Radiocephalic Arteriovenous Fistula

Kwon H, Choi JY, Ko HK, et al (Univ of Ulsan College of Medicine and Asan Med Ctr, Seoul, Korea)

Ann Vasc Surg 28:1840-1846, 2014

Background.—Although dysfunctional radiocephalic arteriovenous fistulas (RCAVFs) are typically treated surgically, the endovascular approach is also considered suitable. The aim of this retrospective study was to compare the cumulative patency rates following surgical and endovascular salvaging of dysfunctional RCAVFs, and to evaluate whether the maturity of vascular access sites at the time of treatment influenced the outcomes.

Methods.—A total of 60 patients underwent surgical or endovascular salvage treatment for juxtaanastomotic stenosis of autogenous wrist RCAVFs: 35 patients underwent proximal neoanastomosis and 25 underwent percutaneous transluminal angioplasty (PTA).

Results.—Clinical and anatomical success rates were, respectively, 100% and 97.1% in the surgery group, and 100% and 96.0% in the angioplasty group ($P = 0.81$). The post-treatment restenosis rate was higher in the angioplasty group ($n = 11$, 46.0%) than in the surgery group ($n = 8$, 22.8%), without reaching statistical significance ($P = 0.15$). In a Kaplan–Meier analysis, the primary and assisted primary patency rates were significantly higher in the surgery group ($P = 0.036$ and $P = 0.026$, respectively), but there was no significant difference in secondary patency rates between the groups ($P = 0.52$). When stratified by RCAVF maturity at the time of

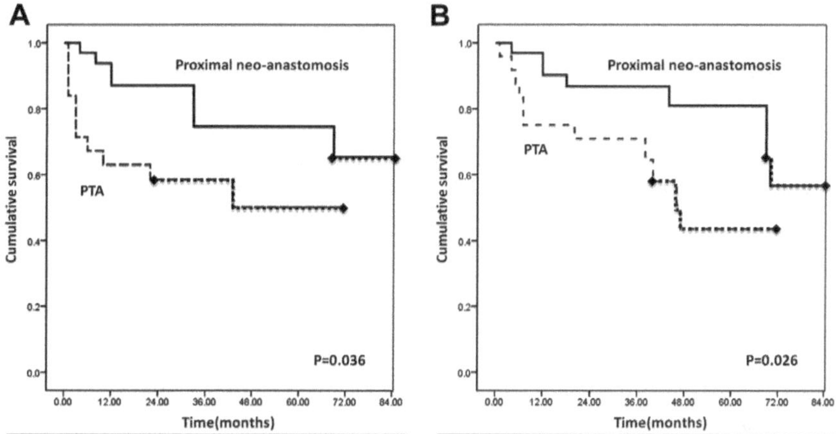

Numbers at risk	0 months	6 months	12 months	24 months	36 months
Surgery	35	31	27	22	16
PTA	25	16	15	12	8

Numbers at risk	0 months	6 months	12 months	24 months	36 months
Surgery	35	31	28	22	18
PTA	25	20	18	15	11

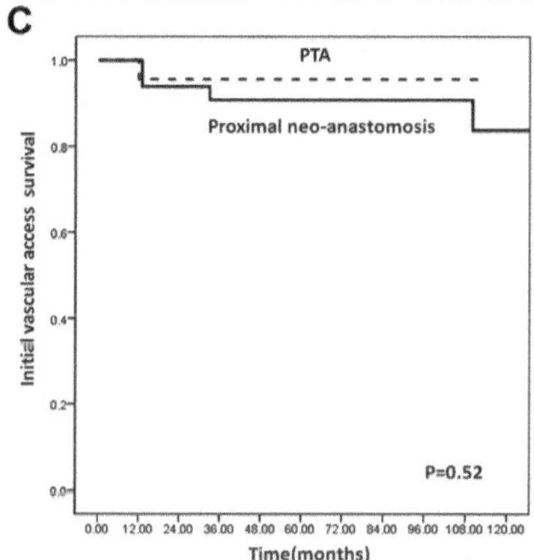

Numbers at risk	0 months	6 months	12 months	24 months	36 months
Surgery	35	35	35	31	29
PTA	25	25	21	20	18

FIGURE 1.—Kaplan–Meier estimates of post-treatment (**A**) primary and (**B**) assisted primary patency rates after salvage treatment, and (**C**) secondary patency rates of the initial vascular access stratified by the type of treatment (surgical: proximal neo-anastomosis; endovascular: PTA). The *dotted lines* (◆··◆) indicate when standard error exceeds 10% of the mean estimate. (Reprinted from the Annals of Vascular Surgery. Kwon H, Choi JY, Ko HK, et al. Comparison of surgical and endovascular salvage procedures for juxta-anastomotic stenosis in autogenous wrist radiocephalic arteriovenous fistula. *Ann Vasc Surg.* 2014;28:1840-1846, Copyright 2014, with permission from Annals of Vascular Surgery, Inc.)

treatment, no significant difference was noted in primary patency rates between the treatment groups. After adjusting for other variables, the relative risk of restenosis was significantly higher in the angioplasty group (hazard ratio 2.56; 95% confidence interval 1.02–6.46; $P = 0.046$).

Conclusions.—Post-treatment primary and assisted primary patency rates after proximal neoanastomosis were significantly higher than after PTA, and RCAVF maturity did not influence the outcomes (Fig 1).

▶ I completely agree with the statement in the background that salvage of failed or failing dialysis access is as important as timely placement. This retrospective review compared redo radiocephalic anastomoses with balloon angioplasty for juxta-anastomotic stenoses in radiocephalic dialysis accesses that were dysfunctional. The authors showed a significant advantage for open revision of the anastomosis in terms of primary and assisted primary patency (Fig 1). Secondary patency was roughly equivalent between the procedures. Interestingly, angioplasty may be more effective in poorly matured fistulas, whereas open surgery may be more effective in mature fistulas. I was confused by the description of the endovascular percutaneous transluminal angioplasty that was performed in these patients. The authors describe antegrade access followed by traversing the lesion with a guidewire and catheter, eventually ending in the antecubital or upper arm veins. The working distance required for such a maneuver indicates to me that the stenosis was at some distance from the anastomosis. If an exact distance between stenosis and anastomosis had been established or if an angiogram had been included, the definition of juxta-anastomotic would be more clearly illustrated. As it is, one wonders if the authors are comparing apples to oranges.

P. W. White, MD, FACS

Value of doppler ultrasonography in the study of hemodialysis peripheral vascular access dysfunction

Moreno Sánchez T, Martín Hervás C, Sola Martínez E, et al (Hosp Juan Ramón Jiménez, Huelva, Spain; Hosp Universitario La Paz, Madrid, Spain)
Radiologia 56:420-428, 2014

Objective.—The main objectives of this study were to evaluate the sensitivity and specificity of duplex Doppler ultrasonography in the study of hemodialysis peripheral vascular access dysfunction and to analyze the resistance index and flow in the afferent artery.

Material and Methods.—We prospectively studied 178 patients with 178 peripheral vascular accesses that were dysfunctional in at least three consecutive hemodialysis sessions. Patients underwent duplex Doppler ultrasonography and clinical and laboratory follow-up for three months (provided angiography findings were negative). We calculated the sensitivity, specificity, predictive values, and coefficients of probability. We studied the morphology of the afferent artery, the arteriovenous anastomosis, and the efferent vein, and we measured the resistance index and the flow of the afferent artery, the diameter of the anastomosis, and the flow and peak systolic velocity in the efferent vein.

Results.—The final sample consisted of 159 patients. The sensitivity, specificity, positive and negative predictive values, and positive and negative coefficients of probability were 0.98 (95% CI: 0.88–1.00), 0.74 (95% CI: 0.66–0.81), 0.96, 0.82, 3.7, and 0.03, respectively. The resistance index was less than 0.5 in 78.5% of the peripheral vascular accesses with normal function and greater than 0.5 in 86.1% of the dysfunctional peripheral vascular accesses. We found aneurysms in 19 of the native peripheral vascular accesses and pseudoaneurysms in 7 of the prosthetic grafts. Inverted flow was seen in 57 peripheral vascular accesses.

Conclusion.—Duplex Doppler ultrasonography is an efficacious method for detecting and characterizing stenosis and thrombosis in peripheral vascular accesses, and it provides information about the morphology and hemodynamics.

▶ With an increasing number of dialysis patients, the maintenance of dialysis access will remain a major part of many vascular surgery practices. Complications of dialysis access are already a leading driver of mortality, morbidity, and cost in the care of dialysis patients. This report reinforces the value of duplex ultrasound scan in the assessment of dialysis access. The reported sensitivity of 98% in detecting significant problems in a poorly functioning dialysis access confirms that duplex ultrasound scan is the ideal first step in evaluating dialysis accesses. I was also intrigued by the authors' use of the resistive index (RI) in the afferent artery. The data in this report, although just preliminary, seem to indicate than an RI of less than 0.5 in the afferent artery is indicative of a functioning access. I look forward to the results of the more thorough study of the RI in the afferent artery that the authors promise to perform.

P. W. White, MD, FACS

In vitro hemodynamic model of the arm arteriovenous circulation to study hemodynamics of native arteriovenous fistula and the distal revascularization and interval ligation procedure

Varble N, Day S, Phillips D, et al (Rochester Inst of Technology, NY; et al)

J Vasc Surg 59:1410-1417, 2014

Background.—Experimental modeling of arteriovenous hemodialysis fistula (AVF) hemodynamics is challenging. Mathematical modeling struggles to accurately represent the capillary bed and venous circulation. In vivo animal models are expensive and labor intensive. We hypothesized that an in vitro, physiologic model of the extremity arteriovenous circulation with provisions for AVF and distal revascularization and interval ligation (DRIL) configurations could be created as a platform for hemodynamic modeling and testing.

Methods.—An anatomic, upper extremity arteriovenous model was constructed of tubing focusing on the circulation from the subclavian artery to subclavian vein. Tubing material, length, diameter, and wall thickness were selected to match vessel compliance and morphology. All branch points were constructed at physiologic angles. The venous system and capillary bed were modeled using tubing and one-way valves and compliance chambers. A glycerin/water solution was created to match blood viscosity. The system was connected to a heart simulator. Pressure waveforms and flows were recorded at multiple sites along the model for the native circulation, brachiocephalic AVF configuration, and the AVF with DR without and with IL (DR no IL and DRIL).

Results.—A preset mean cardiac output of 4.2 L/min from the heart simulator yielded a subclavian artery pressure of 125/55 mm Hg and a brachial artery pressure of 121/54 mm Hg with physiologic arterial waveforms. Mean capillary bed perfusion pressure was 41 mm Hg, and mean venous pressure in the distal brachial vein was 17 mm Hg with physiologic waveforms. AVF configuration resulted in a 15% decrease in distal pressure and a 65% decrease in distal flow to the hand. DR no IL had no change in distal pressure with a 27% increase in distal flow. DRIL resulted in a 3% increase in distal pressure and a 15% increase in distal flow to the hand above that of DR no IL. Flow through the DR bypass decreased from 329 mL/min to 55 mL/min with the addition of IL. Flow through the AVF for both DR no IL and DRIL was preserved.

Conclusions.—Through the construction and validation of an in vitro, pulsatile arteriovenous model, the intricate hemodynamics of AVF and treatments for ischemic steal can be studied. DR with or without IL improved distal blood flow in addition to preserving AVF flow. IL decreased the blood flow through the DR bypass itself. The findings of the AVF as a pressure sink and the relative role of IL with DR bypass has allowed this model to provide hemodynamic insight difficult or impossible to obtain in animal or human models. Further study of these phenomena with this model should allow for more effective AVF placement and maturation while personalizing treatment for associated ischemic steal.

Clinical Relevance.—The complications of arteriovenous fistula (AVF)-associated steal with its concurrent surgical treatments have been clinically described but have relatively little published, concrete hemodynamic data. A further understanding of the underlying hemodynamics is necessary to prevent the occurrence of steal and improve treatment when it occurs. Specific objectives are to study the blood flow through an AVF with varying anatomic and physiologic parameters, determine what factors contribute to the development of arterial steal distal to an AVF, and create optimal interventions to treat arterial steal from an AVF when it occurs. The long-term goal is creation of AVF tailored to patient-specific parameters, resulting in higher rates of functional fistulas with decreases in fistula-related complications. The ability to study fluid dynamics using a unique, in vitro, upper extremity pulsatile arteriovenous circulation simulator creates the ideal platform for this work.

▶ The steal syndrome is a complication that can occur from arteriovenous fistulas (AVF) in patients requiring dialysis. Distal revascularization and interval ligation (DRIL) is a means to salvage both the AVF and the hand in which much of the clinical signs and symptoms occur (pain, nonhealing ulcers, and gangrene). The concept is that the forearm and hand receives direct blood flow proximal to arterial anastomosis of the AVF, and the artery between the AVF and distal anastomosis of the bypass is ligated, referred to as interval ligation. The hemodynamics of flow to the ischemic extremity in the presence or absence of the interval ligation are not well described. In this study, the objective is to study an in vitro model of the flow characteristic in an AVF model that has pulsatile flow and how the DRIL procedure in the presence or absence of the interval ligation affect flow to the hand. The main findings are that an AVF results in a 65% decrease in flow to the hand. Placement of a distal revascularization with or without interval ligation resulted in increased flow to the hand, but higher flow with the interval ligation. Simultaneously, there was no effect on the flow of the AVF. Although this is an important model to study pressure and flow in AVF and the effect of perfusion distally, as well as determining the hemodynamics that lead to distal hand ischemia after AVF, the important principles of a proper pulse examination, a complete ultrasound assessing the venous network and arterial characteristics (diameter, calcium, patency, volume flows), and judicious application of technique in creating the arterial-venous anastomosis so as not to make the arteriotomy too large are paramount and will avoid many complications related to steal.

J. D. Raffetto, MD, FACS, FSVM

Prospective, randomized study of cutting balloon angioplasty versus conventional balloon angioplasty for the treatment of hemodialysis access stenoses

Saleh HM, Gabr AK, Tawfik MM, et al (Ain Shams Univ, Cairo, Egypt)

J Vasc Surg 60:735-740, 2014

Objective.—The aim of this trial was to compare the rates of patency achieved by cutting and conventional balloon angioplasty to treat hemodialysis access stenoses.

Methods.—End-stage renal failure patients (at three tertiary referral centers) with significant hemodialysis access stenoses were prospectively randomized to have percutaneous transluminal angioplasty (PTA) by either cutting or conventional balloons. Patients with more than one hemodynamically significant stenosis were excluded. Kaplan-Meier method was used to compare the primary assisted patency rates for the two groups.

Results.—The study randomized 623 patients into two groups, and the duration of follow-up was 15 ± 3 months. In the cutting balloon angioplasty group, the clinical success rate was 89% (282 of 316 stenoses). In the conventional balloon angioplasty group, the clinical success rate was 86% (265 of 307 stenoses; P =.637). Assisted primary patency for cutting PTA was statistically significantly higher at 6 months and 1 year (86% and 63%) than that for conventional PTA (56% and 37%, respectively; P =.037) in the treatment of stenosis of the graft-to-vein anastomosis. In the venous stenosis subgroup, equivalent primary assisted patency at 6 months and 1 year was observed for cutting PTA (84% and 55%) and

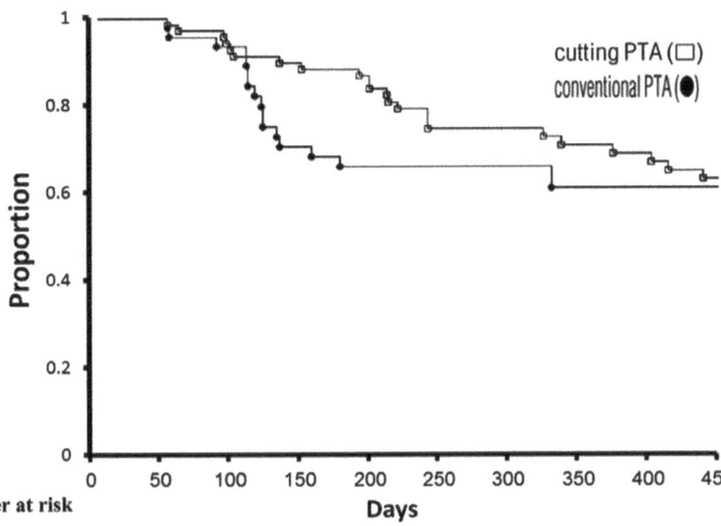

Number at risk

Cutting	95	85	83	81	79	70	61	52	47	40
Conventional	81	68	65	60	56	50	42	37	30	22

FIGURE 1.—Graph shows the Kaplan-Meier survival analysis for assisted primary patency rates in patients with venous stenosis in the cutting and conventional percutaneous transluminal angioplasty (*PTA*) groups. No significant differences in assisted primary patency rates were identified between groups (P =.360). The number of patients at risk in each time period is listed. (Reprinted from the Journal of Vascular Surgery. Saleh HM, Gabr AK, Tawfik MM, et al. Prospective, randomized study of cutting balloon angioplasty versus conventional balloon angioplasty for the treatment of hemodialysis access stenoses. *J Vasc Surg*. 2014;60:735-740, Copyright 2014, with permission from The Society for Vascular Surgery.)

conventional PTA (70% and 46%, respectively; $P = .360$). In the intragraft stenosis subgroup, primary assisted patency was equivalent at 6 months and 1 year for cutting PTA (67% and 39%) and conventional PTA (62% and 49%, respectively; $P = .371$). In the arterial anastomotic stenosis subgroup, assisted primary patency at 6 months and 1 year was equivalent for cutting PTA (70% and 30%) and conventional PTA (75% and 33%, respectively; $P = .921$).

Conclusions.—Cutting balloon angioplasty proved to be a safe and effective treatment of graft-to-vein anastomotic stenosis, with significantly higher patency than that of conventional balloon angioplasty (Figs 1-4).

▶ Maintenance of dialysis access is one growing problem for vascular surgeons. Any tool to assist in prolonging the life span of a dialysis access is

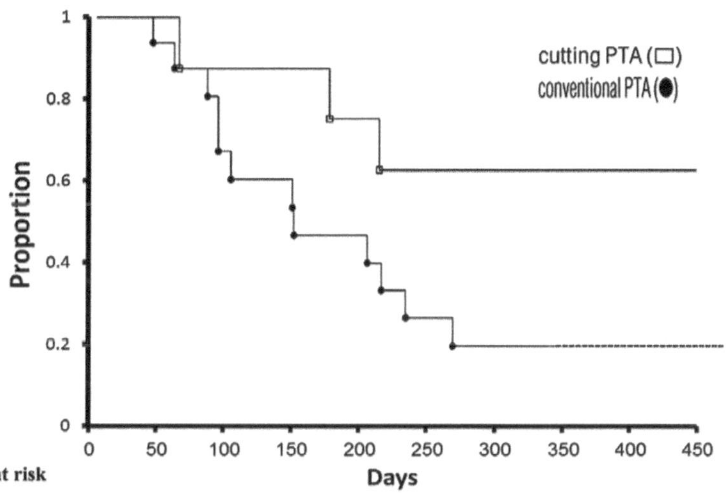

Number at risk

Cutting	80	71	70	69	68	62	55	50	43	30
Conventional	82	70	64	55	45	40	35	30	22	11

FIGURE 2.—Graph shows the Kaplan-Meier survival analysis for assisted primary patency rates in patients with graft-to-vein anastomotic stenosis in the cutting and conventional percutaneous transluminal angioplasty (*PTA*) groups. The assisted primary patency rate was significantly higher in the cutting PTA group than in the conventional PTA group ($P = .037$). Note that the line is interrupted beyond the point at which standard error exceeds 10%. The number of patients at risk in each time period is listed. (Reprinted from the Journal of Vascular Surgery. Saleh HM, Gabr AK, Tawfik MM, et al. Prospective, randomized study of cutting balloon angioplasty versus conventional balloon angioplasty for the treatment of hemodialysis access stenoses. *J Vasc Surg*. 2014;60:735-740, Copyright 2014, with permission from The Society for Vascular Surgery.)

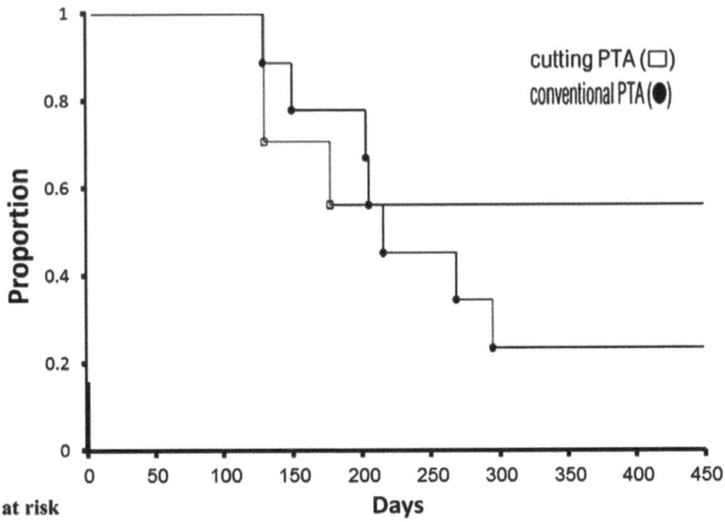

Number at risk

Cutting	61	55	52	48	40	36	30	23	20	15
Conventional	72	63	62	59	54	45	30	23	19	14

FIGURE 3.—Graph shows the Kaplan-Meier survival analysis for assisted primary patency rates in patients with intragraft stenosis in the cutting and conventional percutaneous transluminal angioplasty (*PTA*) groups. No significant differences in assisted primary patency rates were identified between groups ($P = .371$). The number of patients at risk in each time period is listed. (Reprinted from the Journal of Vascular Surgery. Saleh HM, Gabr AK, Tawfik MM, et al. Prospective, randomized study of cutting balloon angioplasty versus conventional balloon angioplasty for the treatment of hemodialysis access stenoses. *J Vasc Surg*. 2014;60:735-740, Copyright 2014, with permission from The Society for Vascular Surgery.)

and will continue to be useful. This prospective analysis between 2 techniques of angioplasty may point to particular niche for cutting balloon angioplasty: outflow stenosis of synthetic AV grafts. The authors divided their patients into 4 groups, and only the stenosis at the graft-venous anastomosis of an AV graft benefited from cutting balloon angioplasty (Figs 1-4). Unfortunately, the primary and primary-assisted patency rates are reported only for subgroups. The authors point out that the subgroups are small but fail to discuss whether the division into subgroups occurred before the initiation of the study and randomization or if it was a result of post hoc analysis. If the subgroup analysis was post hoc, I would hope the authors would consider repeating the study only on patients with an outflow stenosis at the synthetic AV graft-venous outflow

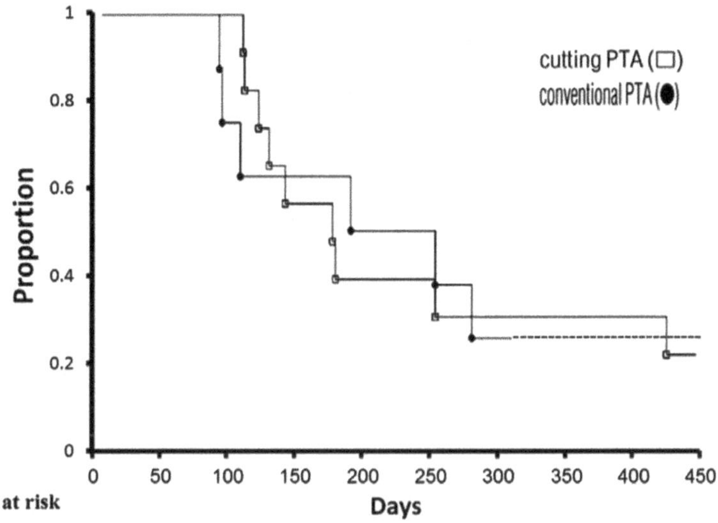

Number at risk

Cutting	**80**	**71**	**68**	**60**	**56**	**45**	**30**	**24**	**20**	**18**
Conventional	**72**	**64**	**60**	**50**	**44**	**40**	**37**	**34**	**28**	**20**

FIGURE 4.—Graph shows the Kaplan-Meier survival analysis for assisted primary patency rates in patients with arterial anastomotic stenosis in the cutting and conventional percutaneous transluminal angioplasty (*PTA*) groups. No significant differences in assisted primary patency rates were identified between groups ($P = .921$). Note that the line is interrupted beyond the point at which standard error exceeds 10%. The number of patients at risk in each time period is listed. (Reprinted from the Journal of Vascular Surgery. Saleh HM, Gabr AK, Tawfik MM, et al. Prospective, randomized study of cutting balloon angioplasty versus conventional balloon angioplasty for the treatment of hemodialysis access stenoses. *J Vasc Surg*. 2014;60:735-740, Copyright 2014, with permission from The Society for Vascular Surgery.)

anastomosis. Perhaps comparing cutting balloon angioplasty to primary stenting as well as conventional angioplasty would be helpful.

P. W. White, MD, FACS

11 Carotid and Cerebrovascular Disease

Treatment of Symptomatic Aberrant Subclavian Arteries

Jalaie H, Grommes J, Sailer A, et al (Univ Hosp of the RWTH Aachen, Germany; Maastricht Univ Med Centre, The Netherlands)

Eur J Vasc Endovasc Surg 48:521-526, 2014

Objective.—The aim of this study is to present experience with 10 patients with symptomatic aberrant subclavian artery (ASA) and aneurysm of ASA who underwent surgical treatment.

Methods.—From 2008 to 2011 10 patients with symptomatic aberrant subclavian artery (mean age 60 years [range 24–90 years]) were studied. Symptoms were dysphagia ($n = 7$), dyspnea ($n = 4$), acute chest pain ($n = 1$), respiratory distress syndrome ($n = 1$), superior cava syndrome, and shock ($n = 1$). Six patients had aneurysm formation of the ASA (mean diameter of 7.1 cm [range 3.0–12.4 cm]; rupture [$n = 1$], dissection [$n = 1$]). All data were analyzed retrospectively.

Results.—Treatment was performed as a hybrid procedure in eight patients. This included thoracic endoluminal graft exclusion with revascularization of the ASA, a pure endovascular procedure with two occluders in one patient, and an open procedure in one patient with ligation of the aberrant artery through a thoracotomy. Three patients died during the early postoperative period owing to pulmonary complications. All three suffered from a symptomatic aneurysm, and two were treated as an emergency procedure. Median follow-up was 20 months (range 12–49 months).

Conclusion.—A symptomatic ASA and its associated aneurysmal formation should be excluded after diagnosis. In most cases, a hybrid procedure consisting of thoracic endografting and revascularization of the ASA is feasible (Fig 1).

► Treatment of aberrant right subclavian arteries (SCA) has become well accepted when aneurysmal change is present or the patient has symptoms. Although open surgical treatment historically dominated repair choice, endovascular solutions are now the mainstay for treatment of the aortic disease with carotid subclavian bypass or transposition done for revascularization

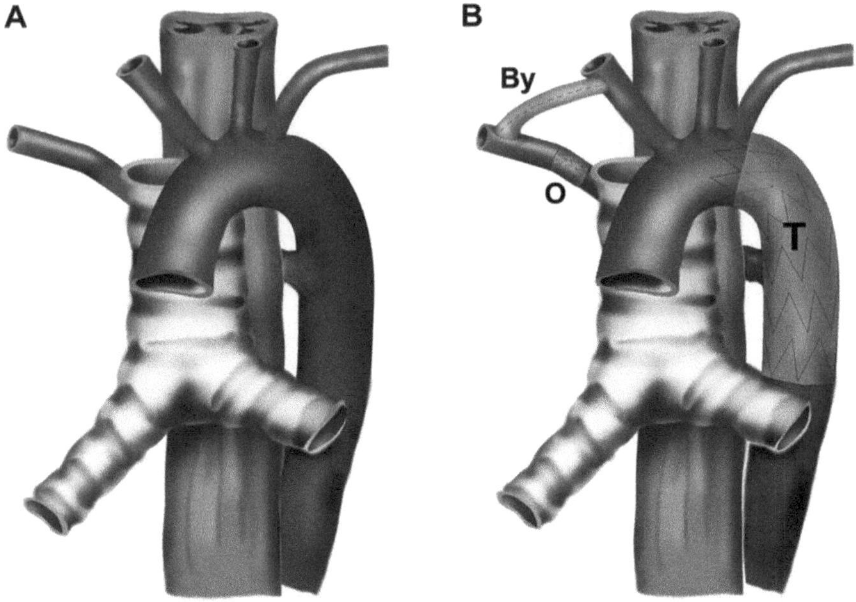

FIGURE 1.—(A) Anatomy of an aberrant right subclavian artery, which arises as the last branch of the aortic arch and crosses the midline between the esophagus and vertebral column. (B) Hybrid procedure: endovascular occlusion of the aberrant right subclavian artery (O) and the origin of the aberrant subclavian artery is covered by a thoracic stentgraft (T). Revascularization is facilitated by carotid subclavian bypass (By) or transposition of the aberrant artery. The vertebral artery (not shown in the figure) has to be preserved in both procedures. (Reprinted from the European Journal of Vascular and Endovascular Surgery. Jalaie H, Grommes J, Sailer A, et al. Treatment of symptomatic aberrant subclavian arteries. *Eur J Vasc Endovasc Surg*. 2014;48:521-526, Copyright 2014, with permission from the European Society for Vascular Surgery.)

(Fig 1). It is well accepted that aberrant right SCA harbor embryologic tissue, predisposing to degeneration. Dysphagia or dyshphagia lusorum is the most common complaint and represents an indication for repair. Technical challenges occur when the right and left SCA orifices are close. In these cases, coverage of the left SCA is accepted with revascularization either by fenestrated repair or open treatment (bypass or transposition). Revascularization of the right SCA is recommended and open treatment predominates. The course of the aberrant subclavian artery in the right supraclavicular fossa runs higher under anterior scalene as it crosses the neck. Following, the proximal SCA should be plugged or ligated, especially in the setting of a Kommerell's diverticulum as retrograde flow is robust. Occlusion plugs should be placed proximal to the vertebral artery, yet attempts should be made to avoid placement directly behind the esophagus. It has been theorized that a plug behind the esophagus can induce dysphagia or potential erosion, which would be a monumental failure. If plug placement is not technically feasible, surgical ligation is recommended. Large aneurysms and ruptures portend poor results as demonstrated within this article. Overall, the hybrid approach to this disease has shortened the hospital course and eliminated the need for thoracotomy. Complex anatomy can usually be addressed with complex endovascular solutions or supra-aortic revascularization.

J. H. Black III, MD, FACS

Predicting Carotid Artery Disease and Plaque Instability from Cell-derived Microparticles

Wekesa AL, Cross KS, O'Donovan O, et al (Waterford Inst of Technology, Ireland; Waterford Regional Hosp, Ireland; et al)

Eur J Vasc Endovasc Surg 48:489-495, 2014

Objectives.—Cell-derived microparticles (MPs) are small plasma membrane-derived vesicles shed from circulating blood cells and may act as novel biomarkers of vascular disease. We investigated the potential of circulating MPs to predict (a) carotid plaque instability and (b) the presence of advanced carotid disease.

Methods.—This pilot study recruited carotid disease patients (aged 69.3 ± 1.2 years [mean ± SD], 69% male, 90% symptomatic) undergoing endarterectomy ($n = 42$) and age- and sex-matched controls ($n = 73$). Plaques were classified as stable ($n = 25$) or unstable ($n = 16$) post surgery using immunohistochemistry. Blood samples were analysed for MP subsets and molecular biomarkers. Odds ratios (OR) are expressed per standard deviation biomarker increase.

Results.—Endothelial MP (EMP) subsets, but not any vascular, inflammatory, or proteolytic molecular biomarker, were higher ($p < .05$) in the unstable than the stable plaque patients. The area under the receiver operator characteristic curve for $CD31^{+}41^{-}$ EMP in discriminating an unstable plaque was 0.73 (0.56–0.90, $p < .05$). $CD31^{+}41^{-}$ EMP predicted plaque instability (OR = 2.19, 1.08–4.46, $p < .05$) and remained significant in a multivariable model that included transient ischaemic attack symptom status. Annexin V^{+} MP, platelet MP (PMP) subsets, and C-reactive protein were higher ($p < .05$) in cases than controls. Annexin V^{+} MP (OR = 3.15, 1.49–6.68), soluble vascular cell adhesion molecule-1 (OR = 1.64, 1.03–2.59), and previous smoking history (OR = 3.82, 1.38–10.60) independently ($p < .05$) predicted the presence of carotid disease in a multivariable model.

Conclusions.—EMP may have utility in predicting plaque instability in carotid patients and annexin V^{+} MPs may predict the presence of advanced carotid disease in aging populations, independent of established biomarkers.

▶ The ability to identify carotid plaques that confer increased risk would greatly assist in the selection of patients for carotid artery endarterectomy or stenting. Simple quantification of carotid artery disease based on the degree of stenosis has limitations; therefore, there is a need to look for physiologic or molecular parameters that may reflect stroke risk. It is believed that plaque characteristics at one vascular site are reflective of plaque at other sites and that plaque instability is influenced by systemic processes. Cell-derived microparticles (MPs) are putative vesicular biomarkers of atherosclerotic disease. MPs are shed from the plasma membrane of vascular cells including platelets, endothelial cells, erythrocytes, and leucocytes. Endothelial microparticles (EMPs), platelet microparticles (PMPs), and leukocyte microparticles have been reported in the plasma of patients with atherosclerotic diseases compared with matched controls. The purpose of this study was to determine the ability of EMP and PMP to predict carotid plaque instability in patients undergoing endarterectomy and the presence of advanced carotid disease in a cohort of cases and matched controls. When patients with stable and unstable carotid plaques were compared, the $CD31^{+}41^{-}$EMP and the mmEMP subsets were higher in the unstable plaque group. $CD31^{+}41^{-}$EMPs were also significantly higher in patients presenting with transient ischemic attack (TIA) than those who were asymptomatic, albeit with a very small sample size of asymptomatic patients. $CD31^{+}41^{-}$EMPs emerged as the single significant biomarker of an unstable plaque in a multivariable analysis and remained significant even after adjusting for TIA symptom status. A clear limitation of the study is the potential confounding effect of prescribed medications on biomarker concentrations. Antilipemic, antiplatelet, and antihypertensive medication use was considerably greater in the group of cases. Nevertheless, these findings provide considerable support for including this kind of analysis in a prospective manner in patients with carotid artery occlusive disease.

M. T. Watkins, MD

Twenty-Four Hour Staged Carotid Endarterectomy Followed by Off-Pump Coronary Bypass Grafting for Patients With Concomitant Carotid and Coronary Disease

Nabagiez JP, Bowman KC, Shariff MA, et al (Staten Island Univ Hosp, NY; Stony Brook Univ Med Ctr, NY)
Ann Thorac Surg 98:1613-1619, 2014

Background.—Carotid artery stenosis and coronary artery disease share common risk factors and often coexist in the same patient. Currently, no consensus exists regarding the optimal treatment strategy for patients with concomitant severe coronary and carotid disease. We reviewed the results of our experience performing off-pump coronary artery bypass grafting (CABG) within 24 hours of carotid endarterectomy (CEA) in this select patient population.

Methods.—In this single institution retrospective study we identified patients who underwent CEA followed by CABG from March 2001 to March 2012. Preoperative, intraoperative, and postoperative data were collected and analyzed.

Results.—Ninety patients underwent CEA followed by off-pump CABG. The duration between CEA and CABG was 1.8 ± 5.6 days with 80 (89%) within 24 hours. Mean age was 69 ± 9 years, 68% male. Perioperative comorbidities included hypertension (87%), diabetes (50%), previous myocardial infarction (24%), peripheral arterial disease (20%), and strokes and transient ischemic attack (16%). Extensive aortic atherosclerosis was noted in 15 patients (17%). The average number of vessels bypassed was 3.4 ± 1.0, and the average number of proximal vein aortotomies was 1.7 ± 0.92. Post-CEA surgical outcomes were myocardial infarction (1%), acute embolic cerebrovascular accident (1%), left upper extremity weakness (1%), and hypoglossal nerve injury (1%). Post-CABG surgical outcomes included atrial fibrillation (34%), anemia (12%), pneumothorax (7%), and postoperative bleeding (4%). No post-CABG cerebrovascular accident was identified. Patients were discharged 7.5 ± 3.5 days after CEA.

Conclusions.—Twenty-four hour staged CEA followed by CABG minimizes myocardial infarction post-CEA while minimizing cerebrovascular accident post-CABG in patients with concomitant severe coronary and carotid artery disease.

▶ The authors sought to understand whether a 24-hour staged approach to combined coronary and carotid disease can decrease the risk of myocardial infarction (MI) post carotid endarterectomy (CEA) while simultaneously reducing risk of cerebrovascular accident in these high-risk patients. Patients with combined disease are typically treated with either synchronous coronary artery bypass grafting (CABG) and CEA or staged CABG and CEA. Synchronous surgery requires prolonged anesthesia, and several studies have suggested higher rates of stroke and mortality as opposed to staged. On the other hand, staged procedures expose the patient to the increased risk of developing a stroke if they undergo CABG with untreated carotid disease or MI if they undergo CEA with untreated coronary artery disease. The authors show that acute stroke and mortality rates for staged intervention was 1.1%, which is substantially less than reports for synchronous operations. A substantial number of carotid stenoses were asymptomatic (94%), thus this aggressive approach may not be warranted as an overall principle. However, in the patient with symptomatic carotid and coronary artery disease, a staged approach might be appropriate to avoid the morbidity and mortality associated with combined CABG and CEA. The retrospective nature of the report and high number of asymptomatic patients likely contribute to the low incidence of stroke in this complex patient population. It is also possible that the lack of aortic cross-clamping during off-pump CABG may additionally benefit patients with atheromatous disease of the ascending aorta and therefore contribute to the decrease in stroke rate compared to simultaneous CEA and CABG.

M. T. Watkins, MD

Female Sex Does Not Influence 30-Day Stroke and Mortality Rates after Carotid Endarterectomy

Guzman RP, Weighell W, Guzman C, et al (Saint Boniface Hosp, Winnipeg, Manitoba, Canada; Univ of Manitoba, Winnipeg, Canada; et al)
Ann Vasc Surg 28:245-252, 2014

Background.—Sex-based differences in outcomes for the treatment of carotid arterial disease remains a controversial topic. The main objective of this study was to determine if gender differences influence 30-day stroke and mortality rates after carotid endarterectomy (CEA) in a large series of patients.

Methods.—This is a retrospective study of all patients undergoing endarterectomy performed by a single surgeon between January 1, 1993 and December 15, 2010. The analysis included data from 1,046 CEAs (683 men and 363 women).

Results.—There were no differences found in 30-day stroke, death, or combined stroke and death rates between women and men. The 30-day stroke rate was 1.6% for women and 1.8% for men ($P = 0.98$), with no significant differences between asymptomatic patients (1.7% for women vs. 1.2% for men; $P = 0.70$) or symptomatic patients (1.6% for women vs. 2.1% for men; $P = 0.74$). The 30-day mortality rate was 0.8% for women and 0.9% for men ($P = 0.85$) with no significant differences between asymptomatic patients (0.8% for women vs. 1.2% for men; $P = 0.77$) and symptomatic patients (0.8% for women vs. 0.7% for men; $P = 0.84$). There was a similar low risk for the combined outcome of stroke and death (1.9% for women vs. 2.2% for men; $P = 0.92$), with no differences between asymptomatic patients (1.7% for women vs. 1.6% for men; $P = 0.89$) or symptomatic patients (2.1% for women vs. 2.5% for men; $P = 0.84$).

Conclusions.—Female sex does not influence 30-day stroke and mortality rates after CEA, regardless of preoperative symptom status.

▶ Guzman et al revisit the ongoing controversy regarding outcomes of carotid revascularization in women and provide yet another compelling study to indicate that carotid endarterectomy (CEA) in women is not associated with inferior outcomes. While citing numerous recent reports that support the noninferiority of CEA in women, the authors appropriately discuss several other studies showing that women experienced less benefit compared with men. The authors make the argument that these studies espousing sex-based differences tend to be older and perhaps not consistent with current antiplatelet and statin therapy.

Although this report may not necessarily lay this established controversy to rest, I believe that the authors' conclusion is fairly settled: that the current evidence from several large series suggests that CEA is associated with low risks regardless of patient sex or presenting symptom status. This, of course, would exclude stroke in evolution or crescendo transient ischemic attack.

K. Hughes, MD, FACS

Effects of Extracranial Carotid Stenosis on Intracranial Blood Flow

Shakur SF, Hrbac T, Alaraj A, et al (Univ of Illinois at Chicago)

Stroke 45:3427-3429, 2014

Background and Purpose.—The hemodynamic effects of extracranial carotid stenosis on intracranial blood flow are not well characterized. We sought to determine the impact of degree of stenosis, stenosis length, and residual lumen on intracranial blood flow in patients with extracranial carotid stenosis.

Methods.—Carotid stenosis patients who had undergone both vessel flow rate measurements using quantitative magnetic resonance angiography and digital subtraction angiography were examined. The impact of the anatomic measurements of the stenosis relative to ipsilateral internal carotid artery (ICA) flow and ipsilateral-to-contralateral middle cerebral artery (MCA) flow ratio were assessed.

Results.—Forty-four patients (mean age, 67 years; 64% symptomatic) were included. Higher percentage stenosis and smaller residual lumen were associated with a significant decrease in ICA flow ($P < 0.01$ and 0.04, respectively). On multivariate analysis, percentage stenosis remained as the primary predictor of ICA flow ($P < 0.001$). MCA flow ratio was not significantly associated with percentage stenosis, stenosis length, or residual lumen. However, mean MCA flow ratio was significantly lower in symptomatic compared with asymptomatic patients (0.92 versus 1.22; $P = 0.001$). In contrast, mean ICA flow ratio was similar among these 2 groups (0.55 versus 0.55; $P = 0.99$).

Conclusions.—Percentage stenosis and residual lumen are significantly associated with ICA but not MCA flow, suggesting that local hemodynamic effects of carotid stenosis do not translate directly to distal vasculature, because intracranial flows can be maintained through collaterals. The lower MCA flow ratio in symptomatic patients highlights the potential importance of distal hemodynamics in symptomatic presentation (Fig 1).

▶ Although it is commonly accepted that the degree of extracranial carotid stenosis does correlate with thromboembolic stroke risk, there is little quantitative data to demonstrate that flow through the middle cerebral artery is or is not affected by the degree of stenosis. In this study, the authors aimed to determine the hemodynamic effects of extracranial carotid artery stenosis on intracranial blood flow using quantitative magnetic resonance angiography. Because magnetic resonance imaging is somewhat unreliable for measuring the degree of stenosis, measurements of degree of stenosis, stenosis length, and residual lumen were made from digital subtraction angiography. To provide an internal control for factors such as age and blood pressure, flow ratios (ipsilateral/contralateral vessel flow) were generated for the internal carotid artery (ICA) and middle cerebral artery (MCA). In Fig 1, the authors clearly show that as the degree of stenosis increases, internal carotid artery (ICA) flow decreased, but MCA flow was not decreased. It seems that MCA flow can be maintained by collateral pathways. The most interesting aspect of this report was the fact that MCA flow ratios were significantly lower in symptomatic versus asymptomatic patients, which may reflect inadequate collateral pathways. It is possible that the thromboembolic nature of the symptomatic stenosis compromises collateral blood flow through the MCA. Based on this data in a small patient population, its indeed possible that with further study, flow rates could potentially

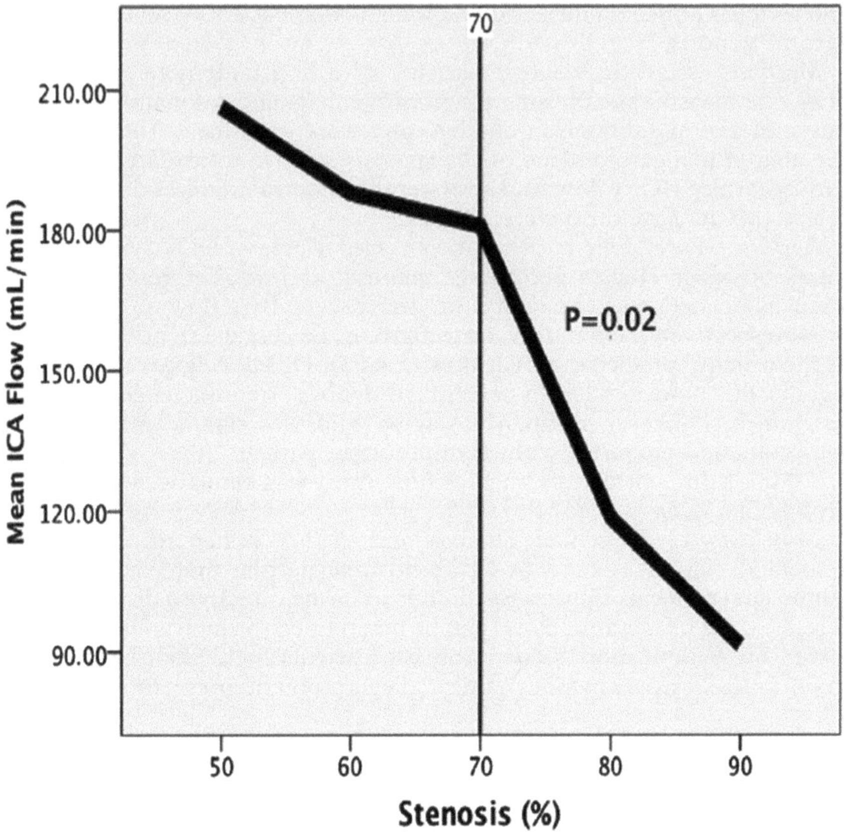

FIGURE 1.—Mean internal carotid artery (ICA) flow for incremental categories of percentage stenosis. The difference in flow between the 70% to 79% and 80% to 89% stenosis groups was statistically significant. (Reprinted from the Stroke. Shakur SF, Hrbac T, Alaraj A, et al. Effects of extracranial carotid stenosis on intracranial blood flow. *Stroke*. 2014;45:3427-3429, Copyright 2014, American Heart Association.)

indicate critical thresholds prognostic of high stroke risk or disclose limited collateral supply that can be used to guide recommendations for revascularization.

M. T. Watkins, MD

Clinical and Imaging Features Associated with an Increased Risk of Late Stroke in Patients with Asymptomatic Carotid Disease

Naylor AR, Schroeder TV, Sillesen H (Leicester Royal Infirmary, Leicester, UK; Univ of Copenhagen, Denmark)

Eur J Vasc Endovasc Surg 48:633-640, 2014

Background.—The 2011 American Heart Association Guidelines on the management of asymptomatic carotid disease recommends that carotid endarterectomy (CEA) (with carotid artery stenting (CAS) as an alternative) may be considered in highly selected patients with 70–99% stenoses. However, no guidance was provided as to what "highly selected" meant. This caveat is, however, important as up to 95% of asymptomatic individuals undergoing prophylactic CEA or CAS will ultimately undergo an unnecessary procedure. Even if the procedural risk following CEA or CAS could be reduced to 0%; 93% of patients would still undergo an unnecessary intervention. This, coupled with growing awareness that the risk of stroke in medically treated patients appears to be diminishing, has led to a renewed drive towards identifying patients with the highest risk of suffering a stroke whilst on medical therapy in whom to target CEA/CAS.

Methods.—Review of clinical and/or imaging based scoring systems, predictive algorithms and imaging parameters that may be associated with an increased (or decreased) risk of stroke in patients with asymptomatic carotid disease.

Results.—Parameters associated with an increased risk of late stroke include: (a) silent infarction on CT/MRI; (b) stenosis progression; (c) hypoechoic plaques or GSM <15; (d) irregular plaques; (e) evidence of spontaneous embolization on TCD; (f) AHA plaque types IV–V, VI; (g) MR diagnosed IPH; (h) plaque area >80 mm^2; (i) juxtaluminal black area >10 mm^2; and (j) tandem intracranial disease.

Conclusions.—A number of imaging parameters have been shown to be predictive of an increased risk of late stroke in previously asymptomatic patients. None have been independently validated, but many could easily be evaluated in natural history studies or randomized trials in order to identify a "high risk for stroke" cohort in whom CEA/CAS could be prioritized.

▶ There is no doubt that a small cohort of "high risk for stroke" patients with asymptomatic carotid stenoses will benefit from carotid endarterectomy/carotid artery stenting (CEA/CAS), but (to date) there have been limited opportunities for defining who these patients are. The aim of this topical review was to first summarize the randomized trial evidence that is used to justify interventions in asymptomatic individuals, before reviewing contemporary clinical, biochemical, and imaging-based strategies that might be used in future natural history or randomized studies to define a higher (or lower) risk cohort of patients who might benefit from CEA/CAS. Subgroup analyses from the European Carotid Surgery Trial and the North American Symptomatic Carotid Endarterectomy Trial showed that stenosis severity (but not near occlusion) was predictive of an increased risk of late stroke in medically treated patients. However, neither the Asymptomatic Carotid Atherosclerosis Study nor the Asymptomatic Carotid Surgery Trial found any evidence that (a) increasing stenosis severity, (b) bilateral severe stenosis, or (c) a severe stenosis and contralateral occlusion were predictive of an increased risk of late stroke in medically treated patients.

There is little evidence that increasing stenosis severity is associated with an increased risk of late stroke. Parameters associated with an increased risk of late stroke in asymptomatic patients with carotid disease include (a) silent infarction on CT/MRI; (b) stenosis progression; (c) hypoechoic plaques or Gray Scale Median (GSM) <15; (d) irregular plaques; (e) evidence of spontaneous embolization on transcranial Doppler ultrasound; (f) American Heart Association plaque types IV–V and VI; (g) magnetic resonance-diagnosed intraparenchymal hemorrhage; (h) plaque area $>80\ mm^2$; (i) juxta-luminal black area $>10\ mm^2$; (j) tandem intracranial disease. Clinical features associated with an increased risk of late stroke include; and (k) a history of previous ipsilateral and contralateral transient ischemic attack/minor stroke. Many of the parameters that have been reported to be associated with a greater (or lesser) risk of suffering a stroke have not been subject to independent validation and most of the patients in the constituent studies were not receiving what would now be considered optimal medical therapy. There is also the unanswered question relating to dynamic plaque changes: Can a single "snapshot" be used to predict late stroke risk or is serial surveillance required? It is, therefore, essential that any new natural history studies or randomized trials in asymptomatic patients include an analysis of 1 or more of these imaging strategies to identify the small cohort of "high risk for stroke" patients who will benefit from CEA/CAS. This is a comprehensive well-referenced analysis of a controversial topic.

M. T. Watkins, MD

Outcomes of urgent carotid endarterectomy for stable and unstable acute neurologic deficits

Barbetta I, Carmo M, Mercandalli G, et al (S. Carlo Borromeo Hosp, Milan, Italy)

J Vasc Surg 59:440-446, 2014

Objective.—The aim of the study was to assess the outcomes of carotid endarterectomy (CEA) performed in an urgent setting on acutely symptomatic patients selected through a very simple protocol.

Methods.—From January 2002 to January 2012, 193 symptomatic patients underwent CEA. Of these, 90 presented with acute symptoms, and after a congruous carotid stenosis was identified, underwent urgent operations (group 1): 27 patients had transient ischemic attack (group 1A), 52 patients had mild to moderate stroke (group 1B), and 11 patients had stroke in evolution (group 1C). The remaining 103 patients with a nonrecent neurologic deficit were treated by elective surgery in the same period (group 2). End points were 30-day neurologic morbidity and mortality.

Results.—The median delay of urgent CEA (U-CEA) from deficit onset was 48 hours (interquartile range, 13-117 hours). Groups 1 and 2 were comparable in demographics. Acute patients showed a higher rate of stroke at presentation (70% vs 37%; $P=.001$) and of history of coronary artery disease (30% vs 13.5%; $P=.007$). Acute patients sustained six postoperative strokes (6.6%). Neurologic outcomes were correlated to clinical presentation: no strokes occurred in group 1A patients, and 5.8% group 1B patients and 27.3% group 1C patients had postoperative stroke ($P < .01$). Postoperative mortality was 4.4% for U-CEA: one fatal myocardial infarction, one intracranial hemorrhage, and two thromboembolic strokes. Elective patients sustained four postoperative strokes (3.9%), with one death (0.9%) as a consequence of hyperperfusion cerebral edema. U-CEAs performed ≤48 hours from symptom onset had a lower postoperative stroke rate than those performed >48 hours (4.4% vs 8.8%; $P = .3$). Among patients presenting with a stroke (group 1B), the National Institutes of Health Stroke Scale (NIHSS) assessment at discharge showed improvement in 79% (although only 25% had ≥4 points in reduction), stability in 17%, and deterioration in 4%. Patients with moderate stroke were slightly better in NIHSS improvement than those with mild stroke (median NIHSS variation at discharge, −3 vs −1; $P = .001$).

Conclusions.—Our results with U-CEA confirm that this population has a higher risk profile compared with elective surgery. The type of acute presentation is correlated with perioperative risk. U-CEA was safe when performed on patients presenting with transient ischemic attack. An acceptable complication rate was achieved for patients with minor to moderate strokes. The poorest outcomes occurred in patients presenting with stroke in evolution: U-CEA in these patients should be offered with extreme caution, although we are aware that a conservative treatment may not grant a better prognosis.

▶ This study is significant because it suggests that not only is it safe to perform carotid endarterectomy (CEA) very early after a patient presents with a neurologic event, but that early CEA may, in fact, lead to improved neurologic outcomes. From a practical standpoint, early operation within 48 hours may, perhaps, be of greater convenience to the patient avoiding either a longer hospitalization (while waiting to perform a CEA) or the need for early readmission for a CEA.

Appropriately, the authors discuss a recent Swedish Vascular Registry Study in which a higher rate of complications is reported for symptomatic patients who underwent CEA within 48 hours from symptom onset compared with those who underwent delayed operation (ie, over 48 hours).[1] This study involving more than 2500 patients (compared with 193 in the current study) reported a combined stroke/death rate of 11.5% versus 3.6% to 5.7%. Barbetta et al, however, rightly emphasize that clinical stratification was not reported in the Swedish study. This is germane, because the current study shows that neurologic outcomes were correlated to clinical presentation with those patients presenting with a single or recurrent transient ischemic attack having no adverse neurologic outcomes.

I find it intriguing that the authors have now adopted a nonoperative approach for stroke in evolution, and I wonder if going forward, the results of nonoperative treatment will remain equally dismal or will turn out to actually be significantly worse when compared with operative treatment. I hope the authors will be so kind as to enlighten the vascular community with a follow-up report regarding the nonoperative management of stroke in evolution. Meanwhile, we look forward to larger studies on this topic.

K. Hughes, MD, FACS

Reference

1. Stromberg S, Gelin J, Osterberg T, et al. Very urgent carotid endarterectomy confers increased procedural risk. *Stroke*. 2012;43:1331-1335.

Statins Reduce Peri-procedural Complications in Carotid Stenting

Reiff T, Amiri H, Rohde S, et al (Heidelberg Univ Hosp, Germany; Hosp of Dortmund, Germany)

Eur J Vasc Endovasc Surg 48:626-632, 2014

Background.—In primary and secondary prevention, statins significantly reduce cardiovascular and cerebrovascular events. Pre-interventional statin medication shows a benefit in carotid artery stenosis patients treated with endarterectomy; however, there are few data available for patients treated with stent-angioplasty. The aim of this study was to investigate whether pre-interventional statin therapy is associated with decreased peri-interventional risk of stroke, myocardial infarction, and mortality in patients undergoing stent-angioplasty for internal carotid stenosis.

Methods.—Data for 344 consecutively documented patients with internal carotid artery stenosis treated with stent-angioplasty in the years 2002–2012 at the same stroke center were collected in a prospectively defined database. Risk factors, medication, and indication for therapy were documented. Univariate and multivariate analysis was performed to investigate independent reduction of peri-interventional stroke, myocardial infarction, or death by statin medication prior to stent-angioplasty.

Results.—The median age was 70 years (p25: 63, p75: 76), 75.5% of patients were male, and the median stenosis was 85% according to ECST criteria (p25: 80%, p75: 90%). 20.1% of patients had asymptomatic stenoses, and 60.2% had statin medication before stenting. As per multivariate analysis, pre-interventional statin medication was a predictor for significant peri-interventional risk reduction regarding primary endpoint ischemic stroke, myocardial infarction (MI), or death (odds ratio (OR) 0.31, $p = .006$). Statins also had a significant protective effect in secondary endpoint ischemic stroke, intracranial bleeding or death (OR 0.39, $p = .014$), and ischemic stroke or myocardial infarction (OR 0.20; $p = .002$).

Conclusions.—This study shows that pre-interventional statin medication has a protective effect against peri-interventional stroke, MI, or death in patients with internal carotid artery stenosis treated with stent-angioplasty. Accordingly, statins could be considered as a standard pre-interventional medical therapy in carotid stenting.

▶ The aim of this study was to investigate the effect of preprocedural statin medication on the risk of periprocedural stroke, myocardial infarction, and mortality in a set of patients at a specialized center treated with stent angioplasty for extracranial carotid stenoses. In patients with atherosclerotic stenoses treated by carotid endarterectomy or percutaneous coronary intervention, the periprocedural risk of stroke, myocardial infarction, and death is lowered by preprocedural treatment with statins. In this analysis of patients undergoing carotid artery stenting, patients with statins had fewer ischemic strokes, less subarachnoid hemorrhage, less myocardial infarction, and fewer fatal outcomes, although the differences were not significant. This finding elicits concern regarding the validity of the combined statistical analysis, which showed statin use before stent angioplasty showed a significant preventive effect both for the primary end point as a combination of peri-interventional ischemic stroke, myocardial infarction, and death, and for secondary end points including intracranial hemorrhage and mortality. Is it possible that the reason the uncombined complication rate was not significantly different from the nonstatin patients might be due to the small number of patients in the study. Furthermore, given the preponderance of data that support the protective effects of statins with respect to vascular complications, it seems as if some consideration should be given to those who should be given a short course of a statin therapy; this is particularly important because the protective effect may be independent of the effect of statins on cholesterol.

M. T. Watkins, MD

Carotid Restenosis After Endarterectomy and Stenting: A Critical Issue?

Setacci F, Sirignano P, Galzerano G, et al (Univ of Siena, Italy)

Ann Vasc Surg 27:888-893, 2013

Background.—Carotid artery stenting (CAS) is currently considered a valid alternative to carotid endarterectomy (CEA) for the prevention of stroke in high-risk patients. One of the most important issues for both of these techniques is carotid restenosis. The aim of our study was to evaluate the incidence of post-CEA and post-CAS restenosis in a large cohort of patients in a single high-volume center.

Methods.—Between December 2000 and December 2010, 2453 CEA and 2628 CAS procedures were performed in the Vascular and Endovascular Surgery Unit at our institution. The mean age of patients was 73.8 years (range 55-89 years), 78% of whom were men. Indications for carotid revascularization were: presence of symptomatic carotid artery stenosis of >70%, or asymptomatic stenosis of at least 80%, especially in patients with vulnerable plaques.

Results.—Mild and long-term results after CEA and CAS were similar. The overall perioperative neurologic complication rate (minor and major stroke) was similar in the 2 groups. At 1-year follow-up the restenosis rate after CEA was 1.58%. In-stent restenosis after CAS occurred in 1.67% of the procedures. All but 3 arteries had been treated for postsurgical restenosis. All lesions were approached secondarily with endovascular procedures. Statistical analysis demonstrated that post-CEA restenosis was the most important predictive factor for the development of in-stent restenosis after CAS.

Conclusions.—This review of our 10-year experience confirms that patients who develop restenosis after CEA are also prone to developing in-stent restenosis after CAS.

▶ In this report from Italy, Setacci et al challenge the oft-quoted restenosis rate of 5% to 10% after carotid revascularization by showing their own restenosis rates of less than 2% for both carotid endarterectomy (CEA) and carotid angioplasty and stenting (CAS). Treating these restenoses with CAS yielded a relatively low stroke/death rate at just more than 1% for both CEA and CAS at 30 days and less than 2% at 1 year. Of note, a large number (44%) of restenotic lesions in this study were symptomatic. Interestingly, the most important predictor of restenosis was prior restenosis; actually, virtually all patients treated for restenosis after CAS had originally undergone the CAS for restenosis after previous CEA. This may, in fact, be the real take-home message from this report.

In the discussion, the authors highlight an article suggesting that cilostazol may reduce the restenosis rate after CAS.[1] I look forward to corroborating studies on this topic to see if cilostazol may, in fact, become a standard part of the post-CAS regimen in the future.

K. Hughes, MD, FACS

Reference

1. Takigawa T, Matsumaru Y, Hayakawa M, Nemoto S, Matsumura A. Cilostazol reduces restenosis after carotid artery stenting. *J Vasc Surg*. 2010;51:51-56.

12 Vascular Trauma

Effectiveness of Collateral Vein Embolization for Salvage of Immature Native Arteriovenous Fistulas

Ahmed O, Patel M, Ginsburg M, et al (Univ of Chicago Medicine, IL; et al)
J Vasc Interv Radiol 25:1890-1894, 2014

Purpose.—To investigate the value of collateral vein embolization (CVE) as a salvage treatment for nonmaturing native arteriovenous fistulae (AVFs) in patients requiring hemodialysis.

Materials and Methods.—A total of 49 patients undergoing CVE (N = 65) for immature native AVFs at a single institution were reviewed. The study included 42 patients treated by 56 embolizations. Average fistula age at time of intervention was 18.2 weeks. Each patient underwent angiographic evaluation for fistula immaturity, with clinical success defined by initiation of single-session hemodialysis through the native fistula.

Results.—Fistula maturity was achieved in 32 of 42 patients (76.2%). No major complications occurred. Average time from CVE to fistula maturity was 38.4 days. Angioplasty done with CVE was found in a statistically higher percentage of patients with fistula success versus failure (31.3% vs 8.3%; $P = .039$). Radiocephalic fistulae were seen in a higher percentage of fistula failures compared with successes, but the results were not statistically significant (83.3% vs 59.4%; $P = .054$). Thirty-four patients underwent CVE without angioplasty, which resulted in successful fistula maturation in 22 cases (64.7%). Radiocephalic fistulae were again seen in a higher percentage of fistula failures compared with successes, but the findings did not meet statistical significance (81.8% vs 54.5%; $P = .052$).

Conclusions.—Coil embolization of competing collateral vessels as a salvage treatment for nonfunctioning autologous AVFs is a viable treatment option in the majority of patients. Patients with radiocephalic fistulae may be at higher risk for primary fistula failure, but the present data are inconclusive.

▶ An important barrier toward increasing fistula prevalence remains primary fistula failure, with rates of failure in North America reported to range between 25% and 33%.[1] In this article, the authors focus on the issue salvaging nonmaturing arteriovenous fistulas using the technique of collateral vein embolization (CVE). Although angioplasty of an underlying stenosis remains an effective technique for fistula salvage, the treatment of competing collateral veins remains controversial, with varying opinions regarding their management. Some other interventionists report that underlying venous stenoses are found 100% of the time, leading to their explanation that collateral veins in this setting are secondary to reflux from the downstream narrowing. Alternatively, others have advocated for treatment of collateral veins with surgical ligation or endovascular embolotherapy.

The findings from the present study support the latter theory because the majority of patients treated by CVE (76.2%) did show a progression to fistula maturity. Additionally, the large majority of CVE procedures in the present study were done without angioplasty (44 of 56; 78.6%) because no clear underlying stenosis was observed. This finding is unique in that it contradicts previous findings of a low overall incidence of collateral veins in patients with immature AVFs without a downstream stenosis. The present data suggest that collateral veins may represent true accessory drainage pathways that return blood to the right atrium and subsequently prevent arterialization of the target outflow vein. In addition, the results show that even when CVE is performed alone without additional diagnostic abnormality, fistula maturity was achieved in the majority of patients (64.7%). Finally, no major complications such as coil migration were seen, supporting the safety of this minimally invasive technique.

D. L. Gillespie, MD, RVT, FACS

Reference

1. Falk A. Optimizing hemodialysis arteriovenous fistula maturation. *J VascAccess.* 2011;12:1-3.

Characteristics and clinical outcome in patients after popliteal artery injury

Lang NW, Joestl JB, Platzer P (Med Univ of Vienna, Austria)

J Vasc Surg 61:1495-1500, 2015

Background.—The treatment of popliteal artery injury (PAI) caused by blunt or penetrating mechanism is demanding. Concomitant injuries and prolonged ischemia are the major causes of lower extremity morbidity and poor rates of limb salvage. This study assessed the amputation rate and, subsequently, the therapeutic management and clinical outcomes regarding the effect of concomitant injuries among patients with PAI in a setting of central European trauma care.

Methods.—Sixty-four patients (20 female and 44 male), with an average age of 44 years (range, 17-79 years) at the time of injury, were evaluated for clinical characteristics, concomitant injuries, complications, amputation rates, and functional outcome after traumatic PAI. The mechanism of injury was blunt trauma in 35 patients (54.7%) and penetrating trauma in 29 (45.3%). The Mangled Extremity Severity Score and the Injury Severity Score were assessed initially and the modified Functional Independence Measure (FIM) Score at 12 months after the primary surgery.

Results.—Thirty patients (47%) returned to their normal activity level within 1 year after trauma, and 16 (25%) were limited in their daily activity or suffered from chronic pain symptoms. Within the blunt trauma group 26 of 35 patients (74%) sustained severe concomitant injuries, whereas two of 29 patients (7%) in the penetrating group showed severe concomitant injuries ($P < .046$). Eleven patients (17%) had to undergo revision surgery due to their associated injuries. The median modified FIM score was 10.3, whereas patients with blunt trauma had significantly lower FIM score ($P < .0082$). The median Mangled Extremity Severity Score was 6 points (range, 6-16 points). Primary or secondary amputation was required in 18 patients (28%) due to failure of revascularization. Patients who sustained blunt trauma had significantly higher amputation rates than those with penetrating injuries ($P < .035$).

Conclusions.—Clinical outcome and limb salvage of patients with PAI were influenced by the mechanism of trauma, concomitant injuries, prolonged ischemia time, and the type of surgical procedure. Patients after blunt trauma had a higher incidence of concomitant injuries, and (comminuted) fractures or knee dislocations and severe soft tissue damage had the highest effect on the amputation rate.

▶ Blunt mechanism of trauma and concomitant injuries, such as (comminuted) fractures and knee dislocations, and severe soft tissue damage, lead to a significantly higher rate of amputation compared with penetrating trauma. Other factors that seem to have a negative effect on limb salvage rates and functional outcome are prolonged times of ischemia and the surgical procedure of arterial repair.

The durability of vein grafts is well documented and seems to be the best option for below-knee revascularization, whereas the use of polytetrafluoroethylene (PTFE) remains controversial. In this series, the authors registered the highest secondary amputation rates among patients who underwent arterial repair by PTFE patches (55.5%), 8 times for thrombosis and 2 times for infection. In contrast to the literature, the authors in this small series had a high rate of direct suture repair (> 90%) in patients after penetrating popliteal artery injury. Nevertheless, they observed the best outcome for limb salvage rates and functional outcome in this group of patients.

B. W. Starnes, MD

Outcomes after endovascular repair of arterial trauma

Desai SS, DuBose JJ, Parham CS, et al (Univ of Texas Med School at Houston)

J Vasc Surg 60:1309-1314, 2014

Background.—Endovascular repair of peripheral arterial trauma using covered stent grafts is a minimally invasive alternative to open surgery in selected patients. Although the technical feasibility of endovascular repair has been established, there are a paucity of data regarding outcomes. The purpose of this study was to evaluate the short-term outcomes of endovascular repair in patients with peripheral arterial trauma.

Methods.—A review of a prospectively collected institutional trauma registry captured all patients with peripheral arterial injury who underwent endovascular repair from August 2004 to June 2012. Data collected included demographics, Injury Severity Score (ISS), mechanism, location and type of injury, imaging modality, intervention type, complications and reintervention, length of stay, and follow-up. Descriptive statistics were used for analysis.

Results.—During the study period, we performed endovascular repair in 28 patients with peripheral arterial injuries. There were 20 male patients (71%) with a median age of 39 years (range, 13-88 years). The mean ISS was 17.2 (range, 9-41). The mechanism of injury was penetrating in 21 (75%) and blunt in seven (25%). The anatomic locations of the 28 arterial injuries were carotid (3 [11%]), subclavian (7 [25%]), axillary (6 [22%]), iliac (3 [11%]), and femoral/popliteal (9 [32%]). Findings consistent with injury on imaging included pseudoaneurysms (9 [32%]), extravasations (9 [32%]), occlusions (6 [22%]), and arteriovenous fistulas (4 [14%]). Technical success was achieved in all patients. The overall complication rate was 21%, with six patients requiring a secondary procedure. Two patients underwent a planned, elective conversion to open repair during the initial hospitalization. Four patients required conversion secondary to stent graft thrombosis. Three conversions were early (<30 days) and one was late (>30 days). The mean length of stay was 18.4 ± 22.9 days (range, 1-93 days), with a median follow-up of 13 months (range, 1-60 months). The overall limb salvage rate was 92% at 45 days and 79% at 93 days.

Conclusions.—The present study outlines our early experience with endovascular repair of peripheral arterial injuries in a variety of anatomic locations. Overall complication rates are appreciable but can be effectively detected and managed with additional intervention. The inclusion of endovascular modalities in algorithms of trauma care holds considerable promise. The need to better define optimal algorithms for utilization and determine long-term outcomes of intervention requires significant additional study (Table 1).

▶ Endovascular repair of peripheral arterial trauma is an attractive minimally invasive alternative to open surgery in selected patients. With the development and adoption of endovascular techniques, management of peripheral vascular injuries with covered stents has become more accepted by trauma care providers. Although the technical feasibility of endovascular repair has been established, hesitation surrounding the use of this modality stems from lack of data regarding short-term and long-term outcomes. Trauma patients tend to be younger, and hence, the durability of the repair becomes most important. The purpose of this study was to evaluate the short-term outcomes of endovascular repair in patients with peripheral arterial trauma at a major urban level 1 trauma center in the United States.

TABLE 1.—Demographics, Mechanism of Injury, Angiography Findings, Injury Severity Score (ISS), Length of Stay, and Findings at Follow-up for All Study Patients

Variable	Result (N = 28)
Age, years	39.2 ± 20.5
Male gender	20 (71)
ISS	17.4 ± 8.7
Length of stay, days	18.4 ± 22.9
Follow-up, months	13 (1-60)
Amputation	2 (7)
Mortality	5 (18)
Mechanism of injury	
Penetrating	21 (75)
Blunt	7 (25)
Angiography finding	
Occlusion	6 (20)
Arteriovenous fistula	4 (14)
Pseudoaneurysm	9 (35)
Extravasation	9 (35)
Vascular injury	
Common carotid	1 (3)
Internal carotid	2 (7)
Subclavian	7 (25)
Axillary	6 (22)
Common iliac	1 (3)
External iliac	1 (3)
Internal iliac	1 (3)
Superficial femoral	1 (3)
Popliteal	8 (30)

SD, Standard deviation.

Continuous data are presented as mean ± standard deviation, and categorical data are presented as number (%) or median (range).

During the study period, 223 patients were admitted to this institution with peripheral arterial injuries, and 108 (48%) underwent a vascular intervention. Of these, 28 patients (13%) had a peripheral arterial injury that was managed with endovascular therapy. In the endovascular intervention group, there were 20 males (71%). The median age of the cohort was 39 years (range, 13-88 years). The mean Injury Severity Score was 17.2 (range, 9-41). There were 21 penetrating injuries (75%) and 7 blunt injuries (25%; Table 1).

The present study outlines an early experience with the application of endovascular therapy in the management of peripheral arterial injury in a variety of anatomic locations. Stent graft repair is applicable to a broad range of injuries, but the rate of short-term failure resulting in open conversion remains high. The need to better define optimal algorithms for use and determine long-term outcomes of intervention requires significant additional study.

There remains an opportunity here for newer technologies in the form of bio absorbable stents or "scaffolds" that would allow immediate treatment but leave no foreign body behind in the long term.

B. W. Starnes, MD

Trends and outcomes of endovascular therapy in the management of civilian vascular injuries

Branco BC, DuBose JJ, Zhan LX, et al (Univ of Arizona, Tucson; Univ of Texas Health Sciences Ctr at Houston)

J Vasc Surg 60:1297-1307, 2014

Objective.—The rapid evolution of endovascular surgery has greatly expanded management options for a wide variety of vascular diseases. Endovascular therapy provides a less invasive alternative to open surgery for critically ill patients who have sustained arterial injuries. The purpose of this study was to evaluate recent trends in the management of arterial injuries in the United States with specific reference to the use of endovascular strategies and to examine the outcomes of endovascular vs open therapy for the treatment of civilian arterial traumatic injuries.

Methods.—A 9-year analysis of the National Trauma Data Bank was performed to identify all patients who sustained arterial injuries. Demographics, clinical data, interventions, and outcomes were extracted. Propensity scores were used to match endovascular patients to those undergoing open operation. Patient outcomes were compared according to treatment approach.

Results.—A total of 23,105 patients were available for analysis. Overall, there was a significant increase in the use of endovascular procedures during 9 years (from 0.3% in 2002 to 9.0% in 2010; $P < .001$), particularly among blunt trauma patients (from 0.4% in 2002 to 13.2% in 2010; $P < .001$). This increase was noteworthy and dramatic for injuries of the internal iliac artery (from 8.0% in 2002 to 40.3% in 2010; $P < .001$), thoracic aorta (from 0.5% in 2002 to 21.9% in 2010; $P < .001$), and common/external iliac arteries (from 0.4% in 2002 to 20.4% in 2010; $P < .001$). A significant decrease was noted for open procedures (49.1% in 2002 to 45.6%; $P < .001$), especially for blunt trauma (42.9% in 2002 to 35.8% in 2010; $P < .001$). There was a stepwise increase in the proportion of patients managed by endovascular therapy as the Injury Severity Score increased (highest in the spectrum Injury Severity Score 31-50). When outcomes were compared between matched patients who underwent endovascular and open procedures, patients who underwent endovascular procedures had significantly lower in-hospital mortality (12.9% vs 22.4%; odds ratio, 0.5; 95% confidence interval, 0.4-0.6; $P < .001$). Endovascular patients also had decreased rates of sepsis (7.5% vs 5.4%; odds ratio, 0.7; 95% confidence interval, 0.5-0.9; $P = .025$).

Conclusions.—The use of endovascular therapy in the United States has increased dramatically during the last decade, in particular among severely injured blunt trauma patients. Endovascular therapy was associated with improved in-hospital mortality and lower rates of sepsis (Figs 1, 2 and 4).

► The purpose of this study was twofold: (1) to evaluate recent trends in management of arterial injuries in the United States with specific reference to the

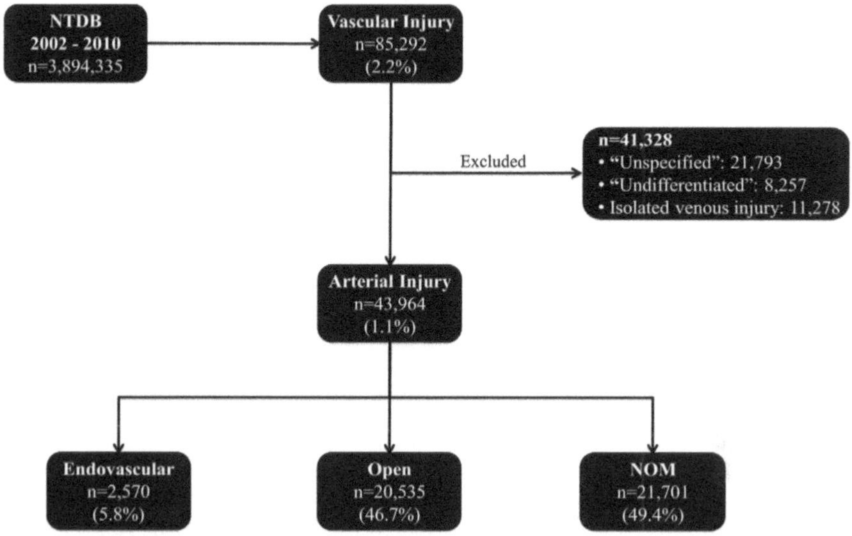

FIGURE 1.—Study outline. A total of 842 patients (1.9%) who sustained arterial injuries underwent hybrid (open and endovascular) procedures. *NOM*, Nonoperative management. *NTDB*, National Trauma Data Bank. (Reprinted from the Journal of Vascular Surgery. Branco BC, DuBose JJ, Zhan LX, et al. Trends and outcomes of endovascular therapy in the management of civilian vascular injuries. *J Vasc Surg*. 2014;60:1297-1307, Copyright 2014, with permission from The Society for Vascular Surgery.)

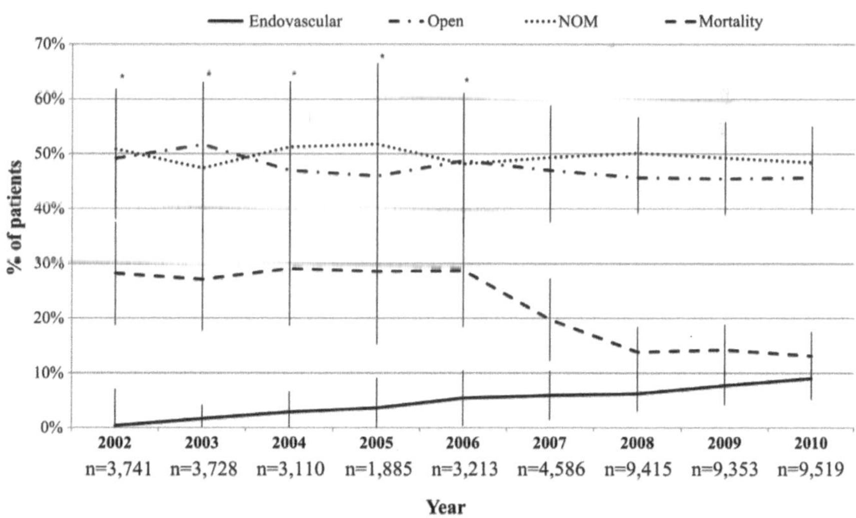

FIGURE 2.—Management trends throughout the study period. There was a significant increase in endovascular management during 9 years ($P < .001$). A significant decrease was noted for the open and nonoperative management (*NOM*) groups ($P < .001$). Mortality significantly decreased during the study period ($P < .001$). *n*, Number of patients per study year. *Standard error exceeds 10%. (Reprinted from the Journal of Vascular Surgery. Branco BC, DuBose JJ, Zhan LX, et al. Trends and outcomes of endovascular therapy in the management of civilian vascular injuries. *J Vasc Surg*. 2014;60:1297-1307, Copyright 2014, with permission from The Society for Vascular Surgery.)

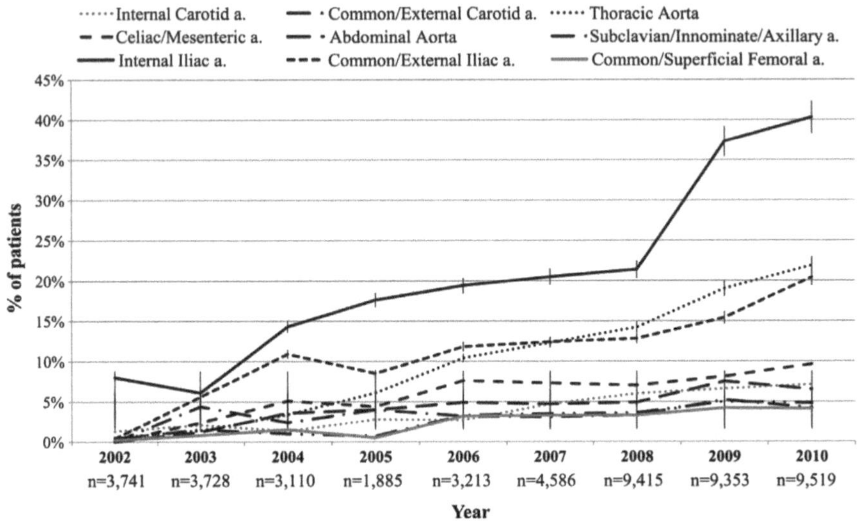

FIGURE 4.—Growth in endovascular procedures during the study period according to the type of arterial injury. Statistically significant growth was achieved for all injuries ($P < .001$). (Reprinted from the Journal of Vascular Surgery. Branco BC, DuBose JJ, Zhan LX, et al. Trends and outcomes of endovascular therapy in the management of civilian vascular injuries. *J Vasc Surg*. 2014;60:1297-1307, Copyright 2014, with permission from The Society for Vascular Surgery.)

use of endovascular strategies and (2) to examine the outcomes of endovascular versus open therapy for the treatment of arterial injuries among civilian trauma patients. The authors hypothesis was that (1) endovascular arterial injury control or repair would be increasing in the United States for the management of both blunt and penetrating arterial injuries—in particular, among severely injured patients—and that (2) endovascular therapy would be associated with lower rates of in-hospital complications and improved survival.

During the 9-year study period, 85 292 (2.2%) of the 3 894 335 National Trauma Data Bank patients sustained a vascular injury. After exclusion of 41 328 patients (48.4%) with "unspecified," "undifferentiated," or isolated venous injuries, 43 964 patients (51.6%) were available for analysis. Of those, 2570 patients (5.8%) underwent endovascular procedures, 20 535 patients (46.7%) underwent open procedures, and 21 701 patients (49.4%) underwent nonoperative management (Fig 1).

This study is the largest examination to date evaluating the role of endovascular therapy in the management of civilian arterial injuries. Trends for endovascular therapies are definitely increasing, especially for blunt aortic injury with associated improvement in outcomes (Figs 2 and 4).

B. W. Starnes, MD

Management and outcomes of blunt common and external iliac arterial injuries

Harris DG, Drucker CB, Brenner ML, et al (Univ of Maryland School of Medicine, Baltimore)

J Vasc Surg 59:180-185, 2014

Objective.—Blunt iliac arterial injuries (BIAI) require complex management but are rare and poorly studied. We investigated the presentation, management, and outcomes of patients with blunt common or external iliac arterial injuries.

Methods.—We identified and reviewed 112 patients with BIAI admitted between 2000 and 2011 at a Level I trauma center. Patients with common/external iliac artery injuries (CE group) were primarily analyzed, with patients with injuries of the internal iliac artery or its major branches (IB group) included for comparison of pelvic arterial trauma.

Results.—Twenty-four patients had CE and 88 had IB injuries. Mean ages (45 ± 19 years) and gender (86% male) were similar between groups. The mean injury severity score was 40 ± 14 (CE, 36 ± 15; IB, 40 ± 14; $P = .19$), indicating severe trauma. Twenty (83%) of the CE patients presented with signs of leg malperfusion. Admission factors associated with CE injury were crush mechanism of injury (37% vs 17%; $P = .03$) and pelvic soft tissue trauma (50% vs 15%; $P < .01$). The CE group had higher early mortality rates, both within 3 hours of admission (50% vs 19%; $P = .04$) and prior to iliac intervention (42% vs 3%; $P < .01$). Among those surviving to management, CE patients were more likely to undergo open repair or revascularization (68% vs 3%; $P < .01$) and had a higher rate of leg amputation (50% vs 6%; $P < .01$), with 8/12 (67%) culminating in hemipelvectomy. Risk factors for amputation included leg malperfusion, high-grade pelvic fractures, pelvic soft tissue trauma, and increasing leg injury severity. Overall mortality was 40%, and was similar between the injury groups. Among CE patients, need for amputation, pelvic fractures, and wounds were associated with inpatient mortality.

Conclusions.—This is the largest series to date of blunt CE injuries and demonstrates distinct clinical features and outcomes for these patients. They have high risk for early death and proximal leg amputation. CE injury is specifically associated with serious open pelvic soft tissue injury, which, along with high-grade pelvic fractures, is a risk factor for amputation and death. On-demand emergent endovascular intervention may play an important role in improving management of these complex injuries.

▶ This study from the University of Maryland R Adams Cowley Shock Trauma Center represents the largest reported single-institution collection of patients with common and external iliac artery (CE) injuries in the setting of blunt trauma. Patients with CE injuries (n = 24) represent 0.04% of all primary blunt trauma admissions at this busy trauma center. Crush mechanism of injury and pelvic soft tissue trauma were associated with CE injuries, and 83% of CE injury patients presented with evidence of malperfusion. Among those patients undergoing revascularization, 80% still required amputation despite patent repairs in 88% of amputees. The overall in-hospital mortality rate for patients presenting with blunt iliac artery injury was 40% and was associated with high-grade pelvic fractures, pelvic soft tissue wounds, and amputation.

One of the interesting points to be taken from this study is that despite technically successful revascularization in those patients presenting with malperfusion, most patients still ultimately required amputation despite patent repairs. As the authors suggest, this finding may suggest a more prominent role for damage control, vascular control, and early amputation in an effort to improve overall survival. Perhaps too, endovascular interventions need to be further evaluated. Only 2 patients (11%) underwent emergent endovascular interventions for CE injuries. The combination of emergent endovascular control with or without revascularization and early amputation may result in improved outcomes in the future.

B. Peterson, MD, FACS

Blunt cerebrovascular injuries in association with craniocervical distraction injuries: a retrospective review of consecutive cases

Vilela MD, Kim LJ, Bellabarba C, et al (Mater Dei Hosp, Belo Hoisonte, Brazil; Univ of Washington, Seattle)

Spine J 15:499-505, 2015

Background Context.—Blunt cerebrovascular injuries (BCVIs) have the potential to cause brain, cerebellar, and/or spinal cord ischemia. Certain subtypes of spine fractures, such as vertebral subluxation, fractures through the foramen transversarium, and C1–C3 fractures have been linked to a higher incidence of BCVI. On the other hand, BCVI in association with craniocervical distraction injuries (CCDs) have been only anecdotally reported.

Purpose.—We hypothesized that because CCD is also caused by a high-energy hyperflexion/hyperextension distraction mechanism, it could also be associated with a high incidence of BCVI.

Study Design/Setting.—Retrospective chart review.

Patient Sample.—Of 46 consecutive patients with unstable craniocervical dissociations treated operatively at a single Level I trauma center from January 1996 to December 2009, 29 of the 46 had vascular studies that comprised the study sample.

Outcome Measures.—Primary outcomes assessed were BCVI subdivided into blunt carotid artery injuries and/or blunt vertebral artery injuries and classified according to the Biffl criteria. Secondary measures included associated strokes and evidence of emboli on transcranial Doppler.

Methods.—All consecutive patients diagnosed with unstable CCD injuries that were surgically treated at a single Level I trauma center during the period of 1996 to 2009 were identified. Those who were adequately screened with a catheter angiogram and/or computed tomography angiogram of the neck so as to rule out BCVI were included in this study. Electronic medical records were used to determine mechanism, demographics, clinical findings, and transcranial Doppler reports. Angiography and computed tomography angiograms were analyzed to assess for BCVI. If a BCVI was identified, these were classified using the Biffl criteria.

Results.—Among the 29 screened patients, 30 BCVIs were identified in 15 patients. According to the Biffl criteria, there were 13 Grade I, eight Grade II, five Grade III, three Grade IV, and one Grade V injuries. Three major strokes were diagnosed in those 15 patients with BCVI, as opposed to none among the other 14 patients without BCVI.

Conclusions.—Blunt cerebrovascular injuries were seen in more than 50% of the patients screened, with major strokes occurring in 20% of the patients. We suggest screening for BCVI in all patients presenting with C0–C1 and/or C1–C2 distraction injuries.

▶ The occurrence of blunt cerebrovascular injuries (BCVIs) is particularly concerning because of the potential deleterious disabilities related to stroke. Recently, screening of certain trauma subpopulations with computed tomography angiograms, magnetic resonance angiograms, or angiography has led to early diagnosis and initiation of treatment, with reported decreases in stroke rates. With advancements in prehospital and hospital care, the number of surviving patients with craniocervical dissociation (CCD) injuries has been increasing. Because BCVI occurs in association with high-energy hyperextension/flexion injuries [6], we hypothesized that patients with CCD injuries would have a high incidence of BCVI because hyperextension/distraction is the primary force responsible for the CCD. These authors investigated the incidence of BCVI in a series of patients treated in a single Level I trauma institution who presented with unstable craniocervical distraction injuries. The authors performed a retrospective review of 29 patients with unstable craniocervical distraction injuries who also had appropriate vascular screening. Approximately half the patients sustained 1 or more BCVIs. Three major strokes occurred among the patients with BCVIs, whereas none were documented in patients without this concomitant injury. The authors advocate for screening for BCVI in all patients with craniocervical distraction injuries. This retrospective study is confounded by selection and indication bias, thus limiting the capacity to determine the true incidence of BCVI after craniocervical trauma. Patients who did not receive appropriate vascular screening may have also had these injuries but could not be included in this analysis. Furthermore, the mere fact that the cohort under consideration had vascular studies performed indicates that they probably were at elevated risk of vascular trauma. Nonetheless, given the rarity of CCD and the severity of vascular sequelae if undetected, the authors' recommendations for universal screening for BCVI are likely well founded.

M. T. Watkins, MD

A Shift Toward Endovascular Repair for Vascular Complications in Lumbar Disc Surgery During the Last Decade

van Zitteren M, Fan B, Lohle PN, et al (St. Elisabeth Hosp, Tilburg, The Netherlands)

Ann Vasc Surg 27:810-819, 2013

Background.—The purpose of this study is to evaluate 2 patients who underwent endovascular repair directly after acute life-threatening vascular injury complicating lumbar disc surgery, and to update an overview of the literature from 2002 to gain insights into characteristics, diagnosis, treatment, and outcomes of this rare, life-threatening complication.

Methods.—PubMed was searched for English language studies on vascular injury (lacerations, arteriovenous fistulas, and pseudoaneurysms) complicating lumbar disc surgery by a posterior approach published from 2002. Two cases from the authors' institute were added to the review. Information on patient characteristics, diagnosis, treatment strategies, and outcomes were extracted by 2 independent reviewers.

> *Case Reports.*—The first case describes a 54-year-old man who underwent lumbar disc surgery through a posterior approach (L5–S1) and became hypotensive intraoperatively. Angiography revealed an injury of the right internal iliac artery. Bleeding was successfully repaired by endovascular repair (acute balloon occlusion followed by coiling). The second case describes a 51-year-old women who suddenly became hypotensive during L4 through L5 discectomy caused by bleeding from a laceration in the right common iliac artery. Angiography confirmed the diagnosis, and the bleeding was successfully treated through endovascular repair with a covered stent.

Results.—A total of 56 cases from 34 articles were found in the literature since 2002, including lacerations, arteriovenous fistulas, and pseudoaneurysms. Two cases from the authors' institute were added to the review. Vascular injury was recognized intraoperatively in 36%, and within 24 hours postsurgery in 28%. The common iliac artery was most frequently affected (51%), followed by the iliac vein (23%). All lacerations were detected during surgery, whereas most arteriovenous fistulas and pseudoaneurysms were detected in the long term. Treatment consisted of open surgical repair (57%) or endovascular repair (43%). All patients survived surgery.

Conclusions.—Publication bias might play a role in the literature of this area because all cases survived surgery, whereas mortality rates for this condition are high. However, early recognition, diagnosis, and prompt surgical repair are essential to prevent fatal outcomes in vascular injuries complicating lumbar disc surgery. Endovascular repair is a minimally invasive, fast, and efficient treatment modality that is increasingly and preferably used because of its low morbidity and mortality.

▶ Vascular injuries, traumatic or iatrogenic, can benefit greatly from endovascular surgery for several reasons. First, endovascular surgery is less physiologically insulting than open surgery in patients who are often bleeding severely. Second, endovascular therapy offers the opportunity to achieve diagnosis and treatment nearly simultaneously. Controlling bleeding from vascular injuries must be accomplished quickly and with a minimum of collateral damage. The authors of this report, in their description of cases and review of the literature, point to how well-suited endovascular therapy is to the treatment of the difficult retroperitoneal vascular injuries that can complicate lumbar spine surgery.

P. W. White, MD, FACS

Applying peripheral vascular injury guidelines to penetrating trauma

Chong VE, Lee WS, Miraflor E, et al (Univ of California, San Francisco—East Bay, Oakland)

J Surg Res 190:300-304, 2014

Introduction.—Treatment of traumatic vascular injury is evolving because of endovascular therapies. National guidelines advocate for embolization of injuries to lower extremity branch vessels, including pseudoaneurysms or arteriovenous fistulas, in hemodynamically normal patients without hard signs of vascular injury. However, patient stability and injury type may limit endovascular applicability at some centers. We hypothesized that for penetrating trauma, indications for endovascular treatment of peripheral vascular injuries, as outlined by national guidelines, are infrequent.

Methods.—We reviewed records of patients sustaining penetrating peripheral vascular injuries treated at our university-based urban trauma center from 2006–2010. Patient demographics and outcomes were analyzed.

Results.—In 92 patients with penetrating peripheral vascular injuries, 82 were managed operatively and 10 were managed nonoperatively. Seventeen (18%) were hemodynamically unstable on arrival, 44 (48%) had multiple vessels injured, and 76 (83%) presented at night and/or on the weekend. No pseudoaneurysms or arteriovenous fistulas were seen initially or at follow-up. Applying national guidelines to our cohort, only two patients (2.2%) met recommended criteria for endovascular treatment.

Conclusions.—According to national guidelines, indications for endovascular treatment of penetrating peripheral vascular injury are infrequent. Nearly two-thirds of patients with penetrating peripheral vascular injuries were hemodynamically unstable or had multiple vessels injured, making endovascular repair less desirable. Additionally, over

80% presented at night and/or on the weekend, which could delay treatment at some centers due to mobilization of the endovascular team. Trauma centers need to consider their resources when incorporating national guidelines in their treatment algorithms of penetrating vascular trauma.

▶ Usually national guidelines and consensus statements lag behind the cutting edge of medical science by several years. This report reviewed a single center's experience with penetrating vascular trauma in light of the current guidelines from the Western Trauma Association and the Eastern Association for the Surgery of Trauma. The current guidelines are rather conservative in their recommendations for endovascular therapy, limiting the indications to embolization of terminal arteries in areas of good collateralization. Endovascular technology and techniques are relatively new and continue to evolve and improve but remain relatively understudied. National guidelines will more generously recommend these techniques, as their utility, safety, and durability are demonstrated in more patients. There can be no doubt that open surgery will always have a significant role in treating vascular trauma. Nevertheless, endovascular surgery has already established superiority over open surgery in treating blunt aortic injury. Penetrating injuries to the subclavian arteries, aorta, and iliac arteries have been successfully treated in many patients. The authors seem to indicate that endovascular surgery is unsuitable for hemodynamically unstable patients. It is reminiscent of arguments against endovascular aortic repair (EVAR) for ruptured abdominal aortic aneurysms. EVAR is clearly equal to or superior to open repair in suitable patients, and many would argue shows the greatest benefit in unstable patients. In my opinion, endovascular surgery has great promise in rapidly controlling vascular injuries, allowing for the stabilization of the polytrauma patient while definitive repair (open or endovascular) is delayed until physiologic parameters are more favorable. In other words, we can use covered stents as endovascularly deployed vascular shunts. This report strikes me as an attempt by trauma surgeons to defend what they view as their "turf" (operating on trauma patients) against vascular surgeons who bring a more varied and technologically advance skillset to the operating table. I found this report reactionary and backward.

P. W. White, MD, FACS

Common Femoral Vein Reconstruction Using Internal Jugular Vein after Blast Injury

Holt AM, West CA, Davis JA, et al (Baylor College of Medicine, Houston, TX)
Ann Vasc Surg 28:1791.e5-1791.e7, 2014

Common femoral vein traumatic injuries are rare. Surgical management is controversial and by nature case specific. In this report, we present an unusual case of an isolated common femoral vein injury from a gunshot blast repaired with an interposition internal jugular vein bypass. To our knowledge, this is the first reported case of an isolated common femoral vein reconstructed in this manner.

▶ This case report of a serious common femoral vein injury demonstrates the importance of venous reconstruction in traumatic vascular injuries. I commend the authors for their flexibility in changing strategies when ligation for life-threatening hemorrhage clearly caused limb-threatening venous congestion. The use of the internal jugular vein as conduit for interposition reconstruction of a large venous structure has been well described in the past, and the authors applied that knowledge in this case. They also provide a succinct review of other potential conduits used for venous repair, discussing the advantages, disadvantages, and other considerations of each potential choice of conduit. Venous repair clearly improves the long-term outcomes after vascular trauma, but this case also demonstrates that attention to the principles of damage control and the immediate control of hemorrhage are prerequisites to vascular reconstruction. Vascular reconstruction, especially venous repair, should only be undertaken if acidosis, hypothermia, and coagulopathy can be avoided during the potentially long period of time required for vascular reconstruction.

P. W. White, MD, FACS

Comparison of military and civilian popliteal artery trauma outcomes

Dua A, Patel B, Desai SS, et al (UT Health, Houston, TX; Med College of Wisconsin, Milwaukee; Univ of Texas Houston Med School; et al)
J Vasc Surg 59:1628-1632, 2014

Objective.—Popliteal artery injury has historically led to high amputation rates in both the military and civilian setting. Military and civilian popliteal injury patterns differ in mechanism and severity of injury, prompting us to compare modern management and report differences in outcomes between these two patient groups. We hypothesized that whereas amputation rates may be higher in the military, this would correlate with worse overall injury severity.

Methods.—Military casualties from 2003-2007 with a popliteal artery injury identified from the Joint Theater Trauma Registry were compared retrospectively with civilian patients presenting to a single level I institution from 2002-2009 with popliteal arterial injury. Demographics, mechanism of injury, coinjuries, Injury Severity Score (ISS), Mangled Extremity Severity Scores (MESS), interventions, and secondary amputation rates were reviewed. Descriptive statistics and unpaired t-tests were used to compare data. Statistical significance was $P < .05$.

Results.—The study group of 110 patients consisted of 46 (41.8%) military and 64 (58.2%) civilians with 48 and 64 popliteal artery injuries, respectively. The military population was younger (28 vs 35 years; $P < .004$), entirely male (46 [100%] vs 51 [80%]; $P < .0001$), and had more penetrating injuries (44 [96%] vs 19 [30%]; $P < .0001$). ISS (18.7 vs 13.9; $P < .005$) and

MESS (7.3 vs 5.1; $P < .0001$) were higher in the military group. Limb revascularizations in both military and civilian populations were mostly by autogenous bypass (65% vs 77%) followed by primary repair (26% vs 16%), covered stent (0% vs 6%), or other procedure (ligation and/or thrombectomy) (9% vs 1%). Fasciotomy (20 [42%] vs 37 [58%]; $P = .14$), compartment syndrome (10 [21%] vs 15 [23%]; $P = .84$), and concomitant venous repair rates (14 [29%] vs 15 [23%]; $P = .42$) were not different between cohorts. There was no difference in the fracture rate (26 [54%] vs 41 [64%]; $P = .43$), but the civilian group had a higher rate of dislocation (1 [2%] vs 19 [30%]; $P < .0001$). Secondary amputation rates were significantly higher in the military (14 [29%] vs 8 [13%]; $P < .03$).

Conclusions.—Although both civilian and military cohorts have high amputation rates for popliteal arterial injury, the rate of amputation appears to be higher in the military and is associated with a penetrating mechanism of injury primarily from improvised explosive devices resulting in a higher MESS and ISS.

▶ The authors present an excellent exploration of the differences in severity, mechanism of injury, and outcome between civilian and military popliteal artery injuries. Their initial inspiration for the study was the higher amputation rates seen in military popliteal injuries compared with civilian popliteal injuries. Many of their findings are straightforward and somewhat predictable, but they synthesize the information well, pointing out that wartime arterial trauma is often the result of blast injuries. Although categorized as "penetrating" trauma, blast injuries often involve injuries to remote anatomic regions or physiologic systems, and blast injuries often involve more extensive local tissue damage. The authors note the higher Injury Severity Score and Mangled Extremity Severity Scores of the military cohort and rightly suggest that this contributes to the higher amputation rate. As I like to point out to my students and residents, limbs only have 5 important components: bones, muscles, skin, nerves, and blood vessels. The authors did find similar fracture rates, so injuries to bone are unlikely to account for the difference, but blast injuries are far more likely to disrupt the other components of muscle, skin, and nerves than blunt or other forms of penetrating trauma. Future studies to elucidate the role of skin, muscle, and nerve of these tissues in vascular injuries would be helpful.

P. W. White, MD, FACS

Endovascular Repair of Acute Traumatic Aortic Injury: Experience of a Level-1 Trauma Center

Asaid R, Boyce G, Atkinson N (The Royal Melbourne Hosp, Victoria, Australia)
Ann Vasc Surg 28:1391-1395, 2014

Background.—Endovascular repair of the thoracic aorta after traumatic rupture is an alternative to open repair and its use is becoming increasingly widespread. We aimed to determine the concurrent injuries sustained in patients who underwent thoracic endovascular aortic repair (TEVAR) as well as their Glasgow Coma Score (GCS) and Injury Severity Score (ISS). We also aimed to identify the intraoperative and early complications of TEVAR grafting up to 6 months after procedure and in addition identify the late postoperative complications occurring after 6 months after stent.

Methods.—Data were collected retrospectively between January 1998 and January 2012. The Australasian Vascular Audit and hospital trauma registry were used to obtain data related to those patients who underwent TEVAR at our center. Their characteristics were analyzed including associated injuries, delays to diagnosis, ISS scores, and early and long-term complications of endovascular repair.

Results.—Forty patients (mean age 41.3 ± 20.1) underwent stent graft repair of traumatic thoracic rupture at the aortic isthmus. Motor vehicle and motorbike accidents were responsible for 82.5% of presentations. Average ISS was 37 ± 13 (range 20–75) with an average GCS of 12.5 ± 3.8 at scene. Intraoperative death occurred in 2 cases (ISS score of 75), with 1 further death from severe head injures within 30 days. Average follow-up time was 5.48 ± 2.89 years (maximum 13 years).

Conclusions.—Endovascular intervention is a safe and effective treatment, with minimal longer term complications seen after 5-year follow-up.

▶ Endovascular aortic repair (EVAR) for rupture abdominal aortic aneurysms (AAA) and thoracic endovascular aortic repair (TEVAR) for blunt thoracic aortic injury (BTAI) are the 2 best examples of endovascular techniques supplanting open surgery in acute surgical care. This retrospective review out of Australia has similarly low rates of mortality for BTAI to previous studies that showed the superiority of TEVAR. I found several aspects of the results interesting. First, 10% of patients (4/40) suffered an access vessel complication. Thoracic aortic grafts often require a large access sheath, and surgeons need to carefully examine preoperative imaging to ensure adequate access vessel diameter. Postoperative vigilance is also necessary to identify these injuries early on. Second, after 6 months, 8 of 40 grafts developed poor apposition to the lesser curvature, 3 of 40 developed localized stent expansion in the area of injury, and 3 more showed expansion along the entire length of the stent graft. An earlier study[1] had shown similar expansion in treated areas of the aorta. I think these late findings indicate that we can still make improvements in stent graft design and sizing techniques. Both these results show the necessity for accurate preoperative imaging, and the utility of adjunctive measures such as intravascular ultrasound.

P. W. White, MD, FACS

Reference

1. Forbes TL, Harris JR, Lawlor DK, DeRose G. Aortic dilatation after endovascular repair of blunt traumatic thoracic aortic injuries. *J Vasc Surg*. 2010;52:45-48.

Intravascular ultrasound is a critical tool for accurate endograft sizing in the management of blunt thoracic aortic injury

Wallace GA, Starnes BW, Hatsukami TS, et al (Harborview Med Ctr, Seattle, WA)

J Vasc Surg 61:630-635, 2015

Background.—Accurate measurement of true aortic luminal diameter (ALD) is critical for endograft sizing in endovascular treatment of blunt thoracic aortic injury (BTAI), but ALD is dynamic and changes with respect to patients' hemodynamic status. This study aimed to characterize how ALD at the time of diagnosis of BTAI compares with ALD at the time of endovascular repair and later at follow-up.

Methods.—This is an Institutional Review Board-approved, single-institution retrospective analysis of prospectively obtained data. Patients were included who presented between July 2007 and December 2012 with computed tomography angiography (CTA)-diagnosed BTAI; who underwent thoracic endovascular aortic repair (TEVAR); and who underwent preoperative CTA, intraoperative intravascular ultrasound (IVUS), and postimplantation CTA. Comparison measurements of the ALD were made among CTA and IVUS images at the level of the left subclavian artery (LSCA) and between initial CTA and postimplantation CTA at 10, 15, and 20 cm distal to the LSCA. Theoretical endograft sizes were determined and compared for each ALD at the LSCA.

Results.—Twenty-two patients were included in the analysis. Mean age was 38 ± 14 years (range, 17-61 years), with 82% men and mean Injury Severity Score of 43 ± 11 (range, 24-66). Mean time from emergency department admission to initial CTA was −1.2 ± 5 hours (range, −13 to 11.5 hours; negative time implies imaging at an outside facility before admission). Mean time from initial CTA to IVUS was 1.2 ± 1.4 days (range, 2.5 hours-5.7 days) and from IVUS to postimplantation CTA 33 ± 45 days (range, 17 hours-169 days). Overall, ALD measured by IVUS was significantly larger than that by initial CTA (Δ2.5 ± 3.1 mm; $P < .05$). ALD was also larger at 10, 15, and 20 cm distal to the LSCA in comparing the postimplantation CTA with the initial CTA (Δ2.4, 2.0, and 2.0 mm, respectively; all $P < .05$). More than half the devices would be sized differently with ALD measured by IVUS at the time of TEVAR vs initial CTA.

Conclusions.—The ALD of patients with BTAI is significantly larger when it is measured by IVUS at the time of TEVAR compared with at the time of initial CTA. This difference in ALD may translate to undersizing of endografts used in TEVAR for BTAI. IVUS at the time of TEVAR provides a more accurate measurement of the actual ALD and should be used for endograft sizing for patients with BTAI.

▶ Thoracic endovascular aortic repair (TEVAR) appears to offer significant advantages over open repair in cases of blunt thoracic aortic injury (BTAI).

Adequate sizing of aortic stent grafts is an essential step in avoiding serious complications with TEVAR and ensuring the durability of the procedure. This article reinforces the utility of intravascular ultrasound (IVUS) as an adjunct to TEVAR. If BTAI occurs in a younger population, then it is normally treated with TEVAR (for degenerative aneurysms or dissection). Presumably younger patients, who have more compliant aortic walls, will have greater changes in aortic luminal diameter (ALD) with changes in physiologic parameters such as intravascular volume, cardiac stroke volume, heart rate, and blood pressure, for example. The initial CT obtained soon after the trauma may not accurately reflect ALD because of derangements in these parameters. The authors show that measurements of ALD with IVUS at the time of surgery more closely reflect a baseline ALD. They also substantiate the clinical relevance of IVUS measurements because in many cases the sizing of stent grafts would change. Considering the mounting evidence supporting the use of IVUS with TEVAR for aortic dissection and the data in this article, I believe IVUS should be used in most endovascular therapies for thoracic aortic pathology.

P. W. White, MD, FACS

Patient-based outcomes and quality of life after salvageable wartime extremity vascular injury

Scott DJ, Arthurs ZM, Stannard A, et al (Lackland Air Force Base, San Antonioa, TX; U.S. Army Inst of Surgical Res, Fort Sam Houston, TX; et al)
J Vasc Surg 59:173-179, 2014

Objective.—To date, contemporary studies on wartime vascular trauma have focused on acute management strategies and early results, with no characterization of enduring functional limb salvage or its relation to quality of life. The objective of this study was to describe long-term, patient-based quality of life and function after extremity vascular injury (EVI).

Methods.—The Joint Theater Trauma Registry was queried for U.S. troops with EVI. Injury and management data was obtained and the Medical Outcomes Study Short Form 36 (SF-36) Health Survey administered after patient contact and consent. Demographic, injury, and management variables were analyzed and examined for correlation with the primary end points of favorable or unfavorable outcome defined by SF-36 Mental (MCS) or Physical Component Summary (PCS) scores of >42 or <42 (effect size ≥0.8).

Results.—Surveys were completed by 214 patients, who were a median age of 25 years (range, 19-52 years). The Injury Severity Score was 15.3 ± 8.6 and the Mangled Extremity Severity Score was 5.65 ± 1.4. Amputation-free survival was 84% at mean follow-up of 61 ± 24 months. Overall SF-36 PCS and MCS scores were 43.0 ± 9.2 and 46.6 ± 12.4, respectively, with 92 respondents (43%) reporting favorable outcomes on both MCS and PCS. On multivariate analysis, older age, severe extremity injury (Mangled Extremity Severity Scores ≥7), and chronic pain were predictive of unfavorable physical outcomes ($P < .05$). Presence of pain, nerve injury, and junior rank (<E7) were predictive of unfavorable MCS scores ($P < .05$). Higher educational background (baccalaureate or above) was associated with favorable outcome ($P < .05$).

Conclusions.—This study reports the first long-term patient-centered outcomes data after wartime EVI. At 5 years after injury, quality-of-life measures are reduced compared with national norms. Understanding high-risk characteristics, both demographic- and injury-specific, that are associated with unfavorable outcomes will help guide future acute management and long-term recovery strategies.

▶ The wars in Afghanistan and Iraq have demonstrated how far medicine has advanced in the past century and a half in the care of acute trauma. More than 95% of casualties who reach a medical treatment facility survive their injuries. The long-term care of these wounded warriors remains a challenge. The critical transition from being a patient, to a wounded soldier, to a productive veteran, to an integrated member of civilian society remains difficult to achieve. This article provides an interesting look at the long-term outcomes after wartime vascular injuries. Many of the findings are not unexpected. For example, increased Injury Severity Scores (ISS) and increased Mangled Extremity Severity Scores (MESS) are predictive of worse physical and mental outcomes as measured by the SF-36 questionnaire. The authors also identify other predictors that have influence, perhaps more influence than injury severity, on these outcomes. Lower educational level, increased age, junior rank, and unemployment status at the time of follow-up all correlate with physical and mental outcomes. Unlike injury severity, we also might mitigate or reduce some of these factors. Interestingly, different strategies for treating these injuries in the acute setting had little influence on outcome. The solutions for these problems are probably outside of the purview of vascular surgery per se. Lieutenant Colonel Daniel Gade, a professor of Public Policy at the US Military Academy in West Point, NY, has written on how our current system of medical care with initial treatment in the Department of Defense and a transition over to the Department of Veterans Affairs for chronic and disability care might potentiate worse outcomes. We as surgeons need to ensure that our care does not leave these heroes trapped in dependency.[1,2] To solve this problem, we, as surgeons, need to work with and provide leadership to other medical specialties, such as physiatry, psychiatry, and orthopedics, as well as ancillary professions, such as social work, physical therapy, occupational therapy, and nursing.

P. W. White, MD, FACS

References

1. Phillips D. Iraq veteran, now a West Point professor, seeks to rein in disability pay. *New York Times*. January 7, 2015, http://mobile.nytimes.com/2015/01/08/us/iraq-veteran-now-a-west-point-professor-seeks-to-rein-in-disability-pay.html?_r=0.
2. Gade DM. A better way to help veterans. National Affairs. 2013 (Summer);No 16. http://www.nationalaffairs.com/publications/detail/a-better-way-to-help-veterans.

Pediatric vascular injury: experience of a level 1 trauma center

Allen CJ, Straker RJ, Tashiro J, et al (Univ of Miami Miller School of Medicine, FL)

J Surg Res 196:1-7, 2015

Background.—Our purpose was to analyze modern major vascular injury (MVI) patterns in pediatric trauma, interventions performed, and outcomes at a level 1 trauma center.

Materials and Methods.—From January 2000–December 2012, all pediatric admissions (≤17 y) were reviewed.

Results.—Of 1928 pediatric admissions, 103 (5.3%) sustained MVI. This cohort was 85% male, age 15 ± 3 y, 55% black, 58% penetrating, injury severity score of 23 ± 15, with a length of stay of 8 (5) days. Firearm-related injury (47%) was the most common mechanism. Location of injuries included the extremities (50.5%), abdomen/pelvis (29.1%), and chest/neck (20.4%). Operative procedures included repair/bypass (71.4%), ligation (12.4%), amputation (10.5%), or temporary shunt (2.9%). Only three injuries (2.9%) were treated endovascularly. MVI patients had a mortality rate of 19.4%, higher than the overall pediatric trauma population of 3.5% ($P < 0.001$). After logistic regression, independent risk factors of mortality were vascular injury to the neck (odds ratio [OR]: 6.5; confidence interval (CI): 1.1–39.3), abdomen/pelvis (OR: 16.3; CI: 3.13–80.2), and chest (OR: 49.0; CI: 3.0–794.5).

Conclusions.—MVI in children more commonly results from firearm-related injury. The mortality rate associated with MVI is profoundly higher than that of the overall pediatric trauma population. These findings underscore the major public health concern of firearm-related injury in children.

► The authors report the demographics and epidemiology of about 100 pediatric vascular injuries over a 10-year period. I was disappointed that despite the 10-year study period, essentially no mid- or long-term outcomes were reported. Because vascular surgery in pediatric patients is rare, I find the unfamiliar prospect of operating on a child unnerving. It would have been nice if the authors investigated and reported on the fate of saphenous vein grafts in children. They could have compared the outcomes of primary repair and interposition grafting. What were the long-term results of the polytetrafluoroethylene grafts that were used? The report does describe many of the injuries in detail but then offers platitudes, such as the fact that mortality is higher in patients with major vascular injuries than in those without or that penetrating trauma has a higher incidence of vascular injury than blunt trauma. The major point of this report seems to be an argument for more gun control. A more appropriate forum for an appeal for gun control would be a political journal with an argument based on a more thorough examination of sociologic, legal, and criminologic facts. Listing epidemiologic and demographic truisms in a medical journal then demanding political and legal solutions is infuriating.

D. L. Gillespie, MD, RVT, FACS

The effect of extremity vascular complications on the outcomes of cardiac support device recipients

Ohman JW, Vemuri C, Prasad S, et al (Washington Univ in St. Louis, MO)

J Vasc Surg 59:1622-1627, 2014

Objective.—To assess the effect of extremity vascular complications (EVCs, including ischemia or vessel trauma) on the outcomes of patients receiving cardiac support devices (CSDs, including ventricular assist device [VAD] and extracorporeal membrane oxygenation [ECMO]).

Methods.—Institutional Review Board-approved, retrospective review of a prospectively maintained database of all temporary and permanent CSD recipients from 7/1/10 to 6/30/12. Patient demographics, procedural data, and outcomes were analyzed. The primary endpoint was all-cause mortality at 30-days post-CSD initiation.

Results.—Of 208 patients who received CSDs, 31 (14.9%) experienced EVC: 13 (8.9%) of the 146 permanent VADs, 10 (26.3%) of the 38 temporary VADs, and 8 (33.3%) of the 24 ECMO patients. The 30-day mortality for CSD-EVC patients was not significantly higher than that of the CSD patients who did not experience EVC for permanent VAD (15.4% vs 4.5%; $P = .15$) and ECMO patients (50.0% vs 68.75%; $P = 1.00$), but was significantly higher for temporary VAD patients (80.0% vs 35.7%; $P = .03$). Within the CSD-EVC cohort, patients who received a temporary VAD had a significantly higher 30-day mortality and decision to withdraw care after EVC compared with those who received a permanent VAD ($P = .01$ and $P < .01$, respectively). Looking beyond the 30-day window, EVC was associated with higher mortality rates in the permanent VAD population (53.8% vs 25.6%; $P = .025$) but not the temporary VAD or ECMO groups.

Conclusions.—In temporary VAD recipients, EVCs result in higher 30-day mortality, more frequent withdrawal of care, and shortened survival time relative to the global temporary VAD group. EVC in permanent VAD recipients did not affect early (30-day) mortality rates, but strongly predicted a higher cumulative mortality risk for the 2-year study period. Overall ECMO mortality rates were high, and not significantly impacted by the occurrence of EVC. The nature of the EVC (cannulation site complication vs embolic injury) did not impact mortality. This data provides quality improvement targets for VAD programs.

▶ This retrospective review shows once again that any complication in a critically ill patient can have dire consequences. Clearly, patients in need of cardiac support devices (CSD) are desperately ill, and the use of CSDs could be characterized as a last ditch effort. In such circumstances, perhaps a higher threshold for complications is inevitable. I would have liked to know the rate of complication for percutaneous access as opposed to surgical cut down, particularly for those complications classified as cannulation injuries. I would also like to know how many devices were placed by which specialties and if there was a difference in complication rate based on specialty. Perhaps vascular surgeons need to be involved in all CSD cases to ensure arterial access is as safe as possible. I did appreciate the authors' emphasis on the prognostic consequences of severe vascular complications in the discussion section. Herbert Ratner, MD, a mentor to my father and grandfather at Loyola University, used to say that prognosis is in many ways more important than diagnosis because it guides our therapeutic decisions. Futile surgery is likely worse than futile medical therapy.

P. W. White, MD, FACS

To Shunt or Not to Shunt? An Experimental Study Comparing Temporary Vascular Shunts and Venous Ligation as Damage Control Techniques for Vascular Trauma

Marinho de Oliveira Góes Junior A, de Campos Vieira Abib S, de Seixas Alves MT, et al (Federal Univ of São Paulo (UNIFESP-Brazil))

Ann Vasc Surg 28:710-724, 2014

Background.—To evaluate vascular flow through temporary vascular shunts inserted into peripheral arteries and veins and the repercussion, on the arterial perfusion, of venous ligation and venous shunt insertion in an experimental model for damage control.

Methods.—Experimental study in pigs. Animals were distributed in 5 groups: group 1, right external iliac artery (EIA) shunting and right external iliac vein (EIV) ligation; group 2, right EIA shunting and right EIV shunting; group 3, right EIV ligation; group 4, right EIV shunting; group 5, no vascular shunting and no venous ligation. Flowmeters were used to measure vascular flow on right and left external iliac vessels, and blood samples were collected from the EIVs for biochemical analysis. A right anterior limb biopsy was performed before shock. Hemorrhagic shock was induced through the external right jugular vein, until the vascular flow through right iliac external artery shunt or right iliac external vein shunt (group 4) ceased or until the animal's death. After the end of the experiments, biopsies of bilateral hind limb were obtained for histologic analysis. For statistical analysis, Microsoft Office Excel 2007 and BioEstat 5.0 (2007) were used.

Results.—In the absence of hemorrhagic shock, venous ligation (group 1) was associated with a 38.8% reduction ($P < 0.05$) and venous shunting with a 28.4% reduction on the vascular flow through the arterial shunt. When associated with hemorrhagic shock, the mean vascular flow on the right EIA was 13 mL/min and on the left EIA was 41.2 mL/min; on group 2, the right EIA flow was 8.5 mL/min and the left EIA flow was 8.1 mL/min. When associated with hemorrhagic shock, the pO_2 was 25.8 mm Hg on right EIV and 33.8 mm Hg on the left EIV for group 1 ($P < 0.05$), whereas for group 2, the pO_2 was 22.6 mm Hg on right EIV and 22.8 mm Hg on the left EIV. On group 1, serum potassium was 3.84 mEq/L on the right EIV and 3.96 mEq/L on the left EIV, whereas on group 2, it was 7.1 mEq/L on the right EIV and 5.88 mEq/L on the left EIV ($P < 0.05$).

Conclusions.—In the developed experimental model, venous shunting, when compared with venous ligation, offered less resistance to vascular flow through the arterial shunt and allowed a more efficient limb venous drainage than simple vein ligature.

► Norman Rich in the 1970s was among the first to argue for a more aggressive approach to repairing venous injuries in cases of vascular trauma. On the other hand, several reports on cohorts of civilian trauma patients failed to show a benefit to venous repair in these cases. Nonetheless, in principle, restoring normal venous continuity should improve venous return, reduce engorgement, and improve the overall physiology of blow flow in an injured extremity. Most surgeons are familiar with the use and benefit of vascular shunts in arterial injuries in damage control situations. The authors of this report developed an animal model to examine the benefits of venous shunting on physiologic parameters. Not surprisingly, they showed some benefit of shunting over ligation in these parameters when an arterial shunt was also used. The benefit of shunting was less clear when there was no induced arterial injury. Restoration of normal anatomy is always a goal, but, in cases of trauma, surgeons need to weigh the benefits of restoring normal anatomy against the risks of increased operating time and blood loss leading to hypothermia, coagulopathy, and acidosis. Certainly shunting offers a quicker solution to restoring flow than does reconstruction, but every surgeon should be prepared to ligate venous injuries if necessary. This model also relied on a full dose of intravenous heparin (>100 IU/kg), which isn't an option in most trauma patients.

P. W. White, MD, FACS

Tourniquet use for peripheral vascular injuries in the civilian setting

Passos E, for the Canadian Trauma Trials Collaborative (McMaster Univ, Canada)

Injury 45:573-577, 2014

Background.—Haemorrhage in peripheral vascular injuries may cause life-threatening exsanguination. Tourniquets are used extensively by the military, with increased interest in the civilian setting to prevent deaths. This is a retrospective study of trauma patients at two large Canadian trauma centres with arterial injury after isolated extremity trauma. We hypothesized that tourniquet use may decrease mortality rate and transfusion requirements if applied early.

Methods.—The study group was all adult patients at two Level 1 Trauma Centres in two Canadian cities in Canada, who had arterial injuries from extremity trauma. The study period was from January 2001 to December 2010. We excluded patients with significant associated injuries. The intervention in this study was prehospital tourniquet use. The main outcome was in-hospital mortality. Secondary outcomes were length of stay, compartment syndrome, amputation, and blood product transfusion.

Results.—190 patients were included in the study, and only 4 patients had a prehospital tourniquet applied. They arrived directly from the scene of injury, had improvised tourniquets by police or bystanders, and showed a trend to be more hypotensive and acidotic. Four other patients had tourniquets applied in the trauma bay within 1 h of injury. There were no differences in age, sex, injury severity or physiologic presentation between patients who had an early tourniquet applied and those who died without a tourniquet. However, six patients died without a tourniquet, and all bled to death. Of the eight patients who had early tourniquets applied, none died.

Conclusions.—Tourniquets may prevent exsanguination in the civilian setting for patients suffering either blunt or penetrating trauma to the extremity. Future studies will help determine the utility of deploying tourniquets in the civilian setting, given the rarity of exsanguinating haemorrhage from isolated extremity trauma in this setting (Table 4).

▶ The use of tourniquets for extremity trauma is one of those controversial therapies whose favorable reception has waxed and waned. I think one of the most interesting points of this article is the difference between military and civilian practice patterns with regard to the use of tourniquets. The use of tourniquets in military trauma is accepted, and its benefits have been well established. In this cohort of 190 patients who suffered isolated extremity injuries, only 4 were treated with a tourniquet in the field and only 4 more had a tourniquet applied in the trauma bay. The article also noted that 6 patients without tourniquets did expire and compared them with the patients who did receive a tourniquet (Table 4). I was disappointed that patients with concomitant injuries were excluded from this study. In my opinion, polytrauma patients with serious neurologic or thoracoabdominal injuries might benefit most from early control of extremity hemorrhage with a tourniquet. Although I understand the desire to limit confounding factors by examining isolated injuries, I believe

TABLE 4.—Comparison of Patients Who Died Without Tourniquet and Patients Who Had Early Tourniquet

	No Tourniquet and Died	Early Tourniquet Applied	*P* Value
Number	6	8	
Age	45.1 (+/−14.0)	44.5 (+/−14.8)	0.9
ISS	23.8 (+/−16.2)	15.4 (+/−12.2)	0.47
Units of PRBC (24 h)	13.5 (+/−12.8)	3.6 (+/−2.1)	0.04
Units of FFP (24 h)	7.7 (+/−8.4)	0.75 (+/−2.1)	0.04
Units of platelets (24 h)	4.7 (+/−6.4)	0.5 (+/−1.4)	0.09
MT (%)	50%	0	0.05
Heart rate	110 (+/−30.3)	89.2 (+/−23.2)	0.2
Blood pressure	97.8 (=/−26.2)	109.4 (+/−33.6)	0.5
pH	7.31 (=/−0.05)	7.29 (+/−0.18)	0.86

MT: massive transfusion (10 or more PRBCs in 24 h).

the authors unnecessarily reduced their cohort and were not able to capture enough patients in whom a tourniquet was used. I think those badly injured patients would have also been the most likely to show a benefit from the use of tourniquets.

P. W. White, MD, FACS

UK combat-related pelvic junctional vascular injuries 2008–2011: Implications for future intervention

Walker NM, Eardley W, Clasper JC (Royal Centre for Defence Medicine, Birmingham, UK; et al)

Injury 45:1585-1589, 2014

In a recent publication, 297 of 6450 (4.6%) military coalition deaths over ten years were reported to be due to junctional bleeding. The authors suggested that some of these deaths could have been avoided with a junctional haemorrhage control device.

Prospectively collected data on all injuries sustained in Afghanistan by UK military personnel from 1 August 2008 to 31 July 2011 period were reviewed, using the UK Joint Theatre Trauma Registry. All fatalities with significant pelvic injuries were identified and analysed, and the cause of death established to assess the potential role for a junctional haemorrhage control device.

Significant upper thigh, groin or pelvic injuries were recorded in 124 casualties, of which 93 died. Of these the pelvic injury was the cause of death in 37, but only 1 casualty with potentially survivable injuries was identified where death was due to a vascular injury below the inguinal ligament, not controlled by a CAT. This represents <1% of all deaths in this period, a lower figure than previously published. We further identified 32 casualties where the cause of death was due to a vascular injury between the aortic bifurcation and the inguinal ligament. Eight of these survived to a medical facility but subsequently died of their wounds. These represent a subset in which vascular control proximal to the inguinal ligament could have altered the outcome.

Some potentially survivable deaths due to exsanguination may be amenable to proximal vascular control. Our study does not substantiate previous conclusions that this can be achieved through use of a groin junctional tourniquet. We believe there may be a role for more proximal vascular control of pelvic bleeding, and this merits further research.

▶ Junctional vascular injuries, that is, vascular injuries near the junction of a limb and the trunk, are among the most difficult to manage, especially in the prehospital setting and in combat. They cannot be controlled with a conventional tourniquet, and surgical control is not available on the battlefield. Several new devices, particularly the Combat Ready Clamp, a device similar to a Femostop, are being proposed as solutions to the preventable deaths caused by junctional vascular injuries because they offer the ability to compress the arterial inflow at the level of the common femoral artery. The authors of this article found a very low incidence of pelvic junctional vascular injuries that would have been affected by proximal control at the common femoral artery. They did find a higher number of patients with injuries in then pelvis who would have benefited from proximal arterial control at the distal aorta. The authors make specific mention of intra-aortic balloon occlusion as a possible solution and of deploying them forward to battalion aid stations with experienced medics or physician assistants. Although balloon occlusion of the aorta can be very useful, I believe it cannot be safely pushed forward beyond surgical capabilities. The lack of imaging equipment, sterile conditions, and experience make the likelihood of significant iatrogenic iliac artery injuries to high. I think efforts to improve body armor and casualty evacuation to capable surgical care will yield the most benefits.

P. W. White, MD, FACS

Vascular Injury Is Associated with Increased Mortality in Winter Sports Trauma

Eun JC, Bronsert M, Hansen K, et al (Univ of Colorado Denver, Aurora; et al)
Ann Vasc Surg 29:109-113, 2015

Background.—Trauma is the leading cause of injury and death for individuals aged 1–44 years. Up to 8% of the US population participates in winter sports, and although vascular injuries are uncommon in these activities, little is published in this area. We sought to identify the incidence, injury patterns, and outcomes of vascular injuries resulting from winter sports trauma.

Methods.—Patients with winter sports trauma and the subset with vascular injuries were identified by accessing the National Trauma Data Bank querying years 2007–2010. Patients with and without vascular injuries were then compared. Admission variables included transport time, emergency department hypotension (systolic blood pressure <90), Glasgow Coma Scale ≤ 8, Injury Severity Score ≥ 25, fractures, solid organ injury, and vascular injury. Outcomes were analyzed and associations with vascular injuries were determined.

Results.—A total of 2,298 patients were identified with winter sports–related trauma and 28 (1.2%) had associated vascular injuries. Overall, the top 3 injuries were head trauma (16.7%), thoracic vertebral fractures (5.5%), and lumbar vertebral fractures (5.1%). The most common associated vascular injures were to the popliteal artery (17.7%), splenic artery (14.7%), and brachial blood vessels (14.7%). In the entire cohort, 1 patient (0.04%) suffered an amputation and 15 patients (0.7%) died. There were no amputations in the vascular injury group. Mortality was 0.6% in patients without a vascular injury compared with 7.1% of those with a vascular injury ($P = 0.01$).

Conclusions.—Although vascular injury is an uncommon associated finding in winter sports trauma, it is associated with a significant increase in mortality. These findings highlight the need for rapid identification of traumatic vascular injuries, which predicts worse overall outcomes in this patient population.

▶ Hemorrhage, after head injury, is the leading cause of death in trauma patients, and thus it stands to reason that patients with vascular injuries would have a higher mortality. Winter sports trauma mostly (likely overwhelmingly) consists of blunt trauma. More than one-third of the vascular injuries in this series occurred within the abdomen. I wish the authors had calculated a separate mortality rate for the intraabdominal vascular injuries and for the extremity vascular injuries. I suspect that patients with extremity vascular injuries would have a mortality rate similar to patients without a vascular injury because blunt extremity vascular injuries are not usually associated with life-threatening hemorrhage. In other words, intraabdominal injuries, not vascular injuries per se, are the real cause of mortality in blunt trauma. Because the number of patients with vascular injury was small, discussing the nature of the vascular injuries in the 2 patients from the vascular injury group who died would have been interesting. I agree with the authors that determining the incidence of blunt aortic injuries in the winter sports cohort would be worthwhile, and it is unfortunate that the limitations of the National Trauma Data Bank prevented study of these data.

P. W. White, MD, FACS

13 Venous Thrombosis and Pulmonary Embolism

Inferior Vena Cava Filter Usage, Complications, and Retrieval Rate in Cancer Patients

Abtahian F, Hawkins BM, Ryan DP, et al (Massachusetts General Hosp, Boston; Univ of Oklahoma College of Medicine; et al)

Am J Med 127:1111-1117, 2014

Background.—Venous thromboembolism contributes significantly to morbidity and mortality in cancer patients. Because cancer patients frequently have contraindications to anticoagulation, inferior vena cava filters are commonly placed. The use, safety, and retrieval of retrievable inferior vena cava filters in cancer patients have not been well studied.

Methods.—A retrospective review of retrievable inferior vena cava filter use at a tertiary referral hospital was conducted between January 1, 2009 and December 31, 2011. Indications for inferior vena cava filter placement, anticoagulation practices, complications, filter retrieval, and patient outcomes were analyzed for patients with and without active cancer and for cancer subtypes, including localized and metastatic cases.

Results.—Of 666 patients receiving retrievable inferior vena cava filters during this time period, 247 (37.1%) had active cancer. Of these, 151 (22.7%) had carcinoma, 92 (13.8%) had sarcoma, and 115 (17.3%) had metastatic disease. Overall, follow-up was available for a median of 401.0 (interquartile range: 107.5-786.5) days. Indwelling filter-related complications occurred in 19.8% of patients without cancer and 17.7% with an active cancer ($P = .50$). Patients with cancer were less likely to have the filter retrieved (28.0% vs 42.0%, $P < .001$). In multivariable analysis, cancer was not associated with filter-related complications but was associated with a lower rate of filter retrieval.

Conclusions.—In a modern cohort of patients undergoing retrievable inferior vena cava filter placement, active diagnosis of cancer is not associated with a significant increase in filter-related complications, but is associated with a reduced rate of filter retrieval.

▶ Defining the appropriate use of vena cava filters remains an important challenge. This retrospective review is helpful in showing that many patients with a malignancy have a significant life expectancy and that the risks of filter placement do not appear to be greater than in patients without cancer. The article also reported that the filter retrieval rate was disappointingly low at 36.6%. The rate of reinitiation of appropriately dosed anticoagulation also surprised me at less than 70%. I think the 2 facts indicate that greater emphasis still needs to be placed on thorough follow-up after filter placement with an aggressive practice of restarting anticoagulation and removing filters. This article studied some patients with metastatic disease, and they had a higher complication rate. I think further analysis of this subgroup will reveal that some patients with metastatic carcinomas would not benefit from inferior vena cava filters, but that remains a topic for future study. The main thrust of this article remains valid: cancer in and of itself is not a sufficient reason to prevent filter placement. Clearly, the patient's entire clinical situation needs to be assessed when weighing the risks and benefits of filter placement.

P. W. White, MD, FACS

Prevalence and Clinical Consequences of Fracture and Fragment Migration of the Bard G2 Filter: Imaging and Clinical Follow-up in 684 Implantations

An T, Moon E, Bullen J, et al (Cleveland Clinic, OH)

J Vasc Interv Radiol 25:941-948, 2014

Purpose.—To investigate the prevalence and clinical sequelae of G2 filter (Bard Peripheral Vascular, Tempe, Arizona) fractures and fragment migration.

Materials and Methods.—Patients who underwent G2 filter placement between October 2005 and February 2010 were assessed for filter fractures and complications. Fracture prevalence was estimated at various time points based on data from patients with known fracture status.

Results.—Among 829 patients who underwent G2 filter placement, 684 had follow-up imaging and qualified for the study (381 men and 303 women; average age, 60.3 y; range, 15.8–95.2 y). For 541 (79%) patients, at least one image was available that contained the filter (imaging follow-up interval, 14.9 mo ± 20.0; range, 0–78.6 mo); images that did not include the filter but may have shown the migrated fracture fragment were available for 143 (21%) patients (follow-up interval, 11.2 mo ± 19.3; range, 0–83.4 mo). There were 16 fractured limbs identified in 13 patients (incidence, 1.9%; follow-up interval, 30.4 mo ± 18.7; range, 5.5–76.5 mo). Fracture fragments were identified in the pulmonary arteries (n = 4), right ventricle (n = 2), pericardium (n = 1), iliac vein (n = 1), and kidney (n = 1). Four fracture limbs remained near the filter; the remaining three could not be located. All patients with filter fracture were asymptomatic. The estimated 5-year fracture prevalence was 38% (95% confidence interval, 22.9%, 54.8%).

Conclusions.—The early occurrence of G2 filter fractures was low, but the incidence increased over time. No life-threatening events occurred in patients with filter fracture during the study time frame.

▶ Inferior vena cava filters were devised to address a difficult and life-threatening problem, thromboembolic disease in patients who could not be anticoagulated. In principle, foreign bodies should be removed once the indication for the device no longer exists, and so retrievable filters were developed. The Bard Recovery and G2 filters have been plagued with problems of fracture and fragment migration. The authors estimated rate of fracture of 38% at 5 years is frightening. Although they report no events of clinical significance, I have personally seen 1 patient with a fractured Bard filter fragment that had embolized to the pericardial space. This patient related an episode of severe chest pain and shortness of breath several weeks before his presentation. He was deployed on a submarine and could only seek basic medical attention onboard at the time of his symptoms. Presumably, the fragment had migrated to the heart, penetrated through the myocardium, and caused either severe pericarditis or a significant pericardial effusion. Other recent reports have indicated that other manufacturers devices are penetrating the caval wall or causing caval thrombosis.[1-3] It is possible that newer designs for filters to gain the needed flexibility and compactness for retrieval have sacrificed too much stability and strength. This is another study that highlights the need for thorough follow-up, an aggressive approach to restarting anticoagulation, and thoughtful attempts at retrieval in all patients without an ongoing indication for retrieval. I also wonder if we shouldn't consider a return to the Greenfield permanent filter, which appears to have a better long-term safety profile.[4]

P. W. White, MD, FACS

References

1. McLoney ED, Krishnasamy VP, Castle JC, Yang X, Guy G. Complications of Celect, Günther tulip, and Greenfield inferior vena cava filters on CT follow-up: a single-institution experience. *J Vasc Interv Radiol.* 2013;24:1723-1729.
2. Durack JC, Westphalen AC, Kekulawela S, et al. Perforation of the IVC: rule rather than exception after longer indwelling times for the Günther Tulip and Celect retrievable filters. *Cardiovasc Intervent Radiol.* 2012;35:299-308.
3. Usoh F, Hingorani A, Ascher E, et al. Prospective randomized study comparing the clinical outcomes between inferior vena cava Greenfield and TrapEase filters. *J Vasc Surg.* 2010;52:394-399.
4. Greenfield LJ, Proctor MC. Twenty-year clinical experience with the Greenfield filter. *Cardiovasc Surg.* 1995;3:199-205.

Comparison of Complication Rates Associated with Permanent and Retrievable Inferior Vena Cava Filters: A Review of the MAUDE Database

Andreoli JM, Lewandowski RJ, Vogelzang RL, et al (Northwestern Univ, Chicago, IL)

J Vasc Interv Radiol 25:1181-1185, 2014

Purpose.—To compare the safety of permanent and retrievable inferior vena cava (IVC) filters by reviewing the U.S. Food and Drug Administration Manufacturer and User Facility Device Experience (MAUDE) database.

Materials and Methods.—The MAUDE database was reviewed from January 1, 2009, to December 31, 2012. Product class search criteria were "filter, intravascular, cardiovascular." Type of device used and specific adverse events (AEs) were recorded.

Results.—For the period January 2009-December 2012, 1,606 reported AEs involving 1,057 IVC filters were identified in the MAUDE database. Of reported AEs, 1,394 (86.8%) involved retrievable inferior vena cava filters (rIVCFs), and 212 (13.2%) involved permanent inferior vena cava filters (pIVCFs) ($P < .0001$). Reported AEs included fracture, migration, limb embolization, tilt, IVC penetration, venous thromboembolism and pulmonary embolism, IVC thrombus, and malfunctions during placement. Each specific AE was reported with significantly higher frequency in rIVCFs compared with pIVCFs. The most common reported complication with rIVCFs was fracture, whereas the most commonly reported complications with pIVCFs were placement malfunctions. For rIVCFs, the most commonly reported AE varied depending on filter brand.

Conclusions.—The MAUDE database reveals that complications occur with significantly higher frequency with rIVCFs compared with pIVCFs. This finding suggests that the self-reported complication rate with rIVCFs is significantly higher than the self-reported complication rate with pIVCFs.

▶ This is an important study, and I recommend anyone placing inferior vena cava (IVC) filters, especially retrievable filters, consider reading it. It is important to note that the MAUDE database is a voluntary, self-reported entry of data by individuals placing IVC filters and in which several observed complications have occurred. This study evaluated the MAUDE database from 2009 to 2012, and it should be noted that approximately 800 000 filters were placed in the United States during the time period of this study. However, only 1057 filters were reported to the MAUDE database with complications. This would indicate that the MAUDE database only represents 0.1% of all filters placed and may not reflect the true complications of IVC filters. Of note, the database searched by the authors resulted in the majority of IVC filters being retrievable (86.8%). The majority of complications occurred with retrievable IVC filters, and filter fracture accounting for 24% of reported complications. The Bard filter had the highest reported fracture rate. It is important to note that in this study, 82% of patients with adverse events noted from the filter had no reported information if symptoms were present. An increasing proportion of IVC filters are placed for venous thromboembolism prophylaxis in patients who are at transient high risk of pulmonary embolism (trauma, before major surgery in high-risk patients for deep vein thrombosis, bariatric surgery). Design modification to allow for retrievability may compromise filter durability and hence the increased complications seen with retrievable filters (IVC penetrations, tilting, fracture, migration). It is imperative that as physicians, we place the retrievable IVC filter for the proper indications, and that once the risk of venous thromboembolism is no longer present, strong consideration should be given to removing the retrievable IVC filter within the appropriate time frame as specified by company manufacturer of the retrievable IVC filter. Future designs in retrievable IVC filters will have to focus on reducing the reported complications, while maintaining their efficacy in preventing pulmonary embolism.

J. D. Raffetto, MD, FACS, FSVM

A multicenter randomized controlled trial evaluating balneotherapy in patients with advanced chronic venous insufficiency

Carpentier PH, Blaise S, Satger B, et al (Centre Hospitalier Universitaire, Grenoble, France; et al)

J Vasc Surg 59:447-454, 2014

Background.—Apart from compression therapy, physical therapy has scarcely been evaluated in the treatment of chronic venous disorders (CVDs). Spa treatment is a popular way to administer physical therapy for CVDs in France, but its efficacy has not yet been assessed in a large trial. The objective was to assess the efficacy of spa therapy for patients with advanced CVD (CEAP clinical classes C4-C5).

Methods.—This was a single-blind (treatment concealed to the investigators) randomized, multicenter, controlled trial (French spa resorts). Inclusion criteria were primary or post-thrombotic CVD with skin changes but no active ulcer (C4a, C4b, or C5). The treated group had the usual 3-week spa treatment course soon after randomization; the control group had spa treatment after the 1-year comparison period. All patients continued their usual medical care including wearing compression stockings. Treatment consisted of four balneotherapy sessions per day for 6 days a week. Follow-up was performed at 6, 12 and 18 months by independent blinded investigators. The main outcome criterion was the incidence of leg ulcers at 12 months. Secondary criteria were a modified version of the Venous Clinical Severity Score, a visual analog scale for leg symptoms, and the Chronic Venous Insufficiency Questionnaire 2 and EuroQol 5D quality-of-life auto questionnaires.

Results.—Four hundred twenty-five subjects were enrolled: 214 in the treatment group (Spa) and 211 in the control group (Ctr); they were similar at baseline regarding their demographic characteristics, the severity of the CVD, and the outcome variables. At 1 year, the incidence of leg ulcers was not statistically different (Spa: +9.3%; 95% confidence interval [CI], +5.6 - +14.3; Ctr: +6.1%; 95% CI, +3.2 - +10.4), whereas the Venous Clinical Severity Score improved significantly in the treatment group (Spa: −1.2; 95% CI, −1.6 - −0.8; Ctr: −0.6; 95% CI, −1.0 - −0.2; $P = .04$). A significant difference favoring spa treatment was found regarding symptoms after 1 year (Spa: −0.03; 95% CI, −0.57 - +0.51; Ctr: +0.87; 95% CI, +0.46 - +1.26; $P = .009$). EuroQol 5D improved in the treatment group (Spa: +0.01; 95% CI, −0.02 - +0.04) while it worsened (Ctr: −0.07; 95% CI, −0.10 - −0.04) in the control group ($P < .001$). A similar pattern was found for the Chronic Venous Insufficiency Questionnaire 2 scale (Spa: −2.0; 95% CI, −4.4 - +0.4; Ctr: +2.4; 95% CI, +0.2 - +4.7; $P = .008$). The control patients showed similar improvements in clinical severity, symptoms, and quality of life after their own spa treatment (day 547).

Conclusions.—In this study, the incidence of leg ulcers was not reduced after a 3-week spa therapy course. Nevertheless, our study demonstrates that spa therapy provides a significant and substantial improvement in clinical status, symptoms, and quality of life of patients with advanced venous insufficiency for at least 1 year.

▶ Compression therapy is a standard of care for chronic venous disease (CVD), and especially for patients with ulcers and for the prevention of recurrent ulcers. Patients with advanced CVD are older and have increased complex patterns of venous insufficiency, and frequently the superficial venous system is involved with incompetent valves. A variety of endovenous ablation therapies that include thermal (laser or radiofrequency), chemical in the form of foam sclerosant, and mechanochemical ablation and glue ablation (the latter 2 do not require tumescent anesthetic) are available. When Conrad Jobst first discovered that his CVD afflicting his lower extremities had significantly improved while in the pool with his limb submerged, he determined that pressure was important in reducing symptoms. He rationalized that the pressure exerted by the water at different depths was a pressure gradient that exerted external pressure on his legs. This was the beginning of the development of compression stockings. In various areas of France, spa therapy is a common modality of treating the symptoms of CVD. However, the actual effects of spa therapy are poorly defined. In this randomized trial of 425 patients with primary or secondary CVD with CEAP clinical class C4ab and C5, patients were randomized to the treatment group of 3 weeks of spa therapy or not receiving spa therapy in addition to wearing compression. After 12 months, the control group also received balneotherapy to decrease the dropout rate. The balneotherapy consisted of an intense and sophisticated protocol: a 15-minute walking session in a specially designed pool with tracks in semideep (80 cm), cool (28°C) water; training of muscle pump function under water compression; a 20-minute whirlpool bath session with automatic air and water massage cycles aimed at relaxation and mobilization of the superficial skin volume flow; a 10-minute bath session with customized strong underwater massaging jets that led to mobilization and softening of the sclerotic subcutaneous tissues; and a 10-minute massage session of the leg and ankle skin areas by a registered physiotherapist under a light spray shower, which aimed at softening of the sclerotic subcutaneous tissues or a 15-minute joint mobilization session in a deep (150 cm), warm 34°C pool under the supervision of a physiotherapist for the improvement of ankle and also knee and hip joint mobility for better ambulation and muscle-pump functioning. The therapy consisted of 4 balneotherapy sessions per day for 6 days a week for a total of 3 weeks. To remain enrolled in the study, none of the study or control patients received any endovenous or surgical treatment for their venous insufficiency. The primary end point was development of venous leg ulcer at 12 months, and secondary outcomes were Venous Clinical Severity Score, a visual analog scale for leg symptoms, and the Chronic Venous Insufficiency Questionnaire 2, and EuroQol 5D quality-of-life questionnaires. The hypothesis was that there would be a reduction of venous ulcers at 1 year with balneotherapy. The main findings were that there was no statistical difference of the primary end point, but the balneotherapy group had significantly improved all 3 aspects of the secondary end points. Importantly, when the control patients also received their therapy after 12 months, they had the same benefits in secondary outcomes. Some unanswered question are as follows: (1) Would increasing the length of time of balneotherapy reduce venous ulcer rates? (2) What are the hemodynamic benefits of balneotherapy? (3) Does the venous filling index, residual volume fraction, and ejection fraction actually improve? (4) Should this form of therapy be offered to patients with primary and/or secondary disease, and who benefits most? (5) What is the cost-effective analysis of such a therapy? Regardless, I must admit that it would be nice to enjoy a pool and spa resort in the beautiful country of France, especially because balneotherapy is partly reimbursed by the French national health insurance system!

J. D. Raffetto, MD, FACS, FSVM

Compression stockings to prevent post-thrombotic syndrome: a randomised placebo-controlled trial

Kahn SR, for the SOX trial investigators (Jewish General Hosp, Montreal, Québec, Canada; et al)

Lancet 383:880-888, 2014

Background.—Post-thrombotic syndrome (PTS) is a common and burdensome complication of deep venous thrombosis (DVT). Previous trials suggesting benefit of elastic compression stockings (ECS) to prevent PTS were small, singlecentre studies without placebo control. We aimed to assess the efficacy of ECS, compared with placebo stockings, for the prevention of PTS.

Methods.—We did a multicentre randomised placebo-controlled trial of active versus placebo ECS used for 2 years to prevent PTS after a first proximal DVT in centres in Canada and the USA. Patients were randomly assigned to study groups with a web-based randomisation system. Patients presenting with a first symptomatic, proximal DVT were potentially eligible to participate. They were excluded if the use of compression stockings was contraindicated, they had an expected lifespan of less than 6 months, geographical inaccessibility precluded return for follow-up visits, they were unable to apply stockings, or they received thrombolytic therapy for the initial treatment of acute DVT. The primary outcome was PTS diagnosed at 6 months or later using Ginsberg's criteria (leg pain and swelling of ≥1 month duration). We used a modified intention to treat Cox regression analysis, supplemented by a prespecified per-protocol analysis of patients who reported frequent use of their allocated treatment. This study is registered with ClinicalTrials.gov, number NCT00143598, and Current Controlled Trials, number ISRCTN71334751.

Findings.—From 2004 to 2010, 410 patients were randomly assigned to receive active ECS and 396 placebo ECS. The cumulative incidence of PTS was 14·2% in active ECS versus 12·7% in placebo ECS (hazard ratio adjusted for centre 1·13, 95% CI 0·73–1·76; $p=0·58$). Results were similar in a prespecified per-protocol analysis of patients who reported frequent use of stockings.

Interpretation.—ECS did not prevent PTS after a first proximal DVT, hence our findings do not support routine wearing of ECS after DVT.

▶ Compression therapy has been the cornerstone to the treatment of chronic venous disorders (CVD), especially with advanced stages of CVD with skin changes, healed ulcerations, and active ulcerations. The etiology of CVD is primary (reflux of the superficial and deep venous system), secondary (from deep venous thrombosis [DVT] resulting in recanalization, valve dysfunction, and reflux), or congenital conditions. Patients affected by DVT are at risk for developing the postthrombotic syndrome (PTS), especially for patients affected by iliofemoral DVT, but can also occur in patients with femoral-popliteal DVT, but at a lower rate. Several randomized controlled trials (RCTs) have demonstrated that there can be up to 50% reduction at 2 years from PTS by wearing 30 to 40 mm Hg elastic compression stockings (ECS) at the time of initial diagnosis. These older trials have recently been challenged by the SOX trial, which is an RCT multicenter placebo controlled trial. Patients with a first episode of iliofemoral and/or femoral-popliteal DVT are randomized to either an active ($n=409$, 30–40 mm Hg) or placebo ($n=394$, <5 mm Hg) ECS. The ECS are worn for 2 years. The primary outcome is PTS at ≥6 months using the Ginsberg Criteria (swelling or pain at 1 month). The major outcome of the trial was that there was no difference in Ginsberg Criteria (active vs placebo, 14.2% vs 12.7%, respectively, $P=.58$) or Villalta score (active vs placebo, 52.6% vs 52.3%, respectively, $P=.96$). In addition, there were no differences in secondary end points of quality of life, venous leg ulcer rate, recurrent DVT, or venous thromboembolism. However, there are significant limitations to this study that must be discussed, and before we discard the compression stocking for preventing PTS. (1) It is difficult to "blind" the active versus placebo stockings because the difference in application will be apparent. (2) The primary endpoint (Ginsberg Criteria) is subjective and left to the discretion of the observer. (3)

Originally PTS was to be assessed at 2 years but changed to cumulative incidence from 6 to 24 months, which may not be reflective of the actual number of patients with PTS. (4) Only 45.5% and 27% of patients evaluable at 2 years for primary and secondary endpoints. (5) Definition and evaluation of compliance was unclear; compliance was checked at 6-month intervals. (6) The timing of ECS application from time of DVT diagnosis unknown. (7) Patients were sized and ECS mailed to patient to wear; there was no training, and it is unclear whether appropriate fitting and wearing was actually performed by participants. Therefore, inadequate fitting among participants may be quite high. (8) By 24 months, only 69.1% (active) and 55.6% (placebo) were wearing ECS. (9) The number of patients lost to follow-up was 114 of 803 (14%). Future studies are required that address the shortcomings of the SOX trial and determine unequivocally if ECS are beneficial in reducing PTS.

J. D. Raffetto, MD, FACS, FSVM

Editor's choice - Efficacy and Safety of the New Oral Anticoagulants Dabigatran, Rivaroxaban, Apixaban, and Edoxaban in the Treatment and Secondary Prevention of Venous Thromboembolism: A Systematic Review and Meta-analysis of Phase III Trials

Kakkos SK, Kirkilesis GI, Tsolakis IA (Univ Hosp of Patras, Greece)

Eur J Vasc Endovasc Surg 48:565-575, 2014

Objectives.—The aim was to perform a review of the efficacy and safety of new oral anticoagulants (NOAs) in the management of venous thromboembolism (VTE).

Methods.—This was a systematic review and meta-analysis. On March 26, 2014, Medline, Embase, and the Cochrane trial register were searched for randomized controlled trials (RCTs) comparing the NOAs dabigatran, rivaroxaban, apixaban, and edoxaban with vitamin K antagonists (VKAs) in VTE treatment and secondary prevention. Two investigators assessed the methodological quality of the RCTs. The main study outcomes (efficacy, safety and net clinical benefit) were expressed as risk ratios (RR) with 95% confidence interval (CI).

Results.—Ten RCTs, mostly with low risk of bias, with nearly 38,000 patients, were identified. In six trials of treatment, NOAs were equally effective as VKAs in preventing recurrent symptomatic VTE (RR 0.89, 95% CI 0.75–1.05), but major bleeding occurred less often (1.08% vs. 1.73% for VKAs, RR 0.63, 95% CI 0.51–0.77), leading net clinical benefit to favor NOAs (RR 0.79, 95% CI 0.70–0.90). Fatal bleeding occurred less often with NOAs (0.09% vs. 0.18% for VKAs), a difference that approached statistical significance (RR 0.51, 95% CI 0.26–1.01). In three secondary prevention trials, NOAs reduced VTE recurrence rates to 1.32% (vs. 7.24% with placebo, RR 0.17, 95% CI 0.12–0.24) and fatal pulmonary embolism (PE) (including unexplained deaths) to 0.1%

(vs. 0.29% for placebo, RR 0.37, 95% CI 0.10–1.38) at the expense of clinically relevant non-major bleeding (4.3% vs. 1.8% for placebo, RR 2.32, 95% CI 1.65–3.35), but not major bleeding. All-cause mortality rate was reduced to 0.41% with NOAs (vs. 0.86% with placebo, RR 0.38, 95% CI 0.18–0.79). Net clinical benefit favored NOAs (RR 0.21, 95% CI 0.15–0.29), and NNT was 18.

Conclusions.—Compared to VKAs, NOAs are not only effective in treating VTE but also safer in terms of bleeding, thereby conferring clinical benefit. Their safety and efficacy was confirmed further in secondary prevention trials.

▶ This is an excellent review of the safety and efficacy of the new oral anticoagulants (NOACs) in the treatment of venous thromboembolism (VTE). The main players are factor IIa (thrombin) inhibitors and factor Xa inhibitors. The study's aim was to identify randomized controlled trials (RCTs) that assessed efficacy, safety, and net clinical benefit. Ten RCTs met the criteria and evaluated the NOACs compared with vitamin K antagonist (VKA), in preventing recurrent VTE and assessed bleeding complications associated with anticoagulation. Recurrent symptomatic VTE, defined as the composite of deep venous thrombosis, nonfatal pulmonary embolism (PE), and fatal PE, was the most commonly used efficacy outcome of the RCTs. Clinically relevant bleeding, a composite of major and clinically relevant nonmajor bleeding, was the mostly frequently used safety outcome, whereas major bleeding was used in others. The overall findings of this well-researched and written article were that NOACs are equally as effective if not superior to VKA in the treatment of VTE and preventing recurrent symptomatic VTE, but importantly, NOACs have a decreased rate of major and fatal bleeding. Major bleeding rates fell from 1.73% with the use of traditional treatment to 1.08% with the use of NOACs (relative risk 0.63, 95% confidence interval 0.51-0.77, $P < .00001$). Importantly, there was little or no heterogeneity in the evaluation of the RCTs with respect to recurrent VTE but some heterogeneity in assessing bleeding. These data clearly favor the NOACs for clinical benefit (the combination of VTE recurrence and major bleeding). The clear advantages of NOACs are that they do not require bridging parental anticoagulation (rivaroxaban and apixaban) or dose response monitoring, and there are no food interactions. Some potential issues with NOACs are the lack of specific reversal agents and the potential for increased risk for bleeding; however, based on this meta-analysis, this latter concern is not supported. In addition, the recently developed factor Xa inhibitor antidote, andexanet alfa (PRT4445, Portola Pharmaceuticals), is expected to resolve concerns over the reversal of NOACs.

J. D. Raffetto, MD, FACS, FSVM

Higher soluble P-selectin is associated with chronic venous insufficiency: The San Diego Population Study

Bryan LJ, Callas PW, Criqui MH, et al (Univ of Vermont, Burlington; Univ of California San Diego)

Thromb Res 130:716-719, 2012

Introduction.—P-selectin is a cell adhesion molecule shown to play a role in venous thromboembolism. We evaluated whether higher P-selectin is associated with chronic venous insufficiency (CVI).

Materials and Methods.—In a cohort of 2408 participants, the San Diego Population Study, peripheral venous disease was established by symptoms, clinical examination, and ultrasound. We measured P-selectin in a subsample of 352 CVI cases frequency matched to controls. Cases included four hierarchical groups of increasing severity of CVI.

Results.—The association of P-selectin with CVI considering all cases was weak, with an age, race and sex-adjusted odds ratio (OR) of 1.3 (95% CI 1.0-2.2) for values in the 3rd versus 1st tertile. The OR for cases in the two most severe groups was 2.3 (95% CI 1.2-4.2). Addition of body mass index to the model reduced this OR to 1.9 (95% CI 1.0-3.6).

Conclusions.—Higher circulating P-selectin was associated with more severe CVI, but not CVI overall. Results support that platelet and endothelial cell activation may be involved in the pathogenesis of CVI.

► Chronic venous insufficiency (CVI) represents impaired venous return in advanced chronic venous disease (CVD). The pathophysiology of CVD is complex and multifactorial. It is true that patients with higher clinical classes have higher venous clinical severity scores and impaired quality of life. It is unclear what, if any, inflammatory circulating markers are correlated with increasing severity of clinical class in Clinical Etiologic Anatomic Pathologic (varicose veins vs skin changes) as well as with the areas of venous insufficiency affecting the superficial and deep venous systems. In this cross-sectional case-control study from a large epidemiologic database, 352 patients were selected with different classes of CVD and involvement of venous insufficiency (superficial or deep veins). Patients were separated into 4 severity groups based on the presence of skin changes or edema versus none and the involvement of CVI in the superficial or deep venous systems and examined for P-selectin levels compared with age-sex-race—matched controls. P-selectin is a protein adhesion molecule important in activation of leukocytes to endothelium during inflammatory conditions and has been studied extensively in its role with deep venous thrombosis and resolution. In this study, the overall levels of P-selectin in the patients with CVI were not statistically different from controls that did not have any evidence of CVI and CVD. A confounder in this study was that increasing body mass index was associated with increasing levels of P-selectin, and, once adjusted, only the more severe forms of CVI (deep venous insufficiency and skin changes) had a weak association with elevated levels of P-selectin (odds ratio = 1.9; 95% confidence interval, 1.0-3.6). This study suggests that platelet and endothelial cell activation and release of P-selectin may be involved in the pathogenesis of CVI. However, when correcting for body mass index, this correlation is weak. A significant limitation of this study is that there were only 49 patients in the most severe group with CVI. Further work in this area is required to determine the impact of circulating inflammatory markers and their association and pathogenesis of CVD and disease progression.

J. D. Raffetto, MD, FACS, FSVM

Low-molecular-weight heparin modulates vein wall fibrotic response in a plasminogen activator inhibitor 1-dependent manner

Obi AT, Diaz JA, Ballard-Lipka NL, et al (Conrad Jobst Vascular Research Laboratories, Ann Arbor, MI; Univ of Michigan Med School, Ann Arbor)

J Vasc Surg Venous Lymphat Disord 2:441-450, 2014

Background.—Treatment with low-molecular-weight heparin (LMWH) favorably alters the vein wall response to deep venous thrombosis (DVT), although the mechanisms remain unclear. Previous studies have suggested that LMWH alters the levels of circulating plasminogen activator inhibitor 1 (PAI-1), a known mediator of fibrosis, and may improve endogenous fibrinolysis. We hypothesized that LMWH favorably alters the vein wall response by binding of PAI-1 and acceleration of fibrinolysis.

Methods.—Wild-type and PAI-$1^{-/-}$ mice underwent treatment with LMWH after induction of occlusive DVT. Vein wall and plasma were harvested and analyzed by enzyme-linked immunosorbent assay, zymography, real-time polymerase chain reaction, and immunohistochemistry.

Results.—Wild-type mice treated with LMWH exhibited diminished vein wall fibrosis (0.6 ± 0.6 vs 1.4 ± 0.2; $P < .01$; n = 5) and elevation of circulating PAI-1 (1776 ± 342 vs 567 ± 104 pg/mL; $P < .01$; n = 5) compared with untreated controls after occlusive DVT. PAI-$1^{-/-}$ mice treated with LMWH were not similarly protected from fibrosis, despite improved thrombus resolution. Treatment with LMWH was associated with decreased intrathrombus interleukin-1β (68.6 ± 31.0 vs 223.4 ± 28.9 pg/mg total protein; $P < .01$; n = 5) but did not alter inflammatory cell recruitment to the vein wall. PAI-1L/L mice exhibited significantly elevated intrathrombus (257.2 ± 51.5 vs 14.3 ± 3.8 pg/mg total protein; n = 5) and vein wall interleukin-13 (187.2 ± 57.6 vs 9.9 ± 1.1 pg/mg total protein; $P < .05$; n = 5) as well as vein wall F4/80 positively staining monocytes (53 ± 11 vs 16 ± 2 cells/5 high-power fields; $P < .05$; n = 4).

Conclusions.—LMWH did not accelerate venous thrombosis resolution but did protect against vein wall fibrosis in a PAI-1-dependent manner in an occlusive DVT model. Lack of PAI-1 correlated with accelerated venous thrombosis resolution but no protection from fibrosis. PAI-1 inhibition as a treatment strategy for DVT is likely to accelerate clearance of the thrombus but may come at the expense of increased vein wall fibrosis.

Clinical Relevance.—The pathophysiologic mechanism of postthrombotic syndrome is not well understood clinically or experimentally. In this study, we evaluated the effect of the prominent fibrinolytic mechanism, plasminogen activator inhibitor 1 (PAI-1), and low-molecular-weight heparin (LMWH) on vein wall injury after thrombosis. We show here that LMWH is protective from vein wall fibrosis, but this is abrogated in PAI-1-deleted mice. This is also correlated with monocyte vein wall influx. These data support the clinical observation that LMWH may be protective from postthrombotic vein wall injury in a PAI-1-dependent manner.

► This is truly a remarkable study with an incredible amount of work; it was systematically well designed, employed an exceptional experimental protocol, and provides important results and interpretation. For basic scientists and those with an interest in deep venous thrombosis pathogenesis and resolution, this is a landmark reference. It is clear from this study that low molecular weight heparin (LMWH) does not expedite thrombus resolution (fibrinolysis), but LMWH does decrease overall thrombus size and significantly decreases vein wall fibrosis in a plasminogen activator inhibitor 1 (PAI-1) dependent manner (increased circulating levels of PAI-1) in wild-type mice, which is critical in maintaining a functional and active endothelium. PAI-1 deletion led to increased thrombus resolution with or without LMWH but at an increased rate of vein wall fibrosis. Interesting from this study is the inflammatory monocyte infiltrate (associated with an increase in monocyte chemoattractant protein-1) and cytokine presence (profibrotic interleukin [IL]-13) in the PAI-1 knockout mice, as well as the increased vein wall fibrosis. Although LMWH did not reduce vein wall fibrosis in PAI-1 knockout mice, it significantly decreased the expression of IL-13 in the vein wall. This would imply that vein wall fibrosis is mediated by multiple different pathways involving inflammation, matrix metalloproteinases (MMPs), cytokines, and monocyte chemoattractant factors. The action of MMPs and vein wall fibrosis is likely due to the absence of PAI-1 and inhibition of uPA, where uPA catalyzes the production of plasmin formation from plasmiogen, and plasmin in turn can activate MMPs, which are involved in vein wall remodeling including fibrosis. Because of the availability of the new oral anticoagulants (NOACs; rivaroxaban, abixaban, dabigatran), future studies should assess the effects of the NOACs on thrombus resolution, vein wall cytokine and MMP expression, vein wall fibrosis, and vein wall function. These studies will be important in determining whether vein wall inflammation and fibrosis are affected by NOACs, and the information gained from basic science studies will have a positive impact on reducing the postthrombotic syndrome in clinical practice.

J. D. Raffetto, MD, FACS, FSVM

Recanalization and flow regulate venous thrombus resolution and matrix metalloproteinase expression in vivo

Chabasse C, Siefert SA, Chaudry M, et al (Univ of Maryland, Baltimore)
J Vasc Surg Venous Lymphat Disord 3:64-74, 2015

Objective.—We examined the role of thrombus recanalization and ongoing blood flow in the process of thrombus resolution by comparing two murine in vivo models of deep venous thrombosis.

Methods.—In CD1 mice, we performed surgical inferior vena cava ligation (stasis thrombosis), stenosis (thrombosis with recanalization), or sham procedure. We analyzed thrombus weight over time as a measure of thrombus resolution and quantified the messenger RNA and protein levels of membrane-type matrix metalloproteinases (MT-MMPs) as well as effectors of the plasmin complex at days 4, 8, and 12 after surgery.

Results.—Despite similar initial thrombus size, the presence of ongoing blood flow (stenosis model) was associated with a 45.91% subsequent improvement in thrombus resolution at day 8 and 12.57% at day 12 compared with stasis thrombosis (ligation model). Immunoblot and real-time polymerase chain reaction analysis demonstrated a difference in MMP-2 and MMP-9 activity at day 8 between the two models ($P = .03$ and $P = .006$, respectively) as well as a difference in MT2-MMP gene expression at day 8 ($P = .044$) and day 12 ($P = .03$) and MT1-MMP protein expression at day 4 ($P = .021$). Histologic analyses revealed distinct areas of recanalization in the thrombi of the stenosis model compared with the ligation model as well as the recruitment of inflammatory cells, especially macrophages, and a focal pattern of localized expression of MT1-MMP and MT3-MMP proteins surrounding the areas of recanalization in the stenosis model.

Conclusions.—Recanalization and ongoing blood flow accelerate deep venous thrombus resolution in vivo and are associated with distinct patterns of MT1-MMP and MT3-MMP expression and macrophage localization in areas of intrathrombus recanalization.

Clinical Relevance.—Incomplete thrombus resolution after deep venous thrombosis is important in the development of post-thrombotic syndrome. This study directly examines the role of ongoing blood flow and recanalization in the resolution of deep venous thrombosis in vivo. We find that the presence of ongoing blood flow enhances thrombus resolution and is associated with expression of key matrix metalloproteinases in areas of recanalization within the thrombus. These findings help define the physiology of thrombus resolution and provide potential therapeutic targets to accelerate this clinically important process for patients with deep venous thrombosis.

► There are a number of inferior cava venous thrombosis models in the mouse. There is a ligation model that ligates the inferior vena cava below the renal veins, as well as all side branches. This model provides significant information regarding the inflammatory mechanisms involved in venous thrombus formation and the fibrinolytic mechanisms involved in thrombus resolution; however, it is not physiologic or seen in humans because ligation is not performed. The stenosis mouse model reduces the luminal diameter of the inferior vena cava, allowing for thrombosis to occur. This model can identify the critical factors involved in inflammation and thrombus resolution but also allows for recanalization to occur with blood flow and is a closer representation to the physiologic occurrence that is present in humans with deep venous thrombosis.

There is also an electrolytic model that damages the intima, causing inferior vena cava thrombosis, and, as in the stenosis model, the events leading to thrombosis and resolution can be studied in a more physiologic and representative manner in relation to human deep venous thrombosis. As this study demonstrated, thrombus resolution, matrix metalloproteinases (MMPs), the membrane-type MMPs, and macrophages in the recanalized segments. Both models are important; however, the ligation model represents deep venous thrombosis that has poor resolution and continued obstructive physiology, leading clinically to a postthrombotic picture, and the stenosis model identifies the steps of recanalization with reestablished flow and a nonobstructive or less obstructive physiology.

J. D. Raffetto, MD, FACS, FSVM

Role of compression stockings after endovenous laser therapy for primary varicosis

Elderman JH, Krasznai AG, Voogd AC, et al (Atrium Med Ctr, Sittard, The Netherlands; Maastricht Univ Med Ctr, The Netherlands; et al)
J Vasc Surg 2:289-296, 2014

Objective.—The objective of this prospective, randomized trial was to evaluate the effect of compression stockings after endovenous laser therapy (EVLT) for insufficiency of the great saphenous vein. Effect evaluation was focused on differences in postoperative pain within 6 weeks.

Methods.—The study randomized 111 patients undergoing EVLT for duplex ultrasound–confirmed great saphenous vein insufficiency ($C_{2\text{-}4}E_PA_SP_R$) to receive either 2 weeks of elastic stockings (class II, thigh length) or no elastic stockings after an initial 24-hour period of wearing bandages. Patients registered pain scores (primary outcome) and use of analgesics in a diary on a visual analog scale. At 2 days, 14 days, and 6 weeks after the procedure, leg circumferences, Aberdeen Varicose Vein Questionnaire scores, RAND 36-Item Health Survey scores, patient satisfaction (5-point scale), time before returning to work, and adverse events (secondary outcomes) were evaluated.

Results.—In the 79 patients (15 men and 64 women; mean age, 52 years) who completed the treatment and follow-up, small but significant differences in pain scores were observed during the first week after laser surgery, with more favorable scores in the group wearing stockings. Patients not wearing stockings used more analgesics than did patients wearing stockings ($P < .05$). Patients wearing stockings reported a statistically significantly higher score of satisfaction at 2 days (4.44 vs 4.15) and

6 weeks (4.59 vs 4.18), although the absolute differences were small. No significant differences were found regarding time to return to work, Aberdeen Varicose Vein Questionnaire scores, RAND 36-Item Health Survey scores, leg circumference measurements, and risk of complications.

Conclusions.—Wearing of postoperative stockings for 2 weeks after an initial 24-hour period of wearing bandages results in a small but significant reduction of postoperative pain and use of analgesics compared with not wearing compression stockings after EVLT for great saphenous vein insufficiency.

▶ Few studies assess the role of compression following endovenous ablation procedures. It is unclear if there is any benefit in wearing compression garments following endovenous ablation to reduce pain, ecchymosis, phlebitis, and edema. There is evidence that compression stockings help reduce pain and ecchymosis in patients undergoing great saphenous vein stripping and ligation; however, given newer less-invasive techniques that use tumescent anesthesia, and also the newer nonthermal nontumescent techniques, ligation and stripping of the great saphenous vein for chronic venous diseases is rarely practiced in the United States. In this small randomized, controlled trial, the authors evaluate the effectiveness of compression stockings (20-30 mm Hg) worn for 2 weeks following endovenous laser ablation following 24 hours of bandages after the procedure in the treatment group (n = 39) or no compression stocking (n = 40) and assess a reduction in pain at 2 days and 2 and 6 weeks. Patients enrolled had varicose veins, edema, and skin changes but no healed or active ulcers. The main outcome was a small but significant reduction in pain in the patients wearing the compression stockings, but this difference was no longer significant after 2 weeks. There were no differences in quality of life, leg circumference, return to work, and adverse events. In this study, it is important to note that the laser energy used was an 810-nm diode. Newer higher frequency lasers require less wattage and target water rather than red blood cells, with the advantage of less pain, ecchymosis, and less tumescent required. In addition, there are endovenous ablative techniques for treating chronic venous disease that are both nonthermal and nontumescent. It would be important to evaluate these newer techniques and the need for postoperative compression stockings. In addition, it should be noted that in patients with healed and active venous leg ulcers following endovenous ablation, compression should always be applied.

J. D. Raffetto, MD, FACS, FSVM

The real cost of treating venous ulcers in a contemporary vascular practice

Ma H, O'Donnell TF Jr, Rosen NA (Tufts Med Ctr, Boston, MA)

J Vasc Surg Venous Lymphat Disord 2:355-361, 2014

Background.—Venous leg ulcers (VLUs) are a prevalent and morbid disease that consumes considerable health care resources. Estimates place the total costs for treatment of VLU at 1% of health care budgets in many industrialized countries. Unfortunately, there is little contemporary information on the total cost of treating VLU in the United States, particularly in a wound center staffed by vascular specialists. The purpose of this study was to define the actual cost of treating VLU and to identify factors influencing costs.

Methods.—A cohort of 84 patients with active VLU (Clinical, Etiologic, Anatomic, and Pathologic class 6 disease) who were treated in a wound center by five vascular surgeons with a minimum follow-up of 6 months (median, 368 days; range, 336-483 days) was retrospectively studied. Actual costs (not charges) were obtained for outpatient and inpatient facility, visiting nurse services, and our physician practice group to yield true cost. The proportion of healed VLUs and time to complete healing were determined to calculate time to healing as well as ulcer-free intervals. Calculations of cost/ulcer-free days and cost to complete healing for the entire follow-up period were carried out as well as univariate analysis of factors affecting cost.

Results.—The mean total cost of treating VLU during this follow-up period was $15,732. A total of 50 patients (60%) healed their VLUs without recurrence in a mean time of 122 days (range, 6-379 days) at a cost of $10,563 (range, $430-$50,967). This translated to $86/day of treatment to heal an ulcer, resulting in a cost of $42/ulcer-free day. In comparison, the total cost was threefold higher at $33,907 (range, $390-$132,730) for the patients ($n = 17$; 20%) who did not heal their VLUs. Significant contributing factors included outpatient facility fees ($10,332) and visiting nurse services ($11,365) related to extended treatment of the open VLU. Patients who had a recurrence of their VLU ($n = 17$; 20%) during the follow-up period had a total cost of $12,760. Inpatient admission for wound-related issues increased total cost to $33,629. Nearly two thirds of admissions were for treatment of cellulitis with intravenous antibiotics. VLUs treated with surgical intervention did not significantly increase total cost ($12,304 vs $19,503; $P > .05$) but significantly reduced recurrence rates (34% vs 5%). There were three outliers who experienced complications after treatment of outflow obstruction that dramatically increased the total cost to $71,526.

Conclusions.—This economic analysis demonstrates the high true costs associated with modern treatment of VLU by aggressive medical and surgical techniques. Inpatient and outpatient facility fees, physician fees, and visiting nurse payments all contribute to the cumulative tally that results in these staggering direct costs for treatment of VLUs. The daily cost of treatment that accrues for the ongoing care of VLU patients until they are healed provides an economic rationale for initiatives that advance approaches seeking to provide more rapid wound healing. Our analysis also highlights the significant costs associated with treatment of infections and complications encountered in aggressive surgical interventions for patients with extensive chronic central venous occlusive disease. More aggressive early outpatient treatment of infections and refined criteria for selection of outflow stenting candidates may reduce total cost by preventing complications while improving outcomes.

▶ Venous leg ulcers (VLUs) have a significant socioeconomic impact. VLUs affect up to 1% of the Western adult population, and in the United States, there are about 0.5 to 1 million active VLUs annually. VLUs are the most common leg ulcer evaluated and treated in wound care centers. The economic impact from VLUs is significant with 2 million workdays per year lost due to the burden of caring for VLU, and the cost of treating VLU is estimated to be about $3 billion per year. There are many factors (direct and indirect) that need to be figured into the overall cost of treating VLU. In this important article, the authors evaluate what are the direct costs of treating VLU, the cost of treating healed VLU versus nonhealing VLU, the cost associated with outpatient and nursing care, the financial impact of hospitalization of patients with complex VLU, and the factors that affect cost in treating VLU. In this series of 84 patients with VLU, 60% healed their VLU, 20% did not, and 20% had a recurrence. The significant findings of this study were as follows: (1) patients with healed VLUs had a cost of $10 563 ± $9132. (2) Patients with nonhealing VLUs had a 3-fold increase in the cost of treatment ($33 907 ± $28 000; $P < .0005$). (3) Patients who did not heal had significant outpatient nursing needs that increased the overall cost of care ($11 365 ± $4116; $P < .05$), as well as outpatient facility costs ($10 332 ± $3477; $P < .05$). (4) Treating VLUs as an outpatient was significantly less expensive than when a patient required hospitalization and inpatient treatment ($10 851 ± $33 629; $P < .001$), the majority of admissions (61%) for VLU was for infection requiring intravenous antibiotics. It is clear that nonhealing VLUs requiring continued nursing support and hospital admissions increased the costs of treating VLU, and recurrent VLU also increases the costs of treatment. It is unclear whether early intervention in correcting venous hemodynamics (reflux) increases VLU healing; studies support reduction in ulcer recurrence but not overall healing rate. However, from our daily practice, we see VLUs heal after correcting the superficial venous insufficiency, and future studies are needed to address early intervention in healing VLU and reducing VLU recurrence to reduce the cost burden that VLUs pose to the health care system.

J. D. Raffetto, MD, FACS, FSVM

Therapeutic Effect of Compression Stockings Versus no Compression on Isolated Superficial Vein Thrombosis of the Legs: A Randomized Clinical Trial

Boehler K, Kittler H, Stolkovich S, et al (Med Univ Vienna, Austria)
Eur J Vasc Endovasc Surg 48:465-471, 2014

Objective/Background.—Leg compression is considered basic treatment for superficial vein thrombosis (SVT), although scientific proof for its efficacy is lacking. The aim of the study was to evaluate the therapeutic effect of compression stockings on isolated SVT of the legs.

Methods.—This was a single-center randomized controlled trial. Eighty patients with isolated SVT of the legs were instructed to wear compression stockings (23–32 mm Hg) (CG) or no compression (NCG) for 3 weeks. All patients received low molecular weight heparin (LMWH) at prophylactic dosage. Non-steroidal anti-inflammatory drugs (NSAIDs) were allowed. The primary outcome variable was the reduction of pain as assessed by a visual analog scale (VAS) and the Lowenberg test. Secondary outcomes were the consumption of analgesics, thrombus length, skin erythema, D-dimer, and quality of life (QoL).

Results.—Seventy-three patients completed the study. Clinical symptoms and QoL significantly improved from baseline to day 21 in both groups ($p < .001$ for VAS, Lowenberg test, thrombus length, and erythema; $p < .006$ for QoL), and consumption of analgesics and D-dimer significantly decreased ($p < .001$). There was no significant difference between the groups for all tested variables. At day 7, patients in the CG revealed a significantly faster thrombus regression ($p = .02$).

Conclusion.—Adding compression stockings for 3 weeks to LMWH and NSAIDs does not bring significant additional benefit in the treatment of isolated SVT. When worn for 1 week, compression stockings stimulate significantly faster thrombus regression.

▶ Superficial venous thrombosis (SVT) can be associated with varicose veins; in nonvaricose veins, SVT is associated with hypercoagulable states and/or malignancies. The treatment of SVT is controversial, and guidelines recommend treating with fondaparinux or low molecular weight heparin (LMWH) for SVT extending greater than 5 cm for 45 days over no anticoagulation (Grade 2B). However, this methodology is not very cost-effective because the rate of venous thromboembolism was 1.3% in untreated patients. This would require a significant number of patients treated (88) to prevent 1 deep venous thrombosis and 300 patients treated to prevent one pulmonary embolism, which is clearly not cost-effective. A more cost-effective means would be to identify high-risk patients with SVT (cancer, a history venous thromboembolism [VTE], severe chronic venous insufficiency, nonvaricose veins, or a shorter treatment duration). The role of compression stocking as an adjunct to treating VTE in addition to LMWH is not known. In this small randomized controlled trial, compression stockings plus LWMH versus LMWH only did not offer any additional advantage in pain or quality of life, but surprisingly increased the resolution of the SVT. The mechanism of this phenomenon is not known. It is known, however, that compression can alter the cytokine, chemokines, and inflammatory cells in patients with venous ulcer. Whether a similar mechanism is in effect with compression and SVT resolution is not known and warrants further study.

J. D. Raffetto, MD, FACS, FSVM

14 Chronic Venous and Lymphatic Disease

A Randomized Trial Comparing Treatments for Varicose Veins

Brittenden J, Cotton SC, Elders A, et al (Aberdeen Royal Infirmary, Aberdeen, Scotland; et al)

N Engl J Med 371:1218-1227, 2014

Background.—Ultrasound-guided foam sclerotherapy and endovenous laser ablation are widely used alternatives to surgery for the treatment of varicose veins, but their comparative effectiveness and safety remain uncertain.

Methods.—In a randomized trial involving 798 participants with primary varicose veins at 11 centers in the United Kingdom, we compared the outcomes of foam, laser, and surgical treatments. Primary outcomes at 6 months were disease-specific quality of life and generic quality of life, as measured on several scales. Secondary outcomes included complications and measures of clinical success.

Results.—After adjustment for baseline scores and other covariates, the mean disease-specific quality of life was slightly worse after treatment with foam than after surgery ($P = 0.006$) but was similar in the laser and surgery groups. There were no significant differences between the surgery group and the foam or the laser group in measures of generic quality of life. The frequency of procedural complications was similar in the foam group (6%) and the surgery group (7%) but was lower in the laser group (1%) than in the surgery group ($P < 0.001$); the frequency of serious adverse events (approximately 3%) was similar among the groups. Measures of clinical success were similar among the groups, but successful ablation of the main trunks of the saphenous vein was less common in the foam group than in the surgery group ($P < 0.001$).

Conclusions.—Quality-of-life measures were generally similar among the study groups, with the exception of a slightly worse disease-specific quality of life in the foam group than in the surgery group. All treatments had similar clinical efficacy, but complications were less frequent after laser treatment and ablation rates were lower after foam treatment. (Funded by the Health

Technology Assessment Programme of the National Institute for Health Research; Current Controlled Trials number, ISRCTN51995477.)

▶ Comparative effectiveness and safety of treatment options for axial reflux involving the saphenous vein and varicose veins is lacking. In this randomized multicenter clinical trial (Comparison of Laser, Surgery, and Foam Sclerotherapy), outcomes of foam sclerotherapy (sodium tetradecyl sulfate 3% for saphenous veins and 1% for varicose veins), endovenous ablation (laser ablation of truncal saphenous veins with foam sclerotherapy of residual varicose veins 6 weeks later), and surgery (proximal ligation and stripping saphenous veins with concurrent phlebectomies) were compared using primary patient-reported measures and secondary measures to assess clinical success. Although overall outcomes were good for all treatment options, foam sclerotherapy had worse disease-specific quality-of-life measures and lower successful ablation rates (54.6%) compared with laser endovenous ablation (83.0%) and surgery (84.4%). Complication rates were statistically lowest in the endovenous ablation group (1.0%) compared with foam (6.2%) and surgery (7.1%). Although limitations including lack of blinded participants and assessors, lack of a sham group, short follow-up, and absence of other methods for endovenous ablation, the study design, and conduct were otherwise reasonable and the observations likely valid. Overall, practitioners may use this evidence to guide therapeutic options across all 3 treatment strategies, but it seems that clinical decision making slightly favors endovenous ablation options based on some differences seen in outcome measures.

M. Passman, MD

Biomechanical comparison between mono-, bi-, and tricuspid valve architectures

Chen HY, Berwick Z, Krieger J, et al (Res Engineering, Bloomington, IN; et al)
J Vasc Surg Venous Lymphat Disord 2:188-193, 2014

Background.—An understanding of the relationship between venous valve architecture and associated fluid and solid mechanical forces will undoubtedly advance prosthesis design and treatments. The objective of the current study was to compare three valve architectures (mono-, bi-, and tricuspid) and the implications of these designs on the fluid and solid mechanics of the valve leaflets. The hypothesis is that the bicuspid valve has the lowest mechanical cost, defined as the ratio of leaflet wall stress and fluid wall shear stress (WSS), for the venous environment as compared with mono- and tricuspid valves.

Methods.—To address this hypothesis, fully coupled, two-way fluid-structure interaction computational models were developed and simulated for the three types of valves.

Results.—The numerical simulations showed that the mean fluid WSS of the bicuspid valve was generally higher than the tricuspid valve, which was further higher than the monocuspid valve. The mean leaflet wall stress of the bicuspid valve was lower than the tricuspid valve, which was further lower than the monocuspid valve. Therefore, the mechanical cost, which was defined as solid wall stress/fluid WSS, of the bicuspid valve was the lowest.

Conclusions.—The lower mechanical cost may be a reason why the bicuspid valve is the dominant design in the venous system. This knowledge provides guidance for the design of novel venous prosthetic valves and may shed light on venous valve disease when the architecture of the valve is altered.

▶ Using a computational model, this study shows that bicuspid valve architecture has a more favorable and efficient profile in terms of fluid and mechanical forces (mechanical cost defined as solid wall stress and fluid wall shear stress) than mono- and tricuspid valve configurations. This fluid dynamic advantage seems to be the result of more optimal anatomic factors in the stasis region at the base of the valve and in the leaflet pocket region that was observed during the full valve opening and closing cycle and may provide less flow stagnation and potential decreased adhesion of thrombotic and inflammatory cells. Although in part this may explain why venous valves have a bicuspid configuration in nature, but it may also have bearing on optimizing novel venous valve design based on bicuspid rather than monocuspid or tricuspid designs. However, the computational model used in this study is mathematical only and represents an idealized concept that has yet to be tested in an in vivo flow model.

M. Passman, MD

Catheter-directed Foam Sclerotherapy of Great Saphenous Veins in Combination with Pre-treatment Reduction of the Diameter Employing the Principals of Perivenous Tumescent Local Anesthesia

Devereux N, Recke AL, Westermann L, et al (Univ of Schleswig-Holstein, Campus Luebeck, Germany; Dermatological Practise, Hamburg, Germany)
Eur J Vasc Endovasc Surg 47:187-195, 2014

Objectives.—The aim of this study was to evaluate occlusion rates of great saphenous veins (GSV) with a diameter between 5–10 mm that received a pre-treatment size reduction via perivenous tumescent application (TA) followed by catheter-directed foam sclerotherapy (CDFS).

Methods.—A prospective blinded randomized clinical trial comparing the occlusion rates of GSV at 1-, 6-, and 12-month follow-up. Fifty patients were included and randomized into two groups. CDFS was performed accessing the GSV at knee level and applying 8 mL of 2% polidocanol-foam (EasyFoam) while the catheter was withdrawn. Strictly perivenous TA was performed in group 1 before applying the sclerosant agent. Occlusion rates and clinical scores were assessed by blinded examiners.

Results.—After 12 months in group 1 full occlusion was achieved in 73.9%, partial occlusion in 8.7%, and 17.4% were classified as treatment failure. In group 2, 75% of the targeted GSV were fully occluded, 20% were partially occluded, and 5% were diagnosed as treatment failure. Both groups showed a significant reduction of the vein diameter. Patient's tolerance and satisfaction with the treatment was high in both groups.

Conclusion.—No benefit could be found using additional TA to reduce the vein diameter before the treatment.

▶ In an effort to optimize contact of foam sclerosant with endothelium in large-caliber veins without exceeding maximum amount of sclerosant agents, this study evaluated the impact of perivenous tumescence on occlusion rates of great saphenous veins (GSV) treated with catheter-directed foam sclerotherapy. As a prospective blinded randomized study, there is no difference in primary outcome of venous occlusion at 12 months. Unfortunately, the presumption that reduced diameter of GSV by pretreatment perivenous tumescence will ensure minimal vessel diameter, increase contact of sclerosant with vein endothelium, and decrease sclerosant volume at the time of treatment is not directly evaluated or proven. Other limitations, including small sample size, tumescence solution with saline only and no lidocaine or epinephrine, and variable distribution of tumescence application, make any further conclusions unsupported. Regardless, the use of saline tumescence pretreatment prior to foam sclerotherapy does not offer any additional benefit in terms of occlusion rates and other measured parameters and is not recommended.

M. Passman, MD

Compression Therapy Versus Surgery in the Treatment of Patients with Varicose Veins: A RCT

Sell H, Vikatmaa P, Albäck A, et al (Univ of Helsinki, Finland; et al)
Eur J Vasc Endovasc Surg 47:670-677, 2014

Objective.—Superficial venous reflux and varicose veins are common. The aim of this randomized controlled trial was to assess effectiveness of compression therapy compared with surgery for superficial venous reflux.

Methods.—153 patients with CEAP class C2–C3 and superficial venous reflux were randomized to receive either conservative treatment (compression stockings) ($n = 77$) or surgery ($n = 76$). Clinical examination including duplex ultrasound (DUS) was performed at entry and 1 and 2 years after randomization (compression group) or surgery (surgery group). Venous Clinical Severity Score without compression stockings (VCSS-S), Venous Segmental Disease Score (VSDS), Venous Disability Score (VDS), and health-related quality of life (HRQoL) were assessed at entry and at the follow-ups. Data were analysed on an intention-to-treat basis and according to the actual treatment performed.

Results.—At 2 years, 70/76 patients in the surgery group and 11/77 patients in the compression group had been operated on. VCSS-S decreased from 4.6 to 3.5 in the compression group ($p < .01$) and from 4.8 to 0.6 in the surgery group ($p < .001$). VSDS decreased from 7.7 to 7.0 in the compression group and from 8.2 to 0.9 in the surgery group ($p < .0001$). HRQoL did not change in the compression group, but improved significantly in the surgery group.

Conclusion.—The surgical elimination of non-complicated superficial venous reflux is an effective treatment when compared with providing compression stockings only.

▶ In this randomized, controlled trial for the treatment of patients with superficial venous reflux and varicose veins (clinical, etiology, anatomy, pathophysiology class 2–3), surgical correction (ligation, stripping, and phlebectomy) was more effective than compression (class II compression stockings) at 2 years in terms of patient-oriented outcome measures. As an intent-to-treat analysis, these findings held up despite 14.3% crossover rate from the compression group to surgery. The results in this trial are in agreement with the only other published randomized trial comparing open ablative surgery and compression therapy for varicose veins.[1] Many health plans and insurance carriers require a trial of nonoperative measures, including compression, prior to approval of operative correction, a requirement that is not supported by evidence including this clinical trial. Although this study compared surgical options and did not include endothermal and nonthermal interventions, elimination of superficial reflux and varicose veins is the key pathophysiologic factor, and there is plenty of other evidence suggesting superiority of these less invasive options over surgery. Based on a growing body of evidence, health policy makers should eliminate compression as a requirement prior to treatment of superficial venous reflux and varicose veins, but obviously this evidence-based decision is still clouded by the financial conflicts of interest of these health carrier providers to restrict financial expenditure.

M. Passman, MD

Reference

1. Michaels JA, Brazier JE, Campbell WB, MacIntyre JB, Palfreyman SJ, Ratcliffe J. Randomized clinical trial comparing surgery with conservative treatment for uncomplicated varicose veins. *Br J Surg*. 2006;93:175-181.

Endovenous Laser Ablation of Great Saphenous Veins Performed Using Tumescent Cold Saline Solution without Local Anesthesia

Cavallini A, Marcer D, Bernardini G, et al (Verona Veins Clinic, Italy)
Ann Vasc Surg 28:951-956, 2014

Background.—In recent years, laser systems with higher wavelengths, associated with new optical fibers, have shown excellent short-term results in treating saphenous veins and reducing the side effects and, in particular, the postoperative pain. However, if the patients are not anesthetized, they may feel pain even when using low energy with the high-wavelength laser; the only tumescent local anesthesia often does not guarantee a complete pain control during endovenous laser ablation (EVLA). Aim of this study was to demonstrate that the local anesthesia during EVLA of great saphenous veins (GSVs) is not essential for the perioperative comfort of the patient if a mild sedation is made.

Methods.—Forty-nine incompetent GSVs were treated by EVLA with a cold saline tumescent solution (CSTS) without local anesthetic drugs. EVLA was performed with a 1540-nm diode laser and a 600-mc ball-tipped fiber. Intraoperative ultrasonography was then used to guide delivery of CSTS (cold saline solution 0.9% at 5°C) using a motor pump under intravenous sedation. The gravity of chronic venous disease was determined according to the clinical-etiology-anatomy-pathophysiology classification. Patients rated surgery global pain according to 4 types: "extremely," "rather," "slightly," and "not at all" painful.

Results.—Twenty-five cases (51%) were classified as C3, 20 (41%) as C2, 6 (13%) as C4, and 1 (2%) as C6. Midazolam 2.5 mg + a mean of 0.16 mg of fentanil (minimum: 0.10; maximum: 0.20; standard deviation [SD]: 0.4) + a mean of 178.21 mg of propofol (minimum: 100; maximum: 300; SD: 47.1) were administrated as intravenous sedation. The total average linear endovenous energy density was 57.7 J/cm. Approximately 250 mL (minimum: 100; maximum: 780) of CSTS was administered. No patient has had pain during the procedure. All patients were discharged 2.5 hrs after surgery.

Conclusions.—EVLA under sedation using CSTS without diluted anesthetic drugs is a suitable technique in an outpatients clinic, especially useful if the ablation of the saphenous vein is combined with an extended phlebectomy or if a bilateral treatment is performed, to eliminate the risks of overdose with local anesthesia and with the aim of improving the comfort of the patient.

▶ The success of endovenous ablation in the office setting has been predicated on the advancement of tumescence techniques that allow for delivery of dilute local anesthetic in the perivascular tissue and the fluid buffer provided to protect adjacent tissue. With concern for need of increased systemic concentrations of local anesthetics, this study showed that with a high wavelength laser fiber (1540-nm diode laser), intravenous sedation, and use of cold tumescence infusion (0.9% normal saline at 5°C) that endovenous ablation was possible with minimal discomfort to the patient. However, enthusiasm should be tempered by lack of a randomized controlled arm of those who received local anesthetic mixed in the cold tumescence, the concomitant use of what was effectively conscious sedation, and the limitations of success based on the higher wavelength fiber. With appropriate tumescence solutions containing a local anesthetic, often endovenous ablation procedures can be performed in an outpatient setting with minimal to no sedation. Although not addressed here, what may be of more interest in this study is the possibility of using cold tumescence with current solutions containing local anesthetics to potentially increase the effect and decrease the volume. Ultimately, as other nonthermal ablation techniques evolve, the entire issue of tumescence may become less of a concern.

M. Passman, MD

Improvement of Venous Pumping Function by Double Progressive Compression Stockings: Higher Pressure Over the Calf is More Important Than a Graduated Pressure Profile

Mosti G, Partsch H (Clinica MD Barbantini, Lucca, Italy; Med Univ of Vienna, Austria)

Eur J Vasc Endovasc Surg 47:545-549, 2014

Background.—Previous studies have shown that so-called progressive elastic compression stockings (PECS) with a negative pressure gradient have a more pronounced effect on venous pump function than conventional, graduated stockings. The aim of this study was to investigate the effect of higher graduated and non-graduated pressures on the venous calf pump in patients with venous disease.

Methods.—The ejection fraction (EF) of the calf pump was measured by plethysmography under a standardized walking test in 20 patients suffering from chronic venous disease (CEAP C2—C5) without compression, (a) with one and (b) two PECS on top of each other, and (c) with one additional conventional stocking covering only the gaiter area to achieve a graduated high pressure profile. Interface pressure was measured in the gaiter area and on the calf.

Results.—A significant improvement of EF compared with baseline was found with all three compression modalities. The two superimposed PECS, providing median pressures of 33 mm Hg in the gaiter area and 46 mm Hg at calf level, increased EF significantly up into the normal range. Increasing the gaiter pressure to 56 mm Hg without changing the calf pressure did not result in further improvement.

Conclusions.—Two PECS applied on top of each other lead to a maximal improvement of the venous pump function, which cannot be further improved by increasing the pressure in the gaiter area thereby restoring a graduated pressure profile.

▶ The benefits of external compression of the leg on venous calf pump function and venous hemodynamics is well established. Most current elastic compression stockings exert a pressure that is higher at the ankle and gradually lowers toward the calf. More recently, progressive elastic compression stockings (PECS) that have a negative pressure gradient with a higher pressure in the calf than the ankle have been shown to have a greater increase in ejection fraction in patients with venous disease.[1] This current study is a follow-up evaluation of higher negative graduated pressure using different stocking configurations. The improvement seen in venous pump function with 2 PECS applied over each other generating 33 mm Hg pressure at the gaiter area and 48 mm Hg at the calf level over a single PECS suggests that the higher reverse pressure gradient has better hemodynamic effect. These findings, as suggested in this study, may reflect the need to augment larger volume of blood in the calf compared with the gaiter area that needs to be ejected by the calf muscle with a stocking that reverses the gradient. Although the physiologic observations in this study and the preceding work from the same authors is interesting and deserves further investigation, the clinical impact of these observations remains unclear.

M. Passman, MD

Reference

1. Mosti G, Partsch H. Compression stockings with a negative pressure gradient have a more pronounced effect on venous pumping function than graduated elastic compression stickings. *Eur J Vasc Endovasc Surg*. 2011;42:261-266.

Incidence and Risk Factors for Venous Reflux in the General Population: Edinburgh Vein Study

Robertson LA, Evans CJ, Lee AJ, et al (Univ of Edinburgh, UK; Univ of Aberdeen, UK; et al)

Eur J Vasc Endovasc Surg 48:208-214, 2014

Objective/Background.—Chronic venous disease (CVD) is common, but the incidence of venous reflux, a precursor to this condition, is unknown. This study measured the incidence of venous reflux and associated risk factors, and examined the association between venous reflux and the incidence of CVD.

Methods.—In the Edinburgh Vein Study, a random sample of 1566 men and women aged 18–64 years were examined at baseline. Eight hundred and eighty of these patients were followed up 13 years and underwent an examination comprising clinical classification of CVD and duplex scanning of the deep and superficial systems to measure venous reflux ≥0.5 s.

Results.—The 13-year incidence of reflux was 12.7% (95% confidence interval [CI] 9.2–17.2), equivalent to an annual incidence of 0.9% (95% CI 0.7–1.3). The 13-year incidence of isolated superficial, isolated deep, and combined deep and superficial reflux was 8.8% (95% CI 5.6–12.0), 2.6% (95% CI 1.2–5.0), and 1.3% (95% CI 0.4–3.2), respectively. The highest incidence was in the great saphenous vein in the lower thigh (8.1%, 95% CI 5.4–11.8). There were no age or sex differences ($p > .050$). The risk of developing reflux was associated with being overweight (odds ratio [OR] 2.1, 95% CI 1.0–4.4) and with history of deep vein thrombosis (OR 11.3, 95% CI 1.0–132.3). Venous reflux at baseline was associated with new varicose veins at follow up ($p < .001$): the age- and sex-adjusted OR was 4.4 (95% CI 1.8–10.8) in those with isolated superficial reflux and 7.3 (95% CI 2.6–22.5) in those with combined deep and superficial reflux.

Conclusion.—For every year of follow-up, around 1% of this adult population developed venous reflux. In two thirds of cases, the superficial system was affected. Venous reflux increased the risk of developing varicose veins, especially when combined deep and superficial reflux was present.

▶ There have been several large population-based epidemiologic studies measuring the prevalence of venous disease, but none have provided longitudinal data on the risk of developing venous reflux over time. Building on the prior Edinburgh Vein Study, this follow-up study provides a snapshot of the incidence of venous reflux 13 years later, which averages out to around 1% per year, and increased risk of developing varicose veins (C2) especially if venous reflux was present at baseline. Although the data from this study provide some insight to risk of developing varicose veins and venous reflux over time, as a longitudinal study, there is considerable variability in preventative measures such as lifestyle modification or compression.[1] Furthermore, the risk of progression to more advanced venous disease (C3-6) is not elucidated and may have been underpowered in this study. That said, this study does provide some important information on the earlier side of the spectrum for risk of developing varicose veins and venous reflux in the future that may be a general baseline regarding future investigations on the impact of preventative measures and advice we provide our patient regarding potential natural history.

M. Passman, MD

Reference

1. Evans CJ, Fowkes FGR, Ruckley CV, Lee AJ. Prevalence of varicose veins and chronic venous insufficiency in men and women in the general population: Edinburgh Vein Study. *J Epidemiol Community Health*. 1999;53:149-153.

Mechanochemical endovenous ablation for the treatment of great saphenous vein insufficiency

van Eekeren RRJP, Boersma D, Holewijn S, et al (Rijnstate Hosp, Arnhem, The Netherlands, St. Antonius Hosp, Nieuwegein, The Netherlands)
J Vasc Surg Venous Lymphat Disord 2:282-288, 2014

Objective.—This study evaluated the feasibility, safety, and 1-year results of mechanochemical endovenous ablation (MOCA) of great saphenous vein (GSV) insufficiency.

Methods.—A consecutive 106 patients were treated for primary GSV insufficiency with MOCA by the ClariVein device and polidocanol. The primary outcome measures were technical success, clinical success, and anatomic success after 1 year of follow-up. Secondary outcome measures were postprocedural pain, complications, general- and disease-specific quality of life, and time to return to work. Patients were evaluated with clinical examination and duplex ultrasonography at 6 weeks, 6 months, and 1 year after treatment.

Results.—The technical success was 99%. The mean postprocedural pain during the first 14 days after treatment was 7.5 mm (interquartile range [IQR], 0.0-10.0 mm) per day on a 0- to 100-mm visual analog scale. The time to return to normal activities and work was 1.0 day (IQR, 0-1.0 day) and 1.0 day (IQR, 1.0-4.0 days), respectively. No major complications were recorded. At 1-year follow-up, the clinical success was 93%. The Venous Clinical Severity Score decreased significantly from 4.0 (IQR, 3.0-5.0) before treatment to 1.0 (IQR, 0-1.0) ($P < .001$) 1 year after MOCA. At 1 year, 88.2% of the treated GSVs remained occluded as measured by duplex ultrasonography. Twelve patients had a recanalization, of which eight were partial. Disease-specific quality of life and the RAND 36-Item Health Survey scores improved significantly at 1-year follow-up.

Conclusions.—MOCA is a safe and effective technique in the treatment of GSV insufficiency with good clinical and anatomic success at 1-year follow-up. The technique is related to low postprocedural pain scores, low complication rate, improved quality of life, and rapid resumption of normal activities and work.

▶ Although the use of endovenous ablation techniques have become standard therapy for treatment of saphenous vein reflux associated with varicose veins, it is limited by thermal effects of laser and radiofrequency catheters and requires tumescence anesthesia. Mechanochemical endovenous ablation (MOCA) uses mechanical damage of the venous endothelium by a rotating catheter that delivers liquid sclerosant as the catheter is withdrawn. In the absence of thermal energy, it has the advantage, over endothermal ablation techniques, of avoiding heat-related complications and the need for tumescence. This study with 1-year follow-up confirms earlier short-term reports that MOCA is safe and effective. Ablation rates were technically successful in 99% of cases on initial follow-up and in 93% at 6 months and 88% at 1 year. Complications were low, and patient satisfaction based on patient-reported outcome measures was high. However, whether MOCA is better or at least equivalent to standard endovenous thermal-based ablation techniques remains uncertain in the absence of prospective randomized controlled investigation.

M. Passman, MD

Patient-reported outcomes 5–8 years after ultrasound-guided foam sclerotherapy for varicose veins

Darvall KA, Bate GR, Bradbury AW (Solihull Hosp, UK)

Br J Surg 101:1098-1104, 2014

Background.—The aim was to determine the long-term (5–8 years) outcomes of ultrasound-guided foam sclerotherapy (UGFS) for varicose veins using health-related quality of life (HRQL), patient-reported outcomes (PROMs), patient satisfaction and retreatment rates.

Methods.—Consecutive patients undergoing UGFS between April 2004 and May 2007 were invited for review at least 5 years after treatment. Patients completed generic (Short Form 12) and disease-specific (Aberdeen Varicose Vein Symptom Severity Score, AVSS) HRQL instruments, and questionnaires enquiring about lower limb symptoms, lifestyle factors and satisfaction with treatment. Data on retreatments were recorded prospectively.

Results.—A total of 391 limbs in 285 patients were included (81·2 per cent response rate) at a median of 71 (i.q.r. 67–78) months following first UGFS treatment. Originally 72·1 per cent had symptomatic, uncomplicated varicose veins, 21·9 per cent had undergone surgery previously, 87·2 per cent had treatment of great saphenous veins and 19·9 per cent treatment of short saphenous veins. Disease-specific HRQL scores improved significantly at long-term follow-up, with 88·5 per cent having an improved AVSS compared with baseline. Regarding lower limb symptoms and lifestyle improvement, 62·7–93·8 per cent of patients had their pretreatment expectations met or exceeded. Overall, 82·0 per cent were very satisfied with their treatment and only 3·3 per cent were dissatisfied; 91·0 per cent would recommend the treatment to others. Some 15·3 per cent of limbs required retreatment by 5 years (Kaplan–Meier analysis).

Conclusion.—UGFS has durable results as reported by PROMs to at least 5 years. Only 15·3 per cent of limbs required retreatment for recurrence during follow-up.

▶ Reports on the durability of ultrasound-guided foam sclerotherapy for varicose veins have been variable. Although many of these studies have focused on technical outcomes, this study reports on long-term follow-up of patient-related outcome measures (PROMs) for patients undergoing ultrasound-guided foam sclerotherapy for varicose veins. In this prospective observational cohort study, most patients had durable results based on PROMs including generic and disease-specific health-related quality of life questionnaires and with high patient satisfaction (82%) and low reintervention rates (15%). Although ultrasound-guided foam sclerotherapy had favorable results in this study, it is difficult to extrapolate how this compares to endovenous ablation or surgery in the absence of another treatment arm, which should be analyzed by a properly conducted randomized trial that also focus on longer term follow-up intervals.

M. Passman, MD

Reflux in the below-knee great saphenous vein can be safely treated with endovenous ablation

Gifford SM, Kalra M, Gloviczki P, et al (Mayo Clinic, Rochester, MN)
J Vasc Surg Venous Lymphat Disord 2:397-402, 2014

Background.—Intervention on the great saphenous vein (GSV) has traditionally been limited to the above-knee (AK-GSV) segment for fear of saphenous neuralgia in spite of incompetence demonstrated in the below-knee (BK-GSV) segment. Residual symptoms and need for reintervention are reported to result in nearly half the patients if the refluxing BK-GSV is ignored. Experience with endovenous ablation of the BK-GSV at the time of AK-GSV treatment is sparsely reported in the literature. The aim of this study was to evaluate the safety of endovenous ablation of the refluxing BK-GSV.

Methods.—Data from consecutive patients treated with superficial venous ablation during a 48-month period from January 2010 to December 2013 were retrospectively reviewed. Demographic and procedure-related outcome and complication data were analyzed specifically for patients undergoing BK-GSV interventions.

Results.—A total of 550 patients were treated with superficial venous ablation during the study period. Of those, 61 (79 limbs) underwent BK-GSV ablation for reflux at this site. There were 36 women and 25 men (mean age, 55 years). Median Clinical, Etiologic, Anatomic, and Pathologic (CEAP) score was 3.4; 43 limbs were treated for symptomatic varicose veins (C 1-3) and 36 for advanced venous insufficiency (C 4-6); 14 limbs (18%) were treated for recurrent symptomatic varicose veins or venous insufficiency after prior superficial venous intervention with AK-GSV ablation, sclerotherapy, or stripping. Comorbidities included obesity (54%) with mean body mass index of 30.7 (range, 19 to 52), obstructive sleep apnea (10%), pulmonary hypertension (3%), and congestive heart failure (3%). Ablation was performed in 77 limbs (99%) with the VenaCure EVLT laser vein treatment (AngioDynamics, Queensbury, NY) and in two limbs by radiofrequency ablation with ClosureFAST system (VNUS Medical Technologies, San Jose, Calif). The mean length of GSV ablated was 51.2 cm (range, 26-67 cm). Endovenous ablation was performed concomitantly on 22 accessory GSVs (28%) and 10 incompetent perforators (13%). Ambulatory stab phlebectomy of branch varicosities was performed simultaneously in 59 limbs (75%). All veins treated were evaluated with ultrasound on postprocedure day 1, and no evidence of endovenous heat-induced thrombosis was detected. Eight patients (10%) went on to have preplanned sclerotherapy treatment for small-branch varicosities. Postoperative paresthesia occurred in three patients (4%) and resolved within 4 weeks. Wound infection in three (4%) stab phlebectomy wounds resolved with oral antibiotic therapy. Follow-up surveillance ultrasound was available in 32 of 79 limbs that were >6 months from the procedure. Partial late recanalization was noted in four of 32 limbs, but no patient had recurrent symptoms requiring repeated endovenous ablation during this period.

Conclusions.—Endovenous ablation of the refluxing BK-GSV segment can be performed safely with minimal complications. Consideration should be given to concomitant ablation of the BK-GSV in treatment of patients with varicose veins with reflux extending to the BK segment of the GSV to improve long-term outcomes.

▶ Because of saphenous nerve proximity to the below-knee (BK) great saphenous vein (GSV) segment, endovenous ablation of GSV is typically recommend for the above-knee segment to avoid potential for saphenous nerve injury. In this series, endovenous ablation of the GSV including BK segments was performed in 79 limbs with 82% first-time treatment of the entire GSV and 18% in those with previous above-knee GSV ablation, plus concomitant varicose procedures in 75%. Postoperative saphenous nerve paresthesia occurred in 4% and was transient, resolving within 4 weeks. It is important to note that success of endovenous ablation of BK segment in this study was based on techniques that included generous tumescence to separate the GSV from the nerve and use of a 1470-nm laser with absorption by water within blood and potential less thermal transfer to adjacent tissue. Also, success seen in this study should be tempered by the retrospective nature and lack of a control group. Furthermore, as a single-arm study, the impact of more extensive GSV endovenous ablation including BK segments on patient-reported venous outcomes remains unclear.

M. Passman, MD

The effect of single phlebectomies of a large varicose tributary on great saphenous vein reflux

Biemans AAM, van den Bos RR, Hollestein LM, et al (Erasmus MC, Rotterdam, The Netherlands; et al)

J Vasc Surg Venous Lymphat Disord 2:179-187, 2014

Objective.—Phlebectomy of varicose tributaries is usually considered an additional treatment after or during saphenous ablation. As phlebectomies alone affect the hemodynamics of the venous system, this treatment can be effective as primary intervention in selected patients. The objective of this study was to analyze hemodynamic, clinical, and patient-reported outcomes after phlebectomies in a prospective multicenter study to determine predictors for treatment success, that is, restoration of great saphenous vein (GSV) competence.

Methods.—Patients with symptomatic GSV and tributary incompetence (reflux > 0.5 second) at the level of the thigh were included. Duplex ultrasound (DUS) was used to assess GSV and tributary characteristics, and a reflux elimination test was performed. Three and 12 months after phlebectomy of the tributary, reflux and GSV diameter were evaluated with DUS. Clinical outcome measures were C class of the Clinical, Etiologic, Anatomic, and Pathologic (CEAP) classification and Venous Clinical Severity Score; patients' reported outcome was determined by the Aberdeen Varicose Vein Questionnaire. To evaluate differences between the success and failure groups, baseline DUS characteristics, Venous Clinical Severity Score, CEAP class, and Aberdeen Varicose Vein Questionnaire score were compared. Multivariable logistic regression including all clinically relevant variables following a backward variable elimination process was used to determine predictors for success. The model was internally validated by 1000 bootstrap samples.

Results.—The study included 94 patients (65 women, 29 men) with a mean age of 53 years. The majority had C2 or C3 disease. One year after treatment, GSV reflux had disappeared in 50% of patients ($P < .01$), and GSV diameter had decreased significantly ($P < .01$). Clinical outcome and Aberdeen Varicose Vein Questionnaire score improved significantly ($P < .01$) and symptoms had disappeared in 66%. Of 47 patients with persisting GSV incompetence, 15 did not receive additional treatment because they were asymptomatic. Independent predictors for success were low C class of the CEAP classification, low number of refluxing GSV segments, small diameter of the GSV above the tributary, and positive reflux elimination test result ($P < .0001$). The reflux elimination test appeared to be an important independent predictor, with >65% chance of success when the result was positive.

Conclusions.—At 1-year follow-up, treatment with single phlebectomies of a large tributary was effective to abolish GSV reflux in 50% of patients and to free 66% of patients from symptoms. Patients with limited disease progression and mild DUS alterations are most likely to benefit from this approach.

▶ There continues to be debate regarding descending concept of superficial venous reflux at an escape point (saphenofemoral junction, saphenopopliteal junction, or perforator vein) downward from the main trunk to the tributary versus the ascending concept from the tributary into the saphenous trunk. This differentiation is important regarding potential treatment strategy addressing saphenous reflux and phlebectomy for descending reflux versus treating the varicose vein tributary first and reassessing need for saphenous reflux. As a prospective multicenter study, patients with symptomatic great saphenous reflux and varicose vein tributary were treated with phlebectomy alone directed at the tributary feeding into the saphenous vein, with reflux in the great saphenous vein eliminated in 50%, significant reduced saphenous diameter, and improved symptoms in 66%. Independent predictors for the disappearance of reflux included C2 disease, short (< 10 cm) refluxing saphenous segment, reflux into a single saphenous segment, small diameter saphenous vein and tributary, and positive reflux elimination test. Based on these and other variables, a prediction model was developed that mathematically suggests that phlebectomy alone would be effective in 90% of patients. Although this study seems to support the ascending concept, lack of external validation of this prediction model limits adoption until better evidence supports these concepts. Until a randomized study testing ascending versus descending treatment strategies is done, the debate will continue.

M. Passman, MD

The Incidence and Outcome of Endothermal Heat-induced Thrombosis after Endovenous Laser Ablation

Kane K, Fisher T, Bennett M, et al (Baylor Univ Med Ctr, Dallas, TX)
Ann Vasc Surg 28:1744-1750, 2014

Background.—Endovenous laser ablation (EVLA) of the saphenous vein has become one of the preferred treatments for treating saphenous vein reflux that has resulted in symptomatic lower extremity venous insufficiency or varicose veins. This procedure was noted during initial reports to have a low incidence of postoperative thrombosis of the femoral or popliteal vein adjacent to the treated great saphenous vein (GSV) or small saphenous vein (SSV). Later clinical experience suggested that the actual incidence of this event is higher and it was subsequently termed endothermal heat-induced thrombosis (EHIT).

Methods.—We reviewed the office records and the pre- and post-treatment ultrasounds of patients undergoing EVLA in our office from 2005 to 2010 to determine the frequency of EHIT in patients we had treated and then graded them according to a previously published classification.

Results.—There were 528 veins treated in 192 men and 336 women. The clinical, etiology, anatomy, pathophysiology (CEAP) class for these patients was 1 (0), 2 (291), 3 (65), 4 (104), 5 (26), and 6 (40), respectively. The GSV was treated in 496 patients, the SSV in 22, and both were treated in 10 patients. EHIT occurred in 29 of the legs treated for an incidence of 5.1%. The EHIT in the femoral vein were of level 3 (3), 4 (7), 5 (12), and 6 (3), respectively. Two patients developed EHIT in the popliteal vein after EVLA of the SSV. Treatment for the EHIT consisted of observation (13), anticoagulation (9), antiplatelet therapy (2), and nonsteroidal anti-inflammatory agents (1). Duration of therapy was usually 1 week, but 7 patients were treated for periods ranging from 1 to 7 weeks. No pulmonary emboli occurred in any of these patients. The EHIT resolved completely in all patients.

Conclusions.—EHIT after EVLA occurs frequently and mainly consists of low-risk level 3, 4, and 5 deep vein thrombosis. The risk of pulmonary embolism is low and the EHIT typically resolves after 1 week. It can be treated with a short course of antiplatelet or anticoagulation therapy, although observation appears to be sufficient as well for lesser grades of EHIT.

▶ The reported incidence of endothermal heat-induced thrombosis (EHIT) has been variable in the literature from 0% to 16%. This study reports an incidence of 5.1%, stratified based on classification as Level 3 (0.6%), Level 4 (1.3%), Level 5 (2.3%), and Level 6 (0.6%), which falls within the reported range. Much of this variability may reflect differences in technique, laser wavelength, timing of postoperative ultrasound, diameter of the saphenous vein at the junction, and other patient-related factors. However, there is no analysis in this study regarding contributing factors. Regardless, with no reported pulmonary embolism, it is clear that EHIT may be of negligible clinical significance, although it is difficult to draw any conclusions from this study given that treatment of EHIT with anticoagulation was not standardized. The debate regarding the need for routine postoperative ultrasound and how best to treat EHIT (observation vs anticoagulation) is not settled by this study.

M. Passman, MD

Characterization of a Bioprosthetic Bicuspid Venous Valve Hemodynamics: Implications for Mechanism of Valve Dynamics

Tien W-H, Chen HY, Berwick ZC, et al (Univ of Washington, Seattle; 3DT Holdings, LLC, Indianapolis, IN; et al)

Eur J Vasc Endovasc Surg 48:459-464, 2014

Background.—Chronic venous insufficiency (CVI) of the lower extremities is a common clinical problem. Although bioprosthetic valves have been proposed to treat severe reflux, clinical success has been limited due to thrombosis and neointima overgrowth of the leaflets that is, in part, related to the hemodynamics of the valve. A bioprosthetic valve that mimics native valve hemodynamics is essential.

Methods.—A computational model of the prosthetic valve based on realistic geometry and mechanical properties was developed to simulate the interaction of valve structure (fluid–structure interaction, FSI) with the surrounding flow. The simulation results were validated by experiments of a bioprosthetic bicuspid venous valve using particle image velocimetry (PIV) with high spatial and temporal resolution in a pulse duplicator (PD).

Results.—Flow velocity fields surrounding the valve leaflets were calculated from PIV measurements and comparisons to the FSI simulation results were made. Both the spatial and temporal results of the simulations and experiments were in agreement. The FSI prediction of the transition point from equilibrium phase to valve-closing phase had a 7% delay compared to the PD measurements, while the PIV measurements matched the PD exactly. FSI predictions of reversed flow were within 10% compared to PD measurements. Stagnation or stasis regions were observed in both simulations and experiments. The pressure differential across the valve and associated forces on the leaflets from simulations showed the valve mechanism to be pressure driven.

Conclusions.—The flow velocity simulations were highly consistent with the experimental results. The FSI simulation and force analysis showed that the valve closure mechanism is pressure driven under the test conditions. FSI simulation and PIV measurements demonstrated that the flow behind the leaflet was mostly stagnant and a potential source for thrombosis. The validated FSI simulations should enable future valve design optimizations that are needed for improved clinical outcome.

► A significant problem after deep venous thrombosis is the development of the postthrombotic syndrome. This can be mild or severe with venous leg ulceration. Valvular destruction resulting in significant reflux and elevated ambulatory venous pressures can be severe, limiting the patient's well-being. Compression therapy is the mainstay of treatment, but compression also has limitations in shortcomings in compliance, application, inappropriate pressure after bandaging, and patient-related factors such as ambulatory status and comorbidities. The limitations of current bioprosthetic valves include neo-intima and fibrosis, as well as high thrombosis rates. The importance of this study is that it evaluates flow and pressure characteristics in a simulation and experimental model of a bioprosthetic venous valve. A key finding is that flow stagnation was seen behind the valve leaflet in the sinus, which could become a source of thrombus formation and eventual thrombosis. Understanding the mechanics of valve function with simulations and in vitro experiments will enable better venous valve designs, and hopefully better durability and relief of symptoms in patients with postthrombotic disease who are not able to be managed with compression therapy.

J. D. Raffetto, MD, FACS, FSVM

Donning Devices (Foot Slips and Frames) Enable Elderly People with Severe Chronic Venous Insufficiency to put on Compression Stockings

Sippel K, Seifert B, Hafner J (Univ Hosp of Zurich, Switzerland; Univ of Zurich, Switzerland)

Eur J Vasc Endovasc Surg 49:221-229, 2015

Objective/Background.—Compression therapy is highly effective in the treatment of post-thrombotic syndrome and venous leg ulcer. On average, 50—60% of the patients cooperate with compression therapy. Therefore, it is necessary to improve the user-friendliness. This prospective study investigated whether the use of donning devices can contribute to improving user-friendliness.

Methods.—Forty patients aged >65 years with severe chronic venous insufficiency (CVI; C4—C6) successively donned compression stockings in a randomized order: one 40 mm Hg (CS40) or two superimposed 20 mm Hg (CS20+20), each with open toe (CS-o-t) and closed toe (CS-c-t), using donning devices (three foot slips for CS-o-t; two foot slips and three frames for CS-c-t). The study endpoint was that the stocking was completely donned and correctly positioned on the patient's leg. The success rate and its association with age, sex, first time versus second time user, body mass index, abdominal circumference, ability to reach the forefoot with the hand, and hand grip strength were analyzed. Additionally, subjective evaluation by the patients was performed.

Results.—Without donning devices, success with CS40-c-t was 60% (24/40 patients) and with CS20+20-c-t 70% (28/40 patients) ($p = .220$). Using donning devices increased success rates significantly. With CS40-o-t the success rate was 88% (35/40 patients; $p = .001$) and with CS40-c-t it was 90% (36/40 patients; $p = .002$). With CS20+20-o-t and

CS20+20-c-t, the success rate was 88% (35/40 patients; $p = .016$). The proportion of patients who successfully used either CS40 or CS20+20 increased from 73% to 93%. Relevant for the patients' success was the ability to reach the forefoot with the hand, and hand grip strength. Subjectively, donning with a device was rated significantly better than without.

Conclusion.—Donning devices significantly improve the ability of elderly patients with CVI to don compression stockings successfully. However, there are differences in user-friendliness among the devices.

▶ One of the most significant barriers for elderly patients' ability to comply with elastic compression stockings is the act of donning the garments. This may be due to many reasons but particularly arthritis in the hands, inability to flex at the waist, obesity, and comorbidities that limit physical function. In fact, several studies have demonstrated that in patients older than age 80 years, 62% would not wear compression garments. In another study of 188 patients with a mean age of 72 years (31% of whom were older than 80 years), the reasons for poor compliance with elastic compression stockings were the following: 12% unsuitable due to limb conditions, 15% could not put them on, and 26% applied with great difficulty. The latter reflects the main issue: because of the compression necessary to treat chronic venous disorders, at a minimum 20 to 30 mm Hg compression is required, but for advanced chronic venous disease with skin changes and healed ulcer, 30 to 40 mm Hg compression is usually required. In this study, the increased effectiveness was demonstrated by using donning assist devices to improve application. The study population studied had chronic venous disease and was older than 65 years, with skin changes or ulcer. Certainly there are other methods to improve compliance with compression by applying custom elastic compression with zippers, using inelastic compression with Velcro straps, or using the mechanical compression pumps that provide pneumatic pressure. The main limitation in these more advanced compression methods is the increased cost. Therefore, any means to improve application of elastic compression stockings with various donning devices in a growing elderly population with chronic venous disease will improve compliance and hopefully control the progression of the disease.

J. D. Raffetto, MD, FACS, FSVM

Endovenous laser ablation versus conventional surgery in the treatment of small saphenous vein incompetence

Roopram AD, Lind MY, Van Brussel JP, et al (Sint Franciscus Gasthuis, Rotterdam, The Netherlands; Polikliniek De Blaak, Leidschendam, The Netherlands; et al)

J Vasc Surg Venous Lymphat Disord 1:357-363, 2013

Introduction.—In this multicenter, randomized controlled trial, endovenous laser ablation (EVLA) is compared with conventional surgery for the treatment of varicose veins based on incompetence of the small saphenous vein and the saphenopopliteal junction (SPJ).

Methods.—In two Dutch hospitals, 189 patients were enrolled and randomized to receive EVLA (810-nm laser) or ligation of the SPJ. End points were success rate measured with duplex ultrasound (6 weeks post-treatment), perioperative pain, quality of life, duration of surgery, difficulty of surgery, complications, cosmetic results, and number of days to resume work and normal activities. Pain was measured on a visual analog scale (VAS). Quality of life was assessed using the Aberdeen Varicose Vein Questionnaire (AVVQ) and Euro Qol-5D. The follow-up duration in this article is 6 weeks.

Results.—One hundred seventy-five patients have been treated and analyzed. One hundred eighteen patients (67%) underwent EVLA, and 57 patients (33%) underwent ligation of the SPJ. The patient characteristics were similar in both groups. In the surgery group, 21% residual incompetence of the SPJ was seen after 6 weeks, compared with 0.9% in the laser group. Both treatment modalities reduced pain after 6 weeks. One week post-treatment, patients in the EVLA group temporarily experienced more pain compared with the surgery group (31 vs 18 on a VAS from 0 to 100). There were no significant differences between the two groups with respect to quality of life. Both treatments did show improvement in quality of life. Also with regard to the cosmetics, there were no differences, aside from the fact that patients rated their scar as more beautiful after EVLA. After EVLA, patients could return to work more quickly. The operation time was longer in the surgery group. After 2 weeks, there were significantly more neurological complications in the surgery group: 18 (31%) vs 16 (17%) patients in the EVLA group. Ten percent of patients in the surgery group developed a surgical site infection vs 0% in the EVLA group.

Conclusions.—EVLA provides an excellent alternative to conventional surgery in the treatment of symptomatic varicose veins due to an incompetent small saphenous vein with SPJ. EVLA has a superior immediate success rate, is easier and faster, and has fewer complications.

▶ This is a 2-center randomized controlled trial assessing ligation of the saphenopopliteal junction (SPJ) with excision of 3 to 5 cm of small saphenous vein versus endovenous laser treatment of the small saphenous vein from the midcalf to just 1 cm of the SPJ. Nearly three-quarters of the patients had C2 disease (varicose veins), and 80% to 85% were a mix of C2 and C3 (edema). Interestingly, pain at 1 week was significantly greater with endovenous laser treatment than surgery, but there was no difference at 6 weeks. Both treatment groups had improvement in quality of life as assessed by the Aberdeen Varicose Vein Questionnaire. What is concerning for this study is the significant neurologic complications (numbness, hyperesthesia, and paraesthesia) for endovenous ablation and surgery of 6.7% and 31%, respectively, at 6 weeks. We should be cautious in the final conclusions of this trial because the follow-up was only 6 weeks. In addition, the role of surgery on the small saphenous vein especially in C2 and C3 disease needs to be further evaluated, given the high rates of neurologic complications. What is unclear is the high rate of neurologic complications of the surgery group because there was no stripping of the small saphenous vein. Clear understanding of the anatomy in the SPJ and the many configurations of the small saphenous vein and the SPJ are needed. In addition, until further guidelines are offered in which patients will benefit from ablating the small saphenous vein in patients with chronic venous disease, this procedure should be limited to patients with skin changes and healed and active ulcers, especially venous leg ulcer on the lateral malleolus.

J. D. Raffetto, MD, FACS, FSVM

Factors that influence perforator thrombosis and predict healing with perforator sclerotherapy for venous ulceration without axial reflux

Kiguchi MM, Hager ES, Winger DG, et al (Univ of Pittsburgh Med Ctr, PA; Univ of Pittsburgh, PA)

J Vasc Surg 59:1368-1376, 2014

Objective.—Refluxing perforators contribute to venous ulceration. We sought to describe patient characteristics and procedural factors that (1) impact rates of incompetent perforator vein (IPV) thrombosis with ultrasound-guided sclerotherapy (UGS) and (2) impact the healing of venous ulcers (CEAP 6) without axial reflux.

Methods.—A retrospective review of UGS of IPV injections from January 2010 to November 2012 identified 73 treated venous ulcers in 62 patients. Patients had no other superficial or axial reflux and were treated with standard wound care and compression. Ultrasound imaging was used to screen for refluxing perforators near ulcer(s). These were injected with sodium tetradecyl sulfate or polidocanol foam and assessed for thrombosis at 2 weeks. Demographic data, comorbidities, treatment details, and outcomes were analyzed. Univariate and multivariable modeling was performed to determine covariates predicting IPV thrombosis and ulcer healing.

Results.—There were 62 patients (55% male; average age, 57.1 years) with active ulcers for an average of 28 months with compression therapy before perforator treatment, and 36% had a history of deep venous thrombosis and 30% had deep venous reflux. At a mean follow-up of 30.2 months, ulcers healed in 32 patients (52%) and did not heal in 30 patients (48%). Ulcers were treated with 189 injections, with an average thrombosis rate of 54%. Of 73 ulcers, 43 ulcers (59%) healed, and 30 (41%) did not heal. The IPV thrombosis rate was 69% in patients whose ulcers healed vs 38% in patients whose ulcers did not heal ($P < .001$). Multivariate models demonstrated male gender ($P = .03$) and warfarin use ($P = .01$) negatively predicted thrombosis of IPVs.

A multivariate model for ulcer healing found complete IPV thrombosis was a positive predictor ($P = .02$), whereas a large initial ulcer area was a negative predictor ($P = .08$). Increased age was associated with fewer ulcer recurrences ($P = .05$). Predictors of increased ulcer recurrences were hypertension ($P = .04$) and increased follow-up time ($P = .02$). Calf vein thrombosis occurred after 3% (six of 189) of injections.

Conclusions.—Thrombosis of IPVs with UGS increases venous ulcer healing in a difficult patient population. Complete closure of all IPVs in an ulcerated limb was the only predictor of ulcer healing. Men and patients taking warfarin have decreased rates of IPV thrombosis with UGS.

▶ This is an important study because it evaluates variables that are independently predictive of venous ulcer failure to heal after perforator vein ablation in the absence of axial reflux. In patients with venous leg ulcer, 60% to 70% will heal their ulcers with compression. To reduce the risk of ulcer recurrence, axial reflux of the saphenous venous system is usually treated with ablation and occasionally ligation and stripping. There is, however, a subset of patients that will persist with venous leg ulcers despite compression and superficial venous reflux treatment. In this group of patients, further consideration should be given in the evaluation of perforator insufficiency in the vicinity of the ulcer. The study findings were that insufficient perforator vein thrombosis rate was 69% in patients whose ulcers healed versus only 38% in patients whose ulcers did not heal ($P < .001$), with overall ulcer healing in 52% of patients. Critical independent factors associated with perforator thrombosis were male gender and anticoagulation use (Coumadin) and that complete perforator thrombosis was a positive predictor for ulcer healing. In this series, all patients had perforators treated under ultrasound-guided foam sclerotherapy. It is not known whether using other modalities such as thermal ablation would have had a greater success, but it is also well known that treated perforators can recanalize at high rates after treatment and that new perforators were not insufficient to develop reflux. There is a lack of randomized trials that assess different treatment modalities in the management of perforator disease associated with healed and active venous ulcers. It is important to keep in mind when we should treat perforators in the setting of chronic venous disease. Until further data determine otherwise, perforator ablation should be limited to patients with healed or active venous leg ulcers, and the pathologic perforator should be at least 3.5 mm in diameter in the vicinity of the ulcer and have a reflux time greater than 0.5 seconds. Because this study demonstrated that prediction of healing was dependent on thrombosis of the perforator, it is important to ensure that the perforator(s) is indeed thrombosed, even if repeat therapy is required; that follow-up is provided in a systematic fashion; and to ensure compliance with compression garments and bandages.

J. D. Raffetto, MD, FACS, FSVM

Progression of varicose veins and chronic venous insufficiency in the general population in the Edinburgh Vein Study

Lee AJ, Robertson LA, Boghossian SM, et al (Univ of Aberdeen, UK; Univ of Edinburgh, UK; et al)

J Vasc Surg Venous Lymphat Disord 3:18-26, 2015

Objective.—The natural history in the general population of chronic venous disease in the legs is not well understood. This has limited our ability to predict which patients will deteriorate and to assign clinical priorities. The aims of this study were to describe the progression of trunk varicose veins and chronic venous insufficiency (CVI) in the general population, to identify important lifestyle and clinical prognostic factors, and to determine the relationship between venous reflux and progression.

Methods.—The Edinburgh Vein Study is a population-based cohort study in which randomly selected adults aged 18 to 64 years had an examination at baseline. This included a questionnaire on lifestyle and clinical factors, standardized assessment and classification of venous disease in the legs, and duplex scan to detect venous reflux in eight segments of each leg. A follow-up examination 13 years later included a reclassification of venous disease to ascertain progression in the development or increase in severity of varicose veins and CVI.

Results.—Among 1566 adults seen at baseline, 880 had a follow-up examination, of whom 334 had trunk varicose veins or CVI at baseline and composed the study sample. The mean (standard deviation) duration of follow-up was 13.4 (0.4) years. Progression was found in 193 (57.8%), equivalent to 4.3% (95% confidence interval [CI], 3.7-4.9) annually. In 270 subjects with only varicose veins at baseline, 86 (31.9%) developed CVI, with the rate increasing consistently with age ($P = .04$). Almost all subjects (98%) with both varicose veins and CVI at baseline deteriorated. Progression of chronic venous disease did not differ by gender or leg, but a family history of varicose veins and history of deep venous thrombosis increased risk (odds ratio [OR], 1.85 [95% CI, 1.14-1.30] and 4.10 [95% CI, 1.07-15.71], respectively). Overweight was associated with increased risk of CVI in those with varicose veins (OR, 1.85; 95% CI, 1.10-3.12). Reflux in the superficial system increased the likelihood of progression, especially in combination with deep reflux (OR, 2.57; 95% CI, 1.55-4.25) and when located in the small saphenous vein (OR, 4.73; 95% CI, 1.37-16.39).

Conclusions.—Nearly half of the general population with chronic venous disease deteriorated during 13 years, and almost one third with varicose veins developed skin changes of CVI, increasing their risk of ulceration. Age, family history of varicose veins, history of deep venous thrombosis, overweight, and superficial reflux, especially in the small saphenous vein and with deep reflux, might influence the risk of progression.

▶ The Edinburgh Vein Study has provided a wealth of information in our understanding of chronic venous disease (CVD), pattern of reflux and associated symptoms, and risks factors for varicose veins and venous disease that has emanated from a longitudinal cross-sectional study of 1566 adults. In this landmark study, a follow-up of 13 years is provided to assess the progression of trunk varicose veins and chronic venous insufficiency (CVI) in the general population. The study also identifies important lifestyle and clinical prognostic factors and determines the relationship between venous reflux and progression. Why is this study so important? First, very few studies have evaluated progression of disease from early clinical class Clinical, Etiological, Anatomical, Pathophysiological (CEAP) to more advanced forms of CVD. The Bonn Vein Study has shown an overall progression of disease of between 20% and 24%. Second, understanding the risk factors that may be associated with progression of disease would allow identification of patients at risk for progression and target early intervention to prevent the more severe clinical classes of CVD (skin changes and venous ulcers). Third, proper identification and treatment would likely reduce health care costs in the treatment and prevention of CVD. The annual rate of progression in patients with trunk varicose vein or chronic venous insufficiency from the Edinburgh Vein Study was 4.3% annually. A family history and a history of deep venous thrombosis were the only 2 independent risk factors that increased the risk of progression. Age, smoking, increased body mass index, mobility at work, and number of pregnancies were not significantly associated with disease progression. However, development of CVI in subjects with varicose veins increased consistently with age and progression of CVI was higher in women. In addition, reflux present in the superficial, both superficial and deep, great saphenous vein in the thigh, and small saphenous vein were all predictors of significant progression. I applaud the authors for their incredible passion to continue the work that began in 1994, which is about the time when the CEAP classification was being developed. Future studies are required to demonstrate benefit and cost-effectiveness of early intervention for patients at risk for disease progression.

J. D. Raffetto, MD, FACS, FSVM

Influence of Manual Lymphatic Drainage on Health-Related Quality of Life and Symptoms of Chronic Venous Insufficiency: A Randomized Controlled Trial

dos Santos Crisóstomo RS, Costa DSA, de Luz Belo Martins C, et al (Universidade de Lisboa, Estrada da Costa, Portugal; Instituto Politécnico de Castelo Branco, Castelo Branco, Portugal; et al)

Arch Phys Med Rehabil 96:283-291, 2015

Objective.—To evaluate the efficacy of manual lymphatic drainage (MLD) in improving health-related quality of life (HRQOL), symptomatology, and physical status in patients with chronic venous insufficiency (CVI).

Design.—Single-blind randomized controlled trial.

Setting.—Health community attendant service.

Participants.—Subjects with CVI (N = 41) were randomly assigned to an experimental group (n = 20; mean age, 54.6 ± 11.3 y) or control group (n = 21; mean age, 46.8 ± 11.1 y).

Interventions.—The experimental group completed 10 lower extremity MLD sessions over 4 weeks and 1 educational session. The control group only attended the educational session. Outcome measures were taken at baseline (t0), at the end of 4 weeks (t1), and after 2 months for follow-up (t2).

Main Outcome Measures.—HRQOL was assessed with the Chronic Venous Insufficiency Quality of Life Questionnaire-20, symptoms (fatigue, heaviness) were assessed with a visual analog scale, severity of the disease was assessed with the Venous Clinical Severity Score (VCSS) (total score, score for each item), leg volumetry was assessed with perimeters, and plantar/dorsiflexion strength and ankle range of motion (ROM) were assessed with dynamometry.

Results.—A significant interaction group × time effect was found for pain on HRQOL ($F_{2,78} = 3.507$; $P = .035$; partial $\eta^2 = .087$), clinical severity ($F_{2,78} = 5.231$; $P = .007$; partial $\eta^2 = .118$), especially for venous edema (assessed with the VCSS), fatigue ($F_{1.67,65.21} = 4.690$; $P = .012$; partial $\eta^2 = .107$), and heaviness ($F_{1.57,61.32} = 9.702$; $P = .001$; partial $\eta^2 = .199$), with the experimental group improving from t0 to t1 and t0 to t2 in all of these outcomes. No effect of MLD treatment could be found for ankle muscle strength, ankle ROM, and leg volume.

Conclusions.—Short-term MLD treatment ameliorates CVI severity and related edema, symptoms, and pain HRQOL in patients with CVI.

▶ This is a small randomized trial assessing manual lymphatic drainage (MLD) treatment (n = 20) versus no treatment (n = 21) in patients with chronic venous insufficiency (CVI) consisting of patients with edema and skin changes, healed venous ulcers, but no active ulcers. The treatment group received 10 treatments of MLD within the first month. The main outcome measure was Chronic Venous Insufficiency Quality of Life Questionnaire—20 (CIVIQ-20) at 4 and 8 weeks. Except for age (treatment group was older), there were no differences in baseline demographics, venous disease clinical class, or medical risk factors. The significant findings were an improvement for the health-related quality of life for pain and Venous Clinical Severity Score (VCSS), especially for edema, which was not seen for the control group at 1- and 2-month follow-up. In addition, fatigue/heaviness and venous edema of the limb improved significantly in the treatment group at 1- and 2-month follow-up, with no difference in the control group. In neither group did ankle range of motion or muscle isokinetics performance (ankle muscle strength) improve, which are important parameters for calf muscle pump function. Although venous edema improved on VCSS, overall measurement of leg volume did not improve in the treatment group, which may be a function that only about 45% of patients wore compression stocking in the study period. It appears that MLD may be of benefit in patients with advanced forms of CVI. Some questions that remain unanswered are as follows: (1) Does the addition of MLD to patients with CVI decrease the rate of progression of chronic venous disease and/or ulcer recurrence? (2) Should MLD be performed for longer than 1 month, and what is the optimal dosage (number of sessions per week)? (3) Does MLD improve venous hemodynamics and also lymphatic function? (4) Does MLD help patients with venous leg ulcer healing?

Additional studies are required to assess the full potential of MLD in patients with CVI.

J. D. Raffetto, MD, FACS, FSVM

15 Visceral and Renal Artery Disease

Anatomic characteristics and natural history of renal artery aneurysms during longitudinal imaging surveillance

Wayne EJ, Edwards MS, Stafford JM, et al (Wake Forest Univ School of Medicine, Winston-Salem, NC)

J Vasc Surg 60:448-453, 2014

Objective.—Renal artery aneurysms (RAAs) are uncommon, and rates of growth and rupture are unknown. Limited evidence therefore exists to guide clinical management of RAAs, particularly small aneurysms that are asymptomatic. To further characterize the natural history of RAAs, we studied anatomic characteristics and changes in diameter during imaging surveillance.

Methods.—Patients evaluated for native RAAs at a single institution during a 5-year period (July 2008 to July 2013) were identified and analyzed retrospectively. Patients with two or more cross-sectional imaging studies (computed tomography or magnetic resonance imaging) more than 1 month apart were included. Demographic and clinical data were collected from medical records, and anatomic data (including aneurysm diameter, calcification, and location) were obtained from electronic images. Changes in RAA diameters over time were evaluated by plots and Wilcoxon signed rank tests.

Results.—Sixty-eight RAAs in 55 patients were analyzed. Median follow-up was 19.4 months (interquartile range, 11.2-49.0 months). Mean age at presentation was 61.8 ± 9.8 years, and 73% of patients were women. Hypertension was prevalent among 73% of patients. Multiple RAAs were present in 18% of patients, and 24% also had arterial aneurysms of other splanchnic or iliac vessels. The majority of RAAs were calcified and located at the main renal artery bifurcation. Mean initial aneurysm diameter was 16.0 ± 6.4 mm. Median annualized growth rate was 0.06 mm (interquartile range, −0.07 to 0.33 mm; $P = .11$). No RAA ruptures or acute symptoms occurred during surveillance, and 10.3% of RAAs were repaired electively.

Conclusions.—Risk of short-term RAA growth or rupture was low. These findings suggest that annual (or less frequent) imaging surveillance

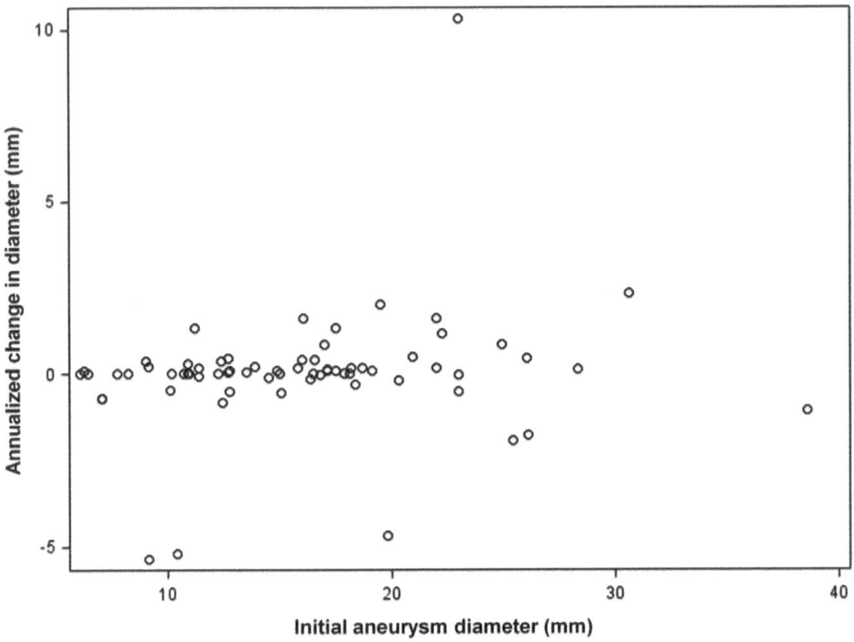

FIGURE 2.—Annualized change in renal artery aneurysm (RAA) diameter based on initial aneurysm diameter. (Reprinted from the Journal of Vascular Surgery. Wayne EJ, Edwards MS, Stafford JM, et al. Anatomic characteristics and natural history of renal artery aneurysms during longitudinal imaging surveillance. *J Vasc Surg*. 2014;60:448-453, Copyright 2014, with permission from The Society for Vascular Surgery.)

is safe in the majority of patients and do not support pre-emptive repair of asymptomatic, small-diameter RAAs (Fig 2).

▶ Renal artery aneurysms (RAA) are a relatively rare occurrence with a incidence of about 0.1%. Because of this, data on growth and rupture risk is sparse. In addition, a majority of the diameter data obtained from older studies is based on conventional angiography, which can underestimate the true diameter because of the presence of mural thrombus. This study is a single-institution retrospective study of RAA over a 5-year period using cross-sectional imaging studies.

The authors followed 68 RAA identified in 55 patients. Mean age at presentation was 61.8 ± 9.8 years and 72.7% of patients were women. Mean diameter at presentation was 16.0 ± 6.4 mm. Over a mean follow-up period of 19.4 months, no RAA ruptured, became acutely symptomatic, or required emergent repair. Seven RAA underwent elective surgical repair and 6 of the 7 measured ≥25 mm in diameter. The median annualized RAA growth was 0.06 mm and no significant annualized change in aneurysm diameter was observed ($P = .11$; Fig 2).

The authors conclude that their results support the recent trend in other publications that small to medium-sized RAA can be safely followed. The strength of their argument is limited by the small number of RAA followed. In addition, because RAA diameter of ≥2.5 cm was used as criterion for elective repair, there is a relatively small size range of aneurysms followed. Therefore, extrapolating this data to include larger RAA may not be accurate.

M. Arnold, MD

Early and Long-term Results after Reconstructive Surgery in 42 Children and Two Young Adults with Renovascular Hypertension due to Fibromuscular Dysplasia and Middle Aortic Syndrome

Sandmann W, Dueppers P, Pourhassan S, et al (Hosp Ev. Klinikum Niederrhein, Duisburg, Germany; Univ Hosp, Dusseldorf, Germany; Heinrich-Heine-Univ Hosp, Dusseldorf, Germany; et al)

Eur J Vasc Endovasc Surg 47:509-516, 2014

Objectives.—This retrospective study presents the early and late results of pediatric patients who underwent reconstructive surgery for renovascular hypertension (RVH) between 1979 and 2009.

Methods.—From 1979 to 2009 44 patients (male 22; mean age 13 ± 5.2 years, range 1–19 years; early childhood 7 [1–6 years], middle childhood 5 [7–10 years]; adolescents 32 [11–19 years]) with renovascular hypertension underwent surgery for abdominal aortic stenoses ($n = 6$), renal artery stenosis (RAS) ($n = 25$) or for combined lesions ($n = 13$). Nineteen aortic stenoses (bypass/interposition 10/5, patch dilatation/thromboendarterectomy 2/2), 51 renal arteries (interposition 36, resection + reimplantation 13, patch dilatation/aneurysmorraphy 1 each), and 10 visceral arteries (resection + reimplantation 6, interposition 3, patch dilatation 1) were reconstructed. Each patient underwent duplex studies and if required intra-arterial digital subtraction angiography. Reoperations within 30 postoperative days were required in four (9%) of the patients for occlusion of four arteries (6%), achieving a combined technical success rate of 94%.

Results.—After 114 ± 81 months 36 patients were re-examined by duplex and magnetic resonance angiography (2 not surgery-related deaths 7/12 years postoperatively, 8 patients lived abroad). Twelve patients had required a second and three a third procedure. Hypertension was cured early/late postoperatively in 27%/56%, improved in 41%/44%, and remained unchanged in 32%/0%. Best late results were obtained in patients with isolated aortic disease and at the age of middle childhood.

Conclusions.—Reconstructive surgery for pediatric RVH yields good results at every age and every type of lesion. However, these children should be followed up closely and to avoid early cardiovascular disease and death in later life, surgery should not be delayed (Fig 3).

▶ Approximately 10% of all pediatric cases of secondary hypertension are caused by renovascular disease. The major player is fibromuscular dysplasia causing renal artery stenosis, but these children also present with midaortic

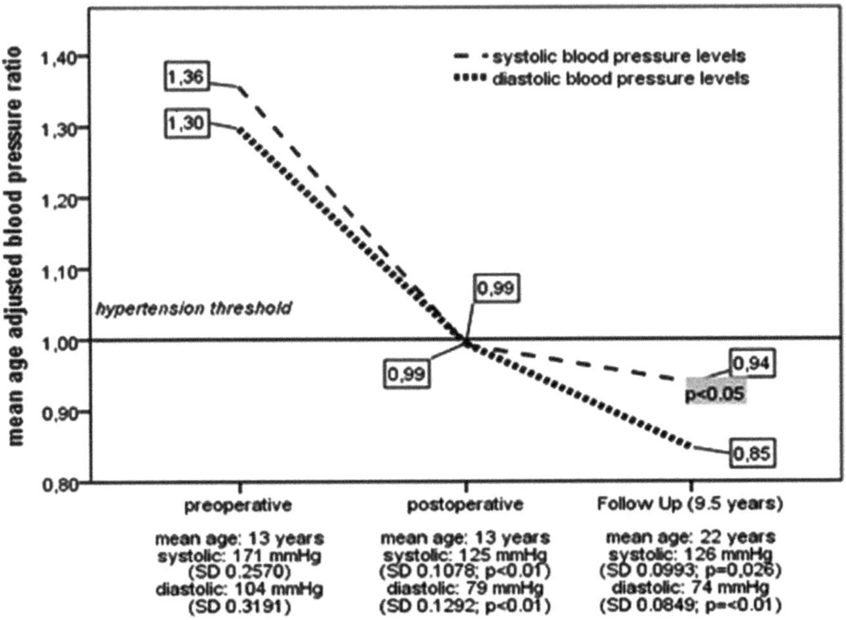

FIGURE 3.—Impact on hypertension over time. Hypertension threshold is equal to 1, which means that ratios above 1 are hypertensive blood pressure values, ratios below 1 are normotensive blood pressure values. (Reprinted from the European Journal of Vascular and Endovascular Surgery. Sandmann W, Dueppers P, Pourhassan S, et al. Early and long-term results after reconstructive surgery in 42 children and two young adults with renovascular hypertension due to fibromuscular dysplasia and middle aortic syndrome. *Eur J Vasc Endovasc Surg*. 2014;47:509-516, Copyright 2014, with permission from the European Society for Vascular Surgery.)

dysplastic syndrome from congenital coarctation or secondarily from vascular neurofibromatosis or Takayasu's or Moyamoya disease. Here is a current large series of children with renovascular hypertension (RVH). The authors skillfully divide the patients into 3 age categories: early childhood (1–6 years), middle childhood (7–10 years), and adolescents (11–19 years). The authors looked at various etiologies, anatomic compositions, and surgical approaches, but all 44 patients underwent an open procedure. Early results were similar to those in previously reported studies; however, long-term results were excellent with 100% showing cure or improvement at a mean of 114-month follow-up. Despite this, their most intriguing finding was centered on age group, depicted nicely in Fig 3. Adolescents showed the best early durability results with minimal revisions, which is not surprising, as they may have completed most of their vascular growth. Patients in "middle childhood," however, presented the best long-term results and required fewer medications overall. Previous works show that in percutaneous transluminal angioplasty, although it has enviable early outcomes in children, restenosis is staggeringly high at 22% to 37%. The exciting discovery here suggests that, when feasible, we may be able to postpone open surgery in the early childhood age with endovascular techniques and find the best advantage for reconstruction during the middle childhood years and before adolescence. RVH is a difficult disease to treat, and many of these children still require multiple revisions throughout their lifetime—amounting to 23% in this work. Clearly we need to be aggressive to prevent prolonged hypertension and preserve renal function in the young patient but balance the definitive surgery until later, if feasible.

K. C. Orion, MD

Ex vivo renal artery reconstruction for complex renal artery disease

Ham SW, Weaver FA (Univ of Southern California, Los Angeles)

J Vasc Surg 60:143-151, 2014

Objective.—The objective of this study was to evaluate long-term outcome of renal revascularization by ex vivo renal artery reconstruction for complex renal artery disease.

Methods.—From 1987 to 2012, 23 patients (17 women; mean age, 45 years) with complex renal artery lesions underwent open renal revascularization by ex vivo technique. Underlying disease included fibromuscular dysplasia with aneurysm (11), atherosclerotic aneurysm (6), Takayasu arteritis (3), and other (3). Outcomes analyzed included primary, primary assisted, and secondary patency rates; antihypertensive medication requirements; renal function and preservation; and mortality. Late graft patency, renal size, and cortical thickness were analyzed by serial renal duplex ultrasound examinations.

Results.—Twenty-four kidneys in 23 patients were revascularized by ex vivo renal artery reconstructive techniques. Perioperative complications were limited to two patients requiring reoperation for bleeding. Renal function did not change, and there were no in-hospital deaths. During a mean follow-up of 44 months, a single bypass graft occluded, requiring repeated bypass, which was performed with renal preservation. Primary, primary assisted, and secondary patency rates were 94% at 5 and 10 years. Compared with preoperative values, systolic and diastolic blood pressure and the number of antihypertensive medications were reduced ($P < .05$) in the 18 patients with hypertension. Late renal function was preserved as measured by no change in both serum creatinine concentration and estimated glomerular filtration rate compared with preintervention values ($P = .25$ and $P = .35$, respectively). In addition, there was no difference in treated kidney size or renal cortical thickness on follow-up compared with preoperative measurements ($P = .15$ and $P = .62$, respectively). No patient required dialysis. There were three late deaths, none related to the renal procedure, providing 5- and 10-year survival of 85% and 68%, respectively.

Conclusions.—Ex vivo renal artery reconstruction for complex renal artery disease confers a benefit in blood pressure while preserving renal mass and function. This technique should be considered a competitive alternative to other open surgical techniques for the management of complex renal artery disease.

▶ This article highlights renovascular revascularization in a young population of patients with nonatherosclerotic disease (fibromuscular dysplasia, aneurysm, arteriovenous fistula, or dissection that involve the distal renal vessels). This population remains a challenge because the surgeon must manage the procedural risk or risk of multiple interventions against long-term durability of a more invasive undertaking. The endovascular approach is the mainstay for treatment of the proximal renal artery but fails when 1 or more branch vessels is involved. The authors nicely describe postembolization syndrome and the concern after loss of segmental flow with endovascular intervention. In the selected cohort, open revascularizations with saphenous vein as the conduit of choice was accomplished with excellent technical success. The technique of ex vivo repair is nicely described with inclusion of operative "pearls," including how to handle the ureter and cold perfusion of the kidney. Of particular interest is reported the long-term durability with primary patency of more than 90% at both 5 and 10 years of follow-up with preserved GFR. What must be considered is whether young healthy patients that have complex renal disease identified early should forgo endovascular attempts knowing that more than 50% will have postembolization syndrome and a third will sustain an ischemic event. Although many have adopted the endovascular-first approach, the authors present compelling arguments that this may worsen future interventions. We have seen similar findings in other arterial beds—namely, tibial level angioplasty before bypass. Although this article does not directly compare open versus endovascular therapy, it highlights a patient population where durability must be underscored during patient counseling. Finally, this patient population was treated at a large hospital with considerable surgical expertise in ex vivo renal vascular repair. It is not clear that the stellar results can be replicated in all centers treating this unique patient population.

B. W. Propper, MD

Management strategy for spontaneous isolated dissection of the superior mesenteric artery based on morphologic classification

Li D-L, He Y-Y, Alkalei AM, et al (Zhejiang Univ, Hangzhou, China)
J Vasc Surg 59:165-172, 2014

Objective.—To explore a therapy strategy for the spontaneous isolated dissection of the superior mesenteric artery (SIDSMA) based on morphologic classification.

Methods.—Forty-two symptomatic patients with SIDSMA presenting with abdominal pain between January 2007 and December 2012 were enrolled in this retrospective study. We proposed a new morphologic classification with subtypes depending on the patency of the true lumen and reviewed the patients' clinical features, risk factors, computed tomography images (morphologic classification, location of entry site, dissection length, and true lumen residual diameter), treatment modalities, and follow-up results.

Results.—Twenty-four patients received only observation treatment, seven received open surgery, and 11 received endovascular therapy. True lumen residual diameter in the observation group (46.6%) was statistically better than that in the surgery group (0%) and the endovascular group (18.3%) ($P < .05$). There was clinical progression in three and imaging progression in seven of the observation group, of which two patients

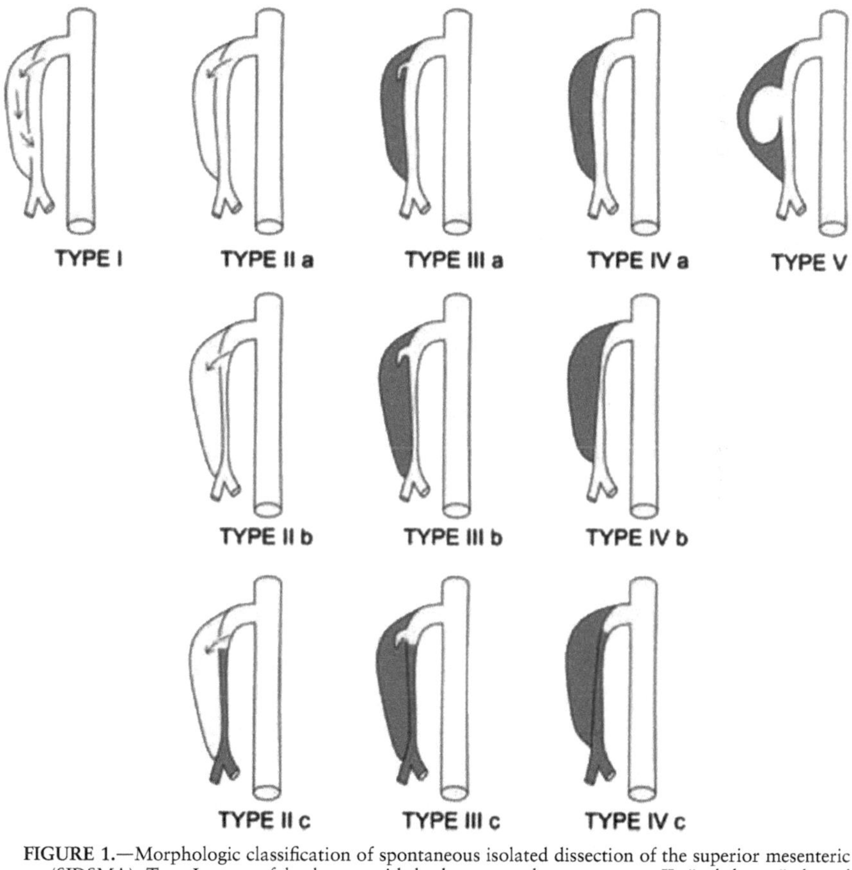

FIGURE 1.—Morphologic classification of spontaneous isolated dissection of the superior mesenteric artery (SIDSMA). Type I, patent false lumen with both entry and re-entry; type II, "cul-de-sac" shaped false lumen without re-entry (subdivided into IIa, patent true lumen; IIb, severe stenosis of the true lumen; and IIc, occlusion of the true lumen); type III, thrombosed false lumen with an ulcer-like projection (ULP) (subdivided into IIIa, patent true lumen; IIIb, severe stenosis of the true lumen; and IIIc, occlusion of the true lumen); type IV, completely thrombosed false lumen without an ULP (subdivided into IVa, patent true lumen; IVb, severe stenosis of the true lumen; and IVc, occlusion of the true lumen); and type V, dissecting aneurysm. (Reprinted from the Journal of Vascular Surgery. Li D-L, He Y-Y, Alkalei AM, et al. Management strategy for spontaneous isolated dissection of the superior mesenteric artery based on morphologic classification. *J Vasc Surg.* 2014;59:165-172, with permission from The Society for Vascular Surgery.)

received endovascular treatment and one patient died of bowel infarction. There were two clinical progressions and one imaging progression in the surgery group, of which two patients received additional surgery and one patient died of bowel infarction. The endovascular group obtained encouraging results with no progressions or complications.

Conclusions.—Symptomatic patients with SIDSMA are at risk of progression. We suggested a morphologic classification to guide the treatment. We recommend observation treatment with close follow-up for patients with patent true lumen flow and endovascular intervention for high-risk patients with true lumen stenosis or occlusion. Surgery is indicated for patients with suspected bowel infarction or arterial rupture (Fig 1).

▶ With the advent and ease of better imaging studies for patients with vague abdominal symptoms, vascular surgeons are more often faced with spontaneous isolated dissections of the superior mesenteric artery (SIDSMA). The potential for a disastrous mesenteric event in a symptomatic patient with SMA dissection is ever-present, and certainly these patients should be watched closely. With any worsening in pain, in this reviewer's position that urgent intervention should be initiated, including laparoscopy and angiography. This article is helpful to consider those patients with initial abdominal discomfort in whom the pain resolves, and we are left with clinical decision making based solely on anatomic features of the dissection and native artery. The authors of this article make an excellent observation that prior classifications of SIDSMA ignore the morphologic patency of the true lumen. In this regard, their classification scheme is helpful and yields clear inference to those patients suitable for stent-graft therapy. Indeed, a parallel consideration of thoracic aortic dissection, many surgeons may lean toward early intervention if the true lumen is < 30% of the total diameter of the vessel. However, the authors do not take a similar stance in prophylactic intervention. To reassure, in the long-term, their experience suggests most SIDSMA run a benign course, with only < 50% requiring long-term intervention.

K. C. Orion, MD

Multiple overlapping uncovered stents as an alternative flow-diverting strategy in the management of peripheral and visceral aneurysms

Zhang Y, Lu Q, Zhao Z, et al (Second Military Med Univ, Shanghai, China)
J Vasc Surg 60:1209-1217, 2014

Objective.—In this study we aimed to report on the midterm outcome of multiple overlapping uncovered stents in the treatment of peripheral and visceral aneurysms, and analyze the possible factors affecting the treatment efficacy.

Methods.—Data of patients who were regularly followed up over 24 months were retrospectively reviewed. Descriptive statistics were applied to present aneurysm thrombosis process and diameter change at each follow-up point, and a comparison with the baseline level was performed. Patients were divided into a totally thrombosed (TT) group and a residual perfusion (RP) group according to the sac thrombosis ratio (thrombus volume to sac volume ratio) at 3, 6, and 12 months of follow-up. Aneurysm shrinkage in the two groups was compared to explore the effect of the initial RP on the treatment outcome. Patients were also grouped based on their aneurysm morphology (saccular/fusiform). The aneurysm sac thrombosis speed (time to thrombosis) and diameter decrease (DD) ratio (percentage of DD) were compared between the two groups to understand the influence of aneurysm shape on the treatment efficacy.

Results.—Of the 64 patients treated, the initial 37 patients (25 male; average age, 55.5 ± 13.0 years) were enrolled into this study. Technical success rate was 100%. All patients were regularly followed up. At 24 months, 94.6% aneurysms (35/37) were TT, and the maximum aneurysm diameter decreased from 36.5 ± 9.7 mm preoperatively to 23.6 ± 7.7 mm ($P < .001$). Overall clinical success rate (complete thrombosis and shrinkage/stabilization of the aneurysm without aneurysm-related mortality) reached 94.6% in the study cohort. Most side branches (31/33) covered by the bare stent stayed patent during follow-up. Initial sac RP at 3, 6, and 12 months might not fully affect the final aneurysm DD ratio (TT group: 0.37 ± 0.09, 0.35 ± 0.09, and 0.35 ± 0.09; compared with the RP group: 0.33 ± 0.09, 0.36 ± 0.11, and 0.36 ± 0.13; $P = .153$, .964, and .418, respectively). At 3 and 6 months follow-up, saccular aneurysms (n = 29) seemed to have a faster thrombosis speed compared with fusiform aneurysms (78.1 ± 26.8% and 83.9 ± 21.8% vs 47.0 ± 24.4% and 63.9 ± 22.6%; $P = .004$ and .013, respectively), but there was no significant difference in aneurysm shrinkage ratio at 24 months between the two groups (0.36 ± 0.10 vs 0.33 ± 0.06; $P = .357$).

Conclusions.—Multiple overlapping uncovered stents could be a feasible option for the endovascular treatment of peripheral and visceral aneurysms. Neither the aneurysm shape nor the initial sac RP would affect the midterm treatment outcome. Further validation of this technique is required to substantiate these results.

▶ An explosion of endovascular techniques in vascular surgery has occurred in the treatment of peripheral and visceral artery aneurysms. The main challenge is no longer the skill to gain access to those aneurysms because of tortuosity or length of wire required, but the ability to exclude the aneurysm while maintaining patency of side branches or adjacent vessels. The authors have elegantly reported their midterm findings after using multiple overlapping uncovered stents (MOUS). Herein, they use a stiff wire and consecutively deploy uncovered stents leaving at least a 10-mm lesion-free landing zone at its proximal and distal neck. The diameter of the stents was oversized by 1 mm, and the specific number was determined intraoperatively by reviewing the angiogram for significantly reduced flow velocity within the aneurysm sac. Previous reports have varied widely in the clinical success rates as well as side branch patency. Excitingly, Dr Zhang and colleagues found an amazingly high percentage of success after 2 years, even if side branches originate directly from the aneurysm sac. At 24 months, 94.6% aneurysms were completely thrombosed with the maximum aneurysm diameter shrinkage from 36.5 ± 9.7 mm to 23.6 ± 7.7 mm. Despite previous belief, there was no difference in thrombosis between saccular versus fusiform aneurysms; the patient simply needed a longer follow-up to determine final outcome. Although the explanation for this phenomenon is still not clear, one might translate what happens in an aortic aneurysm. The degenerating aortic aneurysm builds mural thrombus but still allows patency to the outflow vessels (distal aorta, visceral, and renal). Certainly the diversion of flow into a more laminar stream can slowly decompress the aneurysm over time, but low resistance outflow vessels are able to maintain their blood supply. Thanks to the authors, we may cautiously add MOUS to our armamentarium to approach these difficult aneurysms when surgical exposures are often hazardous or not technically feasible.

K. C. Orion, MD

Open repair, endovascular repair, and conservative management of true splenic artery aneurysm

Hogendoorn W, Lavida A, Hunink MGM, et al (Yale Univ School of Medicine, New Haven, CT; Erasmus Med Ctr, Rotterdam, The Netherlands; et al)

J Vasc Surg 60:1667-1676.e1, 2014

Objective.—True splenic artery aneurysms (SAAs) are a rare but potentially fatal pathology. For many years, open repair (OPEN) and conservative management (CONS) were the treatments of choice, but throughout the last decade endovascular repair (EV) has become increasingly used. The purpose of the present study was to perform a systematic review and meta-analysis evaluating the outcomes of the three major treatment modalities (OPEN, EV, and CONS) for the management of SAAs.

Methods.—A systematic review of all studies describing the outcomes of SAAs treated with OPEN, EV, or CONS was performed using seven large medical databases. The Preferred Reporting Items for Systematic Reviews and Meta-Analyses (PRISMA) guidelines were followed to ensure a high-quality review. All articles were subject to critical appraisal for relevance, validity, and availability of data regarding characteristics and outcomes. All data were systematically pooled, and meta-analyses were performed on several outcomes, including early and late mortality, complications, and number of reinterventions.

Results.—Original data of 1321 patients with true SAAs were identified in 47 articles. OPEN contained 511 patients (38.7%) in 31 articles, followed by 425 patients (32.2%) in CONS in 16 articles and 385 patients (29.1%) in EV in 33 articles. The CONS group had fewer symptomatic patients (9.5% vs 28.7% in OPEN and 28.8% in EV; $P < .001$) and fewer ruptured aneurysms (0.2% vs 18.4% in OPEN and 8.8% in EV;

$P < .001$), but no significant differences were found in existing comorbidities. CONS patients were usually older and had smaller-sized aneurysms than patients in the OPEN and EV groups. The only identified difference in baseline characteristics between OPEN and EV was the number of ruptured aneurysms (18.4% vs 8.8%; $P < .001$). OPEN had a higher 30-day mortality than EV (5.1% vs 0.6%; $P < .001$), whereas minor complications occurred in a larger number of EV patients. EV required more reinterventions per year (3.2%) compared with OPEN (0.5%) and CONS (1.2%; $P < .001$). The late mortality rate was higher in patients treated with CONS (4.9% vs 2.1% in OPEN and 1.4% in EV; $P = .04$).

Conclusions.—EV of SAA has better short-term results compared with OPEN, including significantly lower perioperative mortality. OPEN is associated with fewer late complications and fewer reinterventions during follow-up. Patients treated with CONS showed a higher late mortality rate. Ruptured SAAs are predictors of a significantly higher perioperative mortality compared with nonruptured SAAs in the OPEN and EV groups (Fig 2).

▶ This article is a meta-analysis and, to date, the largest review regarding the treatment of splenic artery aneurysm. The analysis includes articles published

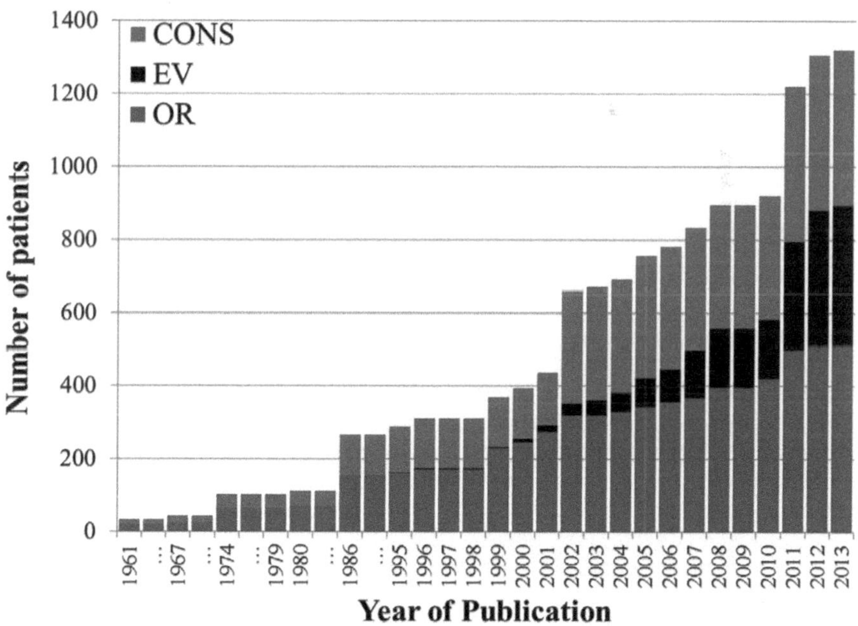

FIGURE 2.—Cumulative number of patients treated with open repair (*OPEN; red*), endovascular repair (*EV; black*), or conservative management (*CONS; blue*) for splenic artery aneurysms (SAAs) by year of publication. For interpretation of the references to color in this figure legend, the reader is referred to web version of this article. (Reprinted from the Journal of Vascular Surgery. Hogendoorn W, Lavida A, Hunink MGM, et al. Open repair, endovascular repair, and conservative management of true splenic artery aneurysm. *J Vasc Surg*. 2014;60:1667-1676, Copyright 2014, with permission from The Society for Vascular Surgery.)

as far back as the 1960s; however, the majority of reporting is after 2005. From Fig 2, one can clearly see a growing trend toward endovascular intervention. No formal treatment conclusions can be reached from this review, because, as the authors identify, details regarding treatment size, type of aneurysm, and type of intervention are lacking from a large meta-analysis. What seems to be clear is that ruptured aneurysms are more often addressed via open repair, and rupture itself portends a high mortality. One area of continued debate is the necessity of splenectomy. The authors show that nearly 60% of patient undergoing open repair had a splenectomy performed. Recent trauma literature for nonselective splenic embolization shows that the majority of patients do not require splenectomy because perfusion is maintained through the short gastrics. Of particular interest is the endovascular group: nearly 95% of patients were treated with embolization, and only 6 (1.6%) of 385 patients required splenectomy. Stent grafting the splenic artery remains challenging for 2 main reasons. Current devices that are equipped to handle an ≥8-mm vessel require large sheath access, and long-term patency likely requires the use of a highly flexible stent graft device. As the authors point out, women develop splenic aneurysm more frequently, and brachial access is advantageous given the celiac angle. Combining the smaller access size of women and the tortuosity of the splenic artery makes coil embolization a far more palatable approach than covered stent grafting or stent assisted coiling. As technology matures, small stent grafts will be available and provide additional options for treatment, yet it is not clear that maintaining inline splenic flow has advantages. Overall, the authors clearly highlight that nearly half of all interventions for splenic aneurysms are now done via an endovascular approach, and this number is rising.

B. W. Propper, MD

Options for treatment of spontaneous mesenteric artery dissection

Garrett HE Jr (Univ of Tennessee-Memphis)

J Vasc Surg 59:1433-1439.e2, 2014

Objective.—Mesenteric artery dissection was once thought to be rare but has been identified more frequently with increasing use of computerized tomographic angiographic imaging. Multiple reports advocate a wide range of treatment including medical therapy, endovascular, and surgical intervention, with no clear guidelines for the application of each treatment.

Methods.—A systematic review of the literature was analyzed and used to create a treatment algorithm that was applied to nine patients in our institution.

Results.—Although medical therapy is adequate for most patients with mesenteric artery dissection, 14% failed medical therapy, sometimes with severe consequences. Asymptomatic status on presentation predicted successful medical therapy for superior mesenteric artery dissection ($P = .0037$).

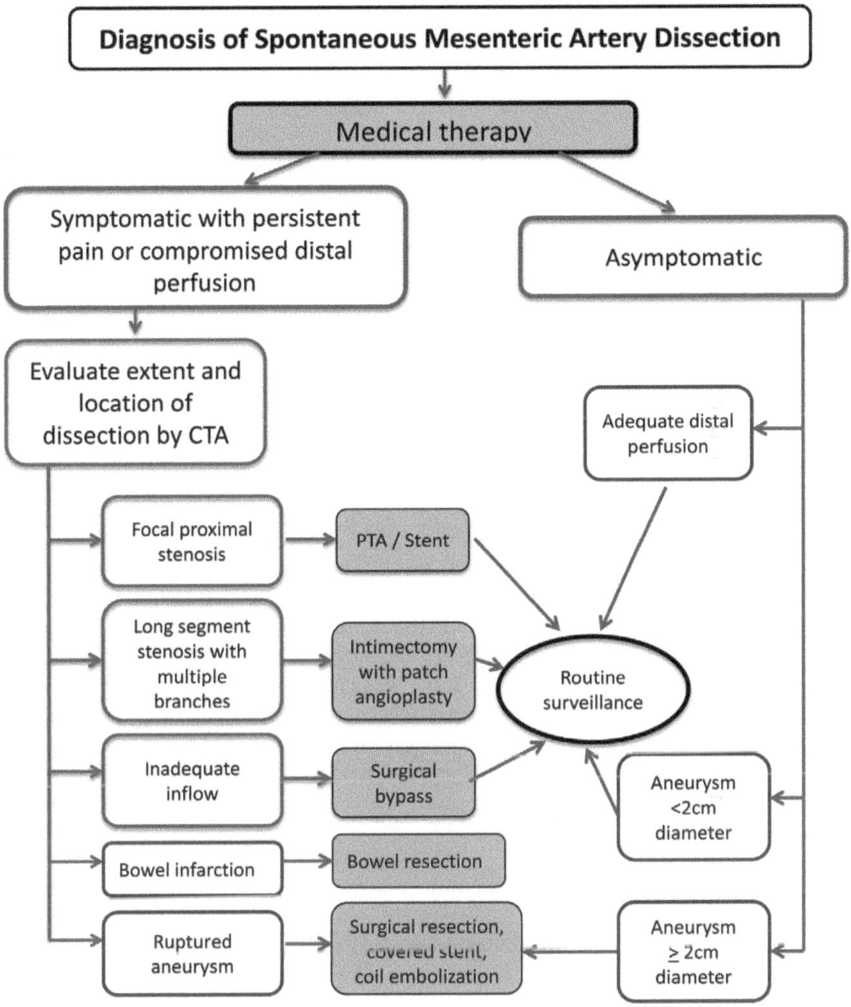

FIGURE 2.—Algorithm for treating mesenteric artery dissection (MAD). *CTA*, Computerized tomographic angiographic imaging; *PTA*, percutaneous transluminal angioplasty. (Reprinted from the Journal of Vascular Surgery. Garrett HE Jr, Options for treatment of spontaneous mesenteric artery dissection. *J Vasc Surg*. 2014;59:1433-1439, Copyright 2014, with permission from The Society for Vascular Surgery.)

Conclusions.—Intensive surveillance is indicated during medical therapy, and invasive intervention may be necessary (Fig 2).

▶ The management of mesenteric artery dissection (MAD) can be confusing. The literature on the topic includes several small series and case reports. Herein, Dr Garrett has assembled a useful synthesis of the data. The article aims to clarify the decision-making process with regard to observation, timing, and method of intervention. Importantly, medical management including anticoagulation, antihypertensive therapy, and surveillance imaging was successful in 86% of patients, and asymptomatic patients had a statistically significant higher rate of success with medical management. It is unclear whether this may reflect a selection bias of retrospective series, but the surgeon and interventionalist can be reassured the chronic MAD will often follow a benign course. Indications for intervention remain bowel ischemia, aneurysm enlargement, and rupture. The methods of intervention were mostly based on anatomic considerations and were well laid out in their treatment algorithm shown in Fig 2. Further study as to the length of anticoagulation therapy as well as the long-term risk of aneurysmal enlargement would help to develop a definitive surveillance protocol in the future.

M. Arnold, MD

Segmental Arterial Mediolysis: A Systematic Review of 85 Cases

Shenouda M, Riga C, Naji Y, et al (Northwick Park Hosp, London, UK)

Ann Vasc Surg 28:269-277, 2014

Background.—Segmental arterial mediolysis (SAM) is a nonatherosclerotic, noninflammatory arteriopathy of unknown etiology with life-threatening manifestations. With advances in endovascular techniques, SAM is increasingly being managed without the need for major surgery.

Methods.—A systematic review of the literature published on SAM between 1976 and 2012 was performed, focusing on arterial involvement, diagnostic imaging modalities, mortality and morbidity rates, and in particular treatment outcomes with open versus endovascular intervention.

Results.—Sixty-two studies reporting on 85 cases of SAM were reviewed. Sixty-nine percent of cases were diagnosed histologically (24% on autopsy). Angiography was the most common form of diagnostic imaging modality (56% of cases). Arterial involvement was largely abdominal or cranial, with splenic arterial involvement being the most prevalent (29% of cases). There was a total SAM-related mortality of 26%. Endovascular intervention, most commonly in the form of coil embolization of aneurysmal vessel(s), was successful in 88% of cases where attempted, with no reported mortality. There was a mortality rate of 9% where open surgery was attempted.

Conclusions.—Catheter-based endovascular techniques can be a successful, minimally invasive treatment option in the management of this potentially life-threatening condition, and may also provide a temporary bailout measure in the acute phase before definitive surgical treatment at a later stage.

▶ The evolution of our understanding of connective tissue disorders is ongoing, and multiple peripheral aneurysms (nonaortic), continue to evade the traditional disease states. Although segmental arterial mediolysis (SAM) is disease that has not been fully understood, this study and others have suggested it is a nonatherosclerotic, noninflammatory, nonimmune arteriopathy that results in dissections, stenosis, occlusions, and ultimately aneurysm formation. Frequently in practice, patients may have vague abdominal pain and a celiac, splenic, or mesenteric aneurysm (or combination thereof) on CT angiography, and we must decide whether to intervene. The authors reviewed 85 cases in the literature and found that most are choosing endovascular intervention with high technical success of 88%. More importantly, there was no mortality in patients undergoing endovascular repair compared with 9% where open surgery was attempted. Interestingly, as more patients are intervened on in endovascular manner, tissue is no longer available for pathologic diagnosis, and therefore, identification depends on patient presentation and imaging. Patients with SAM seem to suffer most commonly from either cranial bed or intraabdominal vessels involved, not both. Radiographically, transmedial mediolysis results in "arterial gaps" as disrupted smooth muscle detaches from the surviving arterial wall or "string of beads" when multiple aneurysms occur with intervening intact arterial segments. What is not reviewed here is follow-up of patients. SAM may fall on the gradation of fibromuscular dysplasia and connective tissue disorders including polyarteritis nodosa and Marfan syndrome. Although we are hesitant to place endovascular stents and stent-grafts in these patients with defined connective tissue disorders because the tissue may continue to degenerate rendering endovascular repair short-lived, the surgical hazard of the mesenteric aneurysms seen in SAM may leave "endo" as the only option.

J. H. Black III, MD, FACS

The contemporary management of renal artery aneurysms

Klausner JQ, for the Vascular Low-Frequency Disease Consortium (Univ of California Los Angeles; et al)

J Vasc Surg 61:978-984, 2015

Background.—Renal artery aneurysms (RAAs) are rare, with little known about their natural history and growth rate or their optimal management. The specific objectives of this study were to (1) define the clinical features of RAAs, including the precise growth rate and risk of rupture, (2) examine the current management and outcomes of RAA treatment using existing guidelines, and (3) examine the appropriateness of current criteria for repair of asymptomatic RAAs.

Methods.—A standardized, multi-institutional approach was used to evaluate patients with RAAs at institutions from all regions of the United States. Patient demographics, aneurysm characteristics, aneurysm imaging, conservative and operative management, postoperative complications, and follow-up data were collected.

Results.—A total of 865 RAAs in 760 patients were identified at 16 institutions. Of these, 75% were asymptomatic; symptomatic patients had difficult-to-control hypertension (10%), flank pain (6%), hematuria (4%), and abdominal pain (2%). The RAAs had a mean maximum diameter of 1.5 ± 0.1 cm. Most were unilateral (96%), on the right side (61%), saccular (87%), and calcified (56%). Elective repair was performed in 213 patients with 241 RAAs, usually for symptoms or size >2 cm; the remaining 547 patients with 624 RAAs were observed. Major operative complications occurred in 10%, including multisystem organ failure, myocardial infarction, and renal failure requiring dialysis. RAA repair for difficult-to-control hypertension cured 32% of patients and improved it in 26%. Three patients had ruptured RAA; all were transferred from other hospitals and underwent emergency repair, with no deaths. Conservatively treated patients were monitored for a mean of 49 months, with no acute complications. Aneurysm growth rate was 0.086 cm/y, with no difference between calcified and noncalcified aneurysms.

Conclusions.—This large, contemporary, multi-institutional study demonstrated that asymptomatic RAAs rarely rupture (even when >2 cm), growth rate is 0.086 ± 0.08 cm/y, and calcification does not protect against enlargement. RAA open repair is associated with significant minor morbidity, but rarely a major morbidity or mortality. Aneurysm repair cured or improved hypertension in >50% of patients whose RAA was identified during the workup for difficult-to-control hypertension (Fig 2).

▶ Because of the rare occurrence of renal artery aneurysms (RAA), an estimated 0.09% of the general population, clear data on risk of rupture and clinical features have not been available. This study used a multiinstitution database to perform a retrospective review on 760 patients with 865 RAA. They evaluated growth rate, rupture risk, and management patterns (see Fig 2).

The mean age at presentation was 61 with a 2:1 women to men predominance. A majority, 75%, of the RAA were asymptomatic at the time of

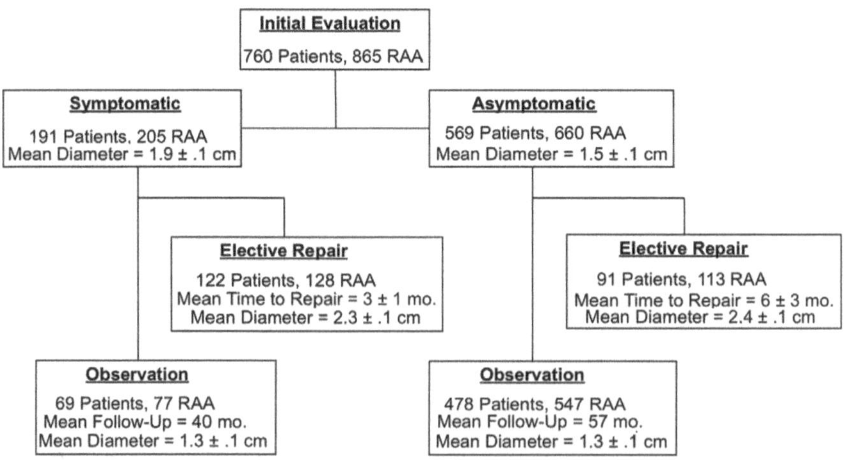

FIGURE 2.—Management used for patients with renal artery aneurysms (*RAAs*). (Reprinted from the Journal of Vascular Surgery. Klausner JQ, for the Vascular Low-Frequency Disease Consortium. The contemporary management of renal artery aneurysms. *J Vasc Surg*. 2015;61:978-984, Copyright 2014, with permission from The Society for Vascular Surgery.)

presentation. The mean diameter at the time of presentation was larger for symptomatic RAA than asymptomatic (1.9 ± 0.1 cm vs 1.5 ± 0.1 cm, $P < .001$). Not surprisingly, management varied by presentation. For symptomatic patients, 128 of 205 RAA were repaired whereas with the asymptomatic group, 113 of 660 RAA were repaired. Treated aneurysms were significantly larger than observed aneurysms. Growth rate for RAA was 0.086 ± 0.08 cm/yr. Calcification of the RAA did not appear to affect growth rate.

Mean follow-up data for patients under surveillance was 49 ± 5 months and no ruptures occurred during this time. In fact, the rupture rate in this study was only 0.3% (3:865 RAA). This includes 88 RAA > 2 cm and 7 RAA > 3 cm. All ruptures occurred in RAA > 3 cm. No patient under observation had acute renal complications as a result of the RAA. The authors conclude that observation and conservative management is safe for 2- to 3-cm asymptomatic RAA. Although this study does have some limitations, namely, that it is a retrospective review with inherent treatment biases, it does provide one of the largest databases of RAA. It challenges current treatment norms of repairing RAA at 2 cm and invites further, prospective study of the natural history of RAA.

M. Arnold, MD

16 Miscellaneous

Radiation-induced skin injury after complex endovascular procedures

Kirkwood ML, Arbique GM, Guild JB, et al (UT Southwestern Med Ctr, Dallas)

J Vasc Surg 60:742-748, 2014

Background.—Radiation-induced skin injury is a serious potential complication of fluoroscopically guided interventions. Transient erythema occurs at doses of 2 to 5 Gy, whereas permanent epilation, ulceration, and desquamation are expected at doses above this level. Complex endovascular procedures (CEPs), such as fenestrated endovascular aortic aneurysm repair (FEVAR), are associated with high radiation doses, yet the prevalence of radiation-induced skin injury is unknown. We hypothesized that skin injury after these exposures is likely to be underrecognized and underreported. This study examined the frequency and severity of deterministic effects and evaluated patient characteristics that might predispose to radiation injury in CEP.

Methods.—CEP was defined as a procedure with a radiation dose ≥5 Gy (National Council on Radiation Protection and Measurements threshold for substantial radiation dose level [SRDL]). Radiation dose and operating factors were recorded for all CEPs performed in a hybrid room during a 30-month period. Patient medical records were retrospectively reviewed for evidence of skin injury. Patients were seen in follow-up daily until discharge and then at weeks 2 and 6, months 3 and 6, and 1 year. Phone interviews were conducted to determine the presence of any skin-related complaints. Peak skin dose (PSD) distributions were calculated for FEVARs with custom software employing input data from fluoroscopic machine logs. These calculations were validated against Gafchromic film (Ashland Inc, Covington, Ky) measurements. Dose was summed for the subset of patients with multiple procedures within 6 months of the SRDL event, consistent with Joint Commission recommendations.

Results.—Sixty-one CEPs reached a reference air kerma (RAK) of 5 Gy (50 FEVARs, six embolizations, one thoracic endovascular aortic repair, one endovascular aneurysm repair, one carotid intervention, and two visceral interventions). The patient cohort was 79% male and had a mean body mass index of 31. The average RAK was 8 ± 2 Gy (5.0-15.9 Gy). Sixteen patients had multiple CEPs within 6 months of the SRDL event, with a mean cumulative RAK of 12 ± 3 Gy (7.0-18.4 Gy). The mean FEVAR PSD was 6.6 ± 3.6 Gy (3.7-17.8 Gy), with a mean PSD/RAK ratio of 0.78. Gafchromic film dose measurements were not statistically different from PSD estimations, with a constant of proportionality of

0.99. Three patients were lost to follow-up before their first postoperative visit. No radiation skin injuries were found.

Conclusions.—This study represents the largest analysis of deterministic skin injury after CEPs, and our results suggest that it is less frequent than expected and not increased in CEPs (Fig 1).

▶ The authors of this article hypothesized that more radiation skin injuries occur during complex endovascular procedures (CEP) with 5 Gy being used as a cutoff indicating high radiation exposure. A total of 784 procedures over 30 months was included, and 61 patients had CEP exceeding 5 Gy. Of this group, none had any radiation-induced skin damage or skin complaints. The average fenestrated repair exceeded 5 Gy with typically 6 to 7 Gy of radiation. Radiation skin injury is an uncommon occurrence, but knowledge of radiation exposure is of utmost importance; Fig 1 is helpful to recall that the image intensifier should be as close as possible to the patient. Although in this subset there

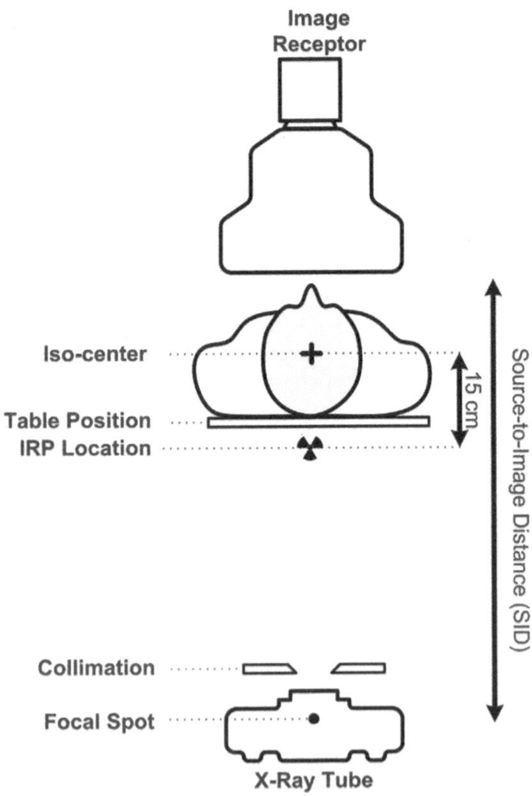

FIGURE 1.—Reference air kerma (RAK). IRP, Interventional reference point. (Reprinted from the Journal of Vascular Surgery. Kirkwood ML, Arbique GM, Guild JB, et al. Radiation-induced skin injury after complex endovascular procedures. *J Vasc Surg*. 2014;60:742-748, Copyright 2014, with permission The Society for Vascular Surgery.)

is no reported injury, the follow-up period is just 1 year, with only 45% of patients being seen back at the 1-year point. Skin cancer may require longer than 1 year to present, so documentation of high radiation exposure is warranted. With that being said, most patients undergoing CEP are not candidates for open procedures, and the underlying indication for the procedure is usually significant. One can take some comfort in knowing that even at high radiation exposures, elderly patients did not present with skin manifestations in the early follow-up period. One area that may be of particular interest is the head and neck. This group consisted mainly of abdominal and chest imaging. Eye and brain exposure to high radiation levels was not evaluated and may present a different level of threat. Although it is important to consider procedures that may cause high radiation exposure and be knowledgeable about dose reduction, this should not deter surgeons from offering CEP for those in need.

B. W. Propper, MD

Arterial Closure Devices for Treatment of Inadvertent Large-Caliber Catheter Insertion Into the Subclavian or Carotid Artery: A Case Series of Five Patients

Stellmes A, Diehm N, Book M, et al (Univ Hosp Berne, Switzerland)
J Cardiothorac Vasc Anesth 28:1319-1322, 2014

Background.—Up to 34% of central venous catheterizations develop iatrogenic complications. Among the treatment options for artery trauma after the inadvertent insertion of large-caliber catheters into the subclavian or carotid artery are arterial closure devices. The results obtained using two specific devices in five patients were reported.

Method.—Five patients required treatment using closure devices when either the subclavian or the carotid artery was injured by inserting a large-caliber catheter. The two devices used were the StarClose and the ExoSeal closure devices. Procedures were performed under biplane digital abstraction angiography with simultaneous endovascular access to the target vessel via the right common femoral artery. After the procedure, ultrasound monitoring and clinical controls were instituted.

Cases and Results.—In a 54-year-old man with hepatocellular carcinoma and hepatitis C, a 7 Fr catheter was inserted into the proximal right subclavian artery rather than the right internal jugular vein. The site was sealed with a StarClose device.

A 77-year-old man having aortic valve replacement and aortocoronary bypass had a 7 Fr venous catheter inserted into the proximal right subclavian artery rather than the right internal jugular vein. A StarClose device sealed the site, and the procedure was completed. A month later, two-dimensional ultrasound found a perfused false aneurysm of the right subclavian artery. Treatment with a thrombin injection was successful.

A 55-year-old woman had multiple bilateral rib fractures, an unstable fractured pelvis, and stable fracture of the twelfth thoracic vertebra. Her right subclavian artery received an 8.5 Fr sheath rather than the subclavian vein. Hemostasis was achieved by inserting an ExoSeal device under fluoroscopy, with 10 minutes of balloon compression to control leakage.

A 78-year-old man with three-vessel disease, limited left ventricular ejection fraction, and pneumonia had a 9 Fr catheter inserted into the right common carotid artery instead of the right internal jugular vein. Endovascular sealing was unsuccessful using the ExoSeal device, but no bleeding was seen after balloon sealing. A stent graft was inserted without complication, permitting the planned extracorporeal circulation to be established.

A woman, age 81 years, with left heart failure caused by severe aortic stenosis and systemic sclerosis with multiple ulcers had a 7 Fr catheter inserted into the right common carotid artery rather than the right internal jugular vein. The puncture site was sealed using the ExoSeal device.

Conclusions.—The complications related to inadvertent insertion of large caliber catheters into smaller vessels can range from hematomas and bleeding complications to pesudoaneurysm, arteriovenous fistula, stroke, or death. For adults, the recommendation is for conservative action, specifically, to leave the catheter in place and consult a general surgeon, vascular surgeon, or interventional radiologist. However, catheter-directed interventions offer an alternative. The puncture site is located, any thrombus identified, and balloon sealing undertaken in case the closure device does not provide an instant seal. This approach also makes it easy to convert to a stent graft or even open surgery. Although this is an off-label use, it appears to have some success. Surgeons should be prepared with endovascular and surgical back-up options should the device fail. Patients should be followed via clinical and ultrasound controls.

▶ Inadvertent puncture of arteries during central venous catheterization remains a dreaded complication even in an era when these procedures are done under ultrasound guidance. In this case series, the authors present 5 instances in which these complications are managed with arterial closure devices. The authors of this case series site ample literature that shows that exploration and primary repair is superior to pulling the line out and compressing the inadvertent arterial puncture site. Open surgical treatment and general anesthesia may be associated with elevated risk in medically frail patients. Closure devices were applied depending on operators' choices through the misplaced catheter or sheath. Importantly, all of these procedures were performed under biplane digital subtraction angiography with simultaneous endovascular access to the target vessel via the right common femoral artery, which allowed backup for bleeding control with balloon catheters or placement of a stent graft if necessary. The percutaneous closures were evaluated by physical examination and duplex ultrasound scan and clinical examination during the postinterventional course. All of the patients in this report had substantial comorbidities such as cirrhosis, intraoperative complex cardiac surgery, multiple trauma, or preoperative severe aortic stenosis, which would have made open repair risky in these patients. Two of the 5 cases in this report did require follow-up treatment with either thrombin injection or a stent graft. Thus, this report shows that with appropriate backup, these puncture sites can be closed with a variety of closure devices provided the appropriate imaging and backup strategies are available. Because cases of arterial embolization caused by closure devices with intraluminal anchorage have been reported, the use of these devices, especially in the carotid artery, is not advisable. Although suture-based closure devices have been described in similar cases to these with good results, they were not used by these authors.

M. T. Watkins, MD

New Aspects on the Metabolic Role of Intestinal Microbiota in the Development of Atherosclerosis

Drosos I, Tavridou A, Kolios G (Democritus Univ of Thrace, Alexandroupolis, Greece)

Metab Clin Exp 64:476-481, 2015

Gut microbiota remains a very interesting, yet largely unexplored ecosystem inside the human organism. The importance of this ecosystem for the physiology and the pathophysiology of the organism is being slowly unraveled. Recent studies reveal a connection between intestinal microbiota and atherosclerosis development. It seems that alterations in the function and composition of this bacterial population lead through complex mechanisms to a high risk for atherosclerosis. Although these mechanisms remain largely unknown, published studies show that microbiota can lead to atherosclerosis either by augmenting known risk factors or via other, more "direct" mechanisms. This review article summarizes the available literature regarding this matter (Fig 1).

▶ There is recent evidence on the association of intestinal microbiota with atherosclerotic cardiovascular disease. Although the exact mechanisms are not yet clear, these authors divide the available literature into 2 categories according to the mechanism that gut microbes lead to an increased risk of atherogenesis. The first category of studies associates microbiota with atherosclerosis "indirectly" by increasing the risk for obesity and diabetes, which are important risk factors for atherosclerosis. The second category contains studies that have shown a "direct" effect of the microbiota on the risk for the development of atheromatous lesions. The authors first quote literature from humans and mice that shows alteration of the bacterial species in association with obesity and systemic inflammation, which can be reversed with low-caloric diets.

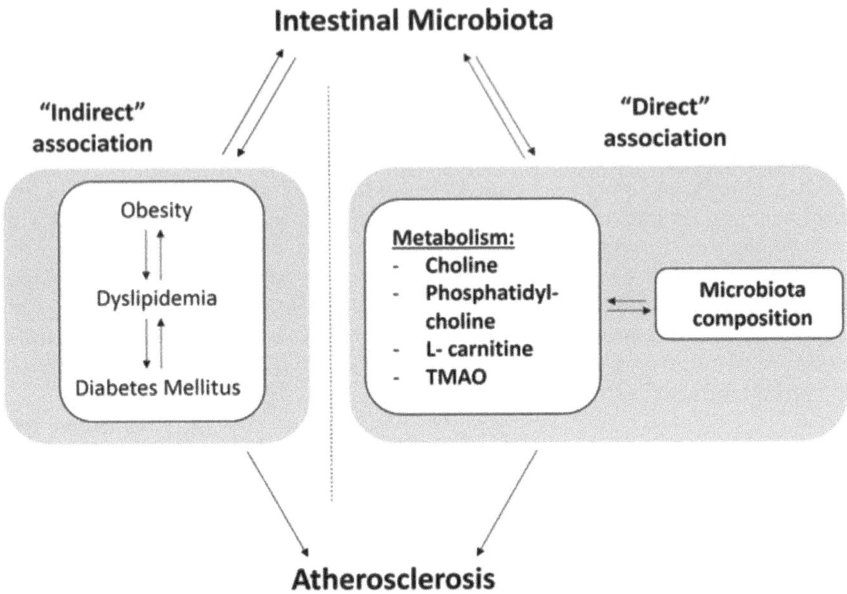

FIGURE 1.—A schematic overview of the observed correlations between features of the intestinal microbiota and the development of atherosclerosis, as presented in the text. (Reprinted from the Metabolism Clinical and Experimental. Drosos I, Tavridou A, Kolios G. New aspects on the metabolic role of intestinal microbiota in the development of atherosclerosis. *Metab Clin Exp*. 2015;64:476-481, with permission from Elsevier.)

A similar alteration in gut microbiotica has also been demonstrated in diabetic mice and humans. To show a potential causal relationship between gut microbiotica and inflammation, the authors show that transfer of the gut microbes between obese and nonobese mice triggers inflammation and obesity in mice. Fig 1 is an excellent schematic overview of the observed direct and indirect correlations between features of the intestinal microbiota and the development of atherosclerosis. This review quotes a connection between the intake of phosphatidylcholine and the formation of trimethylamine-N oxide (TMAO) through the involvement of gut microbiota where gut microbiota participate in the metabolic pathway from choline/phosphatidylcholine to TMAO. This conversion results in increased plasma levels of choline metabolites and betaine. In a recent large study with more than 3900 patients undergoing coronary angiography, higher plasma choline or betaine levels were associated with 1.9-fold and 1.4-fold increased risk for major acute cardiovascular events, respectively. These correlations will need to be studied in patients with aneurysms, carotid occlusive, and peripheral vascular disease.

M. T. Watkins, MD

Article Index

Chapter 1: Basic Considerations

Chapter 2: Epidemiology

Chapter 3: Vascular Laboratory and Imaging

Chapter 4: Perioperative Considerations

Chapter 5: Grafts and Graft Complications

Chapter 6: Aortic Aneurysm

Chapter 7: Nonatherosclerotic Conditions

Chapter 8: Thoracic Aorta

Chapter 9: Aortoiliac Disease and Leg Ischemia

Chapter 10: Upper Extremity Ischemia/Dialysis Access

Chapter 11: Carotid and Cerebrovascular Disease

Chapter 12: Vascular Trauma

Chapter 13: Venous Thrombosis and Pulmonary Embolism

Chapter 14: Chronic Venous and Lymphatic Disease

Chapter 15: Visceral and Renal Artery Disease

Chapter 16: Miscellaneous

Author Index

A

B

C

D

E

L

M

N

O

P

Q

R

S

FSC
www.fsc.org
MIX
Papier | Fördert
gute Waldnutzung
FSC® C083411

Kolibri 360 GmbH
Ferdinand-Jühlke-Straße 7
99095 Erfurt, Deutschland
produktsicherheit@kolibri360.de